table of
contents

Printed in U.S.A.

want a great meal out?

you've come to the right place!

In your hands you have the latest, greatest listing for eating out! That's because these selections come right from YOU, by YOU! Yes, we've scoured our website to collect the eateries and menu items most tracked, and compiled them here. So take a look, choose a restaurant, and enjoy!

Looking for casual dining? Maybe you'll select Olive Garden or Applebee's. Prefer a family restaurant? What about Bob Evans or Denny's. For fast-casual, Panera Bread, Boston Market, and Blaze Pizza are popular choices. In the mood for a sandwich? Try Subway or Jimmy John's. Fine dining? We've included Seasons 52! And there's always McDonald's, Wendy's, or Burger King for a fast food burger. But don't stop there! We have so many more places for you to choose from! Fan these pages—you're in for a delicious ride!

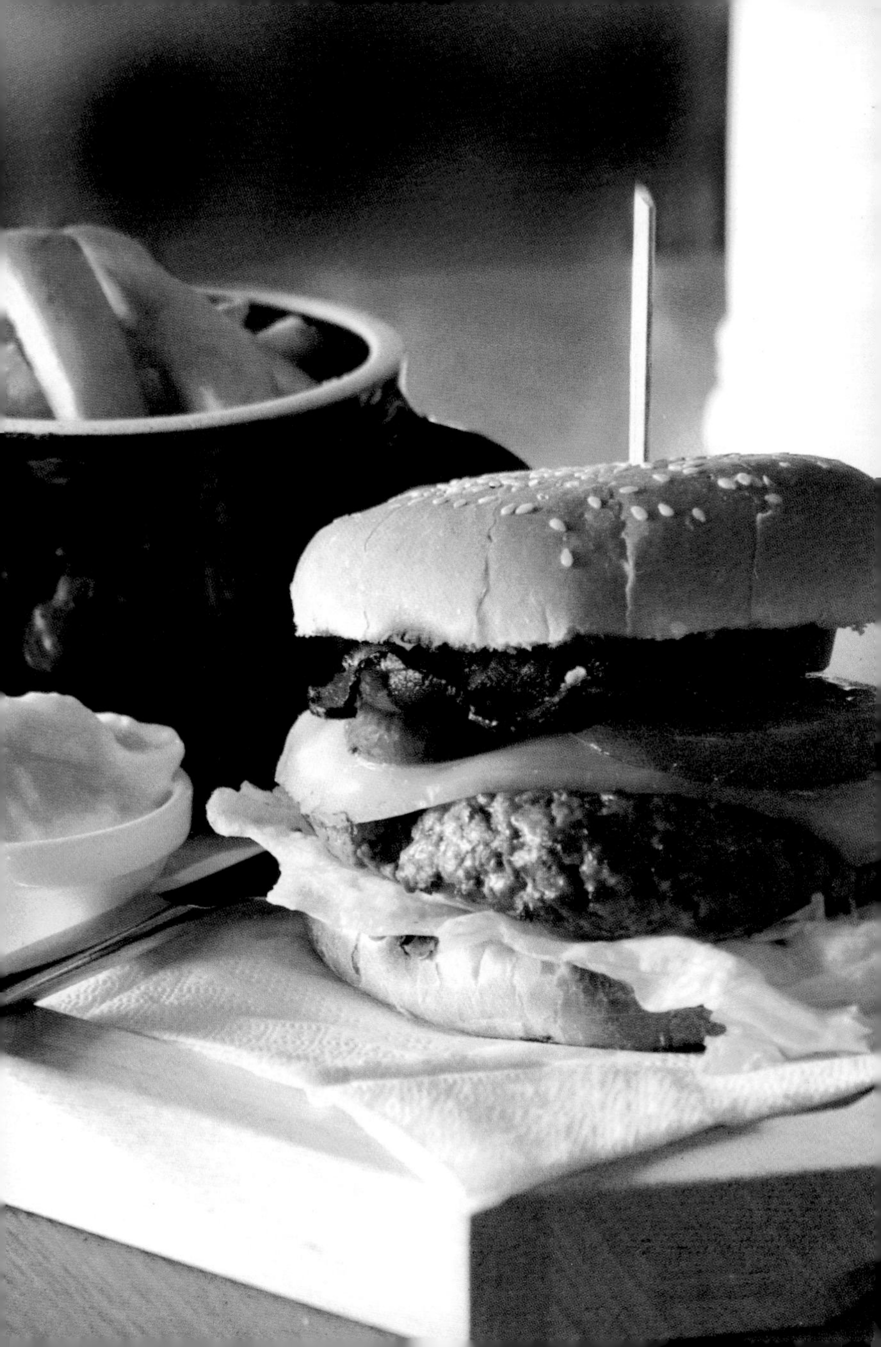

in this book
you will find:

- **SmartPoints® values** for each and every food item listed.
- Our **Restaurant Menus by Cuisine,** a comprehensive general list of restaurant foods, updated to focus on those tracked most on our website. And for those following the **Simply Filling technique,** we've marked no-count foods with an icon (◎) to make finding them easy.
- The latest **Restaurant Menus by National Chain,** now featuring the chains most searched for on our website!! Check out the eateries others are checking out—the popular ones are right here! With lots of locations, lots of choices, and a wide variety of types of eateries, you're bound to find just what you're looking for.
- **"We Like This!" items:** 👍 Some extra support for after you leave your meeting! Not sure what to choose? Think you'll be tempted by those restaurant specialties that are just a bit more than you planned? Just browse the menus for those items shaded in gray. Think of us as a dining companion, giving you ideas to help you stay the course.

What makes something a "We Like This!" item?

- Maybe it's a food item that could help you stay within your SmartPoints Target since these menu items, in general, have a lower SmartPoints value per serving than others from that category in that restaurant. Keep in mind that SmartPoints reflect the serving size, so the SmartPoints listed could change if a different serving size is taken.
- Maybe it's a choice from the kid's menu (ever think of trying one of those? Smaller portions could mean lower SmartPoints values).
- Maybe it's an appetizer (or two), or a side dish and salad, as an entrée.
- Maybe it's something that could satisfy you with just a few bites.

You might decide on something else, and that's fine. **"We Like This!" items** are a way to make it easier to focus on these choices first. Don't want what we suggest? Be creative. Create your own **"We Like This!" item** by splitting an entrée with a friend, or taking half of it home for another day. Keep in mind that SmartPoints values are based on published nutrition information, and sometimes restaurants change their recipes. If you're concerned that you're not going to get what you want, choose something else, or ask the server for help.

A note about restaurant offerings:

Since the restaurants in this book have locations throughout the country, keep in mind that a restaurant chain's offerings may vary by location. And all items featured in each restaurant's menu listings may not be available at every location. Inclusion of the restaurants in this book does not imply endorsement or sponsorship of such restaurants or menu items by Weight Watchers International, Inc. Photographs in this book are depictions of general restaurant offerings and are not necessarily indications of the menu items for any specific restaurants in this book.

A note about the SmartPoints value for each listing:

The SmartPoints values for the foods listed in this book were calculated by Weight Watchers International, Inc. using the most current nutrition information available at the time of the book's publication. Keep in mind that, since restaurants may revise their menus, recipes, or serving sizes from time to time, you should feel free to ask for nutrition information or to check the restaurant's website for specific or updated information.

One more thing to keep in mind:

Note that the alcohol content of certain foods, especially alcoholic beverages, can impact their total SmartPoints values. Because alcohol is not typically included on nutrition labels, you might notice discrepancies with the values of alcoholic beverages you see in these lists and that you calculate with nutrition information. For beverages that contain alcohol, as with all the products in this book, you can feel confident using the SmartPoints values listed here.

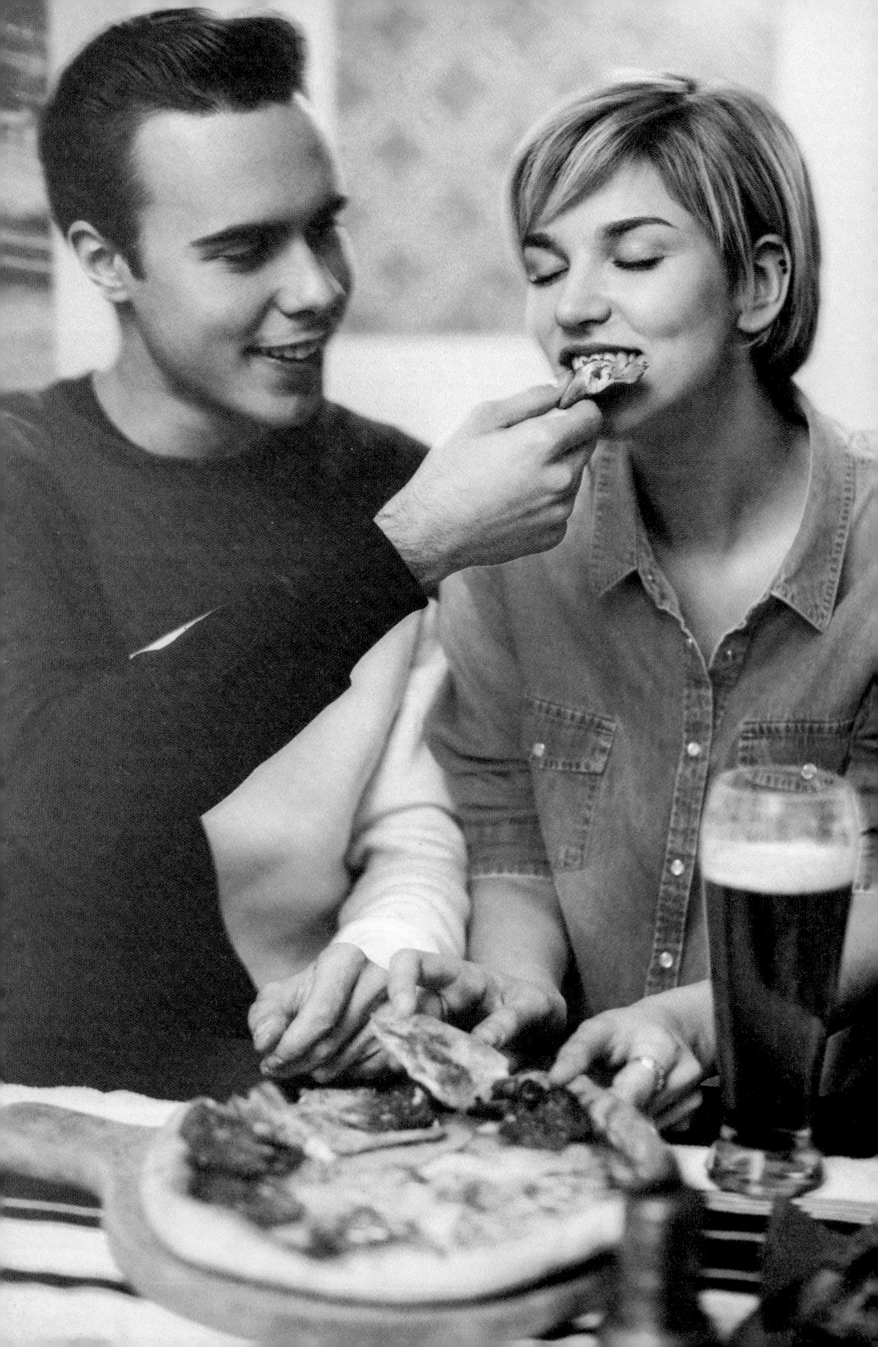

restaurant menus by

cuisine

No Count	SmartPoints® value

African

Couscous	
cooked, 1 cup	5
Curry	
fish, 4 ¼ oz	9
shrimp, 4 ¼ oz	10
Flatbread	
injera, 1 (1 ⅔ oz)	2

Bakery

Banana bread	
with nuts, 1 piece (2 ½ oz)	9
without nuts, 1 piece (2 oz)	8
Boston brown bread	
1 slice (1 ½ oz)	3
Bread	
any type (white, wheat, rye, Italian, French, pumpernickel), 1 slice (1 oz)	2
sourdough, 1 slice (1 ¼ oz)	3
Brownie	
prepared, 1 (2 ½ oz)	15
Cake	
angel food, 1 piece (2 oz)	4
cherry fudge, with chocolate frosting, 1 piece (2 ½ oz)	9
fruit, 1 piece (2 oz)	9
gingerbread, 1 piece (2 ⅔ oz)	10
petit fours, 1 (1 oz)	5
pineapple upside-down (⅑ of 8″ square), 1 piece (4 oz)	16
pound, 1 piece (3 oz)	15
shortcake, strawberry, 1 piece (4 ⅓ oz)	11
Cake, coffee	
1 piece (3 ¼ oz)	14
cheese, 1 piece (2 ¾ oz)	11
crème-filled with chocolate frosting, 1 (3 oz)	12
fruit, 1 piece (1 ¾ oz)	7

"We Like This!" item

No Count	SmartPoints® value
Cheesecake	
plain, 1 piece (4 ½ oz)	18
with fruit topping, 1 piece (5 ¾ oz)	19
Cinnamon bun or roll	
frosted, 1 (2 ⅓ oz)	13
Cookies	
bar, 1 (1 ¼ oz)	5
buttercrunch toffee, 1 (2 oz)	12
chocolate wafers, 2 (½ oz)	2
fruit bar, 1 (½ oz)	3
fudge, cake-type, 1 (¾ oz)	3
gingerbread, 1 (¾ oz)	4
lace, 1 (¼ oz)	2
ladyfinger, 1 (⅓ oz)	2
molasses, 1 (½ oz)	2
rainbow, 1 (⅔ oz)	3
raisin, soft, 1 (½ oz)	3
Danish pastry	
cheese, 1 (2 ½ oz)	9
cinnamon, 1 (2 ⅓ oz)	10
fruit, 1 (2 ½ oz)	11
nut, 1 (2 ⅓ oz)	11
Date-nut bread	
1 slice (2 ½ oz)	11
Doughnut	
cake-type, sugared or glazed, 1 (2 oz)	9
cake-type, wheat, sugared or glazed, 1 (2 oz)	8
cake-type, with icing, 1 (2 oz)	11
with crème filling, 1 (3 oz)	12
yeast, glazed, 1 (2 oz)	10
yeast, with jelly filling, 1 (3 oz)	12
Doughnut holes	
yeast, glazed, 1 (½ oz)	2
Fudge	
1 piece (1 oz)	6
Hot cross buns	
1 (2 ⅓ oz)	9

No Count	SmartPoints® value
Muffin	
any type other than those listed here, 1 (3 ¾ oz)	10
banana-walnut, restaurant-type, 1 (5 oz)	23
blueberry, reduced-fat, restaurant-type, 1 (5 oz)	17
chocolate chip, restaurant-type, 1 (5 oz)	22
corn, restaurant-type, 1 (5 oz)	16
cranberry-orange, restaurant-type, 1 (5 oz)	19
oat bran, 1 (2 oz)	5
orange, 1 (2 oz)	9
pumpkin, restaurant-type, 1 (5 oz)	18
Pie, dessert	
coconut custard, 1 slice (6 oz)	17
cream, with fruit, 1 slice (7 oz)	17
cream, without fruit, 1 slice (6 oz)	17
fruit, one-crust, 1 slice (5 oz)	13
fruit, two-crust, 1 slice (5 ¾ oz)	18
key lime, 1 slice (5 ⅓ oz)	25
meringue, 1 slice (6 ⅓ oz)	21
peach, 1 slice (4 oz)	10
pecan, 1 slice (4 ⅓ oz)	21
pumpkin, 1 slice (6 ⅔ oz)	17
rhubarb, 1 slice (6 oz)	21
Pumpkin bread	
1 slice (3 oz)	13
Sweet roll	
1 (4 oz)	9
cheese, 1 (2 ⅓ oz)	9
Turnover	
fruit, any type, 1 (3 ½ oz)	8

Bar/Pub

No Count	SmartPoints® value
Alcoholic beverages	
bourbon, 1 ½ fl oz	4
brandy, 1 ½ fl oz	3
cognac, 1 ½ fl oz	4
crème de menthe, 1 ½ fl oz	9
gin, 1 ½ fl oz	3
liqueur, any type, 1 ½ fl oz	9
rum, 1 ½ fl oz	3
schnapps, any flavor, 1 ½ fl oz	13
scotch, 1 ½ fl oz	3
tequila, 1 ½ fl oz	3
vodka, 1 ½ fl oz	3
vodka, raspberry-flavored, 1 ½ fl oz	3
whiskey, 1 ½ fl oz	3
Alcoholic mixed drinks	
bay breeze, 5 ½ fl oz	7
bellini, 6 fl oz	6
black Russian, 3 fl oz	11
bloody Mary, 5 fl oz	5
brandy Alexander, 3 fl oz	13
chocolate martini, 2 ½ fl oz	7
citrus vodka and soda, 5 fl oz	3
cosmopolitan, 3 ½ fl oz	7
daiquiri, 3 fl oz	7
gin and diet tonic, 5 fl oz	4
gin and tonic, 5 fl oz	6
gin gimlet, 2 ½ fl oz	5
highball, 5 fl oz	6
Jack and cola, 5 fl oz	6
Jack and diet cola, 5 fl oz	4
kamikazi, 4 ½ fl oz	15
Long Island iced tea, 8 fl oz	18
mai tai, 3 ½ fl oz	11
Manhattan, 4 fl oz	10
Margarita, 6 fl oz	17
martini, 2 fl oz	6
mimosa, 6 fl oz	4
mojito, 12 fl oz	8
old-fashioned, 4 fl oz	12
piña colada, 6 fl oz	16
Rob Roy, 4 fl oz	10
rum and cola, 5 fl oz	6
rum and diet cola, 5 fl oz	3

⭘ No Count	SmartPoints® value
sakatini, 3 fl oz	6
sangria, 5 fl oz	5
screwdriver, 6 fl oz	7
sex on the beach, 6 fl oz	8
Singapore sling, 6 fl oz	8
sour apple martini, 3 fl oz	10
strawberry daiquiri, frozen, 7 fl oz	11
Tom Collins, 6 fl oz	4
vanilla vodka and soda, 5 fl oz	4
vodka and cranberry juice, 5 fl oz	7
vodka and diet soda, 5 fl oz	3
vodka and tonic, 5 fl oz	6
vodka gimlet, 3 fl oz	5
whiskey sour, 4 fl oz	7
white Russian, 3 fl oz	10
Beer	
ginger, 12 fl oz	11
light, 12 fl oz	3
malt, 8 fl oz	5
non-alcoholic, 12 fl oz	7
regular, 12 fl oz	5
Buffalo wings	
1 (1½ oz)	4
Champagne	
5 fl oz	4
Cocktail mix	
daiquiri, 3 fl oz	4
Margarita, 3 fl oz	6
piña colada, 3 fl oz	5
tonic water, 8 fl oz	5
whiskey sour, 3 fl oz	5
Fruit juices and drinks	
cranberry juice cocktail, regular, 8 fl oz	8
Nuts, mixed	
dry-roasted, ¼ cup	6
oil-roasted, ¼ cup	7
shelled, ¼ cup	6

⭘ No Count	SmartPoints® value
Olives	
green, pickled, canned or bottled, 6 (½ oz)	1
pimiento-stuffed, 4 (¾ oz)	1
Peanuts	
¼ cup	6
cooked, shelled, ¼ cup	4
dry-roasted, ¼ cup	7
oil-roasted, ¼ cup	6
raw, ¼ cup	6
Pretzel	
1 oz	3
thins, plain, 1 oz	3
twists, 1 oz	3
Sherry	
dry, 3½ fl oz	5
sweet, 3½ fl oz	7
Soft drink, carbonated	
any flavor other than those listed here, sweetened with sugar, 8 fl oz	7
any flavor, diet, 8 fl oz	0
cola, 12 fl oz	9
ginger ale, 8 fl oz	5
seltzer, plain or flavored, unsweetened, 8 fl oz	0
Wine	
dessert, dry, 3½ fl oz	5
dessert, sweet, 3½ fl oz	7
light, 5 fl oz	2
prosecco, 5 fl oz	4
red, 5 fl oz	4
white, 5 fl oz	4
Wine spritzer	
8 fl oz	3
Wine, non-alcoholic	
5 fl oz	0

"We Like This!" item

○ No Count — SmartPoints® value

Barbecue

Food	SmartPoints® value
Beans, baked	
½ cup	7
Beans, chili, barbecue	
ranch style, cooked, ½ cup	4
Beef	
back rib, barbecued, 3 oz	7
brisket, barbecued, 3 oz	9
shortribs, cooked, barbecued, 3 oz	16
shortribs, lean and fat, cooked, 3 oz	14
shortribs, trimmed, cooked, 3 oz	8
Chicken breast	
barbecued, with skin and bone, 4½ oz	8
rotisserie, barbecue, with skin, 3 oz	3
rotisserie, barbecue, without skin, 3 oz	2
Chicken drumstick	
rotisserie, barbecue, with skin, 1 (2½ oz)	3
rotisserie, barbecue, without skin, 1 (2½ oz)	2
Chicken thigh	
barbecued, with skin and bone, 3 oz	6
rotisserie, barbecue, with skin, 1 (3⅓ oz)	5
rotisserie, barbecue, without skin, 1 (3⅓ oz)	4
Chicken wing	
rotisserie, barbecue, with skin, 1 (1¾ oz)	3
rotisserie, barbecue, without skin, 1 (1¾ oz)	2
Corn	
on the grill, with butter, 1 (4 oz)	8
○ yellow, on the cob, 1 medium (3⅔ oz)	3
Hibachi chicken	
6½ oz	6
Hibachi shrimp	
6½ oz	4
Hibachi steak	
6½ oz	9
Hibachi vegetables	
6"⅔ oz	4
Kabobs	
beef, 3 oz	5
chicken, 4¾ oz	4
fish, 4¾ oz	4
lamb, 4¾ oz	9
Pork	
backribs, cooked, barbecued, 1 rib (3¼ oz)	10
backribs, lean and fat, cooked, 1 rib (2⅔ oz)	6
barbecue, 8½ oz	9
country-style ribs, cooked, 3 oz	6
country-style ribs, loin, lean, bone-in, cooked, 5 oz	7
country-style ribs, loin, lean, boneless, cooked, 5 oz	7
Pulled pork	
in barbecue sauce, 9 oz	15
Rotisserie chicken	
barbecue, with skin, 3 oz	11
Sauce	
barbecue, 2 Tbsp	3
Shrimp	
barbecued, 3 oz	15
Spareribs	
barbecued, 4¼ oz	12
pork, lean and fat, cooked, 3 oz	10

Cajun/Creole

Food	SmartPoints® value
Beans, red, and rice	
6¼ oz	7
Beignet	
¾ oz	3
Blackened chicken	
3 oz	10

Cajun/Creole (cont'd)

○ No Count	SmartPoints® value
Blackened fish	
6 oz	14
Blackened steak	
3 oz	9
Creole, chicken	
without rice, 9⅓ oz	6
Creole, shrimp	
without rice, 9⅓ oz	5
Dirty rice	
12 oz	12
Green rice	
10¾ oz	8
Gumbo	
chicken, 8¾ oz	6
seafood, 1 cup	5
Jambalaya	
chicken, with rice, 12½ oz	12
fish, with rice, 12¾ oz	12
Sandwich	
poor boy, 2¾ oz	8
Sauce	
remoulade, 2 Tbsp	4
Sausage	
andouille, 3 oz	6
Shrimp remoulade	
3¾ oz	10
Soup, vegetable and other	
turtle, 1 cup	3

Canadian

Bacon, Canadian	
○ cooked, 3 slices (1½ oz)	1
Donair	
9 oz	21
Poutine	
12 oz	23
Sauce	
donair, 2 Tbsp	4

"We Like This!" item

○ No Count	SmartPoints® value
Syrup	
maple, ¼ cup	12
Tourtière (Canadian meat pie)	
5 oz	11

Caribbean

Beans, black, and rice	
5¼ oz	6
Chicken and rice	
restaurant-type, 5 oz	6
Chicken asopao	
10¾ oz	10
Chuleta	
1 (6 oz)	13
Conch fritters	
1¾ oz	3
Curry	
goat, 9 oz	5
Deviled crab	
4 oz	6
Enchilada de camarones	
7 oz	5
Jerk chicken breast	
6 oz	3
Lechon asado (roast pork)	
3 oz	4
Macaroni and cheese	
Bahamian, 9¾ oz	13
Peas and rice	
Bahamian-style, 7 oz	10
Jamaican, 7¾ oz	12
Picadillo	
2 Tbsp	2
Plantain	
baked or boiled, 1 cup	8
fried, ½ cup	4
Plátanos maduros (fried sweet plantains)	
1¾ oz	4

No Count	SmartPoints® value
Ropa vieja	
6½ oz	9
Salad	
conch, 5 oz	2
Soup, vegetable and other	
black bean, restaurant-type, 1 cup	7
pigeon pea and dumpling, 1 cup	8
Souse, chicken	
4⅔ oz	9

Chinese/Cantonese

No Count	SmartPoints® value
Beef and broccoli	
6½ oz	4
Bubble tea (milk tea)	
8 fl oz	4
Cashew chicken	
6⅓ oz	7
Char shiu bao (roast pork bun)	
char shiu bao (roast pork bun), 1 (2½ oz)	6
Chicken and broccoli	
6½ oz	3
Chicken breast	
five-spice, 4½ oz	7
Chicken leg	
five-spice, 6 oz	9
Chicken with cashews	
7 oz	11
Chinese lemon chicken	
restaurant-type, 2⅔ oz	6
Chinese orange chicken	
restaurant-type, 2¼ oz	6
Chinese roast pork	
5 oz	5
Chinese vegetables	
with beef, 5¾ oz	6
with chicken, 5¾ oz	5
with pork, 5¾ oz	8
with shrimp, restaurant-type, 1 order (21½ oz)	13
with tofu, 5¾ oz	4

No Count	SmartPoints® value
Chop suey	
beef, 7 oz	5
chicken, 7 oz	3
pork, 7 oz	4
vegetable, 11 oz	3
Chow fun	
beef, 5 oz	10
chicken, 5 oz	10
pork, 5 oz	10
shrimp, 5 oz	10
Chow mein	
beef, 8 oz	4
chicken, 8¼ oz	4
chicken, restaurant-type, 21½ oz	14
pork, 8½ oz	4
subgum chicken, 8¼ oz	3
vegetable, without meat or noodles, restaurant-type, 27¾ oz	12
Cookies	
Chinese almond, 1 (½ oz)	3
fortune, 1 (¼ oz)	1
Crab rangoon	
1 (2¼ oz)	7
Dim sum	
bean curd roll with shrimp and vegetables, 1 (3½ oz)	2
bean curd roll with vegetables, 1 (2½ oz)	2
sesame seed balls, 1 (2 oz)	9
Duck	
tea smoked, 2 oz	3
Dumpling	
beef or pork, fried, 1 (1⅔ oz)	2
beef or pork, steamed, 1 (1½ oz)	2
chicken, fried, 1 (1⅔ oz)	1
chicken, steamed, 1 (1½ oz)	1
shrimp, fried, 1 (1⅔ oz)	1
shrimp, steamed, 1 (1½ oz)	1
vegetarian, fried, 1 (¾ oz)	1

No Count	SmartPoints® value
Egg foo yung	
beef, 1 (3 oz)	5
chicken, 1 (2¾ oz)	5
pork, 1 (3 oz)	5
shrimp, 1 (2¾ oz)	4
Egg roll	
beef, 1 (2½ oz)	7
chicken, 1 (2½ oz)	5
pork, 1 (2½ oz)	6
shrimp, 1 (2½ oz)	5
Fried rice	
beef, 8½ oz	11
chicken, 8½ oz	11
pork, 8½ oz	10
shrimp, 8¼ oz	10
without meat, restaurant-type, 5 oz	7
General Tso's chicken	
restaurant-type, 2 oz	5
Ginger fish	
7⅓ oz	9
Hunan beef	
9 oz	11
Kung pao beef	
11 oz	11
Kung pao chicken	
9¼ oz	8
Kung pao pork	
10½ oz	10
Kung pao shrimp	
10½ oz	9
Lo mein	
beef, 8½ oz	11
chicken, 9 oz	10
pork, 8¾ oz	10
shrimp, 8¾ oz	10
vegetable, 8 oz	9
Lobster Cantonese	
7¾ oz	9

No Count	SmartPoints® value
Mongolian beef	
4⅓ oz	9
Moo goo gai pan	
10 oz	7
Moo shoo	
chicken, 4¾ oz	9
pork, 4¾ oz	9
tofu, 5¼ oz	10
Noodles	
cellophane, cooked, 1 cup	6
fried, 8 oz	8
Oriental (bean thread), cooked, 1 cup	7
Orange-ginger beef	
1 cup	18
Pancake	
Chinese, 1 (1 oz)	2
Peking duck	
5½ oz	13
Pepper steak	
Chinese, 3 oz	3
Pork and broccoli	
6½ oz	3
Pot sticker (filled wontons)	
vegetarian, fried, 3 oz	4
vegetarian, steamed, 3 oz	4
Rice	
white, steamed, restaurant-type, 1 cup	6
Sauce	
Asian stir-fry, 1 Tbsp	1
black bean, 2 Tbsp	2
brown, Chinese, 2 Tbsp	1
duck, 1 Tbsp	2
hoisin, 1 Tbsp	2
hot, Asian, 1 Tbsp	0
kung pao, 1 Tbsp	2
oyster, ¼ cup	1
plum, 2 Tbsp	2
sweet and sour, 1 Tbsp	1

"We Like This!" item

● No Count	SmartPoints® value
Scallion pancake	
1 (2 ¼ oz)	9
Sesame chicken	
7 oz	11
Sesame noodles	
1 cup	9
Shrimp and broccoli	
6 ½ oz	2
Shrimp Cantonese	
7 ¾ oz	9
Shrimp toast	
1 oz	3
Shumai	
fried, 1 (¾ oz)	2
steamed, 1 (¾ oz)	2
Soup, vegetable and other	
egg drop, restaurant-type, 1 cup	2
hot and sour, restaurant-type, 1 cup	2
shark fin, restaurant-type, 1 cup	3
wonton, restaurant-type, 1 cup	2
Spareribs, Chinese	
barbecued, 1 ½ oz	5
Spring roll	
beef or pork, 1 (2 ½ oz)	7
chicken, 1 (2 ½ oz)	5
shrimp, 1 (2 ½ oz)	5
Stir-fried vegetables	
with beef, 1 cup	5
with chicken, 1 cup	3
with pork, 1 cup	4
Stir-fry, mung bean sprouts	
½ cup	1
Stir-fry, with garlic or black bean sauce	
beef, 11 ½ oz	8
chicken, 11 ¾ oz	8
pork, 11 ¾ oz	9
shrimp, 11 ¾ oz	7

● No Count	SmartPoints® value
Sweet and sour	
chicken, restaurant-type, 2 oz	5
pork, restaurant-type, 1 ½ oz	4
Sweet and sour	
shrimp, 8 ½ oz	14
Szechuan pork hotpot	
8 oz	7
Twice-cooked pork	
3 oz	6
Vegetables, Chinese	
prepared with oil, 7 oz	6
prepared without oil, 7 oz	3
Wontons	
boiled, 6 (6 oz)	7
fried, 6 (4 oz)	13
Wrap	
lettuce, beef, 1 (3 oz)	2
lettuce, chicken, 1 (3 oz)	2

Cuban

Bistec de palomilla (Cuban fried steak)	
3 oz	6
Bread	
pan Cubano, 1 (4 ½ oz)	12
Cuban rice	
8 oz	6
Pastelitos de carne (Cuban meat pastry)	
1 (2 ½ oz)	13
Sandwich	
Cuban, 5 ¾ oz	14
Stew	
carne guisado (Cuban beef stew), 1 cup	6

Diner

No Count	Item	SmartPoints® value
	Apple	
	baked, with nuts, butter, and sugar, 1 medium (4 ¾ oz)	9
	Bacon	
	cooked, crisp, 3 slices (1 ¼ oz)	5
	turkey, cooked, 3 slices (¾ oz)	3
	Cereal, hot	
O	cream of rice, cooked, 1 cup	4
O	cream of wheat, cooked, 1 cup	4
O	farina, cooked, 1 cup	4
O	oatmeal, cooked, 1 cup	5
	oatmeal, flavored, cooked, 1 cup	8
	Cereal, ready-to-eat	
	bran flakes, ¾ cup	3
	corn flakes, 1 cup	3
	crisp rice, 1 cup	3
	frosted, 1 cup	7
	nuggets, 1 cup	12
	puffed rice, 1 cup	2
	puffed wheat, 1 cup	1
	raisin bran, 1 cup	8
O	shredded wheat, bite-size, 1 oz	3
	whole-grain, fortified, 1 cup	4
	Cheese	
	cream, regular, 1 Tbsp	2
	cream, whipped, 1 Tbsp	2
	Cheeseburger	
	on bun, plain, without mayonnaise, lettuce, and tomato, 6 ¾ oz	14
	Coleslaw	
	family-style, restaurant-type, 3 ¾ oz	7
	Crackers	
	oyster, 5 (¼ oz)	1
	saltines, 1 oz	4
	Egg	
O	hard-boiled, 1 (1 ¾ oz)	2
	scrambled, with butter and milk, 2 large eggs	6
O	whole, 1	2
	Egg substitute	
O	fat-free, ½ cup	1
O	regular, liquid, ½ cup	1
	Egg white	
O	3	1
	English muffin	
	cinnamon-raisin, 1 (2 oz)	5
	plain, 1 (2 oz)	4
	Fish	
O	salmon, canned, drained, 3 oz	2
	tuna, canned in oil, drained, 3 oz	3
O	tuna, canned in water, drained, 3 oz	1
	French fries	
	20 (5 ⅔ oz)	13
	family-style, restaurant-type, 6 oz	16
	French toast	
	2 slices (4 ⅔ oz)	11
	Fruit juices and drinks	
	grapefruit juice, 8 fl oz	5
	orange juice, fresh, 8 fl oz	6
	Hamburger	
	on bun, plain (without mayonnaise, lettuce, and tomato), 4 ½ oz	11
	Hash browns	
	family-style, restaurant-type, 4 ⅓ oz	8
	Jam	
	any type, 1 Tbsp	3
	Jelly	
	any type, 1 Tbsp	3
	Ketchup	
	1 Tbsp	1

"We Like This!" item

No Count	SmartPoints® value
Marmalade	
orange, 1 Tbsp	3
Meat loaf	
4 oz	8
Melba toast	
plain, 1 oz	3
Mustard	
regular, 1 Tbsp	0
Omelet	
cheese, 4 ⅓ oz	11
ham and cheese, 5 ⅓ oz	12
herb or plain, 3 ⅔ oz	8
vegetable, 12 ¾ oz	8
Onion rings	
fried, 3 oz	8
Pancake	
buttermilk, restaurant-type, with butter and syrup, 2 (6 oz)	17
Potato, home-fried	
5 ¾ oz	7
Preserves	
fruit, 1 Tbsp	3
Rice pudding	
½ cup	7
Salad	
Caesar chicken, grilled, restaurant-type, 6 ½ oz	9
chef's, with dressing, 8 ⅔ oz	11
chef's, without dressing, 8 ⅔ oz	8
chicken, restaurant-type, 3 ½ oz	7
egg, 4 oz	9
○ fruit (mixed fruits without added sugar)	0
garden, restaurant-type, 6 ¼ oz	3
macaroni, 3 ⅔ oz	8
○ mixed greens	0
pasta, 3 ½ oz	5
potato, 3 ⅓ oz	4
shrimp, 2 ⅔ oz	4
three-bean, 5 oz	7
tuna, 3 ⅔ oz	5

No Count	SmartPoints® value
turkey cobb, restaurant-type, 11 ½ oz	11
Sandwich	
bacon, lettuce, and tomato, 9 ¼ oz	16
chicken salad, regular bread, 5 ½ oz	11
egg salad, 6 oz	15
ham and cheese, 4 oz	12
ham and Swiss cheese, restaurant-type, 9 ¼ oz	10
peanut butter and jelly, 3 ⅓ oz	11
peanut butter and jelly, restaurant-type, 4 ⅓ oz	15
roast beef, 7 ¾ oz	10
roast beef, open-face, with gravy, 6 oz	12
shrimp salad, 4 ⅔ oz	9
tuna melt, 5 ¾ oz	11
tuna salad, 6 ⅓ oz	12
turkey, 4 oz	7
Soup, chicken	
○ chicken-noodle, 1 cup	3
Soup, vegetable and other	
broccoli-cheese, 1 cup	10
cream of mushroom, 1 cup	13
cream of potato, restaurant-type, 1 cup	6
cream of tomato, 1 cup	6
vegetable, 1 cup	3
Syrup	
pancake, regular, ¼ cup	8
pancake, with butter, ¼ cup	13
table blend, ¼ cup	10

Eastern European

Beef stroganoff	
with noodles, 15 oz	21
Borscht	
1 cup	6
Cabbage	
stuffed, 11 oz	8

⭘ No Count	SmartPoints® value
Caviar	
any type, 1 Tbsp	1
Chicken paprika	
10 oz	8
Cookies	
chruscik, 1 (¼ oz)	1
kolache (fruit filled), 1 (2 oz)	7
kolache (without filling), 1 (2 oz)	6
Dolma	
4 (3½ oz)	6
Goulash	
Hungarian, 1 cup	9
Kasha (buckwheat groats)	
⭘ cooked, 1 cup	4
Kielbasa	
grilled or pan-fried, 3 oz	10
Polish, turkey and beef, smoked, 3 oz	6
Paprikash	
9⅓ oz	10
Pierogies	
cabbage, 2½ oz	9
cheese, 2½ oz	10
meat, 2½ oz	10
potato, 2½ oz	10
Sausage	
Polish, beef with chicken, hot, 2 oz	5
Polish, pork and beef, smoked, 2 oz	6
Soup, vegetable and other	
cabbage, 1 cup	1

English/Irish

⭘ No Count	SmartPoints® value
Alcoholic beverages	
Irish cream, 1½ fl oz	8
Beef Wellington	
5 oz	15
Beef, corned	
cooked, 3 oz	6
cooked, lean, 3 oz	6
Bubble and squeak	
8 oz	5
Coffee, Irish	
7 fl oz	7
Colcannon	
9 oz	12
Cream	
clotted, 2 Tbsp	7
Crumpet	
2¼ oz	5
Fadge (Irish potato bread)	
1 slice (3⅓ oz)	3
Fish and chips	
11½ oz	17
Irish soda bread	
1 slice (3½ oz)	12
Popover	
1 (1⅔ oz)	3
Pudding	
plum, with 1 Tbsp sauce, ½ cup	20
Sauce	
Worcestershire, 1 Tbsp	1
Scone	
blueberry, restaurant-type, 1 (4¼ oz)	17
chocolate, restaurant-type, 1 (4¼ oz)	20
cinnamon, restaurant-type, 1 (4¼ oz)	20
cranberry, restaurant-type, 1 (4¼ oz)	16
orange, restaurant-type, 1 (4¼ oz)	18
plain, 1 (1½ oz)	5
raspberry, restaurant-type, 1 (4¼ oz)	18

"We Like This!" item

No Count	SmartPoints® value
Shephard's pie	
9 ¾ oz	12
Stew	
burgoo, 1 cup	5
Irish brown, 1 cup	6
lamb, 1 cup	5
Trifle	
½ cup	5
Vegetables, mixed	
carrots and parsnips, 1 cup	1
Yorkshire pudding	
1 (5 oz)	9

Fast Food

No Count	SmartPoints® value
Beans, baked	
6 ⅓ oz	9
Biscuit	
2" square, 1 (2 oz)	11
with egg and bacon, 5 ⅓ oz	15
with egg and ham, 6 ½ oz	13
with egg and sausage, 6 ½ oz	19
with sausage, 4 oz	14
with steak, 5 oz	15
Burrito	
bean, 7 ¾ oz	14
with beans and cheese, 6 ¾ oz	12
with beans and chili peppers, 7 ⅓ oz	14
with beans and meat, 8 ¼ oz	13
with beans, cheese, and beef, 8 ⅔ oz	14
with beans, cheese, and chili peppers, 12 oz	20
with beef and chili peppers, 7 oz	13
with beef, cheese, and chili peppers, 10 ¾ oz	18
with beef, 7 ¾ oz	16
with fruit, 2 ⅔ oz	10

No Count	SmartPoints® value
Cheeseburger	
double, 5 ⅓ oz	15
double, regular patty and bun, with condiments, 5 ½ oz	15
large, with condiments and vegetables, 1 (8 ⅓ oz)	16
single patty, with condiments, 4 ½ oz	12
single, large patty, with condiments, 7 oz	18
small, 1 (3 ¼ oz)	9
small, with condiments and vegetables, 4 oz	10
Cheesecake	
any type, 1 piece (2 ¾ oz)	12
Chicken nuggets	
fried, 6 (3 ¾ oz)	9
Chicken tenders	
3 oz	6
Chicken, breaded and fried	
light meat (from breast or wing), 3 oz	7
Chicken, fried	
breast, with skin, breaded, 3 oz	5
breast, without skin and breading, 3 oz	2
drumstick, with skin and breading, 3 oz	6
drumstick, without skin and breading, 3 oz	3
thigh, with skin, 3 oz	7
thigh, without skin and breading, 3 oz	3
wing, with skin, 3 oz	7
wing, without skin and breading, 3 oz	4
Chili con carne	
9 oz	7
Chili dog on roll	
4 oz	9
Chimichanga	
with beef, 1 (6 ¼ oz)	13

No Count	SmartPoints® value
Cinnamon bun or roll	
mini, 1 (1 oz)	4
Coleslaw	
6 ¾ oz	12
Cookies	
animal crackers, 1 oz	4
chocolate chip, 1 package (2 oz)	8
Corn	
on the cob, with butter, 5 ¼ oz	5
Corn dog	
6 ¼ oz	15
Crab cakes	
fast food, 2 oz	5
Danish pastry	
cheese, 1 (3 ¼ oz)	15
cinnamon, 1 (3 oz)	14
1 (3 ¼ oz)	15
fruit, 1 (3 ⅓ oz)	13
Egg	
scrambled, (2 eggs), 3 ½ oz	7
English muffin breakfast	
with butter, 1 (2 ¼ oz)	6
with cheese and sausage, 4 oz	13
with egg, cheese, and Canadian bacon, 4 ½ oz	9
with egg, cheese, and sausage, 6 oz	16
Fish fillet	
battered or breaded, fried, 3 ¼ oz	6
French fries	
4 oz	11
French toast	
with butter, 2 slices (4 ¾ oz)	13
French toast sticks	
1 (1 oz)	3
Frijoles	
with cheese, 6 oz	7

No Count	SmartPoints® value
Hamburger	
double patty, plain, 1 (4 ¼ oz)	11
double, large patty, with condiments and vegetables, 8 oz	16
large, fast food with condiments, 1 (6 oz)	14
large, plain, 1 (5 oz)	13
single, large patty, with condiments and vegetables, 7 ¾ oz	16
single, with condiments, 3 ½ oz	8
small, 2 ¾ oz	7
small, with condiments and vegetables, 4 oz	9
Hash browns	
1 patty (2 oz)	5
Hush puppies	
1 (¾ oz)	2
Ice cream in cone	
light, vanilla, soft-serve, 4 ¼ oz	9
Ice cream sundae	
caramel, 5 ½ oz	15
hot fudge, 5 ⅔ oz	15
strawberry, 5 ½ oz	13
Muffin	
any type, 4 ¼ oz	14
Nachos	
with cheese, 2 ¾ oz	9
Onion rings	
1 (¼ oz)	1
Oysters	
battered or breaded and fried, 5 oz	11
Pancake	
with butter and syrup, 2 (8 ⅓ oz)	17
Pie, dessert	
fruit, 1 slice (3 ¾ oz)	13
Potato, baked	
topped with cheese sauce and broccoli, 12 oz	15

"We Like This!" item

No Count		SmartPoints® value
	with cheese sauce and bacon, 10⅔ oz	16
	with cheese sauce and chili, 14 oz	17
	with cheese sauce, 10½ oz	17
	with sour cream and chives, 10¾ oz	15
	with vegetables and cheese, 13⅓ oz	14
	Potato, mashed	
	2¾ oz	2
	Quesadilla	
	with chicken, 6½ oz	17
	Salad	
	chef's, 11½ oz	7
	chicken, grilled, without dressing, 12⅓ oz	5
●	side, without dressing, fast food	0
	taco, 7 oz	9
	taco, with chili con carne, 9⅓ oz	10
	taco, without shell and dressing, 14 oz	12
	vegetable, tossed, with pasta and seafood, without dressing, 15 oz	11
	vegetable, with cheese and egg, without dressing, 7¾ oz	3
	vegetable, with chicken, without dressing, 7¾ oz	2
	vegetable, with shrimp, without dressing, 8½ oz	2
	vegetable, with turkey, ham and cheese, without dressing, 11⅔ oz	8
	Sandwich	
	bagel, with ham, egg and cheese, 6¾ oz	15
	chicken fillet, crispy, with lettuce and mayonnaise, 5½ oz	13
	chicken fillet, grilled, with lettuce, tomato, and spread, 8¼ oz	10
	chicken fillet, plain, 6⅔ oz	13
	chicken, fried, 7⅓ oz	14
	chicken, grilled, 6¾ oz	10

No Count		SmartPoints® value
	egg and cheese, 5¼ oz	11
	fish, with tartar sauce and cheese, 4¾ oz	12
	fish, with tartar sauce, 7¾ oz	17
	ham and cheese, 5¼ oz	11
	ham, egg, and cheese, 5 oz	11
	roast beef with cheese, 6¼ oz	15
	roast beef, plain, 5 oz	10
	steak, 7¼ oz	12
	submarine, with cold cuts, 8 oz	15
	submarine, with roast beef, 7¾ oz	12
	submarine, with tuna salad, 9 oz	17
	Sausage biscuit	
	4⅓ oz	15
	Scallops	
	breaded and fried, 3 oz	7
	Shake	
	chocolate, 1 cup	12
	strawberry, 1 cup	13
	vanilla, 1 cup	11
	Shrimp	
	breaded and fried, 3 pieces (1⅓ oz)	4
	Taco	
	hard, 1 (3 oz)	5
	soft, 1 (3½ oz)	4
	Tostada	
	with beans and cheese, 1 (5 oz)	7
	with beef and cheese, 5¾ oz	11
	Turnover	
	fruit, any type, 1 (4 oz)	13

French

	Beef Bourguignon	
	7½ oz	13
	Blanquette of veal	
	5¼ oz	5
	Bread	
	French baguette, 1 piece (2¼ oz)	5

French (cont'd)

No Count	SmartPoints® value
Brioche	
1 (1 oz)	5
Cheese	
brie, 1 oz	4
camembert, 1 oz	3
goat, hard-type, 1 oz	5
goat, semisoft-type, 1 oz	4
goat, soft-type, 1 oz	3
Roquefort, 1 oz	4
Roquefort, crumbled, ¼ cup	4
Chicken cordon bleu	
6 ¾ oz	13
Chocolate mousse	
½ cup	22
Coquilles St. Jacques	
13 ¾ oz	10
Crème brûlée	
½ cup	13
Crème caramel	
½ cup	7
Crème fraiche	
2 Tbsp	5
Crêpe	
6" diameter, 1 (1 ⅓ oz)	3
Crêpes Suzette	
4 ¾ oz	19
Croissant	
apple, 1 (2 oz)	6
butter, 1 (2 oz)	9
cheese, 1 (2 oz)	9
chocolate-filled, 1 (3 ¾ oz)	10
plain, 1 (1 ¾ oz)	9
Croquette	
beef, 5 oz	11
chicken, 5 oz	10
Cruller	
French, glazed, 1 (1 ½ oz)	7

No Count	SmartPoints® value
Duck a l'orange	
17 ¾ oz	17
Eclair	
1 (5 ⅓ oz)	16
Escargots	
3 oz	14
Frog legs	
fried, 1 oz	4
Fruit tart	
with custard, individual, 1 (7 ½ oz)	24
Mussels Marinière	
4 ¼ oz	7
Pâté	
liver, 3 oz	5
Pâté de foie gras	
goose liver, smoked, 1 Tbsp	2
Profiterole	
1 (1 ½ oz)	5
Quiche	
Lorraine, 4 ½ oz	16
vegetable, 6 ⅓ oz	14
Ratatouille	
8 ½ oz	3
Rolls	
French, 1 (1 ⅓ oz)	3
Salad	
Niçoise, without dressing, 16 ½ oz	8
Sandwich	
croque-monsieur, 6 ½ oz	15
Sauce	
Béarnaise, 2 Tbsp	6
hollandaise, 2 Tbsp	6
mornay, 2 Tbsp	3
wine, 2 Tbsp	2
Sorbet	
any flavor, ½ cup	5
Soufflé	
cheese, 3 ⅓ oz	7
fruit, 2 oz	5

"We Like This!" item

No Count		SmartPoints® value
	Soup, seafood	
	bouillabaisse, 1 cup	4
	Soup, vegetable and other	
	French onion au gratin, 1 cup	9
	petite marmite, 1 cup	3
	vichyssoise, 1 cup	4
	Steak au poivre	
	3 oz	7

German

	Cake	
	sachertorte, 1 piece (2¾ oz)	15
	Dumpling	
	potato, 5¾ oz	4
	Fritters	
	apple, restaurant-type, 1 (4 oz)	16
	Peppers, stuffed	
	with beef and rice, 8 oz	11
	Potato pancake	
	3⅓ oz	3
	Salad	
	potato, German, 3¾ oz	4
	Sauerbraten	
	4¾ oz	7
	Sauerkraut	
	fresh	0
	Schaum torte	
	with whipped cream, 1 oz	2
	without whipped cream, 1 oz	2
	Spaetzle	
	1 cup	14
	Strudel	
	any type, 1 (6 oz)	18
	Wiener schnitzel	
	3 oz	10

Greek

No Count		SmartPoints® value
	Baklava	
	1 (2½ oz)	14
	Cheese	
	feta, 1 oz	3
	Chicken pilaf (kotta pilafi)	
	13⅔ oz	12
	Gyro	
	11½ oz	19
	Kataifi	
	1 (2 oz)	11
	Moussaka	
	8⅓ oz	16
	Pastitsio	
	10"⅓ oz	19
	Saganaki	
	1 (2¾ oz)	10
	Salad	
	Greek, restaurant-type, 12¾ oz	13
	Greek, with dressing, 11½ oz	11
	Greek, without dressing, 10 oz	3
	yogurt and cucumber, 3⅓ oz	2
	Sauce	
	tzatziki, 2 Tbsp	1
	Soup, vegetable and other	
	avgolemono, 1 cup	4
O	yogurt and cucumber, 1 cup	4
	Souvlaki	
	chicken, 4½ oz	4
	chicken, in pita bread, 6½ oz	9
	lamb, 4¾ oz	9
	lamb, in pita bread, 6½ oz	11
	Spanakopita	
	5¾ oz	12

Hawaiian

	Chicken hekka	
	8 oz	8
	Chicken long rice	
	7 oz	4
	Haupia (coconut pudding)	
	½ cup	3

No Count		SmartPoints® value
	Huli huli chicken	
	breast, with skin and bone, 7⅓ oz	13
	drumstick, with skin and bone, 2 oz	3
	thigh, with skin and bone, 3 oz	6
	Kahlua pig	
	3 oz	3
	Katsu (4½" x 1½" x ¾" thick)	
	ahi, 4⅓ oz	5
	chicken, 4⅓ oz	5
	pork, 4⅓ oz	7
	Khal bi	
	4 oz	9
	Lau Lau (pork and fish in taro or spinach leaves)	
	7⅔ oz	8
	Lomi lomi salmon	
	3¾ oz	2
	Manapua with char shiu filling	
	1 (3¼ oz)	6
	Poi	
●	½ cup	4
	Salad	
	green papaya, with pork and shrimp, 5 oz	2
●	green papaya, without meat, 8½ oz	0
	poke (Hawaiian fish salad), ahi, 3¼ oz	1
	poke (Hawaiian fish salad), tako, 3¼ oz	2
	Sauce	
	curry, Hawaiian-style, 1 Tbsp	2
	Soup, vegetable and other	
	oxtail, Hawaiian-style, 1 cup	6
	Spam musubi	
	1 (4 oz)	9

Ice Cream Shop

No Count		SmartPoints® value
	Cream, whipped	
	aerosol, 2 Tbsp	1
	Frozen yogurt	
	chocolate, ½ cup	6
	chocolate, fat-free, ½ cup	5
	chocolate, soft-serve, ½ cup	6
	fat-free, no sugar added, ½ cup	3
	low-fat, ½ cup	5
	vanilla, fat-free, ½ cup	5
	Gelato	
	½ cup	7
	Ice cream	
	chocolate, ½ cup	7
	chocolate, light, ½ cup	6
	chocolate, light, no sugar added, ½ cup	5
	chocolate, light, soft-serve, ½ cup	6
	chocolate, rich, ½ cup	9
	chocolate, soft-serve, ½ cup	9
	fat-free, no sugar added, ½ cup	3
	French vanilla, soft-serve, ½ cup	9
	light, any flavor, no sugar added, ½ cup	5
	premium, ½ cup	13
	strawberry, ½ cup	7
	vanilla, ½ cup	7
	vanilla, fat-free, ½ cup	3
	vanilla, light, ½ cup	6
	vanilla, light, soft-serve, ½ cup	5
	vanilla, rich, ½ cup	13
	Ice cream cone only	
	cake or wafer, 1 (1 oz)	4
	plain or sugar, 1 (⅓ oz)	1
	Ice cream in cone	
	sundae cone, 1 (3½ oz)	15
	Ice cream sandwich	
	1 (2½ oz)	7

"We Like This!" item

No Count	SmartPoints® value
cookie-type, 1 (3 oz)	8
light, vanilla, 1 (2 ½ oz)	5
light, vanilla, no sugar added, 1 (2 ½ oz)	5
Ice cream soda	
8 fl oz	15
Sherbet	
½ cup	6
Sprinkles	
any type, 1 Tbsp	1
Topping, dessert	
butterscotch or caramel, 2 Tbsp	5
fruit, 2 Tbsp	5
fudge, regular, 2 Tbsp	7
nuts, in syrup, 2 Tbsp	7

Indian

No Count	SmartPoints® value
Aloo gobi	
1 cup	3
Aloo palak	
8 oz	4
Bhuna gosht	
9 oz	8
Biryani	
chicken, 10 oz	12
lamb, 10 oz	19
Butter chicken	
10¾ oz	9
Chana dal	
9 oz	6
Chicken jalfrezi	
6 oz	6
Chicken tikka	
4 ½ oz	5
Chutney	
2 Tbsp	3
Coconut rice	
Indian, 4 ⅓ oz	8
Curry	
beef, 7 ⅔ oz	13
Bengali fish, 13 ¾ oz	7
chicken, 7 ⅔ oz	12
egg, 7 ½ oz	4
lamb, 7 ⅔ oz	15
Flatbread	
chapati, 1 piece (¾ oz)	3
naan, 1 (3 oz)	6
paratha, 1 (1 ¼ oz)	5
puris, 1 (1 ½ oz)	4
Fritters	
vegetable, 7 oz	13
Kashmiri (lamb meatballs)	
3 ¾ oz	13
Kofta (vegetable balls without sauce)	
3 oz	8
Korma	
vegetable, 14 ¾ oz	12
Malai kofta (vegetable balls in cream sauce)	
7 oz	12
Masala	
beef, 12⅓ oz	9
chana, 8 oz	10
goat, 8 ½ oz	4
lamb, 8 ½ oz	5
Masala dosa	
with filling, 8 oz	16
without filling, 1 (5 ⅓ oz)	14
Mung dal	
9 ⅓ oz	8
Mutter paneer	
9 ⅓ oz	15
Pakora, vegetable	
1 (1 ¾ oz)	4
Palak paneer	
11 oz	15
Palak vada (vegetable dumpling)	
fried, 1 (2 ½ oz)	6
steamed, 1 (2 ¼ oz)	3

No Count	SmartPoints® value
Pesarattu	
6 ¼ oz	8
Raita	
1 cup	7
Rajmah	
1 cup	8
Rice pudding	
kheer, 8 oz	13
Rogan josh	
8 ¾ oz	11
Saag gosht	
8 ½ oz	5
Saag paneer	
9 oz	9
Samosa	
1 (1 oz)	4
Soup, vegetable and other	
mulligatawny, 1 cup	9
○ sambhar (Indian lentil), 1 cup	3
Stew	
bean and lentil stew (dal maharani), 1 cup	9
Tandoori chicken	
breast, without skin, 4 ½ oz	4
thigh, without skin, 1 (3 oz)	4
Tandoori fish	
5 ½ oz	5
Tandoori shrimp	
5 ½ oz	3
Vegetable pulao	
5 oz	5
Vindaloo	
chicken, 8 oz	7
lamb, 8 ⅓ oz	20
pork, 8 ⅓ oz	9
Yogurt drink	
mango lassi, 1 cup	8

"We Like This!" item

Italian, Pizzeria

No Count	SmartPoints® value
Pepperoni	
2 oz	10
Pizza	
14", cheese and pepperoni, regular crust, restaurant-type, 1 slice (4 oz)	10
14", cheese and pepperoni, thick crust, restaurant-type, 1 slice (4 ¼ oz)	11
14", cheese and pepperoni, thin crust, restaurant-type, 1 slice (2 ¾ oz)	9
14", cheese and sausage, regular crust, restaurant-type, 1 slice (4 oz)	11
14", cheese and sausage, thick crust, restaurant-type, 1 slice (4 ½ oz)	12
14", cheese and sausage, thin crust, restaurant-type, 1 slice (3 oz)	9
14", cheese, meat, and vegetable, regular crust, restaurant-type, 1 slice (4 ¾ oz)	11
14", cheese, regular crust, restaurant-type, 1 slice (3 ¾ oz)	9
14", cheese, stuffed crust, restaurant-type, 1 slice (4 oz)	11
14", cheese, thick crust, restaurant-type, 1 slice (4 oz)	10
14", cheese, thin crust, restaurant-type, 1 slice (2 ¾ oz)	8
one-meat topping, deep-dish, restaurant-type, 4 oz	10
one-meat topping, thin crust, restaurant-type, 2 ¾ oz	6
Sicilian, cheese, small, 3 oz	6

Italian, Restaurant

Artichoke	
marinated, 1 cup	6
stuffed, 8 oz	16

○ No Count	SmartPoints® value
Biscotti	
chocolate, 1 (1 oz)	6
plain, 1 (1 oz)	6
Bread, garlic	
1 slice (1½ oz)	8
Bruschetta	
3¼ oz	4
Calamari	
fried, 3½ oz	13
○ grilled, 3 oz	2
Cannelloni	
spinach and cheese, with tomato sauce, 12 oz	14
Cannoli	
1 (3⅓ oz)	13
Capers	
1 Tbsp	0
Caponata (eggplant appetizer)	
6½ oz	5
Cappuccino	
○ made with fat-free milk, 8 fl oz	2
made with reduced-fat (2%) milk, 8 fl oz	3
made with whole milk, 8 fl oz	3
ready-made, from machine, any flavor, 8 fl oz	4
Cavatelli with sausage and broccoli	
5 oz	8
Chai tea latte	
made with fat-free milk, 8 fl oz	4
made with reduced-fat (2%) milk, 8 fl oz	6
Cheese	
asiago, 1 oz	5
gorgonzola, 1 oz	4
mascarpone, 1 oz	6
mozzarella, fresh, 1 oz	3
Parmesan, 1 oz	4
Parmesan, shredded, ¼ cup	3
Parmigiano Reggiano, shredded, ¼ cup	3

○ No Count	SmartPoints® value
Pecorino Romano, grated, ¼ cup	3
Pecorino, grated, 1 Tbsp	1
provolone, 1 oz	4
Romano, 1 oz	4
Chicken cacciatore	
6½ oz	10
Chicken parmigiana	
without sauce, 5½ oz	10
Clams, baked	
2½ oz	11
Clams, fried	
6⅔ oz	12
Cookies	
amaretti, 1 (1 oz)	4
sesame seed, 2 (1 oz)	5
Dip	
artichoke, baked, 2 Tbsp	4
spinach-artichoke, restaurant-type, 2 oz	5
Eggplant	
breaded and fried, 2⅔ oz	3
Eggplant parmigiana	
with sauce, 13¼ oz	16
without sauce, 6¾ oz	12
Focaccia bread	
1 slice (2 oz)	4
Gnocchi	
cheese, 6½ oz	17
potato, 4 oz	7
spinach, 7¼ oz	19
Ices	
Italian, restaurant-type, ½ cup	3
water, pineapple-coconut, 4 fl oz	6
Lasagna	
chicken, 7 oz	8
meat, 7⅔ oz	9
vegetable, 7½ oz	10
vegetarian, with cheese and spinach, 10½ oz	13
with meat sauce, 7½ oz	8

○ No Count		SmartPoints® value
	Latte	
○	made with fat-free milk, 8 fl oz	3
	made with low-fat (1%) milk, 8 fl oz	4
	made with low-fat (1%) milk, 12 fl oz	6
	made with reduced-fat (2%) milk, 12 fl oz	6
	made with whole milk, 8 fl oz	5
	Linguine	
	with red clam sauce, 6 ¾ oz	9
	with white clam sauce, 7 ½ oz	11
	Macchiato	
	caramel, made with fat-free milk, 8 fl oz	6
	caramel, made with reduced-fat (2%) milk, 8 fl oz	7
	Manicotti	
	with tomato sauce, 12 oz	15
	Marsala, chicken	
	10¾ oz	20
	Marsala, veal	
	10½ oz	25
	Meatballs	
	with sauce, 10 oz	15
	without sauce, 1 (1 ¾ oz)	6
	Mozzarella, fried	
	1 piece (1 ¾ oz)	6
	Mushrooms	
	marinated, ½ cup	3
	stuffed, 4 (2 ¾ oz)	4
	Osso bucco	
	10"⅓ oz	12
	Pancetta	
	1 oz	4
	Panettone	
	1 piece (1 ⅔ oz)	10
	Pasta	
	cooked, 1 cup	5
○	whole-wheat, cooked, 1 cup	5
	Pasta e fagioli	
	1 cup	7
	Pasta primavera	
	with cream sauce, 11 ¾ oz	19
	with marinara sauce, 10 oz	7
	Pasta with garlic and oil	
	5 ¾ oz	9
	Penne a la vodka	
	10¾ oz	12
	Polenta	
○	cooked, ½ cup	4
	Prosciutto	
	2 oz	6
	Ravioli	
	cheese, without sauce, 9 oz	20
	meat, with tomato sauce, 13 ⅓ oz	18
	meat, without sauce, 7 oz	16
	mushroom, without sauce, 4 ⅔ oz	9
	Risotto	
	1 cup	15
	Salad	
	tomato and mozzarella, without dressing, 6 ⅓ oz	6
	Sauce	
	a la vodka, ½ cup	5
	Alfredo, ½ cup	14
	arrabbiata, ½ cup	4
	Bolognese, ½ cup	7
	clam, red, ¼ cup	2
	clam, white, ¼ cup	3
	pesto, ½ cup	19
	puttanesca, ½ cup	13
	tomato, Italian, ½ cup	3
○	tomato, with roasted garlic	0
	Sausage	
	Italian, pork, cooked, 3 oz	10
	Soup, seafood	
	cioppino, 1 cup	5

"We Like This!" item

No Count	Item	SmartPoints® value
	Soup, vegetable and other	
	Italian wedding, 1 cup	6
	lentil, 1 cup	5
	minestrone, 1 cup	7
	Spaghetti Bolognese	
	11 oz	13
	Spaghetti with marinara sauce	
	10"½ oz	8
	Spaghetti with meat sauce	
	10 oz	13
	Spaghetti, spinach	
	cooked, 5 oz	5
	Spumoni	
	½ cup	13
	Stromboli	
	2 ¾ oz	6
	Tiramisu	
	1 piece (6 ⅓ oz)	15
	restaurant-type, 1 piece (4 ¾ oz)	20
	Tortellini	
	cheese, without sauce, 3 oz	7
	meat, without sauce, 3 oz	5
	Tortoni	
	2 ½ oz	12
	Veal cutlet	
	breaded, fried, 4 oz	8
	Veal parmigiana	
	with sauce, 13 ¾ oz	14
	without sauce, 5 ½ oz	12
	Veal piccata	
	6 oz	12
	Veal scaloppine	
	4 ⅔ oz	8
	Veal with peppers	
	9 ¾ oz	11
	Zabaglione	
	½ cup	7
	Zeppole	
	1 (3 oz)	9

No Count	Item	SmartPoints® value
	Ziti, baked	
	with meat, 8 ⅔ oz	13
	without meat, 8 oz	9
	Zuppa di pesce	
	14 oz	10

Japanese

No Count	Item	SmartPoints® value
	Alcoholic beverages	
	mirin, 1 fl oz	1
	sake, 1 fl oz	1
	Cabbage	
	Japanese style, fresh, pickled, ¼ cup	0
	Dressing, salad	
	ginger, 2 Tbsp	3
	sesame seed, 2 Tbsp	5
	Edamame	
○	in pods, 1 cup	3
○	shelled, ½ cup	3
	Fish	
	eel, cooked, 3 oz	5
	Gyoza	
	1 (⅔ oz)	1
	Ice cream	
	green tea, ½ cup	6
	Mochi	
	1 (1 ¼ oz)	4
	Natto	
	1 cup	10
	Noodles	
	Japanese, soba, cooked, 1 cup	3
	Japanese, somen, cooked, 1 cup	6
	Noodles and sauce, soba	
	8 oz	13
	Rice	
	sushi, cooked, 3 oz	4
	Salad	
	seaweed, ½ cup	2

◎ No Count		SmartPoints® value
	Sashimi	
◎	all varieties except mackerel and salmon, 2 oz	1
	mackerel, 2 oz	3
	salmon, 2 oz	2
	Sauce	
	soy (shoyu), 1 Tbsp	0
	tamari, 2 Tbsp	0
	teriyaki, 1 Tbsp	1
	teriyaki, gluten-free, 1 Tbsp	1
	teriyaki, reduced-sodium, 1 Tbsp	1
	Shabu shabu	
	9 oz	9
	Shoyu chicken	
	3⅓ oz	7
	Soup, vegetable and other	
	miso, 1 cup	2
	saimin, 1 cup	6
	nebeyaki udon, 1 cup	3
	suimono, 1 cup	2
	Sukiyaki	
	with sauce, 15¼ oz	15
	Sunomono	
	2½ oz	1
	Sushi	
	Alaskan roll, 3 oz	4
	California roll, 5⅓ oz	5
	cone, 2¾ oz	4
	inari, 2¾ oz	4
	kappa maki (cucumber roll), 4 medium pieces (5 oz)	3
	maki (vegetables and rice rolled with seaweed), 1 piece (¾ oz)	1
	nigiri (sliced raw fish over rice), 6 small pieces (4 oz)	2
	nigiri (sliced raw fish over rice), 4½ oz	3
	nori maki (raw fish and rice rolled with seaweed), 4½ oz	3

◎ No Count		SmartPoints® value
	Philadelphia roll, 2¾ oz	4
	rainbow roll, 3 pieces (4 oz)	3
	shrimp tempura roll, 8½ oz	10
	spider roll, 9⅔ oz	10
	tuna roll, 4 oz	3
	tuna roll, spicy, 7 oz	7
	uni maki, 4 oz	3
	vegetable tempura roll, 7⅔ oz	6
	yellowtail roll, 4 oz	3
	Tamago-yaki (omelet roll)	
	1 (1½ oz)	2
	Tempura	
	shrimp, 3¾ oz	13
	Teppan yaki (mixed grill of beef, chicken, shrimp and vegetables)	
	9½ oz	12
	Teriyaki	
	beef, 5½ oz	8
	chicken, 5½ oz	6
	fish (except salmon), 5½ oz	5
	salmon, 5⅓ oz	9
	tofu, 5"⅓ oz	5
	Tofu	
	aburage, bean curd, fried, 3 oz	8
	agedashi, fried, 5 oz	7
	fried, 3 oz	6
	Tonkatsu	
	beef, 3⅔ oz	8
	chicken, 3⅔ oz	7
	pork, 3½ oz	10
	Yaki-soba	
	beef, 5⅔ oz	5
	chicken, 5⅔ oz	5
	pork, 5⅔ oz	6
	Yakitori	
	7½ oz	5
	Yosenabe	
	13¼ oz	3

"We Like This!" item

No Count	SmartPoints® value
Jewish	
Bagel	
any type other than those listed here, 1 large (4 ½ oz)	12
blueberry, restaurant-type, 1 (4 oz)	10
cinnamon-raisin, store-bought, 1 (3 ½ oz)	9
egg, small, 1 (2 ½ oz)	5
multi-grain, restaurant-type, 1 (4 ½ oz)	9
oat bran, small, 1 (2 ½ oz)	5
onion, restaurant-type, 1 (4 oz)	9
poppyseed, restaurant-type, 1 (4 oz)	9
pumpernickel, restaurant-type, 1 (4 oz)	8
salt, restaurant-type, 1 (4 oz)	8
Bagel with cream cheese and lox	
6 ½ oz	17
Beef	
flanken, cooked, 3 oz	7
tongue, cooked, 3 oz	8
Bialy	
1 (3 oz)	8
Blintz	
cheese, 1 (4 ¾ oz)	8
Bread	
challah, 1 slice (1 ½ oz)	3
Cake	
honey, 1 piece (4 oz)	14
Passover sponge, 1 piece (2 ½ oz)	6
Chicken and meatball fricassee	
14 ½ oz	8
Cholent	
4 oz	5
Cookies	
macaroon, 1 (⅔ oz)	3
mandelbrot, 1 (2 oz)	8
rugalach, 1 (1 oz)	6

No Count	SmartPoints® value
Fish	
lox, 3 oz	2
sable, smoked, 3 oz	6
whitefish, smoked, 2 oz	1
Gefilte fish	
3 oz	2
Hamantaschen	
1 (1 ⅓ oz)	4
Haroset	
1 Tbsp	0
Herring fillets	
chopped, 3 oz	5
pickled, 3 oz	7
Kasha varnishkes	
7 ¾ oz	7
Kishke	
¾ oz	3
Knish	
potato, 4 oz	9
Knockwurst	
boiled, 3 oz	9
Kreplach	
boiled, 2 ¾ oz	8
fried, 3 oz	9
Kugel	
lukschen, with fruit, 6 ⅔ oz	12
lukschen, without fruit, 5 ⅔ oz	7
potato, 6 ¼ oz	6
Latkes, potato	
6 ½ oz	8
Liver	
chopped, 3 oz	5
Matzo	
1 board (1 oz)	3
egg, 1 oz	3
egg and onion, 1 oz	3
plain, 1 oz	3
whole-wheat, 1 oz	3
Matzo brei	
3 oz	7

No Count	SmartPoints® value
Pastrami	
beef, 3 oz	3
Pickle	
dill, ¼ cup	0
sour, ¼ cup	0
Soup, chicken	
chicken with matzo balls, 1 cup	4
chicken, without matzo balls (broth only), 1 cup	1
Soup, vegetable and other	
mushroom-barley, 1 cup	4
Tzimmes, vegetable	
6 ⅔ oz	5

Korean

Bulgogi (beef stir-fry)	
4 ⅓ oz	4
Japchae	
beef, 4 oz	8
chicken, 4 oz	9
pork, 4 oz	10
Kim chee	
4 oz	1
Korean barbecue beef	
4 oz	7
Korean barbecue chicken thighs	
5 oz	14
Korean barbecue short ribs	
4 oz	9
Mun doo	
fried, 1 (1 ⅔ oz)	1
steamed, 1 (1 ½ oz)	1
Noodles	
potato (dang myeon), 2 oz	6
Pajun (Korean green onion and shrimp pancake)	
7 oz	9
Soup, vegetable and other	
oxtail, 1 cup	2

"We Like This!" item

No Count	SmartPoints® value

Mexican/Tex-Mex

Arroz con leche (Mexican rice pudding)	
restaurant-type, 10 oz	18
Beans, refried	
½ cup	6
restaurant-type, 1 cup	7
Bunuelos (fried yeast bread)	
restaurant-type, 1 slice (2 ½ oz)	12
Burrito	
bean, 1 (7 ½ oz)	8
beef and cheese, large, 1 (6 oz)	11
beef and cheese, small, 1 (3 ⅔ oz)	7
chicken and cheese, large, 1 (6 oz)	9
chicken and cheese, small, 1 (3 ⅔ oz)	6
vegetable, large, 11 oz	14
vegetable, small, 5 ½ oz	6
Cake	
corn, sweet, 4 oz	16
Carne asada	
5 oz	12
Carnitas	
5 ½ oz	8
Chalupa (pork and bean dish)	
5 ⅓ oz	8
Cheese	
manchego, 1 oz	4
queso anejo, 1 oz	4
queso asadero, 1 oz	4
queso chihuahua, 1 oz	4
queso cotija, 1 oz	4
queso fresco, 1 oz	3
Chicken adobo	
4 oz	6
Chicken mole	
7 oz	7

No Count	SmartPoints® value
Chili con carne	
with beans, 1 cup	8
with beans, family-style, restaurant-type, 6 ½ oz	9
without beans, 1 cup	8
Chimichanga	
beef, 1 (8 ⅓ oz)	13
chicken, 1 (8 ⅓ oz)	11
Chips, tortilla	
12 chips (1 oz)	4
Coffee, Mexican	
6 fl oz	6
Cookies	
Mexican wedding, 2 (½ oz)	3
Cornbread	
Mexican, 1 piece (3 ⅔ oz)	12
Dip	
Mexican 7-layer, 2 Tbsp	1
Empanadas	
2 (1 ¾ oz)	7
restaurant-type, 3 oz	10
Enchilada	
beef, cheese, or chicken, 4 ⅓ oz	8
sour cream, 1 (5 ½ oz)	12
Fajita	
beef, 9 oz	15
chicken, 2 (8 ¾ oz)	9
shrimp, 9 ¼ oz	9
vegetarian, 5 ½ oz	7
Flauta	
beef, 4 oz	14
chicken, 4 oz	13
pork, 4 oz	13
Gordita	
beef, 4 ¼ oz	14
Guacamole	
restaurant-type, 2 Tbsp	1
Huevos rancheros	
10 oz	18

No Count	SmartPoints® value
Ice cream	
fried, ½ cup	17
Jalapeño poppers	
1 (1 ⅔ oz)	5
Menudo	
10 oz	7
Nachos	
beef, 8 ⅔ oz	19
cheese, 3 oz	12
cheese and bean, 6 ½ oz	14
chicken, 8 ½ oz	16
with cheese sauce, 2 ¾ oz	8
Pico de gallo	
● fat-free	0
Pozole (pork and hominy soup)	
1 cup	5
Quesadilla	
beef, 4 oz	9
cheese, 2 ¼ oz	8
chicken, 3 ¾ oz	8
vegetable, 3 ⅔ oz	8
Red snapper Veracruz	
11 ¾ oz	11
Rolls	
bollilo, 1 (3 ½ oz)	9
Salsa	
black bean and corn, 2 Tbsp	1
● fat-free	0
● fat-free, gluten-free	0
mango, 2 Tbsp	1
peach, 2 Tbsp	1
pineapple, 2 Tbsp	1
Salsa verde	
● fat-free	0
Sauce	
mole poblano, 2 Tbsp	3
taco, 2 Tbsp	1
Sopaipillas	
2 (1 oz)	3

No Count	SmartPoints® value
Soup, chicken	
chicken-enchilada, 8 ¾ oz	6
with tortilla strips and shredded cheese, 1 cup	5
Soup, vegetable and other	
tortilla, 1 cup	8
Taco	
beef, 1 (3 ⅔ oz)	7
breakfast, 3 ¾ oz	7
chicken, 1 (3 ⅔ oz)	6
fish, 1 (4 ⅓ oz)	5
pork, 1 (3 ½ oz)	5
Tamales	
corn, restaurant-type, 6 oz	11
pork, restaurant-type, 5 oz	8
Taquitos	
beef, 3 oz	5
chicken, 3 oz	3
Tortilla	
corn, 1 (¾ oz)	2
flour, 1 medium (1 oz)	3
flour, 8", 1 (1 ¾ oz)	5
flour, burrito-size, 1 large (2 ¼ oz)	3
multi-grain, 8", 1 (1 ¾ oz)	5
whole-wheat, 1 (1 ⅓ oz)	2
Tostada	
beef, 1 (8 ½ oz)	13
chicken, 1 (8 ⅓ oz)	11
Tostada shells	
corn, 1 (½ oz)	2

Middle Eastern

No Count	SmartPoints® value
Baba ghanoush	
1 ¼ oz	3
Doro wat	
6 ¾ oz	8
Falafel	
in pita, 6 ¾ oz	15
Falafel patty	
4 (4 ⅔ oz)	10
Fattoush	
8 oz	7
Flatbread	
lavash, 1 (2 ¼ oz)	8
Goulash	
beef, 7 ⅔ oz	10
Hummus	
2 Tbsp	2
Kibbe	
baked, 1 piece (⅓ oz)	1
Pita	
pocketless, 1 (2 oz)	5
white, 1 (1 oz)	2
whole-wheat, 1 (1 oz)	2
Rice pilaf	
7 ⅓ oz	8
Shawarma	
chicken, 2 oz	5
Shish kabob	
4 ¾ oz	9
Tabouli	
3 ¼ oz	7

Salad Bar

No Count	SmartPoints® value
Bacon bits	
imitation, ¼ oz	1
Beans	
○ garbanzo (chickpeas), cooked, ½ cup	3
○ kidney, cooked, ½ cup	3
Beets	
pickled, ½ cup	3
Cheese	
blue, 1 oz	4
cheddar or colby, 1 oz	4
cottage, regular (4%), 1 cup	6
cottage, regular, with fruit, 1 cup	6
cottage, with vegetables, 1 cup	6

"We Like This!" item

No Count		SmartPoints® value
	Corn	
○	kernels, cooked, ½ cup	2
	Croutons	
	plain, 7 (1 oz)	3
	seasoned, 1 cup	6
	Dressing, salad	
	blue cheese, regular, 2 Tbsp	5
	French, 2 Tbsp	6
	Italian-tyle, regular, 2 Tbsp	3
	Italian-type, reduced-calorie, 2 Tbsp	2
	mayonnaise-type, 2 Tbsp	3
	Russian, regular, 2 Tbsp	4
	Thousand Island, 2 Tbsp	5
	vinaigrette, regular, 2 Tbsp	5
	Gelatin dessert	
	fruit-flavored, ½ cup	5
	Olives	
	black, ripe, canned, jumbo, 4 (1 oz)	1
	black, ripe, canned, large, 4 (1¼ oz)	1
	black, ripe, canned, small, 6 (⅔ oz)	1
	black, ripe, canned, super-colossal, 4 (2 oz)	2
	Seeds	
	sunflower seeds, dry-roasted, ¼ cup	6
	sunflower seeds, oil-roasted, ¼ cup	6
	sunflower seeds, toasted, ¼ cup	6

Scandinavian

No Count		SmartPoints® value
	Apple streusel	
	3½ oz	6
	Cheese	
	edam, 1 oz	4
	fontina, 1 oz	4
	gjetost, 1 oz	5
	Cookies	
	kringla, 1 (¾ oz)	3
	Dumpling	
	kroppkakor (potato dumpling), boiled, 1 (2 oz)	5
	kroppkakor (potato dumpling), fried, 1 (2 oz)	5
	Fish	
	salmon, smoked, 3 oz	2
	Flatbread	
	lefse, 1 (4½ oz)	8
	Meatballs, Swedish	
	4 oz	12
	Soup, chicken	
	knefla, 1 cup	8

Seafood

No Count		SmartPoints® value
	Crab cakes	
	5 oz	4
	blue crab, 2 oz	2
	Crab puffs	
	2 oz	6
	Fish	
○	arctic char, cooked, 3 oz	2
○	bass, fresh water, cooked, 1 fillet (2¼ oz)	1
○	bass, striped, cooked, 3 oz	1
○	bluefish, cooked, 3 oz	2
○	butterfish, cooked, 3 oz	3
○	carp, cooked, 3 oz	3
○	catfish, farm-raised, cooked, 3 oz	3
○	catfish, wild, cooked, 3 oz	1
○	cod, Atlantic, cooked, 3 oz	1
○	cod, Pacific, cooked, 3 oz	1
○	flounder, cooked, 3 oz	1
○	grouper, cooked, 3 oz	1
○	haddock, cooked, 3 oz	1
○	halibut, cooked, 3 oz	1
	mackerel, cooked, 3 oz	4
○	mahimahi (dolphinfish), cooked, 3 oz	1
○	monkfish, cooked, 3 oz	1
○	mullet, striped, cooked, 3 oz	2

No Count		SmartPoints® value
○	orange roughy, cooked, 3 oz	1
○	orange roughy, farm-raised, cooked, 6 oz	2
○	perch, cooked, 3 oz	1
○	pollack, cooked, 3 oz	1
	pompano, cooked, 3 oz	4
○	rockfish, cooked, 3 oz	1
	salmon, Atlantic, farmed, cooked, 3 oz	4
○	salmon, wild, cooked, 3 oz	3
○	sea bass, cooked, 3 oz	1
○	snapper, cooked, 3 oz	1
○	sole, cooked, 3 oz	1
○	swordfish, cooked, 3 oz	3
○	tilapia, cooked, 3 oz	1
○	tilefish, cooked, 3 oz	2
○	trout, cooked, 3 oz	3
○	trout, rainbow, farmed, cooked (steelhead), 1 fillet (2 ½ oz)	2
○	trout, rainbow, wild, cooked (steelhead), 3 oz	2
○	tuna, bluefin, cooked, 3 oz	3
○	tuna, cooked, 3 oz	1
○	turbot, European, cooked, 3 oz	2
	Fish fillet	
	battered or breaded, fried, family-style, restaurant-type, 8 oz	13
	grilled, with garlic butter, 3 ¾ oz	2
○	grilled, with lemon-pepper, 3 ¾ oz	2
	Fish, baked, stuffed	
	6 ¾ oz	11
	Oysters	
	fried, 5 ¼ oz	9
	Oysters Rockefeller	
	2 oz	4
	Sauce	
	tartar, ¼ cup	5
	Scallops	
	breaded and fried, 3 oz	5
	fried, 3 oz	5

"We Like This!" item

No Count		SmartPoints® value
	Shellfish	
○	clams, cooked, 3 oz	2
○	clams, raw, 4 oz	1
○	crab, Alaska king, cooked, 3 oz	1
○	crabmeat, cooked, 3 oz	1
○	crabmeat, lump, 3 oz	1
○	crayfish, cooked, 3 oz	1
○	crayfish, wild, cooked, 3 oz	1
○	lobster, cooked, 3 oz	1
○	lobster, spiny, cooked, 3 oz	2
○	lobster, steamed (1 ¼ pounds in the shell), 3 oz shelled	1
○	mussels, cooked, 3 oz	3
○	mussels, raw, in shell, 4 oz	2
○	octopus, common, cooked, 3 oz	2
○	oyster, cooked, 3 oz	2
○	oyster, Pacific, cooked, 3 oz	3
○	oyster, raw, 4 oz	2
○	scallops, cooked, 3 oz	1
○	shrimp, cooked, 3 oz	1
○	squid, cooked, 3 oz	1
	Shrimp	
	breaded and fried, 3 oz	5
	broiled, stuffed, 3 oz	12
	fried, 3 oz	5
	fried, stuffed, 9 ½ oz	9
	Shrimp puffs	
	1 (⅓ oz)	1
	Shrimp scampi	
	3 ⅔ oz	13
	Soup, seafood	
	lobster bisque, 11 oz	7
	lobster bisque, restaurant-type, 1 cup	16
	Manhattan clam chowder, 6 ½ oz	4
	Manhattan clam chowder, restaurant-type, 1 cup	5
	New England clam chowder, 1 cup	6
	New England clam chowder, restaurant-type, 1 cup	11

No Count	Food	SmartPoints® value
	Squid	
	fried, 3 oz	3

Southern U.S./Soul Food

No Count	Food	SmartPoints® value
	Apple brown Betty	
	4 ¾ oz	10
	Biscuit	
	cheese, 1 (1 ¾ oz)	8
	small, 1 (1 ½ oz)	4
	Catfish	
	channel, breaded and fried, 3 oz	5
	Chicken and dumplings	
	cooked, with skin, 5 oz	9
	cooked, without skin, 5 oz	8
	Chicken breast	
	fried, with skin and bone, 4 ½ oz	11
	fried, with skin, without bone, 3 oz	5
	Chicken drumstick	
	fried, with skin and bone, 1 (1 ½ oz)	6
	Chicken thigh	
	fried, with skin and bone, 3 oz	8
	Chitterlings	
	cooked, 3 oz	7
	Corn	
	cream-style, ½ cup	3
	Corn casserole	
	6 ¼ oz	14
	Cornbread dressing	
	6 ⅓ oz	11
	Fritters	
	corn, 4 oz	7
	Gravy	
	brown, 2 Tbsp	2
	cream, 2 Tbsp	3
	giblet, 2 Tbsp	1
	sausage, 2 Tbsp	3
	Greens	
	seasoned with bacon or salt pork, 1 cup	5
	Grits	
●	white, cooked, 1 cup	5
●	yellow, quick, cooked, 1 cup	4
	Hush puppies	
	1 ½ oz	5
	Macaroni and cheese	
	9 ¾ oz	14
	family-style, restaurant-type, 7 ½ oz	11
	Okra	
	fried, 7 oz	11
	Peas, black-eyed	
●	fresh, cooked, ½ cup	3
	Sauce	
	hot, 2 Tbsp	0
	Soup, vegetable and other	
	split pea, 1 cup	4
	Spoon bread	
	1 cup	15
	Stew	
	beef, 7 ½ oz	5
	Brunswick, 1 ½ cups	6
	Succotash	
●	cooked, 1 cup	7
	Sweet potato pie	
	6 ¾ oz	16
	Tomatoes	
	fried green, 2 slices (5 oz)	5

Spanish

No Count	Food	SmartPoints® value
	Arroz con pollo	
	11 ⅓ oz	16
	Ceviche	
	4 ¾ oz	2
	Chorizo	
	3 oz	13
	chicken, 1 oz	1

No Count		SmartPoints® value
	Flan	
	½ cup	11
	Paella	
	8½ oz (We Like This!)	9
	Sauce	
	sofrito, 2 Tbsp (We Like This!)	2
	Spanish, 2 Tbsp (We Like This!)	0
	Soup, vegetable and other	
●	gazpacho, 1 cup	3

Steakhouse

No Count		SmartPoints® value
	Beef	
●	bottom sirloin (tri-tip), trimmed, cooked, 3 oz	3
	chuck, blade roast, cooked, 3 oz	9
	chuck, blade roast, trimmed, cooked, 3 oz (We Like This!)	5
	cube steak, cooked, 3 oz	3
●	cube steak, trimmed, cooked, 3 oz	2
●	eye round, steak or roast, trimmed, cooked, 3 oz	2
	filet mignon, cooked, 3 oz	6
●	filet mignon, lean only, trimmed, cooked, 3 oz	3
●	flank, lean, trimmed, cooked, 3 oz	3
	KC strip, cooked, 3 oz	5
●	KC strip, lean, trimmed, cooked, 3 oz	3
	New York steak, cooked, 3 oz	5
●	New York steak, lean, trimmed, cooked, 3 oz	3
	porterhouse steak, cooked, 3 oz	9
	porterhouse steak, trimmed, cooked, 3 oz	7
	rib eye roast, boneless lean, cooked, 3 oz	4
	rib eye, trimmed, cooked, 3 oz	5
●	round, lean, trimmed, cooked, 3 oz	2
	round, steak or roast, cooked, 3 oz	5
●	rump roast, lean, trimmed, cooked, 3 oz	3
	sirloin, cooked, 3 oz	6
●	sirloin, lean, trimmed, cooked, 3 oz	3
	sirloin, trimmed, cooked, 3 oz	4
	skirt steak, cooked, 3 oz	5
	steak, flat iron, cooked, 3 oz	5
●	steak, lean, cooked (round or loin cuts with all visible fat trimmed), 3 oz	3
	steak, regular, cooked, 3 oz	8
	steak, sirloin, family-style, restaurant-type, 6 oz	7
	steak, skirt, lean and fat, trimmed, cooked, 3 oz	5
	strip sirloin, cooked, 3 oz	6
●	strip sirloin, lean, trimmed, cooked, 3 oz	3
	t-bone steak, cooked, 3 oz	8
	t-bone steak, lean, trimmed, cooked, 3 oz	6
	tenderloin, cooked, 3 oz	6
●	tenderloin, lean only, trimmed, cooked, 3 oz	3
	Beefalo	
●	cooked, 3 oz	3
	Breadsticks	
	any type, 1 (⅓ oz) (We Like This!)	1
	soft, 1 (1⅓ oz)	3
	Cream, sour	
	regular, 2 Tbsp	3
	Lamb	
●	chop, baby, cooked, 3 oz	3
●	chop, cooked, 3 oz	4
	Onion, blooming	
	5 oz	6
	Pepper steak	
	7 oz	16

"We Like This!" item

No Count		SmartPoints® value
	Pork	
○	chop, lean, without bone, cooked, 3 oz	3
	chop, loin, center rib, bone-in, lean, cooked, 3 oz	4
	chop, loin, center rib, boneless, lean, cooked, 3 oz	4
○	chop, sirloin, bone-in, lean, cooked, 3 oz	2
○	chop, top loin, boneless, lean, cooked, 1 (5 oz)	5
	Potato, baked	
○	plain, 1 medium (6 oz)	5
	stuffed with bacon and cheese, 9¾ oz	17
	stuffed with vegetables and cheese, 13½ oz	14
	Potato, mashed	
	garlic, 5 oz	7
	Potato, stuffed	
	stuffed with cheese, 5½ oz	7
	stuffed with sour cream and chives, 5½ oz	6
	Potatoes, scalloped	
	5¾ oz	6
	Rolls	
	dinner, 1 (2 oz)	5
	Salad	
	Caesar, 6 oz	8
	cobb, without dressing, 12¾ oz	12
○	tossed, without dressing	0
	Salisbury steak	
	6 oz	14
	Sauce	
	steak, 1 Tbsp	1
	Spinach, creamed	
	restaurant-type, 4⅓ oz	8
	Veal chop	
	cooked, 3 oz	6
○	lean, cooked, 3 oz	4

Thai

No Count		SmartPoints® value
	Coconut rice	
	Thai, 10"⅓ oz	16
	Curry	
	green chicken (gaeng kheow wan gai), 7⅓ oz	13
	Drunken noodles	
	7⅓ oz	6
	Fried rice	
	kho-phat, 6 oz	10
	Ginger chicken	
	7¾ oz	6
	Noodles	
	rice, cooked, 1 cup	5
	Pad si-iew (stir-fried beef with noodles)	
	7⅓ oz	8
	Pad Thai (rice noodles with chicken and shrimp)	
	8 oz	12
	Pad Thai, chicken	
	restaurant-type, 1¼ cups	14
	Panang curry with beef	
	11 oz	19
	Panang curry with chicken	
	11 oz	18
	Salad	
	beef, Thai, 11 oz	17
	chicken, Thai, 15½ oz	12
	seafood, Thai, 9⅓ oz	11
	Satay	
	beef, with peanut sauce, 2 (6 oz)	15
	beef, without peanut sauce, 2 (3 oz)	5
	chicken, with peanut sauce, 2 (5⅓ oz)	12
	chicken, without peanut sauce, 2 (3 oz)	2

No Count	SmartPoints® value
Sauce	
peanut, spicy, 1 Tbsp	2
sambal oelek, 1 Tbsp	0
satay, 1 Tbsp	1
sriracha, hot, 1 Tbsp	0
Seafood cakes (haw mok thalay)	
5 ¾ oz	14
Soup, chicken	
hot and spicy chicken, 1 cup	3
Thai chicken-coconut, 1 cup	12
Soup, vegetable and other	
Thai coconut ginger, canned, 1 cup	8
Spring roll	
Thai, 1 (2 ½ oz)	5
Tapioca	
Thai, ½ cup	7
Thai chicken with basil	
3 ¾ oz	4
Thai chili beef (neua pad prik)	
8 oz	6
Thai coffee or tea	
8 fl oz	16
Thai crisp noodles	
1 cup	10
Thai grilled beef (nuea nam tok)	
5 ¾ oz	6
Tom yum kung	
9 ⅓ oz	2

Vietnamese

No Count	SmartPoints® value
Beef balls	
Vietnamese (thit bo vien), 6 (1 ¼ oz)	2
Curry	
Vietnamese chicken, 8 oz	11
Imperial roll	
2 oz	5
Lemon grass chicken	
8 ¾ oz	9
Sauce	
nuoc cham, 2 Tbsp	1
Vietnamese spring roll dipping, ½ oz	0
Soup, seafood	
asparagus-crab, 1 cup	2
Soup, vegetable and other	
● Vietnamese beef-noodle, 1 cup	3
Spring roll	
fresh, Vietnamese, 1 (1 ¾ oz)	2
fried, Vietnamese, 1 (2 ½ oz)	5

"We Like This!" item

Restaurant Menus By Cuisine

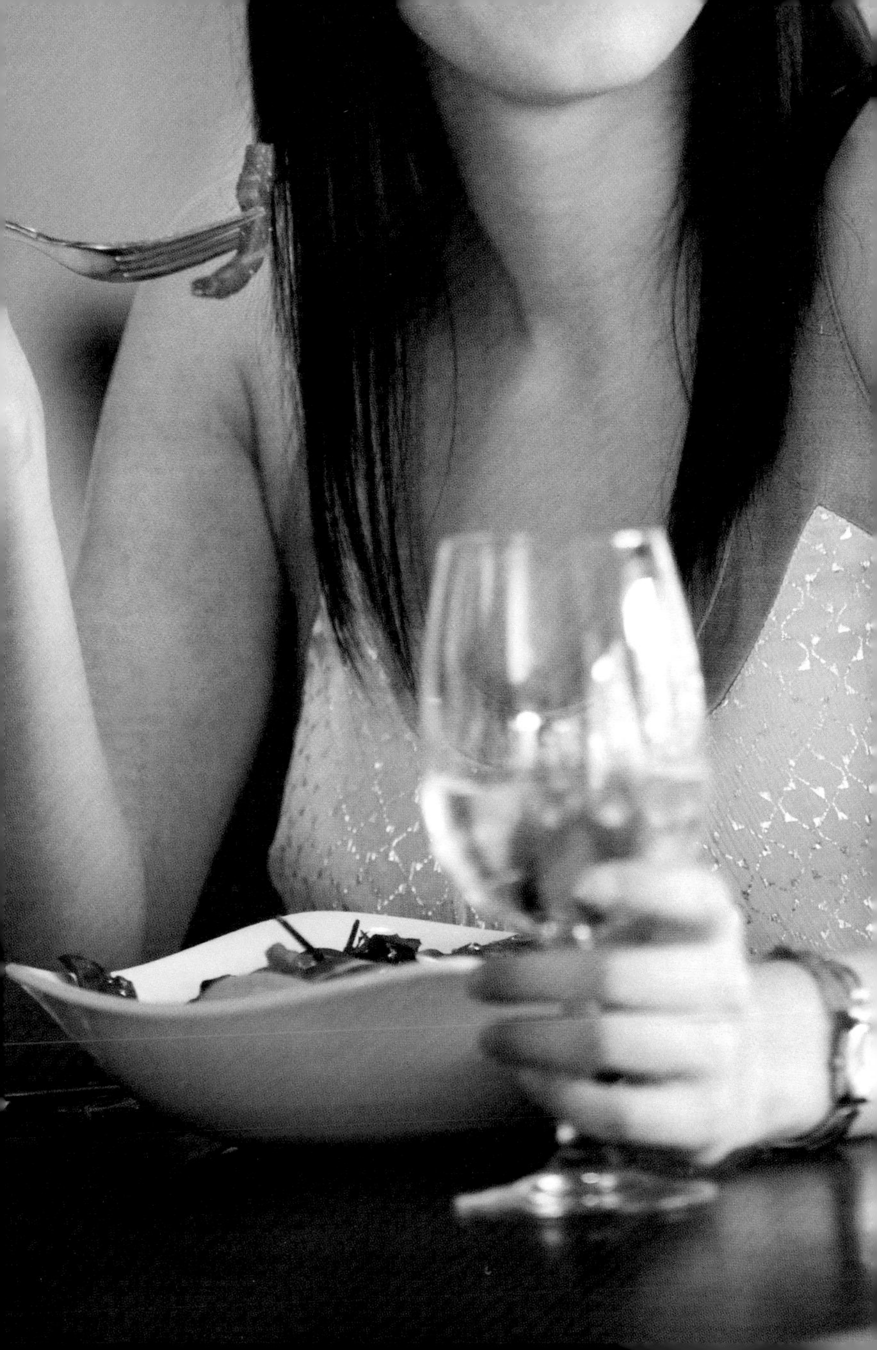

restaurant menus by

national chain

Appetizers & Bar Snacks

	SmartPoints® value
Boneless Wings Sampler (without sauce or dressing), 1 serving	9
Boneless Wings Standard (without sauce or dressing), 1 serving	19
Boneless Wings with Classic Buffalo Sauce and Bleu Cheese Dressing, 1 serving	36
Boneless Wings with Classic Buffalo Sauce and Ranch Dressing, 1 serving	34
Boneless Wings with Honey BBQ Sauce and Bleu Cheese Dressing, 1 serving	40
Boneless Wings with Honey BBQ Sauce and Ranch Dressing, 1 serving	39
Boneless Wings with Hot Buffalo Sauce and Bleu Cheese Dressing, 1 serving	36
Boneless Wings with Hot Buffalo Sauce and Ranch Dressing, 1 serving	34
Boneless Wings with Sweet Asian Chile Sauce and Bleu Cheese Dressing, 1 serving	40
Boneless Wings with Sweet Asian Chile Sauce and Ranch Dressing, 1 serving	39
Cheese Quesadilla, 1 serving	22
Cheeseburger Eggrolls, 1 serving	35
Cheeseburger Eggrolls (sampler), 1 serving	22
Cheesy Bread Pizza (full), 1 serving	22
Cheesy Bread Pizza (half), 1 serving	11
Chicken Quesadilla, 1 serving	33
Chicken Quesadilla (pub plates), 1 serving	32
Chicken Quesadilla Sampler, 1 serving	21
Chips & Salsa, 1 serving	16
Double Crunch Bone-In Wings (without sauce or dressing), 1 serving	18
Double Crunch Bone-In Wings Sampler - Thai, 1 serving	16
Double Crunch Bone-In Wings Sampler (without sauce or dressing), 1 serving	8
Double Crunch Bone-In Wings with Classic Buffalo Sauce & Bleu Cheese Dressing, 1 serving	35
Double Crunch Bone-In Wings with Classic Buffalo Sauce & Ranch Dressing, 1 serving	33
Double Crunch Bone-In Wings with Honey BBQ Sauce & Bleu Cheese Dressing, 1 serving	39
Double Crunch Bone-In Wings with Honey BBQ Sauce & Ranch Dressing, 1 serving	38
Double Crunch Bone-In Wings with Hot Buffalo Sauce & Bleu Cheese Dressing, 1 serving	35
Double Crunch Bone-In Wings with Hot Buffalo Sauce & Ranch Dressing, 1 serving	33
Double Crunch Bone-In Wings with Sweet Asian Chile Sauce & Bleu Cheese Dressing, 1 serving	39
Double Crunch Bone-In Wings with Sweet Asian Chile Sauce & Ranch Dressing, 1 serving	38
Fried Shrimp, 1 serving	7
Green Bean Crispers, 1 serving	18
Grilled Chicken Wonton Tacos, 1 serving	15
Grilled Chicken Wonton Tacos Sampler, 1 serving	11
Housemade Sweet and Spicy Pickles, 1 serving	6
Kobe Style Meatballs, 1 serving	23
Mozzarella Sticks, 1 serving	31

"We Like This!" item

	SmartPoints® value
Mozzarella Sticks Sampler, 1 serving	15
Pot Stickers, 1 serving	23
Pot Stickers (shareables), 1 serving	23
Pot Stickers Sampler, 1 serving	11
Pretzels & Beer Cheese Dip, 1 serving	35
Pretzels & Beer Cheese Dip Sampler, 1 serving	17
Salsa Verde Beef Nachos, 1 serving	64
Salsa Verde Pulled Pork Nachos, 1 serving	39
Salsa Verde Pulled Pork Nachos Sampler, 1 serving	19
Salsa Verde Shredded Brisket Nachos, 1 serving	37
Salsa Verde Shredded Brisket Nachos Sampler, 1 serving	19
Spinach & Artichoke Dip, 1 serving	33
Sriracha Shrimp, 1 serving	22
Sriracha Shrimp Sampler, 1 serving	14
Steak Quesadilla, 1 serving	33
Steak Quesadilla (sampler), 1 serving	21
Sweet Asian Chile Sauce, 1 serving	13
Sweet Asian Chile Sauce (sampler), 1 serving	6
Sweet Chile Brisket Sliders, 1 serving	43
Sweet Chile Brisket Sliders Sampler, 1 serving	19
Sweet Potato Fries & Dips, 1 serving	41

Fire Grilled & Chef Selections

	SmartPoints® value
4 oz Sirloin, 1 serving	3
6 oz USDA Top Sirloin, 1 serving	5
7 oz House Sirloin (ball tip), 1	3
7 oz House Sirloin (tri tip), 1 serving	7
8 oz USDA Top Sirloin, 1 serving	5
9 oz Bourbon Street Steak (ball tip), 1 serving	18
9 oz Bourbon Street Steak (tri tip), 1 serving	22
9 oz House Sirloin (ball tip), 1 serving	4
9 oz House Sirloin (tri tip), 1 serving	8
12 oz New York Strip, 1 serving	11
12 oz Ribeye, 1 serving	13
Bourbon Street Steak (2-4 oz includes side), 1 serving	20
Butcher's Reserve 12 oz Top Sirloin, 1 serving	6
Chicken & Steak (ball tip) Fajitas with Rice, 1 serving	42
Chicken & Steak (tri tip) Fajitas with Rice, 1 serving	43
Crosscut Ribs Platter with Honey BBQ Sauce, 1 serving	53
Crosscut Ribs Platter with Smoky Chipotle Sauce, 1 serving	50
Crosscut Ribs Platter with Sweet Asian Chile Sauce, 1 serving	52
Crosscut Ribs with Honey BBQ Sauce, 1 serving	23
Crosscut Ribs with Smoky Chipotle Sauce, 1 serving	21
Crosscut Ribs with Sweet Asian Chile Sauce, 1 serving	23
Double Glazed Baby Back Ribs Full Rack (without sauce), 1 serving	28
Double Glazed Baby Back Ribs Full Rack with Honey BBQ Sauce, 1 serving	36

Fire Grilled & Chef Selections (cont'd)

	SmartPoints® value
Double Glazed Baby Back Ribs Full Rack with Smoky Chipotle Sauce, 1 serving	35
Double Glazed Baby Back Ribs Full Rack with Sweet Asian Chile Sauce, 1 serving	37
Double Glazed Baby Back Ribs Half Rack (without sauce), 1 serving	14
Double Glazed Baby Back Ribs Half Rack with Honey BBQ Sauce, 1 serving	19
Double Glazed Baby Back Ribs Half Rack with Smoky Chipotle Sauce, 1 serving	17
Double Glazed Baby Back Ribs Half Rack with Sweet Asian Chile Sauce, 1 serving	19
Fried Shrimp-Steak Combo (ball tip), 1 serving	17
Fried Shrimp-Steak Combo (tri tip), 1 serving	21
Full Rack Platter with BBQ Sauce, 1 serving	53
Full Rack Platter with Smoky Chipotle Sauce, 1 serving	52
Full Rack Platter with Sweet Asian Chile Sauce, 1 serving	53
Grilled Onion Sirloin with Stout Gravy, 1 serving	16
Grilled Shrimp-Steak Combo (ball tip), 1 serving	4
Grilled Shrimp-Steak Combo (tri tip), 1 serving	8
Half Rack with BBQ Sauce, 1 serving	35
Half Rack with Smoky Chipotle Sauce, 1 serving	34
Half Rack with Sweet Asian Chile Sauce, 1 serving	35
Hand Cut Bone-In Pork Chop, 1 serving	8

	SmartPoints® value
Honey BBQ Chicken-Steak Combo (ball tip), 1 serving	14
Honey BBQ Chicken-Steak Combo (tri tip), 1 serving	18
Pepper Crusted Sirloin & Whole Grains, 1 serving	10
Riblet & Chicken Tenders Basket with Honey BBQ Sauce, 1 serving	45
Riblet & Chicken Tenders Basket with Smoky Chipotle Sauce, 1 serving	44
Riblet & Chicken Tenders Basket with Sweet Asian Chile Sauce, 1 serving	41
Riblet & Chicken Tenders Platter with Honey BBQ Sauce, 1 serving	59
Riblet & Chicken Tenders Platter with Smoky Chipotle Sauce, 1 serving	57
Riblet & Chicken Tenders Platter with Sweet Asian Chile Sauce, 1 serving	55
Riblets Basket with Honey BBQ Sauce, 1 serving	38
Riblets Basket with Smoky Chipotle Sauce, 1 serving	36
Riblets Basket with Sweet Asian Chile Sauce, 1 serving	34
Riblets Platter with Honey BBQ Sauce, 1 serving	56
Riblets Platter with Smoky Chipotle Sauce, 1 serving	52
Riblets Platter with Sweet Asian Chile Sauce, 1 serving	52
Riblets-Steak Combo, Honey BBQ (ball tip), 1 serving	27
Riblets-Steak Combo, Honey BBQ (tri tip), 1 serving	31
Riblets-Steak Combo, Smoky Chipotle (ball tip), 1 serving	22
Riblets-Steak Combo, Smoky Chipotle (tri tip), 1 serving	25

"We Like This!" item

	SmartPoints® value
Riblets-Steak Combo, Sweet Asian Chile (ball tip), 1 serving	23
Riblets-Steak Combo, Sweet Asian Chile (tri tip), 1 serving	26
Shrimp & Steak (ball tip) Fajitas with Rice, 1 serving	41
Shrimp & Steak (tri tip) Fajitas with Rice, 1 serving	42
Sirloin Stir Fry, 1 serving	23
Sizzling Double Barrel Whisky Sirloins (ball tip), 1 serving	17
Sizzling Double Barrel Whisky Sirloins (tri tip), 1 serving	19
Smokin' Double Steak and Egg, 1 serving	12
Steak (ball tip) Fajitas with Rice, 1 serving	42
Steak (tri tip) Fajitas with Rice, 1 serving	44
Steakhouse Bruschetta Sirloin, 1 serving	16

Burgers

Beer Garden Burger, 1 serving	38
Classic Burger (no cheese or bacon), 1	26
Cowboy Burger, 1	46
Mini Cheeseburger, 1	13
Mini Cheeseburgers, 2	23
Mini Hamburger, 1	11
Mini Hamburgers, 2	21
Mushroom Swiss Burger, 1	37
Quesadilla Burger, 1	48
Sweet Asian Pineapple Burger, 1	36
The All Day Brunch Burger, 1	40
The American Standard Burger, 1	35
The Blazin' Texan Burger, 1	36
Triple Bacon Burger, 1	40
Veggie Burger, 1	16

Chicken

	SmartPoints® value
Bourbon Street Chicken & Shrimp, 1 serving	18
Cedar Grilled Lemon Chicken, 1 serving	16
Cheesy Grilled Chicken, 1 serving	14
Chicken Fajitas with Rice, 1 serving	40
Chicken Griller, 1 serving	2
Chicken Tenders, 1 serving	8
Chicken Tenders Basket, 1 serving	36
Chicken Tenders Platter, 1 serving	46
Crispy Brewhouse Chicken, 1 serving	33
Fiesta Lime Chicken, 1 serving	34
Grilled Chicken Breast, 1 serving	2
Hot Shot Whisky Chicken, 1 serving	18
Napa Chicken & Portobellos, 1 serving	13

Pasta, Seafood & More

Baked Cod, 1 serving	31
Baked Haddock, 1 serving	32
Blackened Tilapia, 1 serving	15
Butcher's Meat and Potatoes, 1 serving	21
Cedar Grilled Salmon, 1 serving	8
Cedar Salmon with Maple Mustard Glaze, 1 serving	18
Chicken and Shrimp Fajitas with Rice, 1 serving	39
Chicken Mac 'n Cheese, 1 serving	20
Double Crunch Shrimp, 1 serving	41
Fish & Chips, 1 serving	47
Four Cheese Mac and Cheese, 1 serving	18
Four Cheese Mac with Honey Pepper Chicken Tenders, 1 serving	57

	SmartPoints® value
Grilled Shrimp, 1 serving	4
Hand Breaded Fish & Chips, 1 serving	49
Loaded Beef Enchiladas, 1 serving	32
Margarita Queso Chicken & Shrimp, 1 serving	28
New England Fish & Chips, 1 serving	64
Northern Walleye, 1 serving	22
Shrimp & Broccoli Cavatappi, 1 serving	17
Shrimp Fajitas with Rice, 1 serving	39
Shrimp 'N Parmesan (steak toppers), 1 serving	8
Shrimp 'N Parmesan Sirloin (8 oz), 1 serving	18
Shrimp 'N Parmesan Sirloin (ball tip), 1 serving	12
Shrimp Scampi Linguini, 1 serving	33
Shrimp Wonton Stir Fry, 1 serving	19
Three Cheese Chicken Cavatappi, 1 serving	42
Three Cheese Chicken Penne, 1 serving	33
Walleye Fish & Chips, Battered, 1 serving	47

Handhelds

American BLT Sandwich, 1	37
Battered Fish Sandwich, 1	25
Brew Pub Philly Sandwich, 1	37
Chicken Fajita Rollup, 1	35
Clubhouse Grille Sandwich, 1	38
Grilled Cheese Sandwich, 1	22
Hot Dog, 1	10
Kickin' Turkey Stacker Sandwich, 1	32
Maple Bacon Chicken Piadini Sandwich, 1	32
Philly Sandwich, 1	39
Triple Hog Dare Ya Sandwich, 1	33

"We Like This!" item

Lunch Combos

	SmartPoints® value
American BLT Sandwich, 1	19
Broccoli & Cheese Soup, 1 serving	16
Caesar Salad, 1 serving	8
Chicken Fajita Rollup, 1 serving	23
Chicken Noodle Soup, 1 serving	3
Chicken Tortilla Soup, 1 serving	6
Clubhouse Grille Sandwich, 1	19
Fiesta Chicken Chopped Salad, 1 serving	10
Four Cheese Mac with Honey Pepper Chicken Tenders (lunch), 1 serving	23
French Onion Soup, 1 serving	14
Fried Chicken Salad, 1 serving	13
Grilled Chicken Caesar Salad, 1 serving	9
Grilled Shrimp 'N Spinach Salad, 1 serving	10
Honey Pepper Chicken Tenders, 1 serving	34
House Salad without dressing, 1 serving	6
Kickin' Turkey Stacker Sandwich, 1	17
New England Clam Chowder, 1 serving	14
Oriental Chicken Salad, 1 serving	15
Potato Soup, 1 serving	17
Shrimp Scampi Linguini, 1 serving	15
Southwest Black Bean Soup, 1 serving	5
Spinach Salad, 1 serving	10
Thai Shrimp Salad, 1 serving	6
Three Cheese Chicken Cavatappi, 1 serving	18
Three Cheese Chicken Penne Pasta, 1 serving	16
Tomato Basil Soup, 1 serving	8

Salads

	SmartPoints® value
Caesar Salad (small), 1 serving	8
Fiesta Chicken Chopped Salad (regular), 1 serving	28
Fried Chicken Salad (regular), 1 serving	39
Green Goddess Wedge Salad, 1 serving	20
Grilled Chicken Caesar Salad (half size), 1 serving	12
Grilled Chicken Caesar Salad (regular), 1 serving	23
Grilled Shrimp 'n Spinach Salad (regular), 1 serving	35
House Salad (without dressing), 1 serving	6
Oriental Chicken Salad (half size), 1 serving	24
Oriental Chicken Salad (regular), 1 serving	48
Oriental Grilled Chicken Salad (half size), 1 serving	24
Oriental Grilled Chicken Salad (regular), 1 serving	44
Pecan Crusted Chicken Salad (regular), 1 serving	48
Thai Shrimp Salad, 1 serving	12

Dressings and Extras

	SmartPoints® value
American Cheese (add on for burger), 1 serving	6
Bacon (add on for burger), 1 serving	3
Bacon Vinaigrette, 1 serving	8
Bacon Vinaigrette (lunch), 1 serving	6
Bleu Cheese Dressing, 1 serving	9
Buttermilk Ranch Dressing, 1 serving	7
Cheddar Cheese (add on for burger), 1 serving	3
Chili Lime Vinaigrette, 1 serving	5
Classic Buffalo Sauce, 1 serving	8
Classic Buffalo Sauce (sampler), 1 serving	4
Crispy Onion Topper (steak toppers), 1 serving	11
Dijon Honey Mustard Dressing, 1 serving	8
Fat Free Italian Dressing, 1 serving	1
Garlic Caesar Dressing, 1 serving	7
Green Goddess Dressing, 1 serving	7
Grilled Onions (steak toppers), 1 serving	2
Guacamole (add on for sizzling entrées), 1 serving	2
Honey Balsamic Dressing, 1 serving	7
Honey BBQ Sauce, 1 serving	13
Honey BBQ Sauce (sampler), 1 serving	6
Honey French Dressing, 1 serving	9
Hot Buffalo Sauce, 1 serving	9
Hot Buffalo Sauce (sampler), 1 serving	5
Lemon Olive Oil Vinaigrette, 1 serving	5
Mexi Ranch Dressing, 1 serving	6
Monterey Jack (add on for burger), 1 serving	3
Oriental Dressing, 1 serving	10
Ranch Dressing, 1 serving	7
Sautéed Garlic Mushrooms (steak toppers), 1 serving	6
Swiss Cheese (add on for burger), 1 serving	6

Sides

	SmartPoints® value
Baked Potato, 1 serving	15
BBQ Spiced Fries, 1 serving	14
Broccoli & Cheese Soup, 1 serving	16
Chicken Noodle Soup, 1 serving	4
Chicken Tortilla Soup, 1 serving	6
Chili, 1 serving	10
Chili Cheese Fries, 1 serving	20
Classic Fries, 1 serving	14
Crispy Cheddar Bacon Potatoes, 1 serving	14
Crunchy Onion Rings, 1 serving	18
Fiesta Corn Chowder, 1 serving	14
French Onion Soup, 1 serving	12
Garlic Fries, 1 serving	21
Garlic Mashed Potatoes, 1 serving	9
Garlicky Green Beans, 1 serving	7
Hearty Grains and Rice, 1 serving	7
House Chips, 1 serving	14
Loaded Baked Potato, 1 serving	17
Loaded Garlic Mashed Potatoes, 1 serving	18
Maple Pecan Mashed Sweet Potatoes, 1 serving	18
New England Clam Chowder, 1 serving	10
Portsmouth Clam Chowder, 1 serving	8
Potato Soup, 1 serving	17
Seasonal Vegetables, 1 serving	0
Southwest Steak and Black Bean Soup, 1 serving	5
Steamed Broccoli, 1 serving	4
Sweet Potato Fries, 1 serving	13
Tomato Basil Soup, 1 serving	8
Tuscan Bean Soup with Chicken & Sausage, 1 serving	5
Wood Fired Grilled Veggies, 1 serving	7

Kid's Menu

	SmartPoints® value
Apple Dippers with Yogurt (sides), 1 serving	4
Apple Juice, 1 serving	5
Baby Carrots with Ranch (sides), 1 serving	9
Chocolate Shake, 1 serving	38
Chocolate Sundae with Chocolate Syrup, 1 serving	20
Corn Dog, 1 serving	7
Fries (sides), 1 serving	14
Fruit Punch, 1 serving	4
Garlic Mashed Potatoes (sides), 1 serving	4
Grape Juice, 1 serving	5
House Salad, without Dressing (sides), 1 serving	7
Lemonade, 1 serving	5
Mozzarella Sticks (sides), 1 serving	12
Orange Tangerine Juice, 1 serving	6
Oreo Cookie Shake, 1 serving	38
Oreo Cookie Sundae, 1 serving	20
Plain Vanilla Sundae, 1 serving	15
Raspberry Iced Tea, 1 serving	3
Steamed Broccoli (sides), 1 serving	0
Strawberry Shake, 1 serving	34
Vanilla Shake, 1 serving	31
Vanilla Yogurt with Strawberries (sides), 1 serving	5
Vinaigrette (sides), 1 serving	8
White Rice (sides), 1 serving	3

"We Like This!" item

Desserts	SmartPoints® value
Apple Chimi Cheesecake, 1 serving	43
Blue Ribbon Brownie, 1	77
Brownie Bite, 1 serving	18
Butter Pecan Blondie, 1	53
Chocolate Chip Cookie Sundae, 1 serving	71
Chocolate Mousse, 1 serving	24
Chocolate Nut Brownie Shorty Shake™, 1 serving	32
Churro S'mores, 1 serving	26
Cracker Jack® Banana Cheesecake, 1 serving	44
Hot Fudge Sundae, 1 serving	23
Salted Caramel Pretzel Bites, 1 serving	35
Salted Caramel Pretzel Bites Mini, 1 serving	18
Salted Caramel Shorty Shake™, 1 serving	25
Strawberry Cheesecake, 1 serving	19
Strawberry Sundae with Strawberry Sauce (kids), 1 serving	17
Triple Chocolate Meltdown Dessert, 1 serving	45

Beverages	SmartPoints® value
Banana Shake, 1	45
Blackberry Honey Quencher Iced Tea, 1 serving	6
Blackberry Quencher Lemonade, 1 serving	10
Brewed Iced Tea, 1 serving	0
Cherry Limeade, 1	12
Chocolate Malt Shake, 1	46
Chocolate Shake, 1	48
Coconut Shake, 1	47
Flavored Mango Lemonade, 1	10
Flavored Strawberry Lemonade, 1	10
Flavored Wildberry Lemonade, 1	10
Fruit Punch, 1	7
Hot Tea, 1 serving	0
Kiwi Iced Tea, 1	2
Kiwi Lemonade, 1 serving	10
Mango Frozen Lemonade, 1	14
Mango Iced Tea, 1 serving	2
Mango Shake, 1	45
Oreo Cookie Shake, 1	49
Peach Quencher Iced Tea, 1 serving	9
Pomegranate Iced Tea, 1 serving	2
Pomegranate Lemonade, 1 serving	10
Raspberry Iced Tea, 1	2
Raspberry Lemonade, 1 serving	10
Strawberry Frozen Lemonade, 1	13
Strawberry Limeade, 1	9
Strawberry Quencher Lemonade, 1	10
Strawberry Shake, 1	43
Sugar Free Lemonade (kids), 1 serving	0
Vanilla Shake, 1	41
Wildberry Frozen Lemonade, 1	14
Wildberry Shake, 1	45

Beef Sandwiches

	SmartPoints® value
Angus Philly, 1	18
Angus Three-Cheese & Bacon Sandwich, 1	20
Arby-Q Sandwich, 1	14
Arby's Melt, 1	10
Beef 'n Cheddar Classic Sandwich, 1	14
Beef 'n Cheddar Mid Sandwich, 1	17
Bourbon Bacon and Brisket Sandwich, 1	23
Bourbon Bacon and Steak Sandwich, 1	18
Corned Beef n Cheese Slider, 1	6
Crispy Onion Mighty Minis - Roast Beef, 2 minis	17
Deluxe Bacon Cheddar, 1	14
French Dip & Swiss Sandwich with Au Jus Sauce, 1	16
Jalapeño Roast Beef n Cheese Slider, 1	7
Jr Bacon Cheddar Melt, 1	9
Jr Deluxe Sandwich, 1	8
Jr Roast Beef Sandwich, 1	7
KING'S HAWAIIAN Roast Beef & Swiss Max Sandwich, 1	25
KING'S HAWAIIAN Roast Beef & Swiss Sandwich, 1	21
KING'S HAWAIIAN Roast Beef Max Sandwich, 1	23
KING'S HAWAIIAN Roast Beef Sandwich, 1	19
Original Mighty Minis - Roast Beef, 2 minis	11
Reuben Sandwich, 1	20
Roast Beef Classic, 1	11
Roast Beef Gyro, 1 serving	17
Roast Beef Max, 1	16
Roast Beef Max with Arby's Sauce, 1	17
Roast Beef Max with Horsey Sauce, 1	19
Roast Beef Mid, 1	14
Roast Beef 'n Cheese Slider, 1	7
Smokehouse Brisket Sandwich, 1	19
Spicy Mighty Minis - Roast Beef, 2 minis	15
Super Roast Beef Sandwich, 1	14

Turkey Sandwiches

	SmartPoints® value
Bourbon Bacon and Turkey Sandwich, 1 serving	18
Crispy Onion Mighty Minis - Roast Turkey, 2 minis	14
Grand Turkey Club, 1 sandwich	15
Jr Turkey & Cheese Sandwich, 1 sandwich	6
Original Mighty Minis - Roast Turkey, 2 minis	9
Roast Turkey & Swiss Sandwich, 1 sandwich	22
Roast Turkey & Swiss Wrap, 1 wrap	16
Roast Turkey Ranch & Bacon Sandwich, 1 sandwich	25
Roast Turkey Ranch & Bacon Wrap, 1 wrap	19
Spicy Mighty Minis - Roast Turkey, 2 minis	13
Turkey Classic Sandwich, 1 sandwich	7
Turkey Gyro, 1 serving	13
Turkey 'n Cheddar Classic Sandwich, 1 sandwich	11

"We Like This!" item

Ham Sandwiches	SmartPoints® value
Ham & Swiss Croissant, 1 sandwich	10
Ham & Swiss Melt, 1 sandwich	9
Ham n Cheese Slider, 1 serving	7
Jr Ham & Cheddar Melt, 1 sandwich	7
Jr Ham & Cheddar Sandwich, 1 sandwich	6
Loaded Italian Sandwich, 1 serving	22

Chicken

Chicken	SmartPoints® value
Buffalo Chicken Slider, 1 serving	8
Chicken Bacon & Swiss Sandwich - Crispy, 1 sandwich	14
Chicken Biscuit, 1 serving	13
Chicken Cordon Bleu Sandwich - Crispy, 1 sandwich	19
Chicken Tender 'n Cheese Slider, 1 serving	8
Cravin' Chicken - Crispy, 1 serving	14
Crispy Chicken Sandwich, 1 serving	15
Jr Chicken Sandwich, 1 sandwich	10
Pecan Chicken Salad Flatbread, 1 serving	22
Prime-Cut Chicken Tenders, 2	6
Prime-Cut Chicken Tenders, 3	9
Prime-Cut Chicken Tenders, 5	15
Roast Chicken Club, 1 sandwich	14
Pecan Chicken Salad Sandwich, 1 serving	27

Salads

Salads	SmartPoints® value
Chopped Farmhouse Chicken Salad, 1 salad	13
Chopped Farmhouse Salad - Crispy Chicken, 1 serving	13
Chopped Farmhouse Salad - Roast Turkey, 1 serving	7
Chopped Side Salad, 1 salad	3

Sauces and Dressings

Sauces and Dressings	SmartPoints® value
Arby's Sauce®, 1 serving	1
Balsamic Vinaigrette Dressing, 1 serving	5
Bronco Berry Sauce, 1 serving	4
Buffalo Dipping Sauce, 1 serving	0
Buttermilk Ranch Dressing, 1 serving	7
Cheddar Cheese Sauce, 1 serving	2
Dijon Honey Mustard Dressing, 1 serving	7
Honey Dijon Mustard Sauce, 1 serving	5
Honey Mustard Dipping Sauce, 1 serving	5
Horsey Sauce, 1 serving	2
Light Italian Dressing, 1 serving	1
Marinara Sauce, 1 serving	1
Ranch Dipping Sauce, 1 serving	4
Spicy Three Pepper Sauce, 1 serving	1
Strawberry Yogurt Dip, 1 serving	2
Tangy Barbeque Sauce, 1 serving	2

	SmartPoints® value
Sides	
Curly Fries, 1 kids	8
Curly Fries, 1 large	20
Curly Fries, 1 medium	17
Curly Fries, 1 small	13
Curly Fries, 1 snack size	8
Homestyle Fries, 1 kids	7
Homestyle Fries, 1 large	18
Homestyle Fries, 1 medium	15
Homestyle Fries, 1 small	11
Jalapeño Bites, 5	10
Jalapeño Bites, 8	17
Loaded Curly Fries, 1 serving	23
Loaded Potato Bites, 5	11
Loaded Potato Bites, 8	18
Mozzarella Sticks, 4	14
Mozzarella Sticks, 6	21
Potato Cakes, 2	8
Potato Cakes, 3	12
Potato Cakes, 4	16
Steakhouse Onion Rings, 5	13
Desserts	
Apple Turnover, 1 serving	20
Cherry Turnover, 1 serving	18
Chocolate Shake, 1 large	43
Chocolate Shake, 1 medium	30
Chocolate Shake, 1 small	23
Chocolate Swirl Shake, 1 serving	36
Chocolate Turnover, 1 serving	23
Gourmet Chocolate Chunk Cookies, 2 cookies	19
Jamocha Oreo Shake, 1 small	24
Jamocha Oreo Swirl Shake, 1 regular	33
Jamocha Shake, 1 large	42
Jamocha Shake, 1 medium	29
Jamocha Shake, 1 small	23
Jr Chocolate Shake, 1 serving	16
Jr Jamocha Oreo Shake, 1 serving	17
Jr Jamocha Shake, 1 serving	16
Jr Vanilla Shake, 1 serving	13
Molten Lava Cake, 1 sandwich	15
Orange Cream Shake, 1 serving	33
Outside-In Cinnamon Bites, 1 serving	11
Salted Caramel and Chocolate Cookie, 1 serving	19
Triple Chocolate Cookie, 1 serving	20
Vanilla Shake, 1 large	35
Vanilla Shake, 1 medium	24
Vanilla Shake, 1 small	19
Breakfast	
Bacon, Egg & Cheese Biscuit, 1 serving	18
Bacon, Egg & Cheese Croissant, 1 sandwich	16
Bacon, Egg & Cheese Sourdough, 1 sandwich	15
Bacon, Egg & Cheese Wrap, 1 wrap	16
French Toast Sticks, 1 serving	12
Ham, Egg & Cheese Biscuit, 1 serving	16
Ham, Egg & Cheese Croissant, 1 sandwich	14
Ham, Egg & Cheese Sourdough, 1 sandwich	14
Ham, Egg & Cheese Wrap, 1 wrap	14
Sausage Biscuit, 1 serving	18
Sausage Gravy Biscuit, 1 serving	18
Sausage, Egg & Cheese Biscuit, 1 sandwich	23
Sausage, Egg & Cheese Croissant, 1 sandwich	22
Sausage, Egg & Cheese Sourdough, 1 sandwich	21
Sausage, Egg & Cheese Wrap, 1 wrap	22

"We Like This!" item

Signature Pizzas	SmartPoints® value
Art Lover Signature Pizza, 1 slice	4
BBQ Chkn Signature Pizza, 1 slice	4
Green Stripe Signature Pizza, 1 slice	4
Link In Signature Pizza, 1 slice	4
Meat Eater Signature Pizza, 1 slice	5
Red Vine Signature Pizza, 1 slice	4
Simple Pie Signature Pizza, 1 slice	3
Veg Out Signature Pizza, 1 slice	4
White Top Signature Pizza, 1 slice	4

Salads	SmartPoints® value
Antipasto Salad (entrée), 1	21
Beet and Goat Cheese Salad, 1	18
Chicken Caesar Salad (entrée), 1	15
Classic Caesar Salad, 1	13
Roasted Veggie and Gorgonzola Salad, 1	17
Tomato Basil Ovaline Salad, 1	11

Dessert

S'more Pie, 1 serving	9

Beverages

Blood Orange Lemonade, 1 serving	18
Lemonade, 1 serving	15

Starters and Soup

	SmartPoints® value
Broccoli Cheddar Soup, 1 cup	7
Broccoli Cheddar Soup and Crackers, 1 bowl	14
Cheddar Baked Potato Soup (with 1 packet saltines), 1 cup	7
Cheddar Baked Potato Soup (with 2 packets saltines), 1 bowl	14
Chicken N Noodles Soup, 1 crock	6
Chicken N Noodles Soup with 1 packet Saltines, 1 cup	3
County Fair Cheese Bites, 1 serving	44
Farm Festival Bean Soup with 1 packet Saltines, 1 cup	3
Farm Festival Bean Soup with 2 packets Saltines, 1 bowl	6
Hearty Beef Vegetable Soup with 1 packet Saltines, 1 cup	3
Hearty Beef Vegetable Soup with 2 packets Saltines, 1 bowl	7
Tomato Basil Soup, 1 bowl	16
Tomato Basil Soup, 1 cup	8
Tomato Basil Soup with 2 packets Saltines, 1 bowl	20

Burgers

Big Farm Bacon Cheeseburger (no French fries or coleslaw), 1	38
Big Farm Hamburger (no French fries or coleslaw), 1	31
The Farm Favorite Burger (no French fries or coleslaw), 1 serving	35
The Smokehouse Burger (no French fries or coleslaw), 1 serving	48
The Three-Cheese Burger (no French fries or coleslaw), 1 serving	38

Chicken

	SmartPoints® value
Blackened Chicken with Cucumber Relish, 1 serving	17
Broasted Chicken Breast, 1	6
Broasted Chicken Leg, 1	3
Broasted Chicken Thigh, 1	4
Broasted Chicken Wing, 1	8
Chicken Tender Crispy (no sides), 4	13
Chicken Tender Crispy Dinner (with garlic herb butter, rolls and margarine), 4	29
Chicken Tender Crispy Dinner (with spicy chipotle sauce, specialty bread and margarine), 4	35
Chicken Tender Grilled (no sides), 4	2
Chicken Tender Grilled Dinner (with garlic herb butter, rolls and margarine), 4	19
Chicken Tender Grilled Dinner (with spicy chipotle sauce, specialty bread and margarine), 4	24
Fried Chicken (rolls and margarine), 1 serving	26
Fried Chicken (specialty bread and margarine), 1 serving	44
Fried Chicken (with sides no bread or sauce), 1 serving	14
Fried Chicken Breast (1 piece, no sides), 1 serving	5
Fried Chicken breast (2 pieces, no sides), 1 serving	11
Fried Chicken Breast Dinner (2 pieces, rolls, and margarine), 1 serving	31
Fried Chicken Breast Dinner (rolls and margarine), 1 serving	25
Fried Chicken Breast Dinner (specialty bread and margarine), 1 serving	38

"We Like This!" item

	SmartPoints® value
Fried Chicken Dinner (2 pieces, specialty bread, and margarine), 1 serving	43
Grilled Chicken (no sides, 2 pieces breast), 1 serving	4
Grilled Chicken (rolls and margarine), 1 serving	22
Grilled Chicken (specialty bread and margarine), 1 serving	41
Grilled Chicken (without bread or sauce), 1 serving	11
Grilled Chicken Dinner (1 breast piece, rolls, and margarine), 1 serving	34
Grilled Chicken Dinner (1 breast piece, specialty bread and margarine), 1 serving	34
Grilled Chicken Dinner (2 pieces, rolls, and margarine), 1 serving	24
Grilled Chicken Dinner (2 pieces, specialty bread, and margarine), 1 serving	36
Grilled Chicken no sides (1 breast), 1 serving	2

Seafood

Blackened Salmon with Cucumber Relish, 1 serving	12
Blackened Whitefish (with tartar sauce), 1 serving	13
Blackened Whitefish (without tartar sauce), 1 serving	7
Grilled Salmon Fillet (no sides), 1 serving	6
Grilled Salmon Fillet with Broccoli and Carrots, 1 serving	11
Potato Crusted Flounder (no sides), 1	6
Potato Crusted Flounder with Broccoli and Carrots, 1 serving	11

Slow Roasted Dinner Entrées

	SmartPoints® value
Slow Roasted Chicken Pot Pie (1 roll and margarine), 1 serving	37
Slow Roasted Chicken Pot Pie (with salad and rolls), 1 serving	45
Slow Roasted Chicken Pot Pie (without bread), 1 serving	31
Slow Roasted Pot Roast (with 2 biscuits and 2 margarine), 1 serving	40
Slow Roasted Pot Roast (with 2 rolls and 2 margarine), 1 serving	33
Slow Roasted Pot Roast (without bread), 1 serving	22
Slow Roasted Turkey Bacon Melt Platter (no fries or coleslaw), 1 serving	18
Slow Roasted Turkey Breast (with 2 biscuits and 2 margarine), 1 serving	50
Slow Roasted Turkey Breast (with 2 rolls and 2 margarine), 1 serving	43
Slow Roasted Turkey Breast (without bread), 1 serving	32
Slow-Roasted Chicken Pot Pie (no sides), 1 serving	31
Slow-Roasted Chicken Pot Pie (with salad and biscuits), 1 serving	57

Dinner

Black Angus Chopped Steak and Portabella Mushroom, 1 serving	29
Blackened Sirloin Steak, 1 serving	9
Chicken N Noodles Crock (no roll or margarine), 1 serving	6
Chicken N Noodles Deep Dish Dinner, 1 serving	21
Country Fried Steak (rolls and margarine), 1 serving	38
Country Fried Steak (specialty bread and margarine), 1 serving	50
Country Fried Steak Dinner (without bread), 1 serving	28

Dinner (cont'd)

	SmartPoints® value
Country Fried Steak Dinner with Cinnamon Bread, 1 serving	49
Country Fried Steak without Bread, 1 serving	27
Country-Fried Steak Dinner (with 2 rolls), 1 serving	36

Sandwiches

Chicken Salad Sandwich, 1	17
Farm Grill Chicken Club Sandwich, Crispy (no fries or coleslaw), 1 serving	17
Farm Grill Chicken Club Sandwich, Grilled (no fries or coleslaw), 1 serving	14
Five Cheese Griddled Cheese Sandwich (full sandwich), 1 serving	34
Five Cheese Griddled Cheese Sandwich (half sandwich), 1 serving	19
Knife and Fork Meat Loaf Sandwich, 1 serving	27
Pot Roast Sandwich Half, 1 serving	13
Pot Roast Sandwich Platter (no fries or coleslaw), 1 serving	21
Slow Roasted Ham and Swiss Cheese Sandwich (full sandwich), 1 serving	29
Slow Roasted Ham and Swiss Cheese Sandwich (half sandwich), 1 serving	15
Slow-Roasted Turkey Knife and Fork Sandwich, 1 serving	26
The Farm Favorite Chicken Sandwich (crispy no fries or coleslaw), 1 serving	16
The Farm Favorite Chicken Sandwich grilled (no fries or coleslaw), 1 serving	13
The Smokehouse Chicken Sandwich grilled (no fries or coleslaw), 1 serving	29
The Smokehouse Chicken Sandwich, crispy (no fries or coleslaw), 1 serving	33
Turkey Bacon Melt (half), 1 serving	8

Add-ons

Bacon, 3 slices	5
Blueberries, 1 serving	0
Chocolate Chips, 1 serving	4
Cinnamon Chips, 1 serving	2
Country Gravy, 1 serving	2
Cranberries, 1 serving	0
Dried Cranberries, 1 side order	3
Garlic Herb Butter, 1 serving	0
Honey Roasted Pecans, 1 serving	2
Pecans, 1 side order	4
Raisins, 1 side order	4
Sour Cream, 1 serving	6

Salads

Apple Cranberry Spinach Salad without dressing (full), 1 serving	10
Apple Cranberry Spinach Salad without dressing (savor), 1 serving	9
Chicken Salad Plate, 1 serving	28
Cranberry Pecan Chicken Salad (with low-fat balsamic vinaigrette and 2 rolls), 1 serving	23
Farmhouse Garden Salad (with Colonial dressing), 1 serving	11
Farmhouse Garden Salad (with low-fat balsamic vinaigrette), 1 serving	5
Farmhouse Garden Salad (without dressing), 1 serving	3
Full Apple Cranberry Spinach Salad (with Colonial dressing and specialty bread), 1 serving	38
Full Apple Cranberry Spinach Salad (with low-fat balsamic vinaigrette and 2 dinner rolls-full), 1 serving	20

"We Like This!" item

	SmartPoints® value
Full Cobb Salad (with Colonial dressing and specialty bread), 1 serving	45
Full Cobb Salad (with low-fat balsamic vinaigrette and 2 rolls), 1 serving	27
Full Cobb Salad Low Calorie (without dressing), 1 serving	17
Full Cranberry Pecan Chicken Salad (with Colonial dressing and specialty bread), 1 serving	50
Full Cranberry Pecan Chicken Salad (with low-fat balsamic vinaigrette and 2 rolls), 1 serving	32
Full Cranberry Pecan Chicken Salad (without dressing), 1 serving	21
Full Heritage Chef Salad (with Colonial dressing and specialty bread), 1 serving	35
Full Heritage Chef Salad (with low-fat balsamic vinaigrette and 2 rolls), 1 serving	23
Full Heritage Chef Salad (without dressing), 1 serving	13
Heritage Chef Salad (with low-fat balsamic vinaigrette and 2 rolls), 1 serving	17
Savor Apple Cranberry Spinach Salad (with Colonial dressing and specialty bread), 1 serving	38
Savor Apple Cranberry Spinach Salad (with low-fat balsamic vinaigrette and 2 dinner rolls-savor), 1 serving	20
Savor Cobb Salad (with Colonial dressing and specialty bread), 1 serving	38
Savor Cobb Salad (with low-fat balsamic vinaigrette and 2 rolls), 1 serving	20
Savor Cobb Salad Low Calorie (without dressing), 1 serving	9
Savor Cranberry Pecan Chicken Salad (with Colonial dressing and specialty bread), 1 serving	41
Savor Cranberry Pecan Chicken Salad (without dressing), 1 serving	13
Savor Heritage Chef Salad (with Colonial dressing and specialty bread), 1 serving	35
Savor Heritage Chef Salad (without dressing), 1 serving	7
Wildfire Fried Chicken Salad (without dressing), 1 serving	20
Wildfire Fried Chicken Salad High Calorie, 1 serving	48
Wildfire Grilled Chicken Salad (without dressing), 1 serving	13
Wildfire Grilled Chicken Salad Low Calorie, 1 serving	24

Dressings

Blue Cheese Dressing, 1 serving	7
Bread and Celery Dressing, 1 side order	9
Buttermilk Ranch Dressing, 1 serving	5
Colonial Dressing, 1 serving	8
French Dressing, 1 serving	7
Lite Ranch Dressing, 1 serving	3
Low-fat Balsamic Vinaigrette (low calorie dressing), 1 serving	2
Reduced Fat Raspberry Vinaigrette, 1 serving	5
Sweet Italian Dressing, 1 serving	6
Wildfire Ranch Dressing, 1 serving	4

Sides

Applesauce, 1 side order	4
Bacon, 1 side order	4
Baked Russet Potato, 1	6
Baked Sweet Potato, 1	14
Breaded Garlic Mushrooms, 1 serving	20
Buttered Sweet Corn, 1 side order	6
Cheesy Hash Brown Casserole, 1 side order	7

	SmartPoints® value
Fresh Fruit Plate, 1 serving	0
Fresh Steamed Broccoli, 1 side order	0
Fresh Steamed Broccoli with Butter, 1 side order	4
Glazed Fresh Baby Carrots, 1 side order	4
Golden Brown Home Fries, 1 side order	6
Green Beans with Ham, 1 side order	1
Hash Browns Loaded, 1 side order	14
Loaded Baked Potato, 1	14
Loaded French Fries, 1 side order	23
Mashed Potatoes (no gravy), 1 side order	7
Mashed Potatoes with Beef Gravy, 1 side order	8
Mashed Potatoes with Chicken Gravy, 1 side order	8
Mashed Potatoes with Country Gravy, 1 side order	9
Potato Baked Loaded, 1 side order	14
Scallions, 1 serving	0
Seasonal Fresh Fruit Dish, 1 side order	0
Signature Coleslaw, 1 side order	9
Special Recipe Macaroni and Cheese, 1 side order	10

Breakfast

	SmartPoints® value
Basted Eggs, 2	4
BE Fit Breakfast (no syrup), 1 serving	12
Belgian Waffle (with margarine and syrup), 1	24
Belgian Waffle Breakfast (with butter/margarine and syrup) and Sausage Links, 1 serving	37
Belgian Waffle Breakfast (with butter/margarine, syrup) and Bacon, 1 serving	29
Blueberry Brioche French Toast (no meat), 1 meal	33
Blueberry Hotcakes (with margarine and syrup), 4	38
Blueberry Topping, 1 serving	8
Brioche French Toast (no syrup or butter), 2 slices	22
Buttermilk Hotcakes (no butter/margarine or syrup), 2	13
Buttermilk Hotcakes (with margarine and syrup), 4	37
Buttermilk Hotcakes Plain, 2	13
Chocolate Chip Hotcakes (with margarine and syrup), 4	43
Cinnamon Hotcakes (with margarine and syrup), 4	42
Cinnamon Supreme Hotcakes (butter/margarine and syrup) with Bacon, 1 serving	49
Cinnamon Supreme Hotcakes (butter/margarine and syrup) with Sausage, 1 serving	57
Cinnamon Supreme Hotcakes (without meat), 4	45
Classic Breakfast (egg lites, homefries, and English muffin), 1 serving	15
Classic Breakfast (eggs, hashbrowns and specialty bread), 1 serving	40
Country Biscuit Breakfast (egg lite, home fries, bacon, and English muffin), 1 serving	23
Country Biscuit Breakfast (fried eggs, grits, sausage, and specialty bread), 1 serving	28
Country Fried Steak and Farm Fresh Eggs (egg lite, home fries, bacon, and English muffin), 1 serving	63
Country Fried Steak and Farm Fresh Eggs (fried eggs, grits, sausage and specialty bread), 1 serving	88

"We Like This!" item

	SmartPoints® value
Double Blueberry Hotcakes (with butter/margarine and syrup) and Bacon, 1 serving	44
Double Blueberry Hotcakes (with butter/margarine and syrup) and Sausage Links, 1 serving	51
Double Blueberry Hotcakes without meat, 4	39
Double Chocolate Hotcakes (with butter/margarine and syrup) and Bacon, 1 serving	51
Double Chocolate Hotcakes (with butter/margarine and syrup) and Sausage Links, 1 serving	58
Double Chocolate Hotcakes (without meat), 4	46
Egg Lites, 2	1
English Muffin Plain, 1	4
Farm Favorite Omelet (egg lite, home fries, bacon, and English muffin), 1 serving	23
Farm Favorite Omelet (eggs, hashbrowns, sausage, and specialty bread), 1 serving	44
Farm Favorite Omelet (no sides), 1 serving	14
Farmer's Choice Breakfast (egg lites, bacon, homefries, French toast, and sugar free syrup), 1 serving	25
Farmer's Choice Breakfast (eggs, sausage, grits, pancakes and syrup), 1 serving	57
Fried Eggs, 2	4
Fruit N Nut Multigrain Hotcakes (with butter/margarine and syrup) and Bacon, 1 serving	38
Fruit N Nut Multigrain Hotcakes (with butter/margarine and syrup) and Sausage Links, 1 serving	47
Fruit N Nut Multigrain Hotcakes (with margarine and syrup), 4	46
Fruit N Nut Multigrain Hotcakes (without meat), 4	34

	SmartPoints® value
Garden Harvest Omelet (egg lite, home fries, bacon, and English muffin), 1 serving	18
Garden Harvest Omelet (eggs, hashbrowns, sausage, and specialty bread), 1 serving	45
Garden Harvest Omelet (no sides), 1 serving	15
Golden Brown Home Fries, 1 side order	6
Golden Cornmeal Mush (3 slices with margarine and syrup), 1 serving	31
Golden Cornmeal Mush Breakfast (egg lites and bacon), 1 serving	37
Golden Cornmeal Mush Breakfast (fried egg and sausage links), 1 serving	48
Griddle Combo (egg lites, bacon, homefries, French toast, and sugar free syrup), 1 serving	22
Griddle Combo (eggs, sausage, grits, pancakes, and syrup), 1 serving	43
Grits, 1 bowl	9
Grits, 1 cup	5
Loaded Home Fries, 1 side order	13
Low Fat Strawberry Yogurt, 1 side order	4
Multigrain Hotcakes (with margarine and syrup), 4	38
Oatmeal, 1 bowl	5
Oatmeal, 1 cup	2
Pancake Syrup, 1 serving	9
Pancake Syrup Sugar Free, 1 serving	1
Pork Ham Steak, 1	2
Sausage Gravy and Biscuits (no potatoes), 1 serving	24
Sausage Gravy Bowl, 1 serving	18
Sausage Gravy Breakfast (hash browns), 1 serving	30
Sausage Gravy Breakfast (home fries), 1 serving	30

Breakfast (cont'd)

	SmartPoints® value
Sausage Gravy Cup, 1 serving	9
Sausage Links, 3	13
Sausage Patties, 2	10
Scrambled Eggs, 2 eggs	4
Seasonal Fresh Fruit Dish, 1 side order	0
Shredded Hash Browns, 1 side order	6
Sourdough Toast, 2 slices	8
Steak and Farm Fresh Eggs (egg lite, home fries, bacon, and English muffin), 1 serving	52
Steak and Farm Fresh Eggs (fried eggs, grits, sausage, and specialty bread), 1 serving	76
Stuffed 3 Egg Omelets Border Scramble (egg lites, home fries, and English muffin), 1 serving	24
Stuffed 3 Egg Omelets Border Scramble (no sides), 1 serving	22
Stuffed 3 Egg Omelets Border Scramble (whole eggs, hashbrowns, and specialty bread), 1 serving	51
Stuffed 3 Egg Omelets Farmers Market (egg lites, home fries, and English muffin), 1 serving	21
Stuffed 3 Egg Omelets Farmer's Market (no sides), 1 serving	18
Stuffed 3 Egg Omelets Farmer's Market (whole eggs, hashbrowns, and specialty bread), 1 serving	48
Stuffed 3 Egg Omelets Western (egg lites, home fries, and English muffin), 1 serving	17
Stuffed 3 Egg Omelets Western (no sides), 1 serving	15
Stuffed 3 Egg Omelets Western (whole eggs, hashbrowns, and specialty bread), 1 serving	44
Sunrise Egg Breakfast High Calorie, 1 serving	34
Sunrise Egg Breakfast Low Calorie, 1 serving	11
Sunshine Skillet (no bread), 1 serving	16
Sunshine Skillet High Calorie (whole egg), 1 serving	37
Sunshine Skillet Low Calorie (egg lites), 1 serving	20
The Big Egg Breakfast High Calorie, 1 serving	11
The Big Egg Breakfast Low Calorie, 1 serving	36
The Homestead Breakfast High Calorie, 1 serving	50
The Homestead Breakfast Low Calorie, 1 serving	35
The Mini Sampler High Calorie (fried egg, grits, links), 1 serving	35
The Mini Sampler Low Calorie (egg lite, home fries, bacon), 1 serving	27
The Rise and Shine High Calorie, serving	47
The Rise and Shine Low Calorie, 1 serving	15
Turkey Sausage Breakfast, 1 serving	10
Turkey Sausage Links, 2	3
Veggie Omelet, 1 serving	9
Wheat Toast, 2 slices	6
White Toast, 2 slices	6

Bread

Banana Nut Bread Plain, 2 slices	13
Blueberry Bread Plain, 1 serving	16
Buttermilk Biscuits Plain, 2	15
Cinnamon Bread, 2 slices	19
Dinner Rolls (no butter or margarine), 2	8
Garlic Ciabatta Bread, 1 slice	7
Texas Toast, 1 slice	4

"We Like This!" item

Condiments	SmartPoints® value
Apple Butter Jelly, 1 packet	2
Blackberry Diet Jelly, 1 packet	0
Butter, 1 packet	2
Buttery Taste Margarine Spread, 1 packet	1
Grape Jelly, 1 packet	2
Honey, 1 packet	3
Honey Mustard Sauce, 1 packet	5
Old Route 35 Sauce, 2 Tbsp	5
Orange Marmalade Jelly, 1 packet	2
Spicy Chipotle Sauce, 2 Tbsp	6
Wildfire Sauce, 1 serving	4

Desserts

Apple Pie, 1 slice	22
Blueberry Blossoms, 1 serving	15
Blueberry Crepe, 1	13
Chocolate Chip M&M's Cookie, 1	18
Chocolate Chunk Cookie, 1	14
Chocolate Peanut Butter Brownie, 1	19
Cinnamon Blossom, 1	13
Coconut Cream Pie, 1 slice	29
French Silk Pie, 1 slice	31
Lemon Blueberry Supreme Pie, 1 slice	35
Lemon Cookie, 1	16
Lemon Supreme Pie, 1 slice	31
Peanut Butter Brownie Bites, 1	40
Pecan Pie (no whip cream), 1 slice	31
Pecan Pie with Whip Cream, 1 slice	33

Beverages

	SmartPoints® value
2% Chocolate Milk, 14 ½ oz	10
2% Chocolate Milk, 7 ½ oz	5
2% Milk, 14 ½ oz	9
2% Milk, 7 ½ oz	4
Apple Juice, 14 ½ oz	12
Apple Juice, 7 ½ oz	6
Caramel Cappuccino, 1 serving	18
Caramel Coffee, 1 serving	1
Caramel Flavoring, 1 serving	4
Caramel Mocha, 1 serving	15
Coffee, 1 serving	0
Decaf Coffee, 1 serving	1
Decaf Earl Grey Tea with Lemon, 1 serving	0
English Breakfast Tea with Lemon, 1 serving	0
French Vanilla Cappuccino, 1 serving	17
French Vanilla Coffee, 1 serving	1
French Vanilla Flavoring, 1 serving	4
Green Tea with Lemon, 1 serving	0
Hot Chocolate, 1 serving	14
Iced Tea, 1 serving	0
Iced Tea Sweet Wildberry, 1 serving	10
Lemonade, 1 serving	8
Orange Juice, 1 large	12
Orange Juice, 1 regular	6
Original Cappuccino, 1 serving	0
Peppermint Tea with Lemon, 1 serving	0
Raspberry Flavoring, 1 serving	3
Raspberry Iced Tea, 1 serving	4
Strawberry Iced Tea, 1 serving	9
Strawberry Smoothie (kids), 1 serving	11
Sweetened Iced Tea, 1 serving	4
Sweetened Raspberry Iced Tea, 1 serving	8
Tomato Juice, 14 ½ oz	4
Tomato Juice, 7 ½ oz	2
Wildberry Lemonade, 1 serving	12

Individual Meals

	SmartPoints® value
BBQ Pulled Pork, 1 serving	22
Dark Chicken - 1 Thigh & 1 Drumstick, 1 serving	6
Meatloaf, 1 large	22
Meatloaf, 1 regular	14
Rotisserie Chicken - Half, 1 serving	10
Rotisserie Chicken - Quarter Dark (1 thigh & 1 drumstick), 1 serving	6
Rotisserie Chicken - Quarter White, 1 serving	5
Rotisserie Chicken - Quarter White, Skinless, 1 serving	3
Rotisserie Chicken - Three Piece Dark, 1 serving	7
Rotisserie Chicken - Three Piece Dark (2 thighs & drumstick), 1 serving	10
Rotisserie Chicken - Three Piece Dark Skinless (2 thighs & drumstick), 1 serving	9
Rotisserie Chicken - Three Piece Dark Skinless (thigh & 2 drumsticks), 1 serving	3
Rotisserie Chicken Carver Sandwich, 1 serving	23
Rotisserie Chicken Pot Pie, 1 serving	30
Slow Braised Pulled Pork, 1 large	10
Slow Braised Pulled Pork, 1 medium	7
Slow Braised Pulled Pork, 1 small	3
St. Louis Style BBQ Ribs - ½ Rack, 1 serving	34
St. Louis Style BBQ Ribs - ¼ Rack, 1 serving	17
Turkey Breast, 1 large	3
Turkey Breast, 1 medium	2
Turkey Pot Pie, 1 serving	28

Sandwiches

	SmartPoints® value
All-White Chicken Salad Sandwich, 1 serving	28
Meatloaf Carver Sandwich, 1 serving	28
Mediterranean Chicken Carver Sandwich, 1 serving	20
Pulled BBQ Chicken Sandwich, 1 serving	21
Roasted Turkey Carver Sandwich, 1 serving	26

Salad Bowls & Soup

	SmartPoints® value
Caesar Salad, Entrée, 1 serving	13
Caesar Side Salad, 1 serving	7
Chicken Noodle Soup, 1 large	6
Chicken Tortilla Soup, 1 serving	10
Mediterranean Salad Entrée, 1 serving	15
Southwest Santa Fe Salad Entrée, 1 serving	15
Turkey Tortilla Soup, 1 serving	9

Extras

	SmartPoints® value
Beef Gravy, 1 serving	0
Citrus Garlic Sauce, 1 serving	4
Cranberry Walnut Relish, 1 serving	7
Honey Habanero (medium hot), 1 serving	4
Poultry Gravy, 1 serving	0
Sweet Thai Chili Garlic Sauce (medium hot), 1 serving	3

"We Like This!" item

	SmartPoints® value

Sides

Cinnamon Apples, 1 serving	14
Cornbread, 1 serving	7
Creamed Spinach, 1 serving	10
Fresh Steamed Vegetables, 1 serving	2
Fresh Vegetable Stuffing, 1 serving	7
Garlic Dill New Potatoes, 1 serving	4
Green Beans, 1 serving	3
Macaroni and Cheese, 1 serving	9
Mashed Potatoes, 1 serving	8
Squash Casserole, 1 serving	9
Sweet Corn, 1 serving	5
Sweet Potato Casserole, 1 serving	21

Kids Menu

Chicken Noodle Soup, 1 serving	2
Cinnamon Apples, 1 serving	8
Corn, 1 serving	3
Creamed Spinach, 1 serving	6
Fresh Steamed Vegetables, 1 serving	1
Green Beans, 1 serving	2
Macaroni and Cheese, 1 serving	8
Mashed Potatoes, 1 serving	4
Meatloaf, 1 serving	7
Squash Casserole, 1 serving	5
Stuffing, 1 serving	4
Sweet Potato Casserole, 1 serving	11
White Chicken 1 Breast & 1 Wing, 1 serving	5

	SmartPoints® value

Desserts

Apple Pie, 1 slice	19
Chocolate Brownie, 1 serving	22
Chocolate Cake, 1 slice	25
Chocolate Chunk Cookie, 1 serving	17
Pecan Pie, 1 slice	27

WHOPPER Sandwiches

	SmartPoints® value
ANGRY WHOPPER® Sandwich, 1 serving	28
ANGRY WHOPPER® Sandwich without Mayo, 1 serving	24
Bacon and Cheese WHOPPER® Sandwich, 1 serving	25
Carolina BBQ WHOPPER JR.®, 1 serving	14
Carolina BBQ WHOPPER®, 1 serving	26
Chipotle WHOPPER JR.®, 1	14
Chipotle WHOPPER®, 1	26
DOUBLE WHOPPER® Sandwich, 1	28
DOUBLE WHOPPER® Sandwich with Cheese, 1	31
DOUBLE WHOPPER® Sandwich with Cheese without Mayo, 1 serving	25
DOUBLE WHOPPER® Sandwich without Mayo, 1 serving	22
Texas DOUBLE WHOPPER® Sandwich, 1	33
Texas WHOPPER® Sandwich, 1	25
TRIPLE WHOPPER® Sandwich, 1	39
TRIPLE WHOPPER® Sandwich no Mayo, 1	28
TRIPLE WHOPPER® Sandwich without Mayo, 1 serving	35
WHOPPER JR.® Sandwich, 1	10
WHOPPER JR.® Sandwich with Cheese, 1	12
WHOPPER JR.® Sandwich with Cheese without Mayo, 1 serving	10
WHOPPER JR.® Sandwich without Mayo, 1 serving	8
WHOPPER® Sandwich, 1	21
WHOPPER® Sandwich with Cheese, 1	24
WHOPPER® Sandwich with Cheese without Mayo, 1	19
WHOPPER® Sandwich without Mayo, 1	15

"We Like This!" item

Burgers

	SmartPoints® value
A.1.® Ultimate Bacon Cheeseburger, 1	25
Bacon Cheddar Stuffed Burger, 1	22
Bacon Cheeseburger, 1	10
Bacon Cheeseburger Deluxe, 1	10
Bacon Double Cheeseburger, 1	12
Big King, 1	18
BK Double Stacker, 1	14
BK Quad Stacker, 1	26
BK Single Stacker, 1	13
BK Triple Stacker, 1	21
BK VEGGIE® Burger, 1	11
BK VEGGIE® Burger without Mayo, 1	9
BK® Bacon Burger, 1	10
Cheeseburger, 1	9
Double Bacon Cheeseburger, 1	12
Double Cheeseburger, 1	12
Double Hamburger, 1	10
Extra Long Buttery Cheeseburger, 1	24
Extra Long Cheeseburger, 1	20
Flame Grilled Chicken Burger, 1	14
French Fry Burger, 1	12
Hamburger, 1	7
King Jr. Cheeseburger, 1	11
Rodeo Burger, 1	10
Rodeo Cheeseburger, 1	12
Turkey Burger, 1	16

Chicken

Buffalo Chicken Strips, 3 pieces	10
Buffalo Chicken Strips, 5 pieces	17
Chicken Fries, 9 pieces	8
Chicken Fries Rings, 6 pieces	9
Chicken Nuggets, 10 pieces	12
Chicken Nuggets, 20 pieces	25
Chicken Nuggets, 4 pieces	5

	SmartPoints® value
Chicken Nuggets, 6 pieces	7
Home-Style Chicken Strips, 2 pieces	6
Home-Style Chicken Strips, 3 pieces	9
Home-Style Chicken Strips, 5 pieces	15
Honey BBQ Chicken Strips, 3 pieces	13
Honey BBQ Chicken Strips, 5 pieces	22

Hot Dogs

Chili Cheese Grilled Dog, 1 serving	11
Classic Grilled Dog, 1 serving	11
WHOPPER® Dog, 1 serving	14

Sandwiches and Wraps

	SmartPoints® value
A.1.® Smoky Bacon TENDERCRISP®, 1 serving	19
Bacon and Cheese TENDERCRISP®, 1 serving	25
Bacon Gouda Muffin Sandwich, 1	12
BBQ Rib Sandwich, 1 serving	15
Big Fish Deluxe, 1 serving	18
Big Fish Sandwich, 1 serving	16
Big Fish Sandwich without Tartar Sauce, 1 serving	10
Bratwurst Sandwich, 1 serving	17
Carolina BBQ TENDERCRISP®, 1 serving	26
Carolina BBQ TENDERGRILL®, 1 serving	21
Chicken Apple and Cranberry Garden Fresh Salad Wrap (crispy), 1 serving	17
Chicken Apple and Cranberry Garden Fresh Salad Wrap (grilled), 1 serving	14
Chicken BLT Garden Fresh Salad Wrap (crispy), 1 serving	15
Chicken BLT Garden Fresh Salad Wrap (grilled), 1 serving	11
Chicken Caesar Garden Fresh Salad Wrap (crispy), 1 serving	13
Chicken Caesar Garden Fresh Salad Wrap (grilled), 1 serving	10
Chicken Crisp Sandwich - Classic, 1	16
Chicken Crisp Sandwich - Spicy, 1	15
Chicken Parmesan Sandwich, 1 serving	20
Chipotle Chicken Wrap (crispy), 1	17
Chipotle Chicken Wrap (grilled), 1	15
Chipotle TENDERCRISP®, 1	29
Chipotle TENDERGRILL®, 1	25
Country Pork Sandwich, 1	26
Crispy Chicken Jr., 1 serving	14
Extra Long Fish Sandwich, 1 serving	18
Honey Mustard Chicken Wrap (crispy), 1 serving	12
Honey Mustard Chicken Wrap (grilled), 1 serving	10
Memphis BBQ Pulled Pork Sandwich, 1 serving	16
Original Chicken Sandwich, 1	20
Original Chicken Sandwich without Mayo, 1 serving	12
Premium Alaskan Fish Sandwich, 1	16
Premium Alaskan Fish Sandwich without Tartar Sauce, 1 serving	10
Ranch Chicken Wrap (crispy), 1 serving	11
Ranch Chicken Wrap (grilled), 1 serving	9
Rib Sandwich, 1 serving	19
Rodeo Crispy Chicken Sandwich, 1 serving	14
Spicy Crispy Chicken Jr., 1 serving	12

	SmartPoints® value
Spicy Original Chicken Sandwich, 1 serving	20
Spicy Original Chicken Sandwich without Mayo, 1 serving	13
TENDERCRISP® Chicken Sandwich, 1	20
TENDERCRISP® Chicken Sandwich without Mayo, 1 serving	12
TENDERGRILL® Chicken Sandwich, 1	11
TENDERGRILL® Chicken Sandwich without Mayo, 1 serving	8

Tacos

Tacos, 2	13

Fries

French Fries, 1 large	13
French Fries, 1 medium	12
French Fries, 1 small	10
French Fries (value), 1 serving	7
Satisfries French Fries (salted), 1 large serving	13
Satisfries French Fries (salted), 1 medium serving	10
Satisfries French Fries (salted), 1 small serving	8
Satisfries French Fries (salted), 1 value serving	6
Sweet Potato Fries, 1 large serving	16
Sweet Potato Fries, 1 medium serving	14
Sweet Potato Fries, 1 small serving	10

Extras

American Cheese Slice (may vary), 1 serving	2
Thick Cut Bacon, 1 serving	1

"We Like This!" item

	SmartPoints® value

Salads

Bacon Cheddar Ranch Chicken Salad with TENDERCRISP® and Dressing, 1 serving	23
Bacon Cheddar Ranch Chicken Salad with TENDERGRILL® and Dressing, 1 serving	18
BBQ Salad - TENDERCRISP® - no dressing, 1 serving	13
BBQ Salad - TENDERGRILL® - no dressing, 1 serving	8
Buttery Garlic Croutons, 1 packet	2
Chicken Apple & Cranberry Garden Fresh Salad with TENDERCRISP® and Dressing, 1 serving	25
Chicken Apple & Cranberry Garden Fresh Salad with TENDERGRILL® and Dressing, 1 serving	18
Chicken BLT Garden Fresh Salad with TENDERCRISP® and Dressing, 1 serving	21
Chicken BLT Garden Fresh Salad with TENDERGRILL® and Dressing, 1 serving	13
Chicken Caesar Garden Fresh Salad with TENDERCRISP® and dressing, 1 serving	20
Chicken Caesar Garden Fresh Salad with TENDERGRILL® and dressing, 1 serving	12
Garden Grilled Chicken Salad with TENDERCRISP® (no dressing), 1 serving	13
Garden Grilled Chicken Salad with TENDERGRILL® (no dressing), 1 serving	8
Garden Side Salad (no dressing), 1 serving	2
Home-style Caesar Croutons, 1 packet	2

	SmartPoints® value
Side Caesar Salad and Dressing, 1 serving	10
Side Garden Salad and Avocado Ranch Dressing, 1 serving	8

Sauces and Dressings

Barbecue Dipping Sauce, 1 oz	2
Buffalo Dipping Sauce, 1 oz	3
Chicken Fry Dipping Sauce, 1 oz	5
French Fry Sauce, 1 oz	3
Honey Mustard Dipping Sauce, 1 oz	4
Ken's Apple Cider Vinaigrette, 1 packet	8
Ken's Avocado Ranch Dressing, 1 serving	6
Ken's Citrus Caesar Dressing, 1 packet	6
Ken's Honey Mustard Dressing, 1 packet	9
Ken's Lite Honey Balsamic, 1 packet	5
Ken's Ranch Dressing, 1 packet	9
Marinara Sauce, 1 oz	1
Picante/Taco Sauce, ½ oz	0
Ranch Dipping Sauce, 1 oz	5
Sweet and Sour Dipping Sauce, 1 oz	3
Zesty Onion Ring Dipping Sauce, 1 oz	5

Sides

Apple Slices, 1 serving	2
Loaded Tater Tots, 8	13
Loaded Tater Tots, 10	16
Loaded Tater Tots, 12	19
Mozzarella Sticks, 4 pieces	9
Onion Rings, 1 large	17
Onion Rings, 1 medium	14
Onion Rings, 1 small	11
Onion Rings (value), 1 serving	5
Pickles, 2	0

	SmartPoints® value

Breakfast

Bacon, Egg, & Cheese Biscuit, 1	12
BK Ultimate Breakfast Platter, 1 serving	41
BK® Breakfast Muffin Sandwich - Sausage and Cheese, 1 serving	13
BK® Breakfast Muffin Sandwich - Sausage, Egg, and Cheese, 1 serving	14
BK® Breakfast Muffin Sandwich - Bacon, Egg, and Cheese, 1 serving	9
BK® Breakfast Muffin Sandwich - Egg and Cheese, 1 serving	8
BK® Breakfast Muffin Sandwich - Ham, Egg, and Cheese, 1 serving	9
Breakfast Syrup, 1 oz	6
Country Ham and Egg Biscuit, 1	16
CROISSAN'WICH® Bacon, Egg, & Cheese, 1	12
CROISSAN'WICH® Egg & Cheese, 1	10
CROISSAN'WICH® Ham, Egg, & Cheese, 1	11
CROISSAN'WICH® Sausage & Cheese, 1	15
CROISSAN'WICH® Sausage, Egg, & Cheese, 1	16
Double CROISSAN'WICH® with Bacon, Egg, & Cheese, 1	16
Double CROISSAN'WICH® with Ham, Bacon, Egg, & Cheese, 1	16
Double CROISSAN'WICH® with Ham, Egg, & Cheese, 1	16
Double CROISSAN'WICH® with Ham, Sausage, Egg, & Cheese, 1	21
Double CROISSAN'WICH® with Sausage, Bacon, Egg, & Cheese, 1	20
Double CROISSAN'WICH® with Sausage, Egg, & Cheese, 1	27
EGG NORMOUS Burrito, 1 serving	27
French Toast Sticks, 3 pieces	8
French Toast Sticks, 5 pieces	13

Breakfast (cont'd)

	SmartPoints® value
Fully Loaded CROISSAN'WICH®, 1 serving	19
Ham, Egg, & Cheese Biscuit, 1	11
Hash Browns, 1 large	22
Hash Browns, 1 medium	17
Hash Browns, 1 small	8
Kids Oatmeal, 1 serving	7
KING CROISSAN'WICH® with Double Sausage, 1 serving	25
KING CROISSAN'WICH® with Ham and Sausage, 1 serving	18
KING CROISSAN'WICH® with Sausage and Bacon, 1 serving	20
NY Ultimate Platter, 1 serving	31
Pancake and Sausage Platter, 1 serving	23
Pancakes (3) and 1 oz Breakfast Syrup, 1 serving	20
Sausage Biscuit, 1	13
Sausage Breakfast Burrito, 1 serving	10
Sausage Egg Cheese and Hash Brown Burrito, 1 serving	12
Sausage, Egg, & Cheese Biscuit, 1	16
Southwestern Breakfast Burrito, 1 serving	20
Supreme Breakfast Sandwich, 1 serving	29

Condiments

Ketchup, 1 packet	1
Mayonnaise, 1 packet	3
Strawberry or Grape Jam, 1 packet	2
SunGlow® Butter blend, 2 pats	3

Desserts

Brownie Sundae, 1 serving	26
Butter Sugar Cookie, 1	7
Caramel Frappe, 12 fl oz	20
Caramel Frappe, 16 fl oz	19
Caramel Frappe, 20 fl oz	28

	SmartPoints® value
Caramel Sundae, 1 serving	14
Carnival Cookie, 1	7
Chocolate Chip Cookie, 1	8
Chocolate Chip Cookies, 2	15
Chocolate Fudge Sundae, 1 serving	14
Chunky Cookie made with Oreo® Pieces, 2	18
Donut Holes, 1 serving	12
Dutch Apple Pie, 1 serving	15
Ginger Spice Cookie, 1	7
HERSHEY®'S Sundae Pie, 1 serving	15
Mini M & M Sundae, 1 serving	23
Mocha Frappe, 12 fl oz	20
Mocha Frappe, 16 fl oz	19
Mocha Frappe, 20 fl oz	29
Oatmeal Raisin Cookies, 2	14
OREO® Sundae, 1 serving	21
Otis Spunkmeyer® Cinnamon Roll, 1	12
Red White and Blue Cookie, 1	7
Reese's Peanut Butter Cup Pie, 1 serving	14
SNICKERS® Pie, 1 serving	14
Soft Serve Cone, 1 serving	9
Soft Serve Cup, 1 serving	8
Strawberry Sundae, 1 serving	10
Warm Oreo®Brownie Sundae, 1 serving	21
White Chocolate Macadamia Nut Cookies, 2	15

Smoothies

Piña Colada Smoothie, 12 fl oz	17
Piña Colada Smoothie, 16 fl oz	27
Piña Colada Smoothie, 20 fl oz	36
Strawberry Banana Smoothie, 12 fl oz	11
Strawberry Banana Smoothie, 16 fl oz	15

"We Like This!" item

	SmartPoints® value
Strawberry Banana Smoothie, 20 fl oz	22
Tropical Mango Smoothie, 12 fl oz	11
Tropical Mango Smoothie, 16 fl oz	18
Tropical Mango Smoothie, 20 fl oz	24

Shakes

Chocolate Milk Shake, 12 fl oz	30
Chocolate Milk Shake, 16 fl oz	31
Chocolate Milk Shake, 20 fl oz	51
Chocolate Oreo® Shake, 1 medium	30
Dr Pepper® Shake, 1 serving	22
Irish Mint Oreo® Shake, 1 serving	30
Oreo® Shake, 1 large	49
Oreo® Shake, 1 medium	36
Oreo® Shake, 1 small	29
Strawberry Milk Shake, 12 fl oz	26
Strawberry Milk Shake, 16 fl oz	33
Strawberry Milk Shake, 20 fl oz	42
Vanilla Milk Shake, 12 fl oz	29
Vanilla Milk Shake, 16 fl oz	29
Vanilla Milk Shake, 20 fl oz	49

Beverages

	SmartPoints® value
1% Low Fat Chocolate Milk, 8 fl oz	8
2% Caramel Latte, 1 large	21
2% Caramel Latte, 1 medium	17
2% Caramel Latte, 1 small	13
2% Latte, 1 large	10
2% Latte, 1 medium	8
2% Latte, 1 small	6
2% Mocha Latte, 1 large	14
2% Mocha Latte, 1 medium	11
2% Mocha Latte, 1 small	8
2% Vanilla Latte, 1 large	21
2% Vanilla Latte, 1 medium	17
2% Vanilla Latte, 1 small	13
Caramel Iced Coffee, 1 large	12
Caramel Iced Coffee, 1 medium	9
Caramel Iced Coffee, 1 small	8
Fat Free Milk, 8 fl oz	3
Frozen Lemonade, 12 oz	4
Frozen Lemonade, 16 oz	5
Frozen Lemonade, 20 oz	6
Frozen Strawberry Lemonade, 12 oz	7
Frozen Strawberry Lemonade, 16 oz	9
Frozen Strawberry Lemonade, 20 oz	12
Hot Chocolate, 1 large	15
Hot Chocolate, 1 medium	12
Hot Chocolate, 1 small	9
Iced Coffee with Milk, 1 medium	8
Mocha Iced Coffee, 1 large	13
Mocha Iced Coffee, 1 medium	9
Mocha Iced Coffee, 1 small	8
Nonfat Caramel Latte, 1 large	18
Nonfat Caramel Latte, 1 medium	15
Nonfat Caramel Latte, 1 small	11
Nonfat Latte, 1 large	7
Nonfat Latte, 1 medium	6
Nonfat Latte, 1 small	5
Nonfat Mocha Latte, 1 large	11
Nonfat Mocha Latte, 1 medium	8
Nonfat Mocha Latte, 1 small	6
Nonfat Vanilla Latte, 1 large	18
Nonfat Vanilla Latte, 1 medium	15
Nonfat Vanilla Latte, 1 small	11
Peach Tea, 20 fl oz	6
Peach Tea, 30 fl oz	8
Peach Tea, 40 fl oz	11
Sweet Tea, 20 fl oz	8
Sweet Tea, 30 fl oz	11
Sweet Tea, 40 fl oz	16
Vanilla Iced Coffee, 1 large	12
Vanilla Iced Coffee with Milk, 1 medium	10

	SmartPoints® value
Classics	
Chargrilled Chicken Club Sandwich, 1 serving	12
Chargrilled Chicken Sandwich, 1 serving	8
Chicken Salad Sandwich, 1 serving	15
Chicken Sandwich, 1 serving	15
Chick-n-Strips, 3 pieces	9
Chick-n-Strips, 4 pieces	12
Chick-n-Strips Kid's Meal, 1 piece	3
Chick-n-Strips Kid's Meal, 2 pieces	6
Deluxe Chicken Sandwich, 1 serving	15
Grilled Chicken Club Sandwich, 1 serving	13
Grilled Chicken Sandwich, 1 serving	8
Grilled Nuggets, 4	1
Grilled Nuggets, 6	2
Grilled Nuggets, 8	2
Grilled Nuggets, 12	3
Nuggets, 8	6
Nuggets, 12	9
Nuggets Kid's Meal (nuggets only), 4 pieces	3
Nuggets Kid's Meal (nuggets only), 6 pieces	5
Spicy Chicken Deluxe Sandwich, 1 serving	17
Spicy Chicken Sandwich, 1 serving	14
Salads and Wraps	
Cobb Salad with Toppings and Avocado Lime Ranch Dressing, 1 serving	25
Cobb Salad with Toppings No Dressing, 1 serving	14
Grilled Chicken Cool Wrap, 1	8
Grilled Market Salad with Toppings and Zesty Apple Cider Vinaigrette Dressing, 1 serving	19
Grilled Market Salad with Toppings no Dressing, 1 serving	9
Side Salad without Dressing, 1 serving	3
Spicy Southwest Salad with Toppings (no dressing), 1 serving	12
Spicy Southwest salad with Toppings and Chili Lime Vinaigrette Dressing, 1 serving	15
Spicy Southwest salad with Toppings and Creamy Salsa Dressing, 1 serving	22
Sides	
Chicken Salad Cup, 1 serving	10
Cole Slaw, 1 large	23
Cole Slaw, 1 medium	14
Fruit Cup, 1 large	0
Fruit Cup, 1 medium	0
Fruit Cup, 1 small	0
Fruit Cup Kids Meals, 1 serving	0
Fruit Cup with Blueberries, 1 large	0
Fruit Cup with Blueberries, 1 medium	0
Hearty Breast of Chicken Soup, 1 large	7
Hearty Breast of Chicken Soup, 1 medium	4
Superfood Side, 1 large	7
Superfood Side, 1 small	6
Waffle Potato Fries, 1 large	16
Waffle Potato Fries, 1 medium	12
Waffle Potato Fries, 1 small	10
Waffle Potato Fries Kids Meal, 1 serving	10

"We Like This!" item

	SmartPoints® value
Sauces and Dressings	
Avocado Lime Ranch Dressing, 1 serving	11
Barbecue Sauce, 1 serving	2
Buffalo Sauce, 1 serving	0
Buttermilk Ranch Dressing, 1 serving	10
Buttermilk Ranch Sauce, 1 serving	4
Chick-fil-A Sauce, 1 serving	6
Chili Lime Vinaigrette Dressing, 1 serving	3
Creamy Salsa Dressing, 1 serving	10
Fat Free Honey Mustard Sauce, 1 serving	5
Garlic and Herb Ranch Dressing, 1 serving	10
Honey Mustard Sauce, 1 serving	3
Honey Roasted BBQ Sauce, 1 serving	2
Honey Sesame Dressing, 1 serving	7
Light Balsamic Vinaigrette Dressing, 1 serving	4
Light Italian Dressing, 1 serving	1
Polynesian Sauce, 1 serving	5
Reduced Fat Berry Balsamic Vinaigrette, 1 serving	5
Spicy Dressing, 1 serving	9
Zesty Apple Cider Vinaigrette, 1 serving	10
Breakfast	
Bacon Platter, 1 serving	20
Bacon, Egg, and Cheese Biscuit, 1 serving	16
Biscuit, 1 serving	12
Chicken Biscuit, 1 serving	15
Chicken Breakfast Burrito, 1 serving	14
Chicken Egg and Cheese Bagel, 1 serving	15
Chicken Platter, 1 serving	22
Chick-n-Minis, 3	9
Chick-n-Minis, 4	11
Greek Yogurt Parfait (no toppings), 1 serving	4
Greek Yogurt Parfait with Harvest Nut Granola, 1 serving	6
Hash Browns, 1 serving	8
Multigrain Oatmeal, 1 serving	5
Multigrain Oatmeal and Toppings, 1 serving	11
Sausage Biscuit, 1 serving	17
Sausage Breakfast Burrito, 1 serving	16
Sausage Platter, 1 serving	28
Sausage, Egg, and Cheese Biscuit, 1 serving	24
Spicy Chicken Biscuit, 1 serving	15
Yogurt Parfait with Chocolate Cookie Crumbs, 1 serving	5
Desserts	
Chick-fil-A Frosted Coffee, 1 large	15
Chick-fil-A Frosted Coffee, 1 small	12
Chocolate Chunk Cookie, 1 serving	15
Chocolate Milkshake, 1 large	37
Chocolate Milkshake, 1 small	29
Cinnamon Apple Sauce, 1 serving	0
Cinnamon Cluster, 1 serving	18
Cookie Sundae, 1 serving	20
Cookies & Cream Milkshake, 1 small	27
Cookies and Cream Milkshake, 1 large	33
Icedream Cone, 1 large	13
Icedream Cone, 1 small	8

Desserts (cont'd)

	SmartPoints® value
Icedream Cup, 1 serving	15
Mini Sundae, 1 serving	9
Mocha Cookies & Cream Milkshake, 1 large	43
Mocha Cookies & Cream Milkshake, 1 small	34
Strawberry Milkshake, 1 large	37
Strawberry Milkshake, 1 small	29
Vanilla Milkshake, 1 large	32
Vanilla Milkshake, 1 small	26

Beverages

	SmartPoints® value
Chocolate Milk, 1 serving	7
Coffee, 1 large	0
Coffee, 1 medium	0
Coffee, 1 small	0
Diet Lemonade, 1 large	1
Diet Lemonade, 1 medium	1
Diet Lemonade, 1 small	1
Diet Lemonade, 1 small kids serving	0
Frosted Lemonade, 1 serving	18
Frosted Lemonade with Diet Soda, 1 serving	13
Iced Coffee-Regular-Large, 1 serving	9
Iced Coffee-Regular-Medium, 1 serving	8
Iced Tea - Sweet, 1 large	14
Iced Tea - Sweet, 1 medium	8
Iced Tea - Sweet, 1 small	6
Iced Tea - Sweet, 1 small kids serving	4
Iced Tea - Unsweetened, 1 large	0
Iced Tea - Unsweetened, 1 medium	0
Iced Tea - Unsweetened, 1 small	0
Iced Tea - Unsweetened, 1 small kids serving	0
Lemonade, 1 large	21
Lemonade, 1 medium	14
Lemonade, 1 small	10
Lemonade, 1 small kids serving	9
Milk, 1 serving	4
Vanilla Iced Coffee, 1 large	10
Vanilla Iced Coffee, 1 small	8

"We Like This!" item

Appetizers

	SmartPoints® value
Boneless Buffalo Wings (for the table), 1 serving	32
Boneless Buffalo Wings (Triple Dipper), 1 serving	20
Boneless Honey Chipotle Wings (Triple Dipper), 1 serving	21
Bottomless Tostada Chips, 1 serving	29
Buffalo Wings (for the table), 1 serving	24
California Grilled Chicken Flatbread (for the table), 1 serving	49
California Grilled Chicken Flatbread (half), 1 serving	25
Chipotle Bacon Jalapeño bites, 4 pieces	10
Chipotle Chicken Flatbread, 1 serving	45
Chipotle Chicken Flatbread (half), ½ serving	23
Classic Beef Nachos (large), 1 serving	53
Classic Chicken Nachos (large), 1 serving	47
Classic Nachos (large), 1 serving	44
Creamy Jalapeño Bone-In Wings, 1 serving	35
Creamy Jalapeño Boneless Wings, 1 serving	42
Creamy Jalapeño Boneless Wings (Triple Dipper), 1 serving	24
Crispy Asparagus (for the table), 1 serving	28
Crispy Cheddar Bites (for the table), 1 serving	35
Crispy Cheddar Bites (Triple Dipper), 1 serving	20

	SmartPoints® value
Crispy Chicken Crispers (no sauce), 1 serving	34
Crispy Honey Chipotle Chicken Crispers (no sauce), 1 serving	45
Crispy Onion & Jalapeño Stack, 1 serving	37
Fresh Guacamole (for the table), 1 serving	38
Fried Cheese, 1 serving	24
Fried Pickles (for the table), 1 serving	22
Fried Pickles (Triple Dipper), 1 serving	14
Honey Chipotle Bone-In Wings, 1 serving	31
Honey Chipotle Boneless Wings, 1 serving	37
Hot Spinach & Artichoke Dip, 1 serving	22
Hot Spinach & Artichoke Dip (for the table), 1 serving	51
Jumbo Soft Pretzels, 1 serving	35
Loaded Boneless Wings (for the table), 1 serving	46
Margherita Flatbread, 1 serving	50
Margherita Flatbread (half), 1 serving	25
Nacho Potatoes with Beef and Bacon, 1 package	12
Original Chicken Crispers (for the table), 1 serving	17
Original Chicken Crispers (no sauce), 1 serving	36
Original Chicken Crispers (Triple Dipper), 1 serving	17
Smoked Bone-In Wings, 1 serving	16
Southwestern Eggrolls (for the table), 1 serving	25

	SmartPoints® value
Southwestern Eggrolls (Triple Dipper), 1 serving	19
Southwestern Style Bites, 5 bites	6
Spiced Panko Onion Rings (for the table), 1 serving	32
Spiced Panko Onion Rings (Triple Dipper), 1 serving	32
Tableside Guacamole, 1 serving	48
Texas Cheese Fries - Full Order, 1 serving	58
Texas Cheese Fries - Half Order, 1 serving	43
White Spinach Queso (for the table), 1 serving	53

Chicken & Seafood

	SmartPoints® value
Ancho Salmon, 1 serving	15
Ancho Salmon (combo), 1 serving	10
Cajun Pasta with Grilled Chicken, 1 serving	40
Cajun Pasta with Grilled Shrimp, 1 serving	39
Chicken and Pasta with Green Chiles, 1 package	11
Chipotle Chicken Bowl with Quinoa (lunch combo), 1 serving	23
Chipotle Chicken Bowl with Rice (lunch combo), 1 serving	23
Creamy Chipotle Chicken and Potatoes, 1 package	8
Grilled Chicken, 1 serving	2
Lighter Choice Grilled Chicken Salad, 1 serving	13
Lighter Choice Margarita Grilled Chicken, 1 serving	14
Lighter Choice Margarita Grilled Chicken (combo) without Sides, 1 serving	4
Mango-Chile Chicken, 1 serving	15
Mango-Chile Tilapia, 1 serving	15
Margarita Chicken Bowl with Quinoa (lunch combo), 1 serving	22
Margarita Chicken Bowl with Rice (lunch combo), 1 serving	22
Parmesan-Crusted Tilapia, 1 serving	19
Pasilla Chile Chicken, 1 serving	11
Seared Shrimp, 1 serving	2
Seared Shrimp (half order), 1 serving	1

Ribs & Steaks

6 oz Ancho Crusted Sirloin, 1 serving	12
6 oz Citrus Chile Avocado Sirloin, 1 serving	10
6 oz Classic Sirloin, 1 serving	6
6 oz Sirloin and Honey Chipotle Shrimp, 1 serving	11
6 oz Sirloin with Grilled Avocado, 1 serving	11
10 oz Ancho Crusted Sirloin, 1 serving	15
10 oz Citrus Chile Avocado Sirloin, 1 serving	13
10 oz Classic Sirloin, 1 serving	9
10 oz Sirloin and Honey Chipotle Shrimp, 1 serving	13
Classic Ribeye, 1 serving	17
Country-Fried Steak, 1 serving	17
Craft Beer BBQ Ribs - Full Rack, 1 serving	30
Craft Beer BBQ Ribs - Half Rack, 1 serving	15
Dr Pepper BBQ Ribs - Full Rack, 1 serving	31
Dr Pepper BBQ Ribs - Half Rack, 1 serving	15

"We Like This!" item

	SmartPoints® value
Grilled Steak, 1 serving	6
Half Rack of Memphis Dry Rub Ribs, 1 serving	18
Half Rack of Original BBQ Ribs, 1 serving	15
Honey Chipotle BBQ Ribs - Full Rack, 1 serving	31
Honey Chipotle BBQ Ribs - Half Rack, 1 serving	16
Memphis Dry Rub Ribs - Full Rack, 1 serving	57
Memphis Dry Rub Ribs - Half Rack, 1 serving	30
Original BBQ Ribs - Full Rack, 1 serving	31
Original Ribs - Full Rack, 1 serving	54
Original Ribs - Half Rack, 1 serving	27
Prime Rib, 1 serving	10
Sweet Bourbon Pork with Rice, 1 package	13

Fajitas & Enchiladas

Beef Enchilada, 1	10
Beef Enchilada Platter, 1 serving	29
Cheese Enchilada, 1	12
Cheese Enchilada Platter, 1 serving	36
Fajita Peppers and Onions, 1 serving	11
Fajita Toppings, 1 serving	13
Green Chile Chicken Enchilada, 1	8
Green Chile Chicken Enchilada Platter, 1 serving	23
Grilled Chicken Fajitas (lunch combo), 1 serving	25
Pork Carnitas, 1 serving	5
Pork Carnitas Fajitas (lunch combo), 1 serving	30
Sizzling Fajita Base, 1 serving	11

	SmartPoints® value
Sour Cream Chicken Enchilada, 1	10
Sour Cream Chicken Enchilada Platter, 1 serving	29

Burritos

Grilled Smoked Chicken Burrito with Quinoa Blend, 1 serving	25
Grilled Smoked Chicken Burrito with Rice, 1 serving	25
Smothered Carnitas Burrito with Quinoa Blend, 1 serving	34
Smothered Carnitas Burrito with Rice, 1 serving	34
Smothered Prime Rib Burrito with Quinoa Blend, 1 serving	32
Smothered Prime Rib Burrito with Rice, 1 serving	32
Smothered Smoked Chicken Burrito with Quinoa Blend, 1 serving	34
Smothered Smoked Chicken Burrito with Rice, 1 serving	34

Tacos & Quesadillas

Bacon Ranch Beef Quesadilla, 1 serving	60
Bacon Ranch Chicken Quesadilla, 1 serving	57
Bacon Ranch Chicken Quesadilla (lunch combo), 1 serving	30
Beef Taco, 1	9
Beef Tostada, 1 serving	12
Chicken Quesadilla, 1	24
Chicken Taco, 1	8
Chicken Tostada, 1 serving	10
Grilled Fish Taco, 1	9
Pork Carnitas Taco, 1	10
Pork Carnitas Tacos (lunch combo), 1 serving	20
Prime Rib Taco, 1	8
Ranchero Chicken Taco, 1	8

	SmartPoints® value
Ranchero Chicken Tacos (lunch combo), 1 serving	16
Smoked Chicken Quesadilla, 1 serving	58
Smoked Chicken Quesadilla (lunch combo), 1 serving	33
Spicy Shrimp Taco, 1	10

Fresh Mex Bowls

Chipotle Fresh Mex Bowl with Quinoa Blend, 1 serving	25
Fresh Mex Chipotle Bowl with Rice, 1 serving	25
Fresh Mex Margarita Bowl with Rice, 1 serving	24
Margarita Fresh Mex Bowl with Quinoa Blend, 1 serving	24
Prime Rib Fresh Mex Bowl with Quinoa Blend, 1 serving	26
Prime Rib Fresh Mex Bowl with Rice, 1 serving	26

Craft Burgers

Big Mouth Bites (lunch combo), 1 serving	20
Big Mouth Bites (Triple Dipper), 1 serving	27
Big Mouth Burger Bites, 1 serving	40
Black Bean Burger Only, 1 serving	5
Cheeseburger, 1 serving	13
Classic Bacon Burger, 1 serving	30
Double Burger, 1 serving	26
Guacamole Burger, 1 serving	30
Mushroom-Swiss Burger, 1 serving	42
Oldtimer Burger with Cheddar Cheese, 1 serving	25

	SmartPoints® value
Southern Smokehouse Burger, 1 serving	39
Sweet and Smoky Burger, 1 serving	37

Sandwiches & Handhelds

Bacon Avocado Chicken Sandwich, 1 serving	35
Bacon Avocado Chicken Sandwich (lunch combo), 1 serving	17
Buffalo Chicken Ranch Sandwich, 1 serving	25
California Turkey Club Toasted Sandwich, 1 serving	36
California Turkey Club Toasted Sandwich (lunch combo), 1 serving	18
Classic Turkey Toasted Sandwich, 1 serving	29
Classic Turkey Toasted Sandwich (lunch combo), 1 serving	16
Grilled Chicken Sandwich, 1 serving	21
Southwestern BLT Toasted Sandwich, 1 serving	14

Salad, Soups & Chili

Boneless Buffalo Chicken Salad, 1 serving	32
Caribbean Salad, 1 serving	25
Caribbean Salad with Grilled Chicken, 1 serving	28
Caribbean Salad with Grilled Shrimp, 1 serving	27
Chicken Caesar Salad, 1 serving	19
Chicken Enchilada Soup, 1 bowl	14
Chicken Enchilada Soup, 1 cup	7

"We Like This!" item

	SmartPoints® value
Fresco Salad, 1 serving	5
Fresco Salad (lunch combo), 1 serving	2
House Salad No Dressing, 1 serving	5
House Salad No Dressing (lunch), 1 serving	2
Loaded Baked Potato Soup, 1 bowl	20
Loaded Baked Potato Soup, 1 cup	10
Quesadilla Explosion Salad, 1 serving	47
Santa Fe Chicken Salad, 1 serving	20
Southwest Chicken Soup, 1 bowl	7
Southwest Chicken Soup, 1 cup	3
Terlingua Chili, 1 bowl	15
Terlingua Chili, 1 cup	8

Dressings and Sauces

Ancho Chile Ranch Dressing, 1½ oz	6
Avocado Ranch Dressing, 1½ oz	5
Black Pepper Gravy, 1 serving	1
Bleu Cheese Dressing, 1 serving	10
Caesar Dressing, 1½ oz	9
Citrus Balsamic Vinaigrette, 1½ oz	9
Honey Chipotle Sauce, 1 serving	5
Honey Lime Dressing, 1½ oz	8
Honey Lime Vinaigrette, 1½ oz	5
Honey Mustard Dressing, 1½ oz	8
Low Fat Ranch Dressing, 1½ oz	2
Original BBQ Sauce, 1 serving	4
Ranch Dressing, 1½ oz	6
Santa Fe Dressing, 1½ oz	7
Thousand Island Dressing, 1½ oz	7

SmartPoints® value

Sides

Asparagus and Garlic Roasted Tomatoes, 1 serving	2
Cinnamon Apples, 1 serving	12
Citrus Chile Rice, 1 serving	4
Fresh Guacamole, 1 large	8
Fresh Guacamole, 1 small	2
Fresh Pineapple, 1 serving	0
Homestyle Fries, 1 serving	12
Homestyle Fries (lunch combo), 1 serving	6
Loaded Mashed Potatoes, 1 serving	13
Loaded Potato Skins, 1 serving	24
Mashed Potatoes with Black Pepper Gravy, 1 serving	10
Quinoa and Wheatberry Blend, 1 serving	4
Rice, 1 serving	5
Sautéed Mushrooms, 1 serving	2
Skillet Mashed Potatoes, 1 serving	14
Southwestern Mac 'N' Cheese, 1 serving	18
Steamed Broccoli, 1 serving	0
Sweet Corn on the Cob, 1 serving	8
Sweet Potato Fries, 1 serving	30

Extras

American Cheese, 1 serving	3
Applewood Smoked Bacon, 1 serving	2
Avocado Slices, 1 serving	3
Black Beans, 1 serving	3
Cheddar Cheese, 1 serving	3
Corn Tortillas, 3	5
Flour Tortillas, 3	9
Provolone Cheese, 1 serving	3

	SmartPoints® value
Rice & Black Beans (Cadi), 1 serving	7
Sour Cream, 1 serving	3
Swiss Cheese, 1 serving	3

Kid's Menu

Apple Juice, 1 serving	7
Burger Bites, 1 serving	14
Burger, 1 serving	11
Celery Sticks, 1 serving	0
Cheese Pizza, 1 serving	20
Cheese Quesadilla, 1 serving	16
Cheeseburger Bites, 1 serving	15
Chocolate Milk, 1 serving	13
Corn Dog, 1 serving	8
Corn Kernels, 1 serving	5
Corn on the Cob, 1 serving	6
Cranberry Juice, 1 serving	5
Crispy Chicken Crispers, 1 serving	9
Electric Blue Blast, 1 serving	14
Grilled Cheese Sandwich, 1 serving	15
Grilled Chicken Bites, 1 serving	9
Grilled Chicken Kids Sandwich, 1 serving	7
Grilled Chicken Platter, 1 serving	2
Homestyle Fries, 1 serving	6
Little Original Chicken Crispers, 1 serving	9
Mandarin Oranges, 1 serving	4
Mashed Potatoes (no gravy), 1 serving	4
Milk, 1 serving	8
Orange Juice, 1 serving	7
Pepperoni Pizza, 1 serving	23
Rockin' Tropical Punch, 1 serving	14
Salad (without dressing), 1 serving	2
Sides Citrus Chile Rice, 1 serving	4

Desserts

Brownie Sundae, 1 serving	53
Cheesecake, 1 serving	35
Mini Molten Chocolate Cake, 1 serving	27
Molten Chocolate Cake, 1 serving	57
Skillet Chocolate Chip Cookie, 1 serving	66
Skillet Toffee Fudge Brownie, 1 serving	61
Triple Berry Crumble, 1 serving	48

Beverages

Iced Tea - Blackberry, 1 serving	5
Iced Tea - Mango, 1 serving	5
Strawberry Lemonade, 1 serving	12
Watermelon Lemonade, 1 serving	12

"We Like This!" item

	SmartPoints® value
Protein	
Barbacoa, 1 serving	3
Carnitas, 1 serving	6
Chicken, 1 serving	3
Sofritas, 4 oz	5
Steak, 1 serving	4
Beans	
Black Beans, 1 serving	3
Pinto Beans, 4 oz	3
Rice & Veggies	
Brown Rice, 1 serving	6
Cilantro-Lime Rice, 1 serving	6
Fajita Veggies, 2½ oz	1
Lettuce, 1 serving	0
Romaine Lettuce (salad), 2½ oz	0
Salsas	
Corn Salsa, 1 serving	3
Green Tomatillo Salsa, 1 serving	0
Red Tomatillo Salsa, 2 oz	1
Tomato Salsa, 3½ oz	0
Sides	
Chips, 1 serving	18
Chips and Fresh Tomato Salsa, 1 serving	19
Chips and Guacamole, 1 serving	26
Chips and Roasted Chili Corn Salsa, 1 serving	21
Chips and Tomatillo Green Chili Salsa, 1 serving	21
Chips and Tomatillo Red Chili Salsa, 1 serving	19

	SmartPoints® value
Extras	
Cheese, 1 serving	4
Chipotle Vinaigrette, 2 fl oz	11
Guacamole, 4 oz	8
Sour Cream, 1 serving	5
Tortillas	
Crispy Taco Shell, 3	7
Flour Tortilla (burrito), 1 serving	9
Soft Corn Tortillas, 3	6
Soft Flour Tortillas, 3	8
Beverages	
Organic Apple Juice, 1 serving	6
Organic Apple Juice, 1 serving	6
Organic Chocolate Milk, 1 serving	6
Organic Milk, 1 serving	4
Patron® Margarita, 1 serving	11
Sauza® Margarita, 1 serving	10

Build Your Own Grand Slam

	SmartPoints® value
Bacon Strips, 2 strips	2
Buttermilk Biscuit, 1 serving	7
Egg Whites, 2	1
Eggs, 1	4
Eggs, 2	8
English Muffin (with margarine), 1 serving	8
English Muffin (without margarine), 1 serving	4
Gluten Free English Muffin (with margarine), 1 serving	9
Gluten Free English Muffin (without margarine), 1 serving	6
Oatmeal with Milk and Brown Sugar, 1 serving	10
Pancakes Buttermilk with Margarine, 1 serving	12
Pancakes Hearty Wheat, 1 serving	9
Sausage Links, 2	6
Slices of Toast with Margarine, 2 slices	9

Slams

All American Slam with hash browns (add bread choice), 1 serving	33
Belgian Waffle Slam, 1 serving	31
Fit Slam, 1 serving	12
French Toast Slam, 1 serving	27
Lumberjack Slam (add bread choice), 1 serving	40
Original Grand Slam, 1 serving	28
The Grand Slamwich with Hash Browns, 1 serving	46

Omelettes

	SmartPoints® value
Fit Fare Loaded Veggie Omelette with Egg Whites Fruit and English Muffin, 1 serving	16
Philly Cheesesteak Omelette with Hash Browns (add bread choice), 1 serving	40
Ultimate Omelette with Hash Browns (add bread choice), 1 serving	28

Breakfast Favorites

Banana Pecan Pancake Breakfast, 1 serving	27
Blueberry Pancake Breakfast with Scrambled Eggs and Hash Brown (add meat choice), 1 serving	28
Cinnamon Pancake Breakfast with Hash Browns and Eggs (add meat choice), 1 serving	37
Country Fried Steak and Eggs with Hash Brown (add bread choice), 1 serving	32
Moons Over My Hammy, 1 serving	32
Pancake Puppies, 10 pieces	36
Pancake Puppies, 6 pieces	21
Peanut Butter Cup Pancake Breakfast with Hash Browns and Eggs (add meat choice), 1 serving	58
T-Bone Steak and Eggs with Hash Browns (add bread choice), 1 serving	23

"We Like This!" item

	SmartPoints® value

Skillets

Fit Fare Veggie Skillet, 1 serving	10
Healthy Breakfast Skillet, 1 serving	36
Hearty Breakfast Skillet, 1 serving	36
Santa Fe Skillet, 1 serving	24
Steak Skewer and Eggs Skillet, 1 serving	30
Ultimate Skillet, 1 serving	24

Breakfast Sides

Bacon Strips, 4 slices	5
Cheddar Cheese Hash Browns, 1 serving	10
Chicken Sausage Patties, 2	7
Everything Hash Browns with Onions Cheddar Cheese and Country Gravy, 1 serving	12
Grilled Ham Slice, 1 serving	3
Grits with Margarine, 4 oz	4
Hash Browns, 1 serving	7
Hearty Breakfast Sausage, 1 serving	10
Tortillas, 3	9
Turkey Bacon Strips, 2 strips	1
Turkey Bacon Strips, 4 strips	3
Whole Grain Rice, 1 serving	6
Yogurt Low Fat, 1 serving	8

Lunch & Dinner Appetizers

	SmartPoints® value
Chicken and Sausage Quesadilla (add ranch dressing), 1 serving	29
Chicken Strips with Buffalo Sauce, 1 serving	21
Chicken Strips with Sweet and Tangy BBQ Sauce, 1 serving	23
Chips and Queso (add dipping sauce), 1 serving	16
Half Size Zesty Nachos, 1 serving	23
Jalapeño Bottle Caps, 1 serving	3
Mozzarella Cheese Sticks (add dipping sauce), 1 serving	17
Sampler Jalapeño Bottle Caps, 1 serving	9
Sampler Jalapeño Bottle Caps (add dipping sauce), 1 serving	9
Sampler Mozzarella Cheese Sticks (add dipping sauce), 1 serving	9
Smothered Cheese Fries with Ranch Dressing, 1 serving	34
Zesty Nachos, 1 serving	45

Sandwiches

Cali Club Sandwich (add choice), 1 serving	35
Chicken Philly Melt (add choice), 1 serving	26
Club Sandwich (add choice), 1 serving	24
Pot Roast Melt (add choice), 1 serving	25
Prime Rib Philly Melt (add choice), 1 serving	30
The Super Bird (add choices), 1 serving	18

Burgers

Bacon Avocado Cheeseburger (add choice), 1 serving	35
Bourbon Bacon Burger (add choice), 1 serving	38
Chicken Bacon Classic (add choice), 1 serving	28
Double Cheeseburger (add choice), 1 serving	36
Slamburger (add choice), 1 serving	34
Spicy Sriracha Burger (add choice), 1 serving	29

Build Your Own Burger

	SmartPoints® value
100% Beef Patty, 1 serving	11
American Cheese, 1 serving	3
Carmelized Onions, 1 serving	2
Cheddar Bun, 1 serving	9
Cheddar Cheese, 1 serving	3
Fresh Avocado, 1 serving	3
Grilled Seasoned Chicken Breast, 1 serving	3
Sauteed Mushrooms, 1 serving	2
Sliced Jalapeños, 1 serving	0
Swiss Cheese, 1 serving	4
Veggie Patty, 1 serving	4
Whole Wheat Bun, 1 serving	6

Dinner

Alaska Salmon (add choices), 1 serving	17
Bourbon Chicken Skillet, 1 serving	24
Brooklyn Spaghetti and Meatballs with Bread, 1 serving	39
Chicken Strips with Bread (add choices), 1 serving	22
Country Fried Steak with Gravy and Bread (add choices), 1 serving	32
Fish and Chips with French Fries (add side), 1 serving	33
Fit Fare Tilapia Ranchero, 1 serving	14
Slow Cooked Pot Roast, 1 serving	42
T-Bone Steak and Shrimp with Bread (add choices), 1 serving	27
T-Bone Steak with Bread (add choices), 1 serving	21
Tilapia Ranchero with Bread, 1 serving	13

55+ Menu

	SmartPoints® value
Belgian Waffle Slam (add meat choice), 1 serving	18
Club Sandwich (add choices), 1 serving	23
Country Fried Steak with Bread (add choices), 1 serving	24
Fit Fare Loaded Veggie Omelette, 1 serving	16
French Toast Slam (add meat choice), 1 serving	11
Grilled Cheese Sandwich (add soup choice), 1 serving	15
Grilled Chicken with Bread (add choices), 1 serving	9
Grilled Tilapia with Bread (add choices), 1 serving	10
Omelette (add choices), 1 serving	15
Scrambled Eggs and Cheddar Breakfast, 1 serving	27
Senior Steak Skewer Dinner (add choices), 1 serving	15
Steak Skewer Dinner (add choices), 1 serving	15

Dinner Sides

Broccoli, 1 serving	1
Cheddar Mashed Potatoes, 1 serving	8
French Fries Salted, 1 serving	16
Fresh Sauteed Zucchini and Squash, 1 serving	2
Fresh Steamed Zucchini and Squash, 1 serving	1
Garlic Toast Dinner Bread, 1 serving	7
Golden Fried Shrimp, 6 pieces	6
Hash Browns, 1 serving	7
Onion Rings, 1 serving	25
Red Skinned Potatoes, 1 serving	6

"We Like This!" item

	SmartPoints® value
Seasonal Fruit, 1 serving	0
Seasoned Fries, 1 serving	21
Sweet Petite Corn, 1 serving	4
Tomato Slices, 1 serving	0

Soups & Salads

Avocado Chicken Caesar Salad, 1 serving	19
Broccoli and Cheddar Soup, 1 bowl	15
Broccoli and Cheddar Soup, 1 cup	10
Caesar Salad without Dressing, 1 serving	8
Chicken Noodle Soup, 1 bowl	4
Chicken Noodle Soup, 1 cup	3
Clam Chowder, 1 bowl	11
Clam Chowder, 1 cup	7
Cranberry Apple Chicken Salad with Balsamic Vinaigrette (no bread), 1 serving	11
Fried Chicken Strips Cobb Salad (add dressing), 1 serving	27
Garden Salad (add dressing), 1 serving	7
Grilled Chicken Cobb Salad (add dressing), 1 serving	18
Loaded Baked Potato Soup, 1 bowl	17
Loaded Baked Potato Soup, 1 cup	12
Prime Rib Cobb Salad (add dressing), 1 serving	20
Vegetable Beef Soup, 1 bowl	5
Vegetable Beef Soup, 1 cup	3

Condiments

	SmartPoints® value
Balsamic Vinaigrette, 3 oz	6
Balsamic Vinaigrette Low Fat, 1½ oz	3
BBQ Sauce, 1 oz	3
BBQ Sweet and Tangy, 1 serving	7
Blue Cheese Dressing, 1½ oz	6
Blue Cheese Dressing, 3 oz	12
Bourbon Sauce, 1 serving	8
Brown Gravy, 1 serving	0
Caesar Dressing, 1½ oz	7
Croutons (for salad), 1 serving	2
Dippable Veggies (with ranch dressing), 1 serving	8
Fat Free Italian Dressing, 1½ oz	1
Fat Free Ranch Dressing, 1½ oz	1
French Dressing, 1½ oz	4
Honey Mustard Dressing, 1½ oz	6
Maple Flavored Syrup, 1 serving	8
Marinara Sauce, 1 serving	1
Pico de Gallo, 1 serving	1
Sour Cream, 1 serving	3
Sugar Free Maple Flavored Syrup, 1 serving	1
Thousand Island Dressing, 1½ oz	6

	SmartPoints® value

Desserts

Banana Split, 1 serving	40
Blackberry Milk Shake, 1 serving	42
Caramel Apple Pie Crisp, 1 serving	35
Caramel Topping, 1 serving	7
Chocolate Ice Cream (build your own sundae), 2 scoops	25
Chocolate Lava Cake, 1 serving	34
Chocolate Peanut Butter Milk Shake, 1 serving	52
Chopped Nuts, 1 serving	6
Glazed Pecans, 1 serving	10
Hot Fudge Topping, 1 serving	5
Ice Cream (chocolate), 1 scoop	25
Ice Cream (strawberry), 1 scoop	23
Milk Shakes (chocolate peanut butter), 1 serving	52
Milk Shakes (chocolate), 1 serving	41
Milk Shakes (Oreo), 1 serving	56
Milk Shakes (strawberry), 1 serving	36
Milk Shakes (vanilla), 1 serving	40
New York Style Cheesecake (plain), 1 serving	23
New York Style Cheesecake (with strawberry topping and whipped cream), 1 serving	29
Oreo Cookie Pieces, 1 serving	4
Oreo Milk Shake, 1 serving	56
Strawberry Ice Cream (build your own sundae), 2 scoops	23
Strawberry Milk Shake, 1 serving	36
Strawberry Topping, 1 serving	2
Vanilla Ice Cream, 1 serving	25
Vanilla Milk Shake, 1 serving	40

	SmartPoints® value

Smoothies

Groovy Mango Smoothie, 1 serving	16
Strawberry Banana Bliss, 1 serving	13

Beverages

Apple Juice, 1 serving	12
Cherry Flavor Shot, 1 serving	0
Chocolate Milk (reduced fat), 1 serving	13
Hot Chocolate, 1 serving	6
Ice Tea (unsweetened), 1 serving	0
Iced Cappuccino, 1 serving	9
Iced Tea (sweet), 1 serving	7
Lemonade, 1 serving	8
Lemonade Iced Tea, 1 serving	4
Mango Lemonade, 1 serving	13
Ruby Red Grapefruit Juice, 1 serving	14
Strawberry Lemonade, 1 serving	12
Tomato Juice, 1 serving	4
Vanilla Flavor Shot, 1 serving	3

"We Like This!" item

American Legends Pizza (Extra Large)

	SmartPoints® value
Buffalo Chicken, Brooklyn Style, ⅙ of pizza	16
Buffalo Chicken, Hand Tossed, ⅛ of pizza	15
Cali Chicken Bacon Ranch, Brooklyn Style, ⅙ of pizza	20
Cali Chicken Bacon Ranch, Hand Tossed, ⅛ of pizza	18
Fiery Hawaiian (with Hot Sauce), Brooklyn Style, ⅙ of pizza	16
Fiery Hawaiian (with Hot Sauce), Hand Tossed, ⅛ of pizza	15
Honolulu Hawaiian, Brooklyn Style, ⅙ of pizza	16
Honolulu Hawaiian, Hand Tossed, ⅛ of pizza	15
Memphis BBQ Chicken, Brooklyn Style, ⅙ of pizza	17
Memphis BBQ Chicken, Hand Tossed, ⅛ of pizza	15
Pacific Veggie, Brooklyn Style, ⅙ of pizza	14
Pacific Veggie, Hand Tossed, ⅛ of pizza	14
Philly Cheese Steak, Brooklyn Style, ⅙ of pizza	16
Philly Cheese Steak, Hand Tossed, ⅛ of pizza	15
Spinach and Feta Brooklyn Style, ⅙ of pizza	16
Spinach and Feta Hand Tossed, ⅛ of pizza	15
Wisconsin 6 Cheese, Brooklyn Style, ⅙ of pizza	16
Wisconsin 6 Cheese, Hand Tossed, ⅛ of pizza	15

American Legends Pizza (Large)

	SmartPoints® value
Buffalo Chicken, Brooklyn Style, ⅙ of pizza	12
Buffalo Chicken, Hand Tossed, ⅛ of pizza	11
Buffalo Chicken, Thin Crust, ⅛ of pizza	7
Cali Chicken Bacon Ranch, Brooklyn Style, ⅙ of pizza	16
Cali Chicken Bacon Ranch, Hand Tossed, ⅛ of pizza	14
Cali Chicken Bacon Ranch, Thin Crust, ⅛ of pizza	10
Fiery Hawaiian Hand Tossed with Hot Sauce, ⅛ of pizza	12
Fiery Hawaiian, Brooklyn Style - with Hot Sauce, ⅙ of pizza	12
Fiery Hawaiian, Thin Crust - with Hot Sauce, ⅛ of pizza	8
Honolulu Hawaiian, Brooklyn Style, ⅙ of pizza	12
Honolulu Hawaiian, Hand Tossed, ⅛ of pizza	12
Honolulu Hawaiian, Thin Crust, ⅛ of pizza	8
Memphis BBQ Chicken, Brooklyn Style, ⅙ of pizza	13
Memphis BBQ Chicken, Hand Tossed, ⅛ of pizza	12
Memphis BBQ Chicken, Thin Crust, ⅛ of pizza	8
Pacific Veggie, Brooklyn Style, ⅙ of pizza	11
Pacific Veggie, Hand Tossed, ⅛ of pizza	11
Pacific Veggie, Thin Crust, ⅛ of pizza	7
Philly Cheese Steak, Brooklyn Style, ⅙ of pizza	11
Philly Cheese Steak, Hand Tossed, ⅛ of pizza	11
Philly Cheese Steak, Thin Crust, ⅛ of pizza	7
Spinach and Feta Brooklyn Style, ⅙ of pizza	12
Spinach and Feta Hand Tossed, ⅛ of pizza	11

	SmartPoints® value
Spinach and Feta Thin Crust, ⅛ of pizza	8
Wisconsin 6 Cheese, Brooklyn Style, ⅙ of pizza	12
Wisconsin 6 Cheese, Hand Tossed, ⅛ of pizza	12
Wisconsin 6 Cheese, Thin Crust, ⅛ of pizza	8

American Legends Pizza (Medium)

Buffalo Chicken, Hand Tossed, ⅛ of pizza	9
Buffalo Chicken, Thin Crust, ¼ of pizza	12
Cali Chicken Bacon Ranch, Hand Tossed, ⅛ of pizza	10
Cali Chicken Bacon Ranch, Thin Crust, ¼ of pizza	16
Fiery Hawaiian, Thin Crust - with Hot Sauce, ¼ of pizza	13
Honolulu Hawaiian, Hand Tossed, ⅛ of pizza	8
Honolulu Hawaiian, Thin Crust, ¼ of pizza	13
Memphis BBQ Chicken, Hand Tossed, ⅛ of pizza	9
Memphis BBQ Chicken, Thin Crust, ¼ of pizza	12
Pacific Veggie, Hand Tossed, ⅛ of pizza	7
Pacific Veggie, Thin Crust, ¼ of pizza	11
Philly Cheese Steak, Hand Tossed, ⅛ of pizza	9
Philly Cheese Steak, Thin Crust, ¼ of pizza	12
Spinach and Feta Hand Tossed, ⅛ of pizza	8
Spinach and Feta Handmade Pan, ⅛ of pizza	11
Spinach and Feta Thin Crust, ¼ of pizza	13

"We Like This!" item

	SmartPoints® value
Wisconsin 6 Cheese, Hand Tossed, ⅛ of pizza	8
Wisconsin 6 Cheese, Thin Crust, ¼ of pizza	13

American Legends Pizza (Small)

Buffalo Chicken Gluten Free, 1 slice	6
Buffalo Chicken, Hand Tossed, 1 slice	8
Buffalo Chicken, Thin Crust, ¼ of pizza	8
Cali Chicken Bacon Ranch Gluten Free, ⅙ of pizza	7
Cali Chicken Bacon Ranch, Hand Tossed, ⅙ of pizza	9
Cali Chicken Bacon Ranch, Thin Crust, ¼ of pizza	10
Fiery Hawaiian Gluten Free with Hot Sauce, ⅙ of pizza	6
Fiery Hawaiian, Hand Tossed - with Hot Sauce, ⅙ of pizza	8
Fiery Hawaiian, Thin Crust - with Hot Sauce, ¼ of pizza	9
Honolulu Hawaiian Gluten Free, ⅙ of pizza	6
Honolulu Hawaiian, Hand Tossed, ⅙ of pizza	8
Honolulu Hawaiian, Thin Crust, ¼ of pizza	9
Memphis BBQ Chicken Gluten Free, ⅙ of pizza	7
Memphis BBQ Chicken, Hand Tossed, ⅙ of pizza	8
Memphis BBQ Chicken, Thin Crust, ¼ of pizza	9
Pacific Veggie Gluten Free, ⅙ of pizza	5
Pacific Veggie, Hand Tossed, ⅙ of pizza	7
Pacific Veggie, Thin Crust, ¼ of pizza	8
Philly Cheese Steak Gluten Free, ⅙ of pizza	6

	SmartPoints® value
Philly Cheese Steak, Hand Tossed, ⅙ of pizza	8
Philly Cheese Steak, Thin Crust, ¼ of pizza	8
Spinach and Feta Gluten Free, ⅙ of pizza	6
Spinach and Feta Hand Tossed, ⅙ of pizza	8
Spinach and Feta Thin Crust, ¼ of pizza	9
Wisconsin 6 Cheese Gluten Free, ⅙ of pizza	6
Wisconsin 6 Cheese, Hand Tossed, ⅙ of pizza	8
Wisconsin 6 Cheese, Thin Crust, ¼ of pizza	8

Build Your Own Pizza (Extra Large)

Brooklyn Crust with BBQ Sauce & Regular Cheese, ⅙ of pizza	11
Brooklyn Crust with Hearty Marinara Sauce & Regular Cheese, ⅙ of pizza	10
Brooklyn Crust with Robust Tomato Sauce - Cheese Only, ⅙ of pizza	11
Brooklyn Crust with Robust Tomato Sauce and Regular Cheese, ⅙ of pizza	10
Brooklyn Crust with White Garlic Parm & Regular Cheese, ⅙ of pizza	12
Hand Tossed Crust with BBQ Sauce & Regular Cheese, ⅛ of pizza	12
Hand Tossed Crust with Hearty Marinara Sauce & Regular Cheese, ⅛ of pizza	12
Hand Tossed Crust with Robust Tomato Sauce - Cheese Only, ⅛ of pizza	12
Hand Tossed Crust with Robust Tomato Sauce and Regular Cheese, ⅛ of pizza	11

	SmartPoints® value
Hand Tossed Crust with White Garlic Parm Sauce & Regular Cheese, ⅛ of pizza	13
Thin Crust with BBQ Sauce & Regular Cheese, ⅛ of pizza	10
Thin Crust with Hearty Marinara Sauce & Regular Cheese, ⅛ of pizza	9
Thin Crust with Robust Tomato Sauce - Cheese Only, ⅛ of pizza	10
Thin Crust with Robust Tomato Sauce and Regular Cheese, ⅛ of pizza	9
Thin Crust with White Garlic Parm Sauce & Regular Cheese, ⅛ of pizza	11

Build Your Own Pizza (Large)

Brooklyn Crust with Hearty Marinara Sauce & Regular Cheese, ¼ of pizza	6
Brooklyn Crust with Robust Tomato Sauce and Regular Cheese, ¼ of pizza	6
Brooklyn Crust with Robust Tomato Sauce Cheese Only, 1 whole pizza	55
Hand Tossed Crust with BBQ Sauce & Regular Cheese, ⅛ of pizza	9
Hand Tossed Crust with Hearty Marinara Sauce & Regular Cheese, ⅛ of pizza	8
Hand Tossed Crust with Robust Tomato Sauce - Cheese Only, ⅛ of pizza	9
Hand Tossed Crust with Robust Tomato Sauce and Regular Cheese, ⅛ of pizza	8
Hand Tossed Crust with White Garlic Parm Sauce & Regular Cheese, ⅛ of pizza	10
Thin Crust with Robust Tomato Sauce - Cheese Only, ⅛ of pizza	8
Thin Crust with Robust Tomato Sauce and Regular Cheese, ⅛ of pizza	7

Build Your Own Pizza (Large) (cont'd)

	SmartPoints® value
Thin Crust with White Garlic Parm Sauce & Regular Cheese, ⅛ of pizza	8

Build Your Own Pizza (Medium)

Hand Tossed Crust with BBQ Sauce & Regular Cheese, ⅛ of pizza	7
Hand Tossed Crust with Hearty Marinara Sauce & Regular Cheese, ⅛ of pizza	6
Hand Tossed Crust with Robust Tomato Sauce - Cheese Only Pizza, ⅛ of pizza	7
Hand Tossed Crust with Robust Tomato Sauce and Regular Cheese, ⅛ of pizza	6
Hand Tossed Crust with White Garlic Parm Sauce & Regular Cheese, ⅛ of pizza	7
Thin Crust with BBQ Sauce & Regular Cheese, ⅛ of pizza	10
Thin Crust with Hearty Marinara Sauce & Reuglar Cheese, ¼ of pizza	10
Thin Crust with Robust Tomato Sauce and Regular Cheese, ¼ of pizza	9
Thin Crust with Robust Tomato Sauce Cheese Only Pizza, 1 whole pizza	44
Thin Crust with White Garlic Parm Sauce & Regular Cheese, ¼ of pizza	12

Build Your Own Pizza (Small)

	SmartPoints® value
Gluten Free Crust with BBQ Sauce & Regular Cheese, ⅙ of pizza	5
Gluten Free Crust with Hearty Marinara Sauce & Regular Cheese, ⅙ of pizza	4
Gluten Free Crust with Robust Tomato Sauce - Cheese Only Pizza, ⅙ of pizza	8
Gluten Free Crust with Robust Tomato Sauce and Regular Cheese, ⅙ of pizza	4
Gluten Free Crust with White Garlic Parm & Regular Cheese, ⅙ of pizza	5
Hand Tossed Crust with BBQ Sauce & Regular Cheese, ⅙ of pizza	6
Hand Tossed Crust with Hearty Marinara Sauce & Regular Cheese, ⅙ of pizza	6
Hand Tossed Crust with Robust Tomato Sauce - Cheese Only Pizza, ⅙ of pizza	7
Hand Tossed Crust with Robust Tomato Sauce and Regular Cheese, ⅙ of pizza	6
Hand Tossed Crust with White Garlic Parm Sauce & Regular Cheese, ⅙ of pizza	7
Thin Crust with BBQ Sauce & Regular Cheese, ¼ of pizza	7
Thin Crust with Hearty Marinara Sauce & Reuglar Cheese, ¼ of pizza	7
Thin Crust with Robust Tomato Sauce - Cheese Only Pizza, ¼ of pizza	5
Thin Crust with Robust Tomato Sauce and Regular Cheese, ¼ of pizza	7
Thin Crust with White Garlic Parm Sauce & Regular Cheese, ¼ of pizza	8

Feast Pizzas - America's Favorite - with Hand Tossed Crust

Extra Large, ⅛ of pizza	15
Large, ⅛ of pizza	11
Medium, ⅛ of pizza	8
Small, ⅙ of pizza	8

"We Like This!" item

	SmartPoints® value

Feast Pizzas - America's Favorite - with Thin Crust

Extra Large, ⅛ of pizza	13
Large, ⅛ of pizza	9
Medium, ¼ of pizza	14
Small, ¼ of pizza	10

Feast Pizzas - Bacon Cheeseburger - with Hand Tossed Crust

Extra Large, ⅛ of pizza	16
Large, ⅛ of pizza	12
Medium, ⅛ of pizza	9
Small, ⅙ of pizza	9

Feast Pizzas - Bacon Cheeseburger - with Thin Crust

Extra Large, ⅛ of pizza	14
Large, ⅛ of pizza	10
Medium, ¼ of pizza	15
Small, ¼ of pizza	11

Feast Pizzas - Deluxe - with Hand Tossed Crust

Extra Large, ⅛ of pizza	13
Large, ⅛ of pizza	10
Medium, ⅛ of pizza	8
Small, ⅛ of pizza	8

Feast Pizzas - Deluxe - with Thin Crust

Extra Large, ⅛ of pizza	11
Large, ⅛ of pizza	8
Medium, ¼ of pizza	13
Small, ¼ of pizza	9

	SmartPoints® value

Feast Pizzas - ExtravaganZZa - with Hand Tossed Crust

Extra Large, ⅛ of pizza	17
Large, ⅛ of pizza	13
Medium, ⅛ of pizza	10
Small, ⅙ of pizza	10

Feast Pizzas - ExtravaganZZa - with Thin Crust

Extra Large, ⅛ of pizza	15
Medium, ¼ of pizza	16
Small, ¼ of pizza	12

Feast Pizzas - MeatZZa - with Hand Tossed Crust

Extra Large, ⅛ of pizza	17
Large, ⅛ of pizza	12
Medium, ⅛ of pizza	9
Small, 1 slice	9

Feast Pizzas - MeatZZa - with Thin Crust

Extra Large, ⅛ of pizza	15
Large, ⅛ of pizza	10
Medium, ¼ of pizza	16
Small, ¼ of pizza	11

Feast Pizzas - Ultimate Pepperoni - with Hand Tossed Crust

Extra Large, ⅛ of pizza	15
Large, ⅛ of pizza	12
Medium, ⅛ of pizza	9
Small, 1 slice	9

Feast Pizzas - Ultimate Pepperoni - with Thin Crust

Extra Large, ⅛ of pizza	13
Medium, ¼ of pizza	15
Small, ¼ of pizza	11

Handmade Pan Pizza

	SmartPoints® value
12" Handmade Pan Pizza with Alfredo Sauce and Extra Cheese (cheese only), 1 whole pizza	93
12" Handmade Pan Pizza with Alfredo Sauce and Extra Cheese with Toppings, 1 whole pizza	89
12" Handmade Pan Pizza with Alfredo Sauce and Light Cheese (cheese only), 1 whole pizza	83
12" Handmade Pan Pizza with Alfredo Sauce and Light Cheese with Toppings, 1 whole pizza	83
12" Handmade Pan Pizza with Alfredo Sauce and Regular Cheese (cheese only), 1 whole pizza	89
12 Handmade Pan Pizza with Alfredo Sauce and Regular Cheese with Toppings, 1 whole pizza	85
12" Handmade Pan Pepperoni Pizza, 1 slice	11
12" Handmade Pan Pizza with BBQ Sauce and Extra Cheese (cheese only), 1 slice	11
12" Handmade Pan Pizza with BBQ Sauce and Extra Cheese with Toppings, 1 slice	11
12" Handmade Pan Pizza with BBQ Sauce and Light Cheese (cheese only), 1 slice	10
12" Handmade Pan Pizza with BBQ Sauce and Light Cheese with Toppings, 1 slice	10
12" Handmade Pan Pizza with BBQ Sauce and Regular Cheese (cheese only), 1 slice	11
12" Handmade Pan Pizza with BBQ Sauce and Regular Cheese with Toppings, 1 slice	10
12" Handmade Pan Pizza with Marinara Sauce and Extra Cheese (cheese only), 1 slice	11
12" Handmade Pan Pizza with Marinara Sauce and Extra Cheese with Toppings, 1 slice	10
12" Handmade Pan Pizza with Marinara Sauce and Light Cheese (cheese only), 1 slice	10
12" Handmade Pan Pizza with Marinara Sauce and Light Cheese with Toppings, 1 slice	10
12" Handmade Pan Pizza with Marinara Sauce and Regular Cheese (cheese only), 1 slice	10
12" Handmade Pan Pizza with Marinara Sauce and Regular Cheese with Toppings, 1 slice	10
12" Handmade Pan Pizza with Robust Tomato Sauce and Extra Cheese (cheese only), 1 slice	11
12" Handmade Pan Pizza with Robust Tomato Sauce and Extra Cheese with Toppings, 1 slice	10
12" Handmade Pan Pizza with Robust Tomato Sauce and Light Cheese (cheese only), 1 slice	10
12" Handmade Pan Pizza with Robust Tomato Sauce and Light Cheese with Toppings, 1 slice	10
12" Handmade Pan Pizza with Robust Tomato Sauce and Regular Cheese (cheese only), 1 slice	10
12" Handmade Pan Pizza with Robust Tomato Sauce and Regular Cheese with Toppings, 1 slice	10
12" Handmade Pan Pizza with White Garlic Parm Sauce and Extra Cheese (cheese only), 1 slice	12
12" Handmade Pan Pizza with White Garlic Parm Sauce and Extra Cheese with Toppings, 1 slice	12
12" Handmade Pan Pizza with White Garlic Parm Sauce and Light Cheese (cheese only), 1 slice	11
12" Handmade Pan Pizza with White Garlic Parm Sauce and Light Cheese with Toppings, 1 slice	11

"We Like This!" item

	SmartPoints® value
12" Handmade Pan Pizza with White Garlic Parm Sauce and Regular Cheese (cheese only), 1 slice	12
12" Handmade Pan Pizza with White Garlic Parm Sauce and Regular Cheese with Toppings, 1 slice	11

Specialty Chicken

Classic Hot Buffalo Specialty Chicken, 12 pieces	15
Crispy Bacon and Tomato Specialty Chicken, 12 pieces	21
Spicy Jalapeño Pineapple Specialty Chicken, 12 pieces	17
Sweet BBQ Bacon Specialty Chicken, 12 pieces	19

Chicken Sides

Boneless Chicken, 8 pieces	10
Boneless Chicken, 14 pieces	18
Boneless Chicken, 40 pieces	50
Wings: BBQ, 8 pieces	16
Wings: BBQ, 14 pieces	28
Wings: BBQ, 40 pieces	79
Wings: Fire, 8 pieces	11
Wings: Fire, 14 pieces	19
Wings: Fire, 40 pieces	55
Wings: Hot, 8 pieces	11
Wings: Hot, 14 pieces	19
Wings: Hot, 40 pieces	55
Wings: Mild, 8 pieces	11
Wings: Mild, 14 pieces	19
Wings: Mild, 40 pieces	55
Wings: Plain, 8 pieces	10
Wings: Plain, 14 pieces	18
Wings: Plain, 40 pieces	52
Wings: Sweet Mango Habanero, 8 pieces	16
Wings: Sweet Mango Habanero, 14 pieces	28

	SmartPoints® value
Wings: Sweet Mango Habanero, 40 pieces	81

Pastas

Chicken Alfredo in Tin, 1 serving	20
Chicken Carbonara in Tin, 1 serving	22
Italian Sausage Marinara in Tin, 1 serving	23
Pasta Primavera in Tin, 1 serving	20

Domino's Breadbowl Pasta™

Chicken Alfredo In Breadbowl (2 servings), 1 serving	22
Chicken Carbonara In Breadbowl (2 servings), 1 serving	23
Italian Sausage Marinara In Breadbowl (2 servings), 1 serving	24
Pasta Primavera In Breadbowl (2 servings), 1 serving	44

Oven Baked Sandwiches

Buffalo Chicken with Blue Cheese, 1 sandwich	26
Chicken Bacon Ranch, 1 sandwich	27
Chicken Habanero Oven Baked Sandwich, 1 sandwich	26
Chicken Parmesan, 1 sandwich	23
Extra Cheese Sandwich Topping, 1 serving	3
Extra Chicken Sandwich Topping, 1 serving	2
Extra Italian Meat Sandwich Topping, 1 serving	4
Extra Philly Meat Sandwich Topping, 1 serving	1
Extra Veggies Italian Sandwich Topping, 1 serving	0
Extra Veggies, Philly Sandwich Topping, 1 serving	0
Italian, 1 sandwich	27
Italian Sausage & Peppers, 1 sandwich	29

	SmartPoints® value
Mediterranean Veggie, 1 sandwich	23
Philly Cheese Steak, 1 sandwich	22

Stuffed Cheesy Bread

Bacon & Jalapeño, 1 serving	41
Cheese Only, 1 serving	36
Spinach & Feta, 1 serving	37

Freshly Made Bread

Breadsticks, 1 serving	28
Cinna Stix®, 4 pieces	16
Parm Bites, 16 pieces	18
Parm Bites, 32 pieces	36

Dipping Cups

BBQ Sauce, 1 container	3
Blue Cheese, 1 container	9
Garlic, 1 container	9
Kicker Hot Sauce, 1 container	2
Marinara, 1 container	1
Ranch, 1 container	7
Sweet Icing, 1 container	14
Sweet Mango Habanero, 1 container	4

Salads & Dressings

Balsamic Dressing, 1 serving	5
Blue Cheese Dressing, 1 package	8
Buttermilk Ranch Dressing, 1 package	8
Chicken Apple Pecan Salad, 1 serving	7
Classic Garden Salad, 1 serving	5
Fat Free Raspberry Dressing, 1 serving	3
Golden Italian Dressing, 1 package	8
Italian Dressing, 1 serving	5
Ranch Dressing, 1 serving	8

"We Like This!" item

	SmartPoints® value

Amazin' Greens

Blue Cheese Dressing, 1 package	8
Buttermilk Dressing, 1 package	8
Creamy Caesar Dressing, 1 package	8
Croutons, 1 package	3
Garden Fresh Salad (serves 2), 1 serving	3
Golden Italian Dressing, 1 package	7
Greek Dressing, 1 package	8
Greek Salad (serves 2), 1 serving	4
Grilled Chicken Caesar Salad (serves 2), 1 serving	5
Light Italian Dressing, 1 package	1

Desserts

Chocolate Lava Crunch Cakes, 1 serving	33
Marbled Cookie Brownie, piece	9

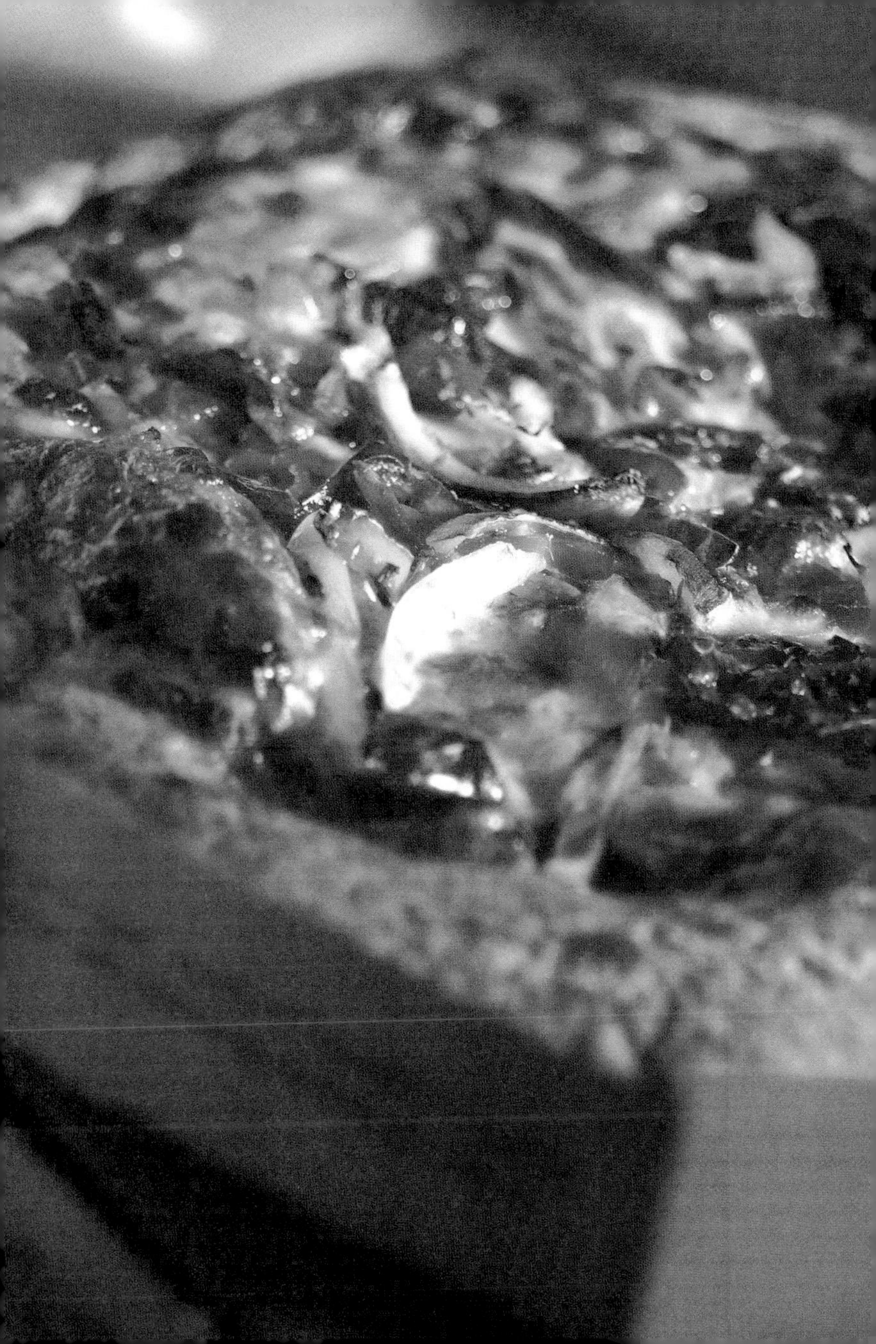

Donuts

	SmartPoints® value
Apple Crumb Donut, 1	14
Apple n Spice Donut, 1	10
Bavarian Kreme Donut, 1	11
Boston Kreme Donut, 1	13
Bow Tie Donut, 1	11
Cherry Blossom Donut, 1	15
Chocolate Coconut Donut, 1	18
Chocolate Dipped Cherries Donut, 1	15
Chocolate Dulce de Leche Donut, 1	14
Chocolate Frosted Cake Donut, 1	15
Chocolate Frosted Cocoa Donut, 1	11
Chocolate Frosted Donut, 1	11
Chocolate Frosted Donut with Sprinkles, 1	12
Chocolate Glazed Donut, 1	15
Chocolate Iced Bismark, 1	16
Chocolate Kreme Filled Donut, 1	13
Cinnamon Donut, 1	13
Cinnamon Stick, 1	16
Cocoa Boston Kreme Donut, 1	13
Cocoa Butternut Donut, 1	12
Cocoa Coconut Donut, 1	12
Cocoa Confetti Donut, 1	12
Cocoa Glazed Donut, 1	11
Cocoa Jelly Donut, 1	13
Cocoa Kreme Puff Donut, 1	14
Dad's Star Donut, 1	13
Double Chocolate Cake Donut, 1	15
Double Cocoa Kreme Donut, 1	13
Double Cocoa Kreme Puff Donut, 1	13
Dulce de Leche Donut, 1	12
Glazed Cake Donut, 1	16
Glazed Chocolate Stick, 1	17
Glazed Donut, 1	11
Glazed Jelly Donut, 1	12
Glazed Stick, 1	18
Guayaba Burst Donut, 1	12
Holiday Star Donut, 1	13
Jelly Donut, 1	11
Jelly Filled Donut, 1	11
Jelly Stick, 1	19
Key Lime Donut, 1	15
Lemon Filled Donut, 1	11
Lemonade Donut, 1	15
Maple Frosted Cocoa Donut, 1	11
Maple Frosted Donut, 1	12
Marble Frosted Cocoa Donut, 1	12
Marble Frosted Donut, 1	11
Mom's Heart Donut, 1	13
Old Fashioned Cake Donut, 1	13
Pina Boom Donut, 1	11
Piña Colada Donut, 1	14
Plain Stick Donut, 1	15
Powdered Cocoa Donut, 1	9
Powdered Donut, 1	13
Powdered Stick, 1	17
Red Velvet Donut, 1	19
Red Velvet Drizzle Donut, 1	18
Reverse Boston Kreme Donut, 1	14
Spring Fling Donut, 1	12
Spring Showers Donut, 1	14
Strawberry Frosted Cocoa Donut, 1	11
Strawberry Frosted Donut, 1	12
Sugar Raised Donut, 1	9
Sugared Cocoa Donut, 1	7
Triple Cocoa Donut, 1	10
Vanilla Cocoa Kreme Donut, 1	13
Vanilla Creme Donut, 1	14
Vanilla Frosted Cocoa Donut, 1	10

Muffins

	SmartPoints® value
Banana Chocolate Chip Muffin, 1 serving	22
Blueberry Muffin, 1	19
Chocolate Chip Muffin, 1	24

"We Like This!" item

	SmartPoints® value
Coffee Cake Muffin, 1	26
Corn Muffin, 1	18
Honey Bran Raisin Muffin, 1	18
Lemon Poppy Seed Muffin, 1	21
Raspberry White Chocolate Muffin, 1	24
Reduced Fat Blueberry Muffin, 1	17

Munchkins

Blueberry Munchkin, 1	3
Boston Kreme Munchkin, 1	3
Butternut Munchkin, 1	4
Chocolate Butternut Munchkin, 1	4
Cinnamon Munchkin, 1	2
Cocoa Glazed Munchkin, 1	1
Cocoa Kreme Puff Munchkin, 1	2
Coconut Munchkin, 1	4
Double Cocoa Kreme Puff Munchin,	12
Glazed Cake Munchkin, 1	3
Glazed Chocolate Munchkin, 1	3
Glazed Munchkin, 1	3
Glazed Old Fashioned Munchkin, 1	3
Jelly Filled Munchkin, 1	3
Old Fashioned Munchkin, 1	2
Plain Cake Munchkin, 1	2
Powdered Munchkin, 1	2
Red Velvet Munchkin, 1	2
Sugared Munchkin, 1	2
Toasted Coconut Munchkin, 1	4

Other Baked Goods

	SmartPoints® value
Apple Cheese Danish, 1	17
Apple Fritter, 1	17
Biscuit, 1	12
Blueberry Coffee Cake, 1 serving	8
Brownie, 1	20
Cheese Danish, 1	18
Chocolate Chip Coffee Cake, 1 serving	10
Chocolate Frosted Coffee Roll, 1	16
Cocoa Coffee Roll, 1	12
Coffee Roll, 1	15
Double Cocoa Coffee Roll, 1	13
Double Cocoa Fritter, 1	18
Eclair, 1	16
English Muffin, 1	4
Flatbread, 1 serving	5
French Cruller, 1	11
French Roll, 1 serving	7
Glazed Fritter, 1	17
Maple Frosted Coffee Roll, 1	16
Oatmeal Raisin Cookie, 1	10
Original Coffee Cake, 1 serving	10
Plain Croissant, 1	13
Reverse Chocolate Chunk Cookie, 1	16
Strawberry Cheese Danish, 1	17
Triple Chocolate Chunk Cookie, 1	16
Vanilla Cocoa Fritter, 1	19
Vanilla Frosted Coffee Roll, 1	16

Sandwiches and Sides

Bacon Ranch Chicken Sandwich, 1	20
BBQ Chicken Sandwich, 1	18
Chicken Salad on a Croissant, 1	20
Chicken Salad Wrap, 1	16
Chicken, Bacon, and Cheese on a Croissant, 1	24
Hash Browns, 6	4
Roast Beef on a French Roll, 1	13
Snack N' Go Chicken Wrap, 1 serving	10
Texas Toast Grilled Cheese, 1	17
Tuna Melt on a Croissant, 1	22
Tuna Salad Sandwich on a Plain Bagel, 1	17
Tuna Salad Sandwich on an English Muffin, 1	12
Tuna Salad Wrap, 1	16
Turkey Cheddar Bacon on a French Roll, 1	14

	SmartPoints® value

Breakfast

Bacon, Egg, and Cheese on a Plain Bagel, 1	14
Bacon, Egg, and Cheese on Biscuit, 1	17
Bacon, Egg, and Cheese on Croissant, 1	17
Bacon, Egg, and Cheese on English Muffin, 1	9
Bacon, Egg, and Cheese Wake Up Wrap, 1	6
Big n Toasted, 1	18
Brown Sugar Flavored Oatmeal with Dried Fruit Topping, 1 serving	12
Chicken Biscuit, 1	18
Egg and Cheese on a Plain Bagel, 1	12
Egg and Cheese on Biscuit, 1	15
Egg and Cheese on Croissant, 1	16
Egg and Cheese on English Muffin, 1	7
Egg and Cheese Wake Up Wrap, 1	5
Egg White Turkey Sausage Wake Up Wrap, 1	5
Egg White Veggie Flatbread, 1	10
Egg White Veggie Wake Up Wrap, 1	6
Glazed Donut Breakfast Sandwich, 1	13
Ham and Cheese on a French Roll, 1	13
Ham, Egg, and Cheese on a Plain Bagel, 1	13
Ham, Egg, and Cheese on Biscuit, 1	16
Ham, Egg, and Cheese on Croissant, 1	16
Ham, Egg, and Cheese on English Muffin, 1	8
Ham, Egg, and Cheese Wake Up Wrap, 1	5
Hot and Spicy Wake Up Wrap, 1	6
Original Oatmeal with Dried Fruit Topping, 1 serving	10
Sausage Biscuit, 1	20
Sausage, Egg, and Cheese on a Plain Bagel, 1	20
Sausage, Egg, and Cheese on Biscuit, 1	23
Sausage, Egg, and Cheese on Croissant, 1	23
Sausage, Egg, and Cheese on English Muffin, 1	15
Sausage, Egg, and Cheese Wake Up Wrap, 1	9
Smoked Sausage Breakfast Sandwich, 1	19
Sweet Black Pepper Bacon Wake Up Wrap, 1 serving	7
Turkey Sausage Breakfast Sandwich, 1	11
Turkey Sausage Flatbread Sandwich, 1	13
Turkey Sausage Wake Up Wrap, 1 serving	8

Bagels

Blueberry Bagel, 1	12
Cheddar Cheese Bagel Twist, 1	12
Chocolate Chip Bagel, 1	11
Chocolate Chip Bagel Twist, 1	12
Cinnamon Raisin Bagel, 1	10
Cinnamon Raisin Bagel Twist, 1	12
Everything Bagel, 1	10
Garlic Bagel, 1	10
Multigrain Bagel, 1	10
Onion Bagel, 1	9
Plain Bagel, 1	9
Poppy Seed Bagel, 1	10
Pretzel Salt Bagel, 1	9
Sesame Seed Bagel, 1	11
Sour Cream and Onion Bagel, 1	10
Whole Wheat Bagel, 1	10

"We Like This!" item

	SmartPoints® value
Spreads	
Plain Cream Cheese, 1 serving	7
Reduced Fat Blueberry Cream Cheese Spread, 1 serving	7
Reduced Fat Onion and Chive Cream Cheese Spread, 1 serving	6
Reduced Fat Plain Cream Cheese, 1 serving	4
Reduced Fat Smoked Salmon Cream Cheese Spread, 1 serving	6
Reduced Fat Strawberry Cream Cheese Spread, 1 serving	7
Reduced Fat Veggie Cream Cheese Spread, 1 serving	5
Coffee	
Blueberry Coffee, 1 small	0
Butter Pecan Coffee, 1 small	6
Butter Pecan Coffee with Cream, 1 small	9
Butter Pecan Iced Coffee, 1 small	6
Butter Pecan Iced Coffee with Cream, 1 small	9
Caramel Coffee, 1 small	0
Caramel Mocha Coffee, 1 small	6
Caramel Mocha Coffee with Cream, 1 small	9
Caramel Mocha Iced Coffee, 1 small	6
Caramel Mocha Iced Coffee with Cream, 1 small	9
Caramel Swirl Coffee with Cream, 1 small	9
Caramel Swirl Iced Coffee, 1 small	6
Caramel Swirl Iced Coffee with Cream, 1 small	9
Coconut Coffee, 1 small	0
Coffee, 1 small	0
Coffee with Cream, 1 small	3
Coffee with Cream and Sugar, 1 small	7
Coffee with Milk, 1 small	1
Coffee with Milk and Sugar, 1 small	5

	SmartPoints® value
Coffee with Skim Milk, 1 small	1
Coffee with Skim Milk and Splenda, 1 small	1
Coffee with Skim Milk and Sugar, 1 small	4
Coffee with Splenda, 1 medium	1
Coffee with Sugar, 1 small	4
Cookie Dough Swirl Hot Coffee, 1 small	6
Cookie Dough Swirl Hot Coffee with Cream, 1 small	9
Cookie Dough Swirl Iced Coffee, 1 small	6
Cookie Dough Swirl Iced Coffee with Cream, 1 small	9
French Vanilla Coffee, 1 small	0
French Vanilla Swirl Iced Coffee, 1 small	6
French Vanilla Swirl Iced Coffee with Cream, 1 small	9
Hazelnut Coffee, 1 small	0
Hazelnut Swirl Iced Coffee, 1 small	6
Hazelnut Swirl Iced Coffee with Cream, 1 small	9
Iced Coffee, 1 small	0
Iced Coffee with Almond Milk, 1 small	1
Iced Coffee with Cream, 1 small	3
Iced Coffee with Cream and Sugar, 1 small	7
Iced Coffee with Milk, 1 small	1
Iced Coffee with Milk and Sugar, 1 small	5
Iced Coffee with Skim Milk, 1 small	1
Iced Coffee with Skim Milk and Splenda, 1 small	1
Iced Coffee with Skim Milk and Sugar, 1 small	5
Iced Coffee with Sugar, 1 small	4
Iced Dunkin Dark Roast Coffee with Cream and Sugar, 1 small	7
Iced Dunkin Dark Roast Coffee with Skim Milk and Splenda, 1 small	1

Coffee (cont'd)

	SmartPoints® value
Irish Cream Iced Coffee, 1 small	6
Irish Creme Coffee, 1 small	6
Irish Creme Coffee with Cream, 1 small	9
Irish Creme Iced Coffee with Cream, 1 small	9
Mint Chocolate Chip Coffee, 1 small	6
Mint Chocolate Chip Coffee with Cream, 1 small	9
Mint Chocolate Chip Iced Coffee, 1 small	6
Mint Chocolate Chip Iced Coffee with Cream, 1 small	9
Mocha Coffee, 1 small	6
Mocha Swirl Coffee, 1 small	6
Mocha Swirl Coffee with Cream, 1 small	9
Mocha Swirl Iced Coffee with Cream, 1 small	9
Pistachio Swirl Hot Coffee, 1 small	6
Pistachio Swirl Hot Coffee with Cream, 1 small	9
Pistachio Swirl Iced Coffee, 1 small	6
Pistachio Swirl Iced Coffee with Cream, 1 small	9
Raspberry Coffee, 1 small	0
Toasted Almond Coffee, 1 small	0

Cappuccino, Macchiato, Espresso, & Latte

	SmartPoints® value
Butter Pecan Iced Latte with Milk, 1 small	12
Butter Pecan Iced Latte with Skim Milk, 1 small	9
Butter Pecan Latte with Milk, 1 small	12
Butter Pecan Latte with Skim Milk, 1 small	9
Butter Pecan Swirl Hot Macchiato with Skim Milk, 10 fl oz	9
Butter Pecan Swirl Hot Macchiato with Whole Milk, 10 fl oz	9
Butter Pecan Swirl Iced Macchiato with Skim Milk, 1 small	8
Butter Pecan Swirl Iced Macchiato with Whole Milk, 1 small	9
Cappuccino, 1 small	4
Cappuccino with Sugar, 1 small	7
Caramel Latte Lite, 1 small	3
Caramel Mocha Latte with Milk, 1 small	11
Caramel Mocha Latte with Skim Milk, 1 small	9
Caramel Swirl Hot Macchiato with Skim Milk, 10 fl oz	8
Caramel Swirl Hot Macchiato with Whole Milk, 10 fl oz	10
Caramel Swirl Iced Macchiato with Skim Milk, 1 small	8
Caramel Swirl Iced Macchiato with Whole Milk, 1 small	10
Caramel Swirl Latte with Skim Milk, 1 small	9
Cookie Dough Swirl Hot Latte with Skim Milk, 1 small	9
Cookie Dough Swirl Hot Latte with Whole Milk, 1 small	12
Cookie Dough Swirl Hot Macchiato with Skim Milk, 10 fl oz	8
Cookie Dough Swirl Hot Macchiato with Whole Milk, 10 fl oz	10
Cookie Dough Swirl Iced Latte with Skim Milk, 1 small	9
Cookie Dough Swirl Iced Latte with Whole Milk, 1 small	12
Cookie Dough Swirl Iced Macchiato with Skim Milk, 1 small	8
Cookie Dough Swirl Iced Macchiato with Whole Milk, 1 small	10
Espresso, 1 small	0
Espresso with Sugar, 1 small	2
French Vanilla Swirl Hot Macchiato with Skim Milk, 10 fl oz	9
French Vanilla Swirl Hot Macchiato with Whole Milk, 10 fl oz	11
French Vanilla Swirl Iced Macchiato with Skim Milk, 1 small	8

"We Like This!" item

	SmartPoints® value
French Vanilla Swirl Iced Macchiato with Whole Milk, 1 small	10
Hazelnut Swirl Hot Macchiato with Skim Milk, 10 fl oz	9
Hazelnut Swirl Hot Macchiato with Whole Milk, 10 fl oz	11
Hazelnut Swirl Iced Macchiato with Skim Milk, 1 small	8
Hazelnut Swirl Iced Macchiato with Whole Milk, 1 small	10
Hot Macchiato with Skim Milk, 10 fl oz	2
Hot Macchiato with Whole Milk, 10 fl oz	4
Iced Caramel Latte Lite, 1 small	3
Iced Caramel Mocha Latte with Milk, 1 small	11
Iced Caramel Mocha Latte with Skim Milk, 1 small	13
Iced Caramel Swirl Latte with Milk, 1 small	17
Iced Caramel Swirl Latte with Skim Milk, 1 small	9
Iced Latte, 1 small	5
Iced Latte Lite, 1 small	3
Iced Latte with Skim Milk, 1 small	3
Iced Latte with Skim Milk and Sugar, 1 small	7
Iced Latte with Sugar, 1 small	9
Iced Macchiato with Skim Milk, 1 small	2
Iced Macchiato with Whole Milk, 1 small	4
Iced Mocha Swirl Latte with Milk, 1 small	11
Iced Vanilla Latte Lite, 1 small	3
Irish Creme Iced Latte with Milk, 1 small	12
Irish Creme Iced Latte with Skim Milk, 1 small	9
Irish Creme Latte with Milk, 1 small	12
Irish Creme Latte with Skim Milk, 1 small	9
Latte, 1 small	5

	SmartPoints® value
Latte Lite, 1 small	3
Latte with Skim Milk and Sugar, 1 small	7
Latte with Sugar, 1 small	9
Mint Chocolate Chip Iced Latte with Milk, 1 small	12
Mint Chocolate Chip Iced Latte with Skim Milk, 1 small	9
Mint Chocolate Chip Latte with Milk, 1 small	12
Mint Chocolate Chip Latte with Skim Milk, 1 small	9
Mocha Swirl Hot Macchiato with Skim Milk, 10 fl oz	8
Mocha Swirl Hot Macchiato with Whole Milk, 10 fl oz	9
Mocha Swirl Iced Latte with Skim Milk, 1 small	9
Mocha Swirl Iced Macchiato with Skim Milk, 1 small	8
Mocha Swirl Iced Macchiato with Whole Milk, 1 small	9
Mocha Swirl Latte, 1 small	11
Mocha Swirl Latte with Milk, 1 small	11
Mocha Swirl Latte with Skim Milk, 1 small	9
Pistachio Swirl Hot Latte with Skim Milk, 1 small	9
Pistachio Swirl Hot Latte with Whole Milk, 1 small	12
Pistachio Swirl Hot Macchiato with Skim Milk, 10 fl oz	8
Pistachio Swirl Hot Macchiato with Whole Milk, 10 fl oz	10
Pistachio Swirl Iced Latte with Skim Milk, 1 small	9
Pistachio Swirl Iced Latte with Whole Milk, 1 small	12
Pistachio Swirl Iced Macchiato with Skim Milk, 1 small	8
Pistachio Swirl Iced Macchiato with Whole Milk, 1 small	10
Vanilla Latte Lite, 1 small	3

Coolatta	SmartPoints® value
Berry Blast Coolatta, 1 small	10
Blue Raspberry Coolatta, 1 small	15
Cherry Coolatta, 1 small	15
Frozen Butter Pecan Coffee Coolatta with Cream, 1 small	26
Frozen Butter Pecan Coffee Coolatta with Milk, 1 small	19
Frozen Butter Pecan Coffee Coolatta with Skim Milk, 1 small	17
Frozen Caramel Coffee Coolatta with Cream, 1 small	26
Frozen Caramel Coffee Coolatta with Milk, 1 small	19
Frozen Caramel Coffee Coolatta with Skim Milk, 1 small	17
Frozen Coffee Coolatta with Cream, 1 small	21
Frozen Coffee Coolatta with Milk, 1 small	14
Frozen Coffee Coolatta with Skim Milk, 1 small	12
Frozen Cookie Dough Swirl Coffee Coolatta with Cream, 1 small	26
Frozen Cookie Dough Swirl Coffee Coolatta with Skim Milk, 1 small	17
Frozen Cookie Dough Swirl Coffee Coolatta with Whole Milk, 1 small	19
Frozen French Vanilla Swirl Coffee Coolatta with Cream, 1 small	26
Frozen French Vanilla Swirl Coffee Coolatta with Skim Milk, 1 small	17
Frozen French Vanilla Swirl Coffee Coolatta with Whole Milk, 1 small	19
Frozen Hazelnut Swirl Coffee Coolatta with Cream, 1 small	26
Frozen Hazelnut Swirl Coffee Coolatta with Skim Milk, 1 small	17
Frozen Hazelnut Swirl Coffee Coolatta with Whole Milk, 1 small	19
Frozen Irish Creme Coffee Coolatta with Cream, 1 small	29
Frozen Irish Creme Coffee Coolatta with Milk, 1 small	22
Frozen Irish Creme Coffee Coolatta with Skim Milk, 1 small	20
Frozen Lemonade Coolatta, 1 small	15
Frozen Mint Chocolate Chip Coffee Coolatta with Cream, 1 small	29
Frozen Mint Chocolate Chip Coffee Coolatta with Milk, 1 small	21
Frozen Mint Chocolate Chip Coffee Coolatta with Skim Milk, 1 small	20
Frozen Mocha Coffee Coolatta with Cream, 1 small	26
Frozen Mocha Coffee Coolatta with Milk, 1 small	18
Frozen Mocha Coffee Coolatta with Skim Milk, 1 small	17
Frozen Pistachio Swirl Coffee Coolatta with Cream, 1 small	26
Frozen Pistachio Swirl Coffee Coolatta with Skim Milk, 1 small	17
Frozen Pistachio Swirl Coffee Coolatta with Whole Milk, 1 small	19
Fruit Punch Coolatta, 1 small	15
Minute Maid Orange Coolatta, 1 small	13
Oreo Coffee Coolatta with Cream, 1 small	24
Oreo Coffee Coolatta with Milk, 1 small	17
Oreo Coffee Coolatta with Skim Milk, 1 small	15
Oreo Vanilla Bean Coolatta, 1 small	23
Raspberry Lime Coolatta, 1 small	15
Strawberry Fruit Coolatta, 1 small	15
Strawberry Lemonade Coolatta, 1 small	15
Vanilla Bean Coolatta, 1 small	24

Dunkaccino	SmartPoints® value
Dunkaccino, 1 small	12
Frozen Dunkaccino, 1 small	22

"We Like This!" item

	SmartPoints® value
Hot Chocolate	
Hot Chocolate, 1 small	12
Hot Chocolate Frozen, 1 small	22
Mint Hot Chocolate, 1 small	11
Mint Hot Chocolate Frozen, 1 small	22
S'mores Hot Chocolate, 1 small	12
S'mores Hot Chocolate Frozen, 1 small	22
Salted Caramel Hot Chocolate, 1 small	12
Salted Caramel Hot Chocolate Frozen, 1 small	22
Turbo Hot Chocolate, 1 small	12
Turbo Shot	
Turbo Shot, 1 small	0
Tea	
Black Tea with Milk, 1 small	1
Black Tea with Milk and Sugar, 1 small	5
Black Tea with Skim Milk, 1 small	0
Black Tea with Skim Milk and Sugar, 1 small	4
Black Tea with Sugar, 1 small	4
Decaffeinated Tea, 1 small	0
Decaffeinated Tea with Milk, 1 small	1
Decaffeinated Tea with Milk and Sugar, 1 small	5
Decaffeinated Tea with Skim Milk, 1 small	0
Decaffeinated Tea with Skim Milk and Sugar, 1 small	4
Decaffeinated Tea with Sugar, 1 small	4
Earl Grey Tea, 1 small	0
Earl Grey Tea with Milk, 1 small	1
Earl Grey Tea with Milk and Sugar, 1 small	5
Earl Grey Tea with Skim Milk, 1 small	0
Earl Grey Tea with Skim Milk and Sugar, 1 small	4

	SmartPoints® value
Earl Grey Tea with Sugar, 1 small	4
English Breakfast Tea, 1 small	0
English Breakfast Tea with Milk, 1 small	1
English Breakfast Tea with Milk and Sugar, 1 small	5
English Breakfast Tea with Skim Milk, 1 small	0
English Breakfast Tea with Skim Milk and Sugar, 1 small	4
English Breakfast Tea with Sugar, 1 small	4
Freshly Brewed Sweetened Iced Tea, 1 small	4
Freshly Brewed Unsweetened Iced Tea, 1 small	0
Frozen Vanilla Chai, 1 small	22
Green Tea, 1 small	0
Green Tea with Milk, 1 small	1
Green Tea with Milk and Sugar, 1 small	5
Green Tea with Skim Milk, 1 small	0
Green Tea with Skim Milk and Sugar, 1 small	4
Green Tea with Sugar, 1 small	4
Peach Flavored Iced Tea, 1 small	0
Peach Flavored Sweetened Iced Tea, 1 small	4
Raspberry Flavored Iced Tea, 1 small	0
Raspberry Flavored Sweetened Iced Tea, 1 small	4
Sweet Tea, 1 small	10
Smoothies	
Strawberry Banana Smoothie, 1 small	15
Tropical Mango Smoothie, 1 small	16
Apple Cider	
Apple Cider, 1 small	7
Iced Apple Cider, 1 small	7

Bagels

	SmartPoints® value
9-Grain Bagel, 1	9
Asiago Cheese Bagel, 1	9
Black Russian Bagel, 1	8
Blueberry Bagel, 1	9
Chocolate Chip Bagel, 1	9
Cinnamon Raisin Bagel, 1	9
Cinnamon Sugar Bagel, 1	10
Cranberry Bagel, 1	9
Dutch Apple Bagel, 1	12
Egg Bagel, 1	9
Everything Bagel Thin Singles, 1	5
Everything Classic Bagel, 1	8
Garlic Bagel, 1	8
Good Grains Bagel, 1	8
Green Chile Bagel, 1	11
Honey Whole Wheat Bagel Thin Singles, 1	4
Honey Whole Wheat Classic Bagel, 1	8
Onion Bagel, 1	8
Plain Bagel Thin Singles, 1	4
Plain Classic Bagel, 1	8
Poppy Bagel, 1	8
Potato Bagel, 1	8
Power Bagel, 1	10
Power Protein Bagel, 1	9
Pumpernickel Classic Bagel, 1	7
Salt Bagel, 1	8
Sesame Bagel, 1	8
Six-Cheese Bagel, 1	10
Spinach Florentine Bagel, 1	11

Spreads

	SmartPoints® value
Blueberry Reduced Fat Schmear, 1 serving	6
Butter Blend, 1 serving	7
Creamy Mustard Spread, 1 serving	3
Creamy Peanut Butter, 1 serving	11
Garden Vegetable Reduced Fat Schmear, 1 serving	5
Garlic Herb Reduced Fat Schmear, 1 serving	5
Honey Almond Reduced Fat Schmear, 1 serving	6
Honey Butter, 1 serving	6
Hummus, 1 serving	2
Jalapeño Salsa Reduced Fat Schmear, 1 serving	5
Onion and Chive Schmear, 1 serving	6
Plain Reduced Fat Schmear, 1 serving	5
Plain Schmear, 1 serving	6
Plain Whipped Light Cream Cheese Shmear, 1 serving	3
Smoked Salmon Schmear, 1 serving	5
Spicy Roasted Tomato Spread, 1 serving	7
Strawberry Reduced Fat Schmear, 1 serving	6
Sundried Tomato Basil Reduced Fat Schmear, 1 serving	5
Sweet Cream Cheese, 1 serving	17

"We Like This!" item

Muffins

	SmartPoints® value
Banana Nut Muffin, 1	19
Blueberry Muffin, 1	16
Blueberry Muffin Poppers, 1 serving	41
Chocolate Chip Muffin, 1	17

Other Breads

	SmartPoints® value
Challah Roll, 1	8
Ciabatta Bread, 1 serving	7

Sandwiches

	SmartPoints® value
Albacore Tuna Salad Deli Sandwich, 1	11
Asiago Hebrew National Bagel Dog, 1	19
Asparagus, Mushroom & Swiss Bagel Thin Sandwich, 1	8
Bacon & Cheddar Egg Sandwich, 1	16

Item	SmartPoints® value
Bagel Thin Club, 1	9
BLT with Avocado Bagel Thin Sandwich, 1	13
Chicken & Mozzarella Sandwich, 1	15
Chicken and Cheddar Bagel Wrapper, 1 serving	7
Chicken Mozzarella for Open Face Deli, 1 serving	15
Chicken Salad Deli Sandwich, 1	14
Club Mex on Challah Sandwich, 1	15
Deli Ham Sandwich, 1	11
Double Double Egg Sandwich, 1	24
Egg Mixture Sandwich, 1	4
Ham & Swiss Bagel Melt, 1	15
Ham & Swiss Egg Sandwich, 1	14
Ham & Swiss for Open Face Deli, 1 serving	13
Ham Sandwich, 1	16
Nova Lox & Bagel, 1	16
Original Hebrew National Bagel Dog, 1	18
Roasted Turkey Sandwich, 1	10
Southwest Turkey Sausage Egg Sandwich, 1	11
Spinach, Mushroom & Swiss Egg Sandwich, 1	15
Tasty Turkey on Asiago Bagel, 1	17
Tuna Bagel Thin Sandwich, 1	8
Turkey & Cheddar Sandwich, 1	14
Turkey Bagel Thin Sandwich, 1	7
Turkey BAT Sandwich, 1	18
Turkey Breast Sandwich, 1	13
Turkey Club Sandwich, 1	18
Turkey Sausage & Cheddar Egg Sandwich, 1	16
Turkey Sausage with Salsa Bagel Thin Sandwich, 1	6
Tuscan Chicken Pesto Sandwich, 1	10
Veg Out on Sesame Seed Bagel, 1	16

Pizza Bagel

Pepperoni Pizza Bagel, 1	14

Wraps & Paninis

Bacon & Cheese Bagel Thin Panini, 1	12
Bacon & Cheese Egg White Panini, 1	10
BBQ Chicken Artisan Panini, 1	24
Buffalo Chicken Wrap, 1	20
California Chicken Wrap, 1	21
Chicken Caesar Wrap, 1	19
Chicken Cuban Panini, 1	20
Chicken Salad Wrap, 1	13
Chipotle Turkey Wrap, 1	20
Club Mex Wrap, 1	17
Green Chile & Turkey Sausage Panini, 1	19
Italian Chicken Panini, 1	20
Santa Fe Breakfast Wrap, 1	21
Spicy Elmo Breakfast Wrap, 1	21
Spinach & Bacon Egg Panini, 1	23
Turkey Club Panini, 1	23
Turkey Tornado Wrap, 1	9

Condiments

Ancho Lime Salsa, 1 serving	0
Ancho Mayo, 1 serving	11
Deli Mustard, 1 serving	0
Whole Kosher Pickle, 1	0
Yellow Mustard, 1 serving	0

Soups and Salads

Albacore Tuna Salad, 1 serving	11
Bagel Croutons, 1 serving	3
Broccoli Cheese Soup, 1 bowl	18
Broccoli Cheese Soup, 1 cup	11
Bros Bistro Salad, 1	30
Bros Bistro Salad with Chicken, 1 serving	32
Caesar Salad, 1 serving	21
Caesar Salad with Chicken, 1 serving	22
Caesar Salad with Chicken, Half, 1 serving	11
Caesar Salad, Half, 1 serving	10

	SmartPoints® value
Chicken Caesar Salad, Full, 1 serving	8
Chicken Caesar Salad, Half, 1 serving	7
Chicken Noodle Soup, 14 oz	5
Chicken Noodle Soup, 8 oz	3
Chicken Salad, 1 serving	12
Chipotle Chicken Salad, Full, 1 serving	6
Chipotle Chicken Salad, Half, 1 serving	5
Chipotle Salad, 1 serving	18
Chipotle Salad with Chicken, 1 serving	20
Chipotle Salad with Chicken, Half, 1 serving	10
Chipotle Salad, Half, 1 serving	9
Deluxe Chef Salad, 1 serving	17
Garden Salad, 1 serving	8
Half Bros Bistro Salad, 1 serving	15
Half Bros Bistro Salad with Chicken, 1 serving	16
Potato Salad, 1 serving	6
Southwest Veggie with Quinoa Soup, 14 oz	11
Southwest Veggie with Quinoa Soup, 8 oz	7
Strawberry Chicken Salad, Full, 1 serving	12
Strawberry Chicken Salad, Half, 1 serving	9
Turkey Chili Soup, 8 oz	5

Dressings

Caesar Dressing, 1 serving	15
Chipotle Vinaigrette, 1 serving	11
Raspberry Vinaigrette, 1 serving	17

Eggs

Egg Mixture, 1 serving	6
Egg White Only, 2 oz	0
Egg White Only, 4 oz	1

"We Like This!" item

SmartPoints® value

Cappuccino & Macchiato

Cappuccino (nonfat milk), 12 fl oz	2
Cappuccino (reduced fat milk), 12 fl oz	4
Cappuccino (whole milk), 12 fl oz	5
Caramel, Macchiato (nonfat milk), 12 fl oz	10
Caramel, Macchiato (reduced fat milk), 12 fl oz	12
Caramel, Macchiato (whole milk), 12 fl oz	13
Iced Caramel Macchiato (nonfat milk), 16 fl oz	17
Iced Caramel Macchiato (reduced fat milk), 16 fl oz	19
Iced Caramel Macchiato (whole milk), 16 fl oz	21

Latte

Cafe Latte (nonfat milk), 12 fl oz	3
Cafe Latte (reduced fat milk), 12 fl oz	5
Cafe Latte (whole milk), 12 fl oz	6
Chai Tea Latte (nonfat milk), 12 fl oz	6
Chai Tea Latte (reduced fat milk), 12 fl oz	8
Chai Tea Latte (whole milk), 12 fl oz	9
Frozen Caramel Latte, 18 fl oz	21
Frozen Vanilla Hazelnut Latte, 18 fl oz	17
Iced Latte (nonfat milk), 16 fl oz	3
Iced Latte (reduced fat milk), 16 fl oz	6
Iced Latte (whole milk), 16 fl oz	7
Iced Sugar Free Vanilla Hazelnut Latte, 16 fl oz	6
Iced Sugar Free Vanilla Latte, 16 fl oz	6
Iced Vanilla Hazelnut Latte (nonfat milk), 16 fl oz	11
Iced Vanilla Hazelnut Latte (reduced fat milk), 16 fl oz	13
Iced Vanilla Hazelnut Latte (whole milk), 16 fl oz	14
Iced Vanilla Latte, 16 fl oz	17

	SmartPoints® value
Soy Latte, 12 fl oz	2
Sugar Free Vanilla Hazelnut Latte, 12 fl oz	5
Sugar Free Vanilla Latte, 12 fl oz	5
Vanilla Hazelnut Latte, 12 fl oz	10
Vanilla Latte, 12 fl oz	8

Hot Chocolate & Mochas

Cafe Mocha, 12 fl oz	11
Dark Chocolate Mocha (nonfat milk), 12 fl oz	15
Dark Chocolate Mocha (reduced fat milk), 12 fl oz	16
Dark Chocolate Mocha (whole milk), 12 fl oz	18
Hot Chocolate (nonfat milk), 12 fl oz	15
Hot Chocolate (reduced fat milk), 12 fl oz	16
Hot Chocolate (whole milk), 12 fl oz	18
Hot Dark Chocolate, 12 fl oz	16
Iced Dark Chocolate Mocha (nonfat milk), 16 fl oz	23
Iced Dark Chocolate Mocha (reduced fat milk), 16 fl oz	25
Iced Dark Chocolate Mocha (whole milk), 16 fl oz	26
Iced White Chocolate Mocha (nonfat milk), 16 fl oz	20
Iced White Chocolate Mocha (reduced fat milk), 16 fl oz	21
Iced White Chocolate Mocha (whole milk), 16 fl oz	23
White Chocolate Mocha (nonfat milk), 12 fl oz	19
White Chocolate Mocha (reduced fat milk), 12 fl oz	16
White Chocolate Mocha (whole milk), 12 fl oz	22
White Hot Chocolate, 12 fl oz	16

Tea

Green Tea, 16 fl oz	3

Smoothies & Juices

	SmartPoints® value
Blackberry Lemonade, 16 fl oz	16
Lemonade, 16 fl oz	9
Mixed Berry Smoothie, 1 serving	18
Orange Juice, 16 fl oz	12
Strawberry Banana Smoothie, 1 serving	16
Strawberry Frozen Blended Drink, 18 fl oz	25

Desserts

Apple Cinnamon Coffee Cake, 1 serving	30
Blueberry Scone, 1	23
Brownie, 1	14
Candied Walnuts, 1 serving	8
Cherry Pastry, 1	15
Chocolate Chip Coffee Cake, 1 serving	35
Chocolate Chip Cookie, 1	16
Chocolate Chunk Cookie, 1	18
Chocolate Chunk Cookie Bites, 1 serving	44
Chocolate Mudslide Cookie, 1	16
Cinnamon Chip Scone, 1	26
Cinnamon Sugar Popper, 1	15
Cinnamon Twist, 1	15
Cinnamon Walnut Strudel, 1	26
Fruit and Yogurt Parfait, 1 serving	7
Fruit Cup, 1 serving	0
Iced Popper, 1	18
Iced Sugar Cookie, 1	25
Low Fat Yogurt Parfait, 1 serving	8
Marshmallow Crispy Treat, 1 serving	17
Mixed Berry Coffee Cake, 1 serving	31
Oatmeal Raisin Cookie, 1	14
Snickerdoodle Cookie, 1	18
Wildberry Yogurt, 18 fl oz	14
Wildberry Yogurt, 24 floz	21

Beef Entrées

	SmartPoints® value
Asian Beef, 1 cup	8
Baby Back Ribs, piece	6
Bacon Wrapped Sirloin, 1 serving	5
BBQ Beef, 1 serving	2
Beef Enchiladas, 1	6
Beef Italian Meatballs, 2 pieces	8
Beef Pot Pie, 1 serving	6
Beef Pot Roast, ½ cup	4
Beef Quesadilla, 1	5
Creamed Chipped Beef, ½ cup	5
Fajita Steak, 3 oz	3
Grilled Chopped Steak, 1 serving	9
Grilled Corned Beef Hash, ½ cup	7
London Broil Beef, 1 serving	3
Macaroni and Beef Casserole, ½ cup	4
Machaca Beef, 3 oz	4
Marinated Beef Tips, 3 oz	3
Marinated Sirloin Beef Tips, 1 serving	4
Meatloaf, 1 serving	7
Mini Hot Dogs, 1	6
Mongolian Beef, 1 cup	9
Oriental Pepper Beef, 1 cup	9
Salisbury Steak, 1 serving	6
Sirloin, 3 oz	3
Sirloin Steak Strips, 3 oz	3
Smoked Beef Brisket, 3 oz	7
Smothered Chopped Steaks, 1	9
Teriyaki Beef, 1 cup	8

Turkey Entrées

	SmartPoints® value
Carved Turkey Breast, 1 serving	2
Turkey Breast with Wing, 3 oz	1
Turkey Slices with Poultry Gravy, 1 serving	2
Whole Carved Turkey (dark meat with skin), 3 oz	4
Whole Carved Turkey (white meat with skin), 3 oz	3

Seafood and Chicken Entrées

	SmartPoints® value
Baked Fish, 1	3
Baked Fish with Shrimp and Lemon Herb Sauce, 3 oz	4
Baked Florentine Fish, 1 serving	5
Baked New Orleans Style Fish, 1 serving	2
BBQ Chicken (leg quarter), 1 piece	15
Bone-In Catfish, 3 oz	6
Bourbon Street Chicken, 3 oz	4
Bourbon Street Chicken Wings, 3 wings	6
Breaded Bay Scallops, 10 pieces	4
Breaded Catfish, 2 pieces	5
Breaded Fried Fish, piece	2
Buffalo Chicken Tenders, 1 serving	4
Buffalo Shrimp, 6 pieces	6
Chicken Breast Strips, 3 oz	1
Chicken Enchiladas, 1	6
Chicken Fried Steak, 1 serving	6
Chicken Parmesan, 1 serving	7
Chicken Pastry Noodles, ½ cup	3
Chicken Piccata, 1 serving	6
Chicken Pot Pie (scratch), 1 serving	5
Chicken Quesadilla, 1 serving	4
Chicken Tenders, 1	4
Chicken Wings, 3 wings	6
Clam Strips, 10 pieces	5
Cold Shrimp, ¼ cup	1
Crab Cakes, 1	6
Fajita Chicken, 3 oz	2
Fish Piccata, 1	4
Fried Chicken - Piece Variety, 3 oz	6

"We Like This!" item

	SmartPoints® value
Fried Chicken Livers, 3 pieces	6
Fried Chicken Wings, 3 pieces	6
Golden Delicious Shrimp, 6 pieces	6
Grilled Chicken Breast, 1	1
Honey Sesame Chicken, 2 pieces	11
Jalapeño Glazed Tilapia, 1 serving	5
Machaca Chicken, 3 oz	3
Mini Chicken Pot Pie, 1 pie	14
Orange Chicken, 1 cup	14
Popcorn Shrimp, 15 pieces	4
Rotisserie Chicken (breast and wing), 1 serving	7
Salmon Lemonata, 3 oz	4
Seafood Newburg (½ cup with 1 pastry triangle), 1 serving	8
Spicy Sweet Pagoda Chicken, 1 cup	8
Sweet and Sour Chicken, 1 cup	8
Sweet and Sour Shrimp, 1 cup	9
Whole Carved Salmon, 3 oz	3

Pasta Entrées

Lasagna (scratch), 1 serving	15
Linguini with Lemon Butter Herb Sauce, 1 cup	9
Lo Mein, 1 cup	7
Macaroni and Cheese, ½ cup	6
Penne Pasta, 1 cup	6
Spaghetti Bake, ½ cup	5
Spaghetti Noodles, ½ cup	4
Steamed Linguini Pasta, 1 cup	8
Stir Fry Pagoda, 1 cup	5
Stir Fry Vegetables, ½ cup	2

Pork Entrées

	SmartPoints® value
BBQ Pork, 3 oz	5
BBQ Pork Ribs, 1 serving	6
Boneless BBQ Pork Ribs, 1 serving	4
Glazed Ham, 1 serving	4
Grilled Ham Steaks, 2 pieces	3
Ham Strips, 3 oz	3
Italian Roped Sausage, 3 oz	6
Mandarin Orange Pork, 1 cup	13
North Carolina BBQ Pork, 3 oz	4
Pork Fillet, piece	7
Pork Posole, 1 cup	4
Pork Ribs, 1 serving	5
Smoked Ham (Spiral Cut, Pit Style), 3 oz	3
Smoked Pork Sausage, piece	7
Southern Style Boneless Pork Chops, 3 oz	7
Spare BBQ Pork Ribs, piece	9
Spinach with Ham, ½ cup	1
Split Pork Sausage, 1	8
Sweet and Sour Pork, 1 cup	7

Sandwiches

BBQ Pork Sandwich, 1 serving	8
Buffalo Chicken Sandwich, 1	7
Chicken Bistro Melt, 1 serving	10
Ham and Cheese Bistro Melt, 1	11
Mini BBQ Brisket Sandwich, 1	5
Mini Chicken Sandwich, 1	6
Patty Melt, 1	13
Philly Steak Sandwich, 1	12
Steakburger Sandwich, 1	9
Turkey and Bacon Bistro Melt, 1 serving	9

Pizza

Cheese Pizza, 1 slice	6
Pepperoni Pizza, 1 slice	7
Sausage Pizza, 1 slice	8

Taco Bar

	SmartPoints® value
Flour Tortillas (scratch), 1	5
Salsa, 2 Tbsp	0
Shredded Lettuce, 1 cup	0
Sour Cream, 2 Tbsp	3
Taco Meat (scratch), ½ cup	4
Taco Shells, 1	2
Tamales, 1	4

Salad Bar

	SmartPoints® value
Artichoke Hearts, ¼ cup	0
Baby Corn, 5 pieces	0
Bacon Bits, 2 Tbsp	1
Beets, ¼ cup	0
Beets, Pickled, ¼ cup	0
Black Olives, 2 Tbsp	1
Blue Cheese Crumbles, 2 Tbsp	2
Broccoli Florets, ¼ cup	0
Celery Sticks, 1 serving	0
Cherry Tomatoes, 5 pieces	0
Chickpeas, ¼ cup	2
Cold Cherry Peppers, 3 pieces	0
Cold Green Peas, ½ cup	2
Cold Kidney Beans, ¼ cup	1
Cold Lima Beans, ¼ cup	2
Cold Pepperoncini, 3 pieces	0
Collard Greens, ½ cup	0
Cranberries, 2 Tbsp	3
Croutons, 2 Tbsp	1
Cucumbers, ¼ cup	0
Cut Kernel Corn, ½ cup	5
Diced Onions, ¼ cup	0
Diced Tomatoes, ¼ cup	0
Dill Spears Pickles, 1 serving	0
Dried Onions, 2 Tbsp	2
Escalloped Apples, ½ cup	7
Flame Broiled Mixed Vegetables, ½ cup	0
Fresh Onion Rings, 3 pieces	0
Garbanzo Beans, ¼ cup	2
Green Beans, ½ cup	1
Green Grapes, 10 pieces	0
Green Olives, 2 Tbsp	1
Green Pepper Rings, 3 pieces	0
Homemade Croutons, 5 pieces	4
Iceberg Lettuce, 1 cup	0
Julienne Carrots, ¼ cup	0
Machaca Beans, ½ cup	2
Onions and Peppers, ¼ cup	1
Oyster Crackers, 1 package	2
Pepperjack Cubes Cheese, 5 pieces	6
Pepperoni, 5 pieces	2
Pico de Gallo, ¼ cup	0
Pimento Cheese, ¼ cup	5
Pine Nuts, 2 Tbsp	4
Radishes, ¼ cup	0
Raisins, ¼ cup	3
Ranch Style Beans, ½ cup	4
Raw Baby Carrots, 5 pieces	1
Raw Cauliflower, ¼ cup	0
Raw Zucchini, 5 pieces	0
Roasted Peppers, ½ cup	3
Romaine Lettuce, 1 cup	0
Seasoned Black Eyed Peas, ½ cup	3
Seasoned Northern Beans, ½ cup	3
Seasoned Pinto Beans, ½ cup	3
Sesame Sticks, 2 Tbsp	4
Shredded Cheddar Cheese, 2 Tbsp	2
Shredded Parmesan, 2 Tbsp	2
Sliced Almonds, 2 Tbsp	2
Sliced Jalapeños, ¼ cup	0
Sliced Mushrooms, ¼ cup	0

"We Like This!" item

	SmartPoints® value
Southern Style Black Eyed Peas, ½ cup	6
Southern Style Lima Beans, ½ cup	5
Southern Style Northern Beans, ½ cup	5
Southern Style Pinto Beans, ½ cup	5
Soy Nuts, 2 Tbsp	1
Spinach, 1 cup	0
Spring Mix Lettuce, 1 cup	0
Steamed Broccoli, ½ cup	0
Steamed Cauliflower, ½ cup	0
Steamed Sauerkraut, 2 Tbsp	0
Sugar Snap Peas, ½ cup	3
Sunflower Seeds, 2 Tbsp	3
Sweet Chips Pickles, 8 pieces	0
Tomato Wedges, 5 pieces	0
Tomatoes and Okra, ½ cup	2
Wasabi Peas, 2 Tbsp	1
Water Chestnuts, ¼ cup	1
Yellow Squash, 5 pieces	0

Soups and Salads

Apple Salad, ½ cup	9
Asian Salad, 1 cup	3
Beet and Onion Salad, ½ cup	2
BLT Salad, 1 cup	3
Broccoli Cheese Soup, 1 cup	8
Broccoli Salad, ½ cup	4
Caesar Salad, 1 cup	4
Cajun Chicken Soup, 1 cup	2
Cajun Potato Salad, ½ cup	8
Carrot Raisin Salad, ½ cup	4
Chicken and Pasta Soup (scratch), 1 cup	3
Chicken Noodle Soup, 1 cup	2
Chicken Salad, ½ cup	7
Clam Chowder, 1 cup	6

	SmartPoints® value
Egg Salad, ½ cup	6
Green Chili Stew, 1 cup	7
Kidney Bean Salad, ½ cup	6
Macaroni Salad, ½ cup	10
Marinated Garden Salad, ½ cup	3
Marinated Mushroom Salad, ½ cup	3
Marinated Vegetable Salad, ½ cup	1
Pasta Salad, 1 cup	5
Pea Salad, ½ cup	8
Potato with Bacon Soup, 1 cup	7
Seafood Salad, ½ cup	5
Seven Seas Shrimp Salad, ½ cup	4
Southern Broccoli Salad, ½ cup	12
Southern Style Chicken Salad, ½ cup	9
Spinach Bacon Salad, 1 cup	4
Steakhouse Potato Salad, ½ cup	6
Strawberry Spinach Salad, 1 cup	1
Summer Marinated Salad, ½ cup	3
Three Bean Salad, ½ cup	4
Timberline Chili, 1 cup	7
Tomato and Onion Salad, ½ cup	1
Tuna Salad, ½ cup	5
Vegetable Beef Soup, 1 cup	2
White Bean and Ham Soup, 1 cup	5

Dressings and Sauces

Alfredo Sauce, ¼ cup	5
Asian Ginger Dressing, 2 Tbsp	5
Au Jus Gravy, 1 serving	1
Bacon Dressing, 2 Tbsp	6
Balsamic Vinaigrette Dressing, 2 Tbsp	1
Balsamic Vinegar, 2 Tbsp	1
BBQ Sauce, 2 Tbsp	2
Blue Cheese Dressing, 2 Tbsp	5

	SmartPoints® value
Brown Gravy, 2 oz	1
Brown Gravy with Mushrooms, 2 oz	1
Caesar Dressing, 2 Tbsp	5
Catalina Dressing, 2 Tbsp	5
Cheese Sauce, ¼ cup	3
Cocktail Sauce, 2 Tbsp	2
Cranberry Sauce, 2 Tbsp	3
Fat Free Catalina Dressing, 2 Tbsp	2
Fat Free Ranch Dressing, 2 Tbsp	2
Fat Free Thousand Island Dressing, 2 Tbsp	2
Honey Mustard Dressing, 2 Tbsp	5
Italian Red Sauce, ¼ cup	2
Lite Olive Oil Vinaigrette, 2 Tbsp	3
Olive Oil, 1 Tbsp	4
Poultry Gravy, 2 oz	1
Queso Cheese Sauce, ¼ cup	3
Ranch Dressing, 2 Tbsp	4
Red Wine Vinegar, 1 Tbsp	0
Salad Oil, 1 Tbsp	4
Sausage Gravy, 2 oz	2
Tartar Sauce, 2 Tbsp	5
Thousand Island Dressing, 2 Tbsp	5
White Gravy, 2 oz	2

Sides

	SmartPoints® value
Asian Green Beans, ½ cup	3
Asparagus, 5 pieces	0
Baked Potatoes, 1	5
Baked Sweet Potato, 1	4
Battered Onion Rings, 2	5
BBQ Baked Beans, ½ cup	7
Breaded Okra, 10 pieces	4
Broccoli & Rice Casserole, ½ cup	4
Broccoli Coleslaw, ½ cup	4
Broiled Corn on the Cob, piece	3
Broiled Pineapple, 1 slice	3
Bruschetta Bread, 1 serving	4
Brussels Sprouts in Sauce, ½ cup	4
Buffalo Wings, 1 serving	6
Cheese Enchiladas, 1	8
Coleslaw, ½ cup	4
Corn on the Cob, 1 serving	2
Country Breaded Wings, 1 serving	9
Creamed Corn, ½ cup	5
Creamed Spinach, ½ cup	6
Deviled Eggs, 1	2
French Fried Potatoes, 20 pieces	5
Fresh BBQ Potato Chips, 20 pieces	4
Fresh Potato Chips, 20 pieces	4
Fried Cubed Potatoes, ½ cup	5
Fried Green Tomatoes, 2 pieces	6
Garlic Cheese Breadsticks, 1	4
Garlic Parmesan Cheese Knots, 1	7
Green Bean Casserole, ½ cup	3
Grilled BBQ Wings, 1 serving	6
Guacamole, ¼ cup	2
Hand Breaded and Fried Mushrooms, 7 pieces	5
Homestyle Yeast Rolls, 1	6
Italian Vegetable Medley, ½ cup	3
Kettle Cooked Cabbage, ½ cup	2
Kettle Cooked Collards, ½ cup	3
Kettle Cooked Lima Beans, ½ cup	5
Kettle Cooked Turnip Greens, ½ cup	3
Marinated Asparagus, 5 pieces	0
Mashed Potatoes, ½ cup	5
Mexican Rice, ½ cup	5
Multigrain Rolls, 1	5
Pagoda Fried Rice, ½ cup	5
Piña Colada Dip, 2 Tbsp	3
Puff Pastry, 1	9

"We Like This!" item

⭘ No Count	SmartPoints® value
Red Beans and Rice, ½ cup	5
Red Bliss Potatoes, ½ cup	2
Refried Beans, ½ cup	6
Rice Noodles, 2 Tbsp	1
Rice Pilaf, ½ cup	4
Saltines, 1 package	1
Sautéed Mushrooms, ½ cup	2
Sautéed Spinach, ½ cup	4
Sautéed Zucchini, ½ cup	2
Scalloped Potatoes, ½ cup	6
Seasoned Potato Chips, 20 chips	4
Seasoned Wedge French Fries, 6 pieces	5
Skillet Cornbread, 1 serving	6
Smokey Cheese Potato Bake, ½ cup	5
Sourdough Rolls, 1	3
Spinach Artichoke Dip, ¼ cup	4
Spring Rolls, 1 serving	4
Squash Medley, ½ cup	6
Steak House Fries, 6 pieces	6
Steamed Baby Carrots, ½ cup	4
Steamed Baby Lima Beans, ½ cup	5
Steamed Brussel Sprouts, ½ cup	3
Steamed Green Beans, ½ cup	3
Steamed Green Peas, ½ cup	4
Stuffed Peppers, 1	6
Sweet Homestyle Cornbread Stuffing, ½ cup	4
Sweet Potato Casserole, ½ cup	9
Tempura Battered Onion Rings, 2 pieces	5
Tempura Battered Squash, 3 pieces	5
Tempura Battered Tilapia, 1 serving	6
Tempura Battered Zucchini, 3 pieces	5
Teriyaki Wings, 1 serving	6
Texas Toast, 1 serving	7
Tortilla Bowl, 1 serving	7
Tortilla Chips, 10 pieces	4
Turnip Greens, ½ cup	2
White Hominy, ½ cup	3
White Rice, ½ cup	4
Yellow Rice, ½ cup	4

Fresh Fruit

Bananas, 1	0
Blueberries, ¼ cup	1
Cantaloupe, ½ cup	0
Cut Apples, ¼ cup	0
Grapefruit, 1	0
Grapefruit Sections, ¼ cup	2
Honeydew Melon, ½ cup	0
Kiwifruit, ½ cup	0
Lemon Wedges, 2 pieces	0
Mandarin Oranges, ¼ cup	0
Mango, ¼ cup	1
Orange Slices, ½ cup	0
Papaya, ¼ cup	1
Pineapple, ½ cup	0
Pineapple Tidbits, ¼ cup	0
Red Grapes, 10 pieces	0
Strawberries, 5 pieces	0
Watermelon, ¼ cup	1

Condiments

Brown Sugar, 1 Tbsp	3
Honey Butter, 1 Tbsp	3
Strawberry Jam, 1 Tbsp	3
Whipped Margarine, 1 Tbsp	3

Golden Corral Buffet & Grill

Breakfast

	SmartPoints® value
Banana Nut French Toast, 1 serving	12
Cajun Sausage, 1 serving	12
Cheese Grits, ½ cup	6
Cottage Cheese, ½ cup	3
Grits, ½ cup	3
Hash Brown Casserole, ½ cup	4
Plain French Toast, 1 serving	7
Skillet Hash Browns, ½ cup	8
Split Smoked Sausage, 1	10
Sugar Free Oatmeal Bars, 1	3
Turkey Sausage, 1	2
Waffles, 1	2
Apple Fruit Topping, 2 Tbsp	2
Bacon, 3 pieces	2
Bacon and Cheese Quiche, 1 serving	10
Biscuits, 1	7
Blueberry Muffins, 1	18
Blueberry Pancakes, 1	3
Blueberry Syrup, 2 Tbsp	7
Breakfast Bacon, 2 pieces	2
Breakfast Pizza, 1 serving	12
Breakfast Pork Steaks, 3 oz	6
Breakfast Sausage Links, 1	4
Canadian Turkey Bacon, 2 pieces	1
Candied Bacon, 2 pieces	5
Cherry Fruit Topping, 2 Tbsp	2
Chocolate Chip Pancakes, 1	7
Chocolate Syrup, 1 oz	4
Chorizo and Egg Breakfast Burrito, 1	11
Corn Muffins, 1	9
Diced Eggs, ¼ cup	1
Down Home Fried Bacon, 2 pieces	4
Garlic Cheese Biscuits, 1	6
Jalapeño Corn Muffin, 1	9
Maple Syrup, 2 Tbsp	7
Mini Bacon and Cheese Quiche, 1	9
Mini Spinach Quiche, 1	8
Pancakes, 1	3
Peach Fruit Topping, 2 Tbsp	2
Pecan Syrup, 2 Tbsp	4
Pineapple Fruit Topping, 2 Tbsp	2
Pork Sausage, piece	10
Pork Sausage Patty, 1	3
Sausage and Egg Breakfast Burrito, 1	11
Scrambled Eggs, ½ cup	6
Spinach Quiche, 1 serving	8
Strawberry Cheesecake French Toast, piece	9
Strawberry Fruit Topping, 2 Tbsp	2
Strawberry Syrup, 2 Tbsp	6
Sugar Free Pancake Syrup, 1 Tbsp	0
Thick Cut Bacon, 2 pieces	2
Whipped Topping, 2 Tbsp	2
Whole Eggs, 1	2

Desserts

	SmartPoints® value
Apple Cobbler, 1 piece	7
Apple Pie, 1 serving	13
Apple Turnover, 1	10
Banana Nut Bread, 1 piece	9
Banana Pudding, ½ cup	12
Boston Cream Cake, 1 slice	9
Bread Pudding, ½ cup	13
Brownies, 1	5
Butter Pecan Ice Cream, ½ cup	7
Candied Orange Slices, 10 pieces	9
Candy Corn, 10 pieces	4
Canned Peaches, ¼ cup	2

"We Like This!" item

	SmartPoints® value
Caramel Chocolate Cheesecake, 1 piece	13
Caramel Pecan Shooters, 1	14
Carrot Cake, 1 serving	14
Carrot Soufflé, ½ cup	8
Checkerboard Bars, 1	4
Cherry Cobbler, 1 serving	8
Cherry Pie, 1 serving	13
Cherry Turnover, 1	10
Chocolate Cake with Cherries, 1 slice	11
Chocolate Cake with Chocolate Frosting, 1 serving	16
Chocolate Chess Pie, 1 serving	18
Chocolate Chip Cookie, 1	3
Chocolate Chips, 2 Tbsp	8
Chocolate Covered Banana (with peanuts), 1	7
Chocolate Covered NY Cheesecake, 1	17
Chocolate Covered Raisins, 2 Tbsp	6
Chocolate Covered Rice Krispy Treats, 1	13
Chocolate Cupcakes, 1	9
Chocolate Fountain Chocolate, 2 Tbsp	11
Chocolate Fudge, 1 serving	6
Chocolate Molten Volcano Cake, ½ cup	13
Chocolate Soft Serve, ½ cup	5
Chocolate White Chip Cookies, 1	3
Chopped Peanuts, 2 Tbsp	3
Cin a Gold Rolls, 1	10
Cinnamon Spice Shooters, 1	10
Cinnamon Sugar, 1 Tbsp	3
Coconut Cookies, 1	3
Coconut Macaroon Cookies, 1	5

	SmartPoints® value
Coconut Macaroon Cookies, Chocolate Covered, 1	10
Cookies and Cream Ice Cream, ½ cup	8
Cotton Candy, 1	6
Crêpes (cherry), 1	6
Crêpes (strawberry), 1	6
Fruit Cocktail, ½ cup	4
German Chocolate Bars, 1 serving	11
German Chocolate Cake, 1 serving	13
Glazed Donuts, 1	7
Gummy Bears, 10 pieces	4
Honey Buns, 1	13
Hot Caramel, 1 oz	4
Hot Fudge, 1 oz	5
Hushpuppies (scratch), 3 pieces	8
Jellybeans, 10 pieces	6
Lemon Bars, 1	7
Luscious Lemon Cake, 1 serving	7
Marshmallows (large), 3 pieces	3
Mini Billionaire's Pie, 1	11
Mini Cheesecake, piece	16
Mini Chocolate Chess Tarts, 1	15
Mini Coconut Cream Tarts, 1	11
Mini Fruit Tarts, 1	9
Mini Lemon Cream Pie, 1	11
Mini Peanut Butter Cream Tarts, 1	13
Mini Pecan Tarts, 1	12
Mini Pumpkin Cupcakes, 1	8
Mini Pumpkin Tarts, 1	9
Mini Strawberry Pie, 1	10
Mint Chocolate Chip Ice Cream, ½ cup	9
No Sugar Added Blueberry Pie, 1 serving	10

Desserts (cont'd)

	SmartPoints® value
No Sugar Added Chocolate Pudding, ½ cup	5
No Sugar Added Mocha Cake, 1 slice	7
No Sugar Added Peach Pie, 1 serving	13
No Sugar Added Peanut Butter Cup Fudge Ice Cream, ½ cup	5
No Sugar Added Pistachio Cake, 1 slice	7
No Sugar Added Pistachio Pudding, ½ cup	4
No Sugar Added Strawberry Cheesecake, 1 serving	9
No Sugar Added Vanilla Nonfat Frozen Yogurt, ½ cup	2
NY Style Cheesecake, 1 serving	12
Oatmeal Cookies, 1	3
Orange Sherbet, ½ cup	6
Peach Cobbler, 1 serving	8
Peanut Butter Cookie, 1	2
Peanut Butter Fudge Tart, 1 serving	9
Peanut Butter Shooters, 1	13
Pecan Pie, 1	17
Pecan Pieces, 2 Tbsp	3
Pineapple Supreme Cake, 1 slice	13
Praline Pecan Pieces, 2 Tbsp	4
Pumpkin Pie, 1 serving	15

	SmartPoints® value
Rainbow Nonfat Sherbet, ½ cup	6
Red Velvet Cake, 1 serving	11
Rice Krispy Treats, 1	3
Shadow Cake, 1 serving	16
Snackums, 10 pieces	2
Sprinkles, 2 Tbsp	8
Strawberry Shortcake, 1	6
Strawberry Shortcake Shooters, 1	8
Strawberry Supreme Cake, 1 slice	13
Sugar Free Chocolate Cookies, 1	2
Sugar Free Oatmeal Cookie, 1	3
Sugar Free Red Gelatin, ½ cup	0
Sugar Free Vanilla Cake, 1 serving	5
Sweet Corn Pudding, ½ cup	12
Truffles with Peanuts, 1	13
Truffles with Sprinkles, 1	14
Turtle Cheesecake Bars, 1	10
Turtle Tart, 1 serving	9
Vanilla Cupcakes, 1	10
Vanilla Soft Serve, ½ cup	6
Yams and Apple Casserole, ½ cup	9
Yogurt Raisins, 2 Tbsp	4

"We Like This!" item

Entrées

	SmartPoints® value
Au Jus, 1 serving	0
Baked Fish, piece	2
Baked Mostaccioli, 1 spoon	5
BBQ Baked Chicken Pizza, 1 slice	8
BBQ Beef, 1 serving	3
BBQ Beef Ribs, 1 serving	11
BBQ Pork Ribs, 1 rib	5
BBQ Smoked Sausage with Peppers and Onions, 1 spoon	8
Beef and Broccoli Stir-Fry, 1 spoon	4
Beef Patties, 1 patty	3
Beef Stroganoff, 1 spoon	5
Buffalo Chicken Poppers, 1 spoon	4
Butter Crumb Alaskan Pollock, piece	2
Butterfly and Popcorn Shrimp, 1 spoon	4
Butterfly Shrimp, 1 shrimp	1
Carved Grilled Pork Loin, 1 serving	4
Carved Ham, 1 serving	2
Carved Roast Beef, 1 serving	7
Carved Salmon Filet, 1 serving	4
Carved Sirloin Steak, 1 serving	4
Cheese Pizza, 1 slice	5
Cheeseburger, 1 burger	9
Cheeseburger Sliders, 1 burger	7
Chicken & Dumplings, 1 spoon	4
Chicken Alfredo, 1 spoon	7
Chicken Sliders, 1 burger	8
Chicken Strips or Tenders, 1 spoon	5
Chicken Zucchini Stir-Fry, 1 spoon	3
Chinese Chicken Livers, 1 spoon	5
Clam Strips, 1 serving	10
Coconut Shrimp, 1 spoon	4

	SmartPoints® value
Corn Dog, 1	8
Country BBQ Chicken Breast, 1 breast	7
Country BBQ Chicken Drumstick, 1 drumstick	3
Country BBQ Chicken Thigh, 1 thigh	5
Country BBQ Chicken Wing, 1 wing	2
Country Fried Steak with Gravy, piece	7
Country Fried Steak without Gravy, piece	7
Country Pasta Gratine, 1 spoon	5
Country-Style BBQ Pork Ribs, 1 rib	5
Creamy Penne Carbonara, 1 spoon	9
Crispy Noodles, 1 spoon	1
Fire Grilled Chicken Alfredo, 1 spoon	7
Fried Catfish, piece	2
Fried Fish, piece	2
Fried Rice with Ham, 1 spoon	4
Fried Shrimp, 11 shrimp	4
Grilled BBQ Pork Steak, 1 steak	4
Grilled BBQ Smoked Sausage, 1 spoon	7
Grilled Cheese Sandwich, ½ sandwich	10
Grilled Ham and Cheese Sandwich, ½ sandwich	11
Grilled Italian Sausage Penne, 1 spoon	6
Grilled Pork Steak, 1 steak	4
Grilled Smoked Sausage, 1 link	7
Grilled Teriyaki Pineapple Chicken, 1 spoon	4
Hand Breaded Fried Chicken Breast, 1 breast	9

Entrées (cont'd)

	SmartPoints® value
Hand Breaded Fried Chicken Drumstick, 1 drumstick	3
Hand Breaded Fried Chicken Thigh, 1 thigh	5
Hand Breaded Fried Chicken Wing, 1 wing	2
Honey BBQ Pork Riblets, 1 rib	4
Honey Glazed Baked Ham, 1 slice	3
Italian Sausage, 1 spoon	5
Jambalaya, 1 spoon	4
King's Ranch Chicken, 1 spoon	6
Kung Pao Beef, 1 spoon	4
Lasagna, piece	5
Lo Mein, 1 spoon	5
Macaroni & Cheese, 1 spoon	3
Meatloaf, 1 serving	6
New Orleans Bourbon Street Chicken, 1 spoon	4
Orange Chicken, 1 spoon	11
Orzo Pasta with Feta Cheese, 1 spoon	5
Oven Roasted Rotisserie Style Turkey, 3 oz	2
Parmesan Crusted Tilapia, piece	4
Pasta Florentine with Creamy Marinara, 1 spoon	5
Pasta Primavera, 1 spoon	5
Peel & Eat Shrimp, 1 shrimp	0
Pepperoni and Sausage Calzone, piece	5
Pepperoni Pizza, 1 slice	6
Perfect Pot Roast, 1 spoon	4
Popcorn Shrimp, 1 spoon	4
Pot Roast Stroganoff, 1 spoon	4
Potatoes O'Brien, 1 spoon	5
Roasted Jerk Chicken Breast, 1 breast	7

	SmartPoints® value
Roasted Jerk Chicken Drumstick, 1 drumstick	3
Roasted Jerk Chicken Thigh, 1 thigh	4
Roasted Jerk Chicken Wing, 1 wing	2
Rotisserie Chicken Breast, 1 breast	7
Rotisserie Chicken Drumstick, 1 drumstick	2
Rotisserie Chicken Thigh, 1 thigh	3
Rotisserie Chicken Wing, 1 wing	2
Salisbury Steak, piece	5
Salmon with Creole Shrimp, piece	3
Seafood Patties, 1 patty	4
Shrimp Alfredo, 1 spoon	6
Shrimp Scampi, 1 spoon	7
Sizzling BBQ Beef Brisket, 3 oz	4
Spaghetti and Meat Sauce, 1 spoon	4
Spaghetti and Meatballs, 1 spoon	4
Steak Fajita, 1 spoon	3
Traditional Baked Chicken Breast, 1 breast	7
Traditional Baked Chicken Drumstick, 1 drumstick	2
Traditional Baked Chicken Thigh, 1 thigh	4
Traditional Baked Chicken Wing, 1 wing	2
Turkey Hot Dogs, 1	4
Wood Seared Salmon, piece	6

Taco Bar

Beef Taco Meat, 1 spoon	1
Black Beans with Ham, 1 spoon	2
Chicken Chilaquiles, 1 spoon	8
Chicken Fajita, 1 spoon	4
Chicken Quesadillas, 1 wedge	4
Chicken Taco Meat, 1 spoon	2

"We Like This!" item

	SmartPoints® value
Diced Onions, 1 spoon	0
Diced Tomatoes, 1 spoon	0
Enchiladas (all), 1	9
Flour Tortilla, 1	4
Fried Jalapeños, 1 serving	0
Guacamole, 1 spoon	1
Jalapeños, 1 spoon	0
Lettuce, Shredded, 1 cup	0
Mexican Rice, 1 spoon	2
Nacho Chips, 1 serving	2
Pico de Gallo, 1 serving	0
Pinto Beans with Bacon, 1 spoon	2
Potatoes Con Queso, 1 spoon	4
Queso Dip, 1 serving	2
Red Beans with Ham, 1 spoon	1
Refried Beans, 1 spoon	2
Salsa, 1 serving	0
Sautéed Bell Peppers, 1 spoon	1
Sautéed Jalapeños & Onions, 1 spoon	1
Sautéed Onions, 1 spoon	1
Shredded Cheddar Cheese, 1 spoon	1
Sliced Tomatoes, 1 spoon	0
Sour Cream, 1 spoon	1
Taco Shell Baskets, 1 basket	5
Taco Shells, 1 shell	2
Tostadas, 1	3

Salads & Toppings

	SmartPoints® value
Ambrosia Salad, 1 spoon	9
Artichokes, 1 spoon	0
Asian Chopped Salad, 1 spoon	4
Bacon Bits, Imitation, 1 spoon	1
Bacon Bits, Real, 1 spoon	1
Banana-Strawberry Salad, 1 spoon	4
BLT Salad, 1 spoon	4
Broccoli Apple Salad, 1 spoon	6
Broccoli Bacon Salad, 1 spoon	7
Bruschetta Tomato Pasta Salad, 1 spoon	5
Bruschetta Tomato Salad, 1 spoon	3
Caesar Salad, 1 cup	2
Carrot and Raisin Salad, 1 spoon	6
Carrots, Matchsticks, 1 spoon	0
Cherry Tomatoes, 1	0
Chicken Breast, Diced, 1 serving	0
Chicken Caesar Salad, 1 cup	3
Chicken Pasta Salad, 1 spoon	8
Craisins, 1 spoon	1
Creamy Pea Salad, 1 spoon	7
Croutons, 7 pieces	1
Crushed Red Pepper, 1 tsp	0
Cucumber Tomato Salad, 1 spoon	1
Cucumbers (sliced), 1 slice	0
Diced Bacon, 1 serving	7
Diced Ham, 1 serving	1
Dilled Potato Salad, 1 spoon	4
Feta Cheese, 1 spoon	5
Garbanzo Beans, 1 spoon	0
Greek Salad, 1 spoon	4
Ham (diced or julienne), 1 serving	1
Imitation Shredded Cheese, 1 spoon	1
Italian Chopped Salad, 1 spoon	3
Italian Pasta Salad, 1 spoon	7
Kidney Beans, 1 spoon	0
Macaroni Vegetable Salad, 1 spoon	8
Marinated Green Bean Salad, 1 spoon	4
Mushrooms, 1 spoon	0
Olives, Black, 1 spoon	0
Olives, Green, 1 spoon	1

	SmartPoints® value
Oriental Chicken Salad (no dressing), 1 spoon	1
Oriental Pasta Salad, 1 spoon	4
Parmesan Cheese, 1 spoon	1
Pepperoncini, 1 spoon	0
Pickled Beets, 1 spoon	4
Pickles, Sweet, 1 spoon	1
Potato Salad, 1 spoon	4
Radishes, 1 spoon	0
Red Onions (sliced), 1 ring	0
Roasted Red Pepper, 1 spoon	0
Romaine Lettuce (chopped), 1 cup	0
Seafood Salad, 1 spoon	10
Seven Layer Salad, 1 spoon	7
Shredded Monterey Jack Cheese, 1 spoon	1
Shredded Mozzarella Cheese, 1 spoon	1
Sicilian Pasta Salad, 1 spoon	5
Sliced Ham, 1 slice	3
Southwest Salad, 1 spoon	2
Spinach Leaves, 1 cup	0
Spinach Salad, 1 cup	3
Spring Mix, 1 cup	0
Strawberry Walnut Salad, 1 spoon	3
Sunflower Seeds, 1 spoon	2
Tarragon Potato Salad, 1 spoon	4
Three Bean Salad, 1 spoon	3
Tossed Green Salad, 1 cup	0
Waldorf Salad, 1 spoon	5

Dressing & Sauces

	SmartPoints® value
Beef Gravy, 1 serving	1
Blue Cheese Dressing, 1 serving	5
Cheese Sauce, 1 serving	2
Chicken Gravy, 1 serving	1
Cocktail Sauce, 1 serving	2
Corn Salsa, 1 spoon	2
Country Gravy, 1 serving	2
Cranberry Sauce, 1 fl oz	3
Creamy Italian Dressing, 1 serving	4
Fat Free Creamy Italian Dressing, 1 serving	1
Fat Free French Dressing, 1 ladle	2
French Dressing, 1 serving	5
Greek Vinaigrette, 1 ladle	5
Horseradish Sauce, 1 fl oz	3
Hot Sauce, 1 tsp	0
Hummus, 1 spoon	2
Italian Dressing, 1 ladle	4
Italian Dressing, Fat Free, 1 ladle	1
Italian Dressing, Low Fat, 1 serving	1
Marinara Sauce, 1 serving	1
Meat Sauce, 1 serving	1
Oriental Sesame Dressing, 1 serving	4
Ranch Dressing, 1 serving	5
Ranch Dressing, Fat Free, 1 serving	1
Raspberry Vinaigrette, Fat Free, 1 serving	2
Reduced Fat Ranch Dressing, 1 serving	2
Sausage Gravy, 1 serving	1
Soy Sauce, 1 tsp	0
Tartar Sauce, 1 fl oz	5
Thick Cheese Sauce, 1 serving	2
Thousand Island Dressing, 1 serving	5
Turkey Gravy, 1 serving	1
White Gravy, 1 serving	2

"We Like This!" item

	SmartPoints® value

Soups

Chicken Noodle Soup, 1 ladle	2
Chicken RIce Soup, 1 ladle	1
Chicken Tortilla Soup, 1 ladle	1
Chili Bean Soup, 1 ladle	2
Corn Chowder, 1 ladle	3
Cream of Broccoli Soup, 1 ladle	3
Creamy Tomato Basil Soup, 1 ladle	3
French Onion Soup, 1 ladle	1
Hearty Seafood Stew, 1 spoon	3
Italian Sausage & Bean Soup, 1 ladle	2
Minestrone Soup, 1 ladle	2
Navy Bean Soup with Ham, 1 ladle	1
New England Clam Chowder, 1 ladle	6
Potato Cheese Soup, 1 ladle	5
Vegetable Beef Soup, 1 ladle	2

Sides

AuGratin Potatoes, 1 spoon	4
Baked Potatoes, 1	4
BBQ Baked Beans, 1 spoon	6
Bread Dressing, 1 spoon	5
Broccoli, 1 spoon	0
Broccoli Florets, 1 spoon	0
Broccoli Florets and Cheese Sauce, 1 spoon	2
Broccoli/Cauliflower Medley, 1 spoon	0
Buttered Noodles, 1 spoon	4
Cajun Rice, 1 spoon	3
California Coleslaw, 1 spoon	6
Candied Yams, 1 spoon	6
Cauliflower, 1 spoon	0

	SmartPoints® value
Cauliflower AuGratin, 1 spoon	2
Cheesy Hashbrowns, 1 spoon	5
Cheesy Twice Baked Potato, 1 spoon	6
Collard Greens with Bacon, 1 spoon	1
Corn, 1 spoon	0
Corn on the Cob, piece	3
Cornbread Dressing, 1 spoon	8
Dill Pickles, 1 spoon	0
Dirty Rice, 1 spoon	3
French Fries, 22	5
Fried Okra, 1 spoon	7
German Boiled Cabbage, 1 spoon	1
Green Bean Casserole, 1 spoon	4
Green Beans, 1 serving	0
Green Beans El Greco, 1 spoon	1
Green Cabbage, 1 spoon	3
Grilled Cowboy Potatoes, 1 spoon	6
Grilled Vegetables, 1 spoon	1
Jo Jo Potatoes, 1 serving	5
Joe's Cracked Pepper Green Beans with Bacon, 1 spoon	2
Marinated Vegetables, 1 spoon	2
Mashed Potatoes, 1 spoon	2
Montreal Vegetable Medley, 1 spoon	2
Onion Rings, 1 serving	8
Peas, 1 spoon	0
Potato Skins, 1 serving	2
Ranch Red Potatoes, 1 spoon	3
Risotto Style Rice, 1 spoon	3
Rissotto Style Rice with Chicken, 1 spoon	3
Sautéed Zucchini, 1 spoon	2
Seasoned Cabbage, 1 spoon	2

Sides (cont'd)

	SmartPoints® value
Seasoned Collard Greens, 1 spoon	1
Seasoned Green Beans, 1 spoon	1
Seasoned Turnip Greens, 1 spoon	1
Smokey Red Beans & Rice, 1 spoon	3
Spaghetti, 1 spoon	4
Spanish Rice, 1 spoon	5
Spinach Marie, 1 spoon	7
Squash, 1 spoon	6
Steamed Carrots, 1 spoon	2
Steamed Corn, 1 spoon	3
Steamed Red Potatoes, 1 spoon	3
Sweet Potatoes, ½ potato	3
Topped Baked Potatoes, ½ potato	5
Vegetable Rice Pilaf, 1 spoon	2
Vegetable Stir-Fry, 1 spoon	2
White Rice, 1 spoon	3

Breads

Buns, Hot Dog, 1	4
Cinnamon Bread, 1 slice	6
Cornbread, piece	6
Dinner Rolls, 1 roll	4
Dinner Rolls, White-Pull-A-Part, 1 roll	4
French Bread Loaf, 1 slice	2
Garlic Bread, piece	2
Garlic Cheese Biscuit, 1 biscuit	8
Honey Cornbread, piece	7
Hot Dog Bun, 1 roll	4
Jalapeño Cornbread, piece	6
Pumpernickel Bread Loaf, 1 slice	2
Rye Bread Loaf, 1 slice	2
Wheat Bread Loaf, 1 slice	2
White Bread Loaf, 1 slice	2

	SmartPoints® value

Condiments

Bacon Cheddar Butter, 1 Tbsp	5
Bacon Cheddar Butter Blend, 1 Tbsp	5
Brown Sugar, 1 Tbsp	2
Butter, 1 packet	2
Honey, 1 packet	2
Jelly, 1 packet	2
Ketchup, 1 packet	1
Lemons, 1 slice	0
Margarine, 1 packet	1
Mayonnaise, 1 Tbsp	3
Melted Butter, 1 ladle	21
Melted Margarine, 1 ladle	15
Mustard, 1 packet	0
Non-Dairy Creamers, 1 packet	0
Peanut Butter, 1 Tbsp	3
Pickle Relish, 1 Tbsp	1
Sauerkraut, 1 spoon	0

Breakfast

Apple Walnut Muffin, 1 muffin	9
Bacon, 1 slice	1
Banana Walnut Muffin, 1 muffin	10
Biscuits, 1 biscuit	4
Blueberry Muffin, 1 muffin	9
Blueberry Pancakes, 1 pancake	4
Buttermilk Pancakes, 1 pancake	4
Carved Rope Sausage, 1 serving	11
Cherry Muffin, 1 muffin	9
Cinnamon Granola Cereal, ¾ sup	8
Coconut Almond Muffin, 1 muffin	9
Corn Muffin, 1 muffin	12
Cottage Cheese, 1 spoon	0
Cranberry Walnut Muffin, 1 muffin	10

"We Like This!" item

	SmartPoints® value
Crisp Rice Cereal, 1 ¼ cups	4
English Muffins (dry), ½ muffin	2
French Toast, 1 slice	8
Frosted Fruit Flavored Cereal, 1 cup	6
Frozen Nutrasweet® Vanilla Nonfat Yogurt, 4 fl oz	3
Frozen Orange Sorbet Nonfat Yogurt, 4 fl oz	5
Grits, 4 ladles	2
Hashbrown Patties, piece	4
Hollandaise Sauce, 1 serving	5
Maple Flavored Syrup, 1 serving	11
Oatmeal, 1 serving	2
Oatmeal Raisin Muffin, 1 muffin	10
Peach Muffin, 1 muffin	10
Piña Colada Muffin, 1 muffin	9
Plain Bagel, 1 bagel	7
Plain Omelet, 1 omlette	4
Poached Eggs, 1	2
Poppy Seed Muffin, 1 muffin	8
Pumpkin with Raisins Muffin, 1 muffin	10
Rum Raisin Muffin, 1 muffin	10
Sausage Links, 1 link	4
Scrambled Eggs, 1 spoon	4
Strawberry Muffin, 1 muffin	11
Toasted Oat Cereal, 1 cup	3
Turkey Sausage, 1 patty	1
Waffle, 1	4
Zucchini Muffin, 1 muffin	8

Desserts

	SmartPoints® value
Apple Spice Cake, piece	8
Applesauce, 1 spoon	1
Banana Nut Cake, piece	12
Banana Pudding, 1 spoon	7
Banana Split, 1 serving	16
Bananas, 1 spoon	0
Black Forest Cake, piece	6
Black Forest Cupcake, 1	10
Bread Pudding, 1 spoon	8
Butterfinger Pieces, 1 spoon	3
Butterscotch Brownie, 1 brownie	7
Butterscotch Topping, 2 Tbsp	6
Cantaloupe, 1 spoon	0
Cappuccino Cake, piece	8
Caramel Apple Crisp, 1 spoon	9
Caramel Rolls, 1 roll	5
Caramel Topped Cupcake (all varieties), 1	14
Carrot Cake, piece	10
Cheesecake, piece	11
Cheesecake, Cherry, piece	11
Cherry Cobbler, 1 spoon	8
Cherry Crisp, 1 spoon	6
Chewy Bears, 9 pieces	3
Chocolate Cake, piece	7
Chocolate Chess Pie (scratch), 1 slice	16
Chocolate Chip Cookie, 1 cookie	5
Chocolate Chip Cookie Bar, 1 bar	13
Chocolate Chip Cookie Pizza, 1 slice	7
Chocolate Chips, 1 spoon	5
Chocolate Cookie Pieces, 1 spoon	1
Chocolate Cream Pie, 1 slice	8
Chocolate Cupcake, 1	13
Chocolate Decadence Cake, piece	9
Chocolate Drizzle Crispy Rice Bar, 1 bar	6
Chocolate Haystacks, piece	7
Chocolate Marble Cake, piece	8
Chocolate Pudding, 1 spoon	6

Desserts (cont'd)

	SmartPoints® value
Chocolate Syrup, 2 Tbsp	5
Cinnamon Rolls, 1 roll	6
Coconut Cream Pie, 1 slice	12
Coconut Cream Pie (scratch), 1 slice	13
Cookies and Cream, piece	14
Cookies and Cream Cheesecake, piece	13
Crispy Rice Bar, 1 bar	5
Crushed Pineapple, 1 spoon	1
Decorated Cookie, 1 cookie	5
Dessert Pizza, 1 slice	5
Dutch Apple Cake, 1 slice	10
Fudge, piece	2
Fudge Brownie, 1 brownie	10
Fun E Chips, 1 spoon	4
Fun E Chips Crispy Rice Bar, 1 bar	5
Gelatin (all flavors), 1 spoon	2
Gelatin Whip (all flavors), 1 spoon	4
German Chocolate Cake, piece	11
Grapes, 1 spoon	0
Heath Bar Bits, 1 spoon	4
Honey Nut Topping, 1 spoon	6
Honeydew, 1 spoon	0
Hot Fudge Chocolate Chip Muffin, 1 muffin	12
Hot Fudge Sundae Cake, 1 spoon	8
Hot Fudge Sundae Muffin, 1 muffin	12
Hot Fudge Topping, 2 Tbsp	6
Ice Cream Cone, 1 cone	1
Iced Decorated Cookie, 1 cookie	9
Key Lime, piece	8
Key Lime Pie (scratch), 1 slice	10
Ko Ko Bits, 1 spoon	3

	SmartPoints® value
Lemon Bar, 1 bar	9
Lemon Cake, piece	8
Lemon Cream Pie, 1 slice	8
Lemon Meringue Pie, 1 slice	6
Lemon Pie (scratch), 1 slice	10
Lemon Reduced Sugar Pie, piece	7
Lime Reduced Sugar Pie, piece	8
Malted Milk Balls, Ground, 1 spoon	4
Maple Walnut Cake, piece	10
Nestle Crunch® Pieces, 1 spoon	21
Nutrasweet Vanilla Frozen Nonfat Yogurt, 1 serving	3
Oatmeal Raisin Cookie, 1 cookie	5
Orange Dreamsicle, piece	12
Orange Sorbet Frozen Nonfat Yogurt, 1 serving	5
Orange Wedges, 1 spoon	0
Peach Cobbler, 1 spoon	17
Peach Cupcake, 1	11
Peach Topping, 1 ladle	2
Peaches (sliced), 1 spoon	1
Peanut Butter Cookie, 1 cookie	5
Pecan Pie, 1 slice	12
Pineapple, 1 spoon	0
Pumpkin Pie, 1 slice	9
Raisin Fluff, 1 spoon	5
Raisins, 1 spoon	2
Reduced Sugar Appie Pie, piece	9
Reduced Sugar Banana Cream Pie, piece	8
Reduced Sugar Cherry Pie, piece	7
Reduced Sugar Chocolate Cream Pie, piece	8
Reduced Sugar Lemon Pie, piece	7
Reduced Sugar Lime Pie, piece	7

"We Like This!" item

	SmartPoints® value
Reduced Sugar Orange Pie, piece	7
Reduced Sugar Raspberry Pie, piece	7
Reduced Sugar Strawberry Pie, piece	7
Reduced Sugar/Calorie Chocolate Pudding, 1 spoon	2
Reduced Sugar/Calorie Vanilla Pudding, 1 spoon	2
Rocky Road Cupcake, 1	14
Rocky Road Pudding, 1 spoon	7
Scotcheroo, 1 bar	8
Seven Layer Bar, 1 bar	11
Snickerdoodle Cookie, 1	5
Snickerdoodle Cookie Pizza, 1 slice	8
Soft Serve, Chocolate, 1 serving	6
Soft Serve, Vanilla, 1 serving	6
Sprinkles, 1 spoon	4
Sprinkles Crispy Rice Bar, 1 bar	5
Stewed Prunes, 1 spoon	5
Strawberries, 1 spoon	0
Strawberry Marble Cake, piece	9
Strawberry Mousse Cake, piece	10
Strawberry Shortcake, piece	10
Strawberry Topping, 2 Tbsp	4
Strawberry Whip, 1 spoon	11
Sugar Free Ranger Cookies, 1 cookie	3
Supreme Cake, piece	8
Sweet Potato Pie, piece	11
Tapioca Pudding, 1 spoon	5
Tres Leches, piece	12
Turtle Brownie, 1 brownie	6
Vanilla Pudding, 1 spoon	6
Vanilla Soft Serve Flurrie (no mix-ins), 8 fl oz	12

	SmartPoints® value
Watermelon, 1 spoon	0
Whipped Topping, 1 spoon	3
White Cupcake, Decorated, 1	14

Beverages

Cappuccino (all flavors), 1 serving	9
Carbonated Beverages (all flavors), 1 serving	10
Chocolate Milk (1% reduced fat), 1 serving	12
Coffee Creamers, 1	0
Coffee, decaffeinated or regular, 1 serving	0
Hi C® Fruit Punch, 1 serving	10
Hot Chocolate (all flavors), 1 serving	8
Hot Tea, 1 serving	0
Icee®, all flavors, 1 serving	7
Lemonade (all flavors), 1 serving	6
Orange Juice, 1 serving	9
Peanut Butter Mocha, 1 cookie	10
Sweetened Iced Tea (all flavors), 1 serving	6
Unsweetened Iced Tea, 1 serving	0

Build Your Own Sandwich

	SmartPoints® value
9 Grain Artisan Bread, 2 slices	7
All Butter Croissant, 1	10
American Cheese, 1 serving	3
Asiago Cheese, 1 serving	3
Cheddar Cheese, 1 serving	3
Hot Corned Beef, 1 serving	2
Mozzerella Cheese, 3 slices	13
Muenster Cheese, 1 serving	3
Onion Bun, 1	8
Premium Ham, 1 serving	1
Provolone Cheese, 1 serving	3
Roast Beef, 1 serving	2
Roasted Turkey Breast, 1 serving	1
Rye Bread, 2 slices	7
Smoked Turkey Breast, 1 serving	1
Swiss Cheese, 1 serving	3
Telera Bread, 1	7

Sandwiches

	SmartPoints® value
Amy's Turkey-O (half), 1 serving	7
Amy's Turkey-O (whole), 1 serving	15
Asiago Pot Roast Sandwich (half), 1 serving	8
Asiago Pot Roast Sandwich (whole), 1 serving	16
Beefeater (half), 1 serving	13
Beefeater (lighter portion), 1 serving	22
Beefeater (whole), 1 serving	26
California Club (half), 1 serving	12
California Club (whole), 1 serving	26
Caprese Panini, 1 serving	26
Carolina Club (half), 1 serving	9
Carolina Club (whole), 1 serving	18
Chicago Club (half), 1 serving	9
Chicago Club (whole), 1 serving	18
Chicken Panini (half), 1 serving	10
Chicken Panini (whole), 1 serving	19
Chicken Veracruz (half), 1 serving	9
Chicken Veracruz (whole), 1 serving	17
Club Royale (half), 1 serving	11
Club Royale (whole), 1 serving	21
Cuban Press (half), 1 serving	8
Cuban Press (whole), 1 serving	16
Deli Club (half), 1 serving	8
Deli Club (whole), 1 serving	19
Grilled Cheese (wheat), 1 serving	16
Grilled Cheese (white), 1 serving	18
Ham & Cheese (wheat), 1 serving	10
Ham & Cheese (white), 1 serving	13
Ham & Cheese (wrap), 1	7
Hot Pastrami, 1 serving	11
Johnny Cashew's Pork Sandwich (half), 1 serving	13
Johnny Cashew's Pork Sandwich (whole), 1 serving	27
MeataBalla (half), 1 serving	18
MeataBalla (whole), 1 serving	37
Mediterranean Wrap, 1	10
Mediterranean Wrap (half), 1 serving	5
New York Yankee (half), 1 serving	14
New York Yankee (lighter portion), 1 serving	17
New York Yankee (whole), 1 serving	28
Organic Wheat Wrap, 1	6
Peanut Butter & Jelly (wheat), 1 serving	15
Peanut Butter & Jelly (white), 1 serving	17
Ranchero Wrap, 1	14
Ranchero Wrap (half), 1 serving	7
Rueben the Great (half), 1 serving	10
Rueben the Great (lighter portion), 1 serving	14
Rueben the Great (whole), 1 serving	20
Santa Fe Chicken Sandwich (half), 1 serving	10

"We Like This!" item

	SmartPoints® value
Santa Fe Chicken Sandwich (whole), 1 serving	19
Smokey Jack Panini (half), 1 serving	11
Smokey Jack Panini (whole), 1 serving	22
Spinach Veggie Wrap, 1	12
Spinach Veggie Wrap (half), 1 serving	6
The Papa Joe (half), 1 serving	10
The Papa Joe (whole), 1 serving	19
The Plain Jane, 1 serving	54
The Plain Jane (lighter portion), 1 serving	33
Tuna Melt (half), 1 serving	15
Tuna Melt (whole), 1 serving	30
Turkey & Cheese (wheat), 1 serving	10
Turkey & Cheese (white), 1 serving	13
Turkey & Cheese (wrap), 1	7
Turkey Wrap, 1	11
Turkey Wrap (half), 1 serving	6
Wild Salmonwich (half), 1 serving	10
Wild Salmonwich (whole), 1 serving	19

Pizza

Cheese Pizza, 1	15

Muffalettas

Ham Muffaletta (half), 1 serving	36
Ham Muffaletta (whole), 1 serving	72
Muffaletta Bun, 1	5
Muffaletta Mix, 1 serving	8
Quarter Ham Muffaletta, 1 serving	18
Quarter Turkey Muffaletta, 1 serving	17
Turkey Muffaletta (half), 1 serving	35
Turkey Muffaletta (whole), 1 serving	70

Meatless Eats

	SmartPoints® value
Cup of Fruit, 1 serving	0
Fruit Bowl, 1 serving	0
Zucchini Garden Pasta, 1 serving	38
Zucchini Grillini, 1 serving	20
Zucchini Grillini (half), 1 serving	10

Salads

American Potato Salad, 1 serving	8
Black Bean Taco Salad (lighter), 1 serving	23
Black Bean Taco Salad (lite), 1 serving	23
Black Bean Taco Salad (original), 1 serving	38
Caprese Salad, 1 serving	4
Chicken Caesar Salad, 1 serving	28
Chicken Caesar Salad (lighter portion), 1 serving	14
Chicken Club Salad, 1 serving	15
Chicken Club Salad (lighter portion), 1 serving	9
Corn and Black Bean (salad bar portion), 1 serving	2
Corn and Black Bean Salad, 1 serving	7
Green Chili Potato Salad (salad bar portion), 1 serving	6
Green Chili Potato Salad (side portion), 1 serving	12
Homemade Chicken Salad with Almonds and Pineapple, 1 serving	6
Homemade Tuna Salad with Eggs, 1 serving	6
Italian Pasta Salad, 1 serving	6
MDA Quinoa Shrimp & Mango Salad, 1 serving	9
Mighty Wild Salmon Salad, 1 serving	18
Mixed Salad Greens, 1 cup	0
Nutty Mixed-Up Salad, 1 serving	21

Salads (cont'd)

	SmartPoints® value
Nutty Mixed-Up Salad (lighter portion), 1 serving	13
Quinoa Mango Salad, 1 serving	3
Taco Salad, 1 serving	42
Taco Salad - Southwest, 1 serving	38
Taco Salad - Southwest (lighter portion), 1 serving	22
Taco Salad (lighter portion), 1 serving	26
The Chef Salad, 1 serving	12
The Chef Salad (lighter portion), 1 serving	6

Salad Bar

	SmartPoints® value
Broccoli Florets, 1 serving	0
Diced Almonds, 1 serving	3
Extra Virgin Olive Oil, 1 serving	4
Feta Cheese, 1 serving	2
Garlic Horseradish Sauce, 1 serving	1
Grape Tomatoes, 4 pieces	0
Grapes, 1 serving	0
Green Peas, 1 serving	1
Guacamole, 1 serving	9
Hard Boiled Egg, 1	2
Hard Salami, 1 serving	1
Homemade Guacamole, 1 serving	1
Homemade Ranch Dressing, 1 serving	2
Honey Mustard, 1 serving	1
Italian Dressing, 1 serving	2
Italian Peppers, 1 serving	0
Jalapeño Pepper Jack Cheese, 1 serving	3
Jalapeño Pepper Jelly, 1 serving	3
Jalapeños, 1 serving	0
Kalamata Olives, 1 piece	0
Leafy Lettuce, 1 serving	0
Leo's Fat Free Italian Dressing (bottle), 1 serving	0
Light Raspberry Cabernet Vinaigrette (bottle), 1 serving	1
Lo Fat Ranch Dressing, 1 serving	1
Marinated Red Onions, 1 serving	6
Natural, Grilled Chicken Breast, 1 serving	1
Olive Oil Blend - Zucchini, 1 serving	1
Organic Baby Carrots, 5	0
Organic Balsamic Vinegar (bottle), 1 serving	1
Organic Field Greens, 1 serving	0
Organic Red Apples, 5	0
Organic Spinach, 1 serving	0
Red Bell Pepper, 1 piece	0
Red Onion Rings, 1 serving	0
Red Wine Vinegar (bottle), 1 serving	0
Roasted Herb Tomatoes, 1 serving	1
Roasted Red Pepper Hummus, 1 serving	8
Roasted Zucchini, 1 serving	0
Roma Tomato Slice, 1 serving	0
Salsa, 1 serving	0
Shredded Cheddar Cheese, 1 serving	2
Sliced Avocado - Half, 1 serving	4
Sliced Avocado - Quarter, 1 serving	2
Sliced Bacon, 2 pieces	2
Sliced Mushrooms, 1 serving	0
Southwest Spices, 1 serving	0
Spicy Cajun Mix, 1 serving	4
Spicy Giardinera, 1 serving	4
Steamed Veggies, 1 serving	0
Strawberry, 2 pieces	0
Stuffed Green Olives, 1 piece	0
Sunflower Seeds, 1 serving	4
Thousand Island Dressing, 1 serving	2
Tomato Slice, 1 serving	0
Whole Beets, 1 piece	0
Wild Alaskan Sockeye Salmon, 1 serving	5
Yellow Bell Pepper, 1 piece	0

"We Like This!" item

Pastas, Potatoes, & More

	SmartPoints® value
Bowtie Pasta & Chicken Alfredo, 1 serving	20
Bowtie Pasta & Meatballs, 1 serving	20
Chicken Alfredo (lighter portion), 1 serving	27
Chicken Alfredo Pasta, 1 serving	47
Chicken Nuggetz, 1 serving	4
Chicken Pasta Primo, 1 serving	41
Chicken Pasta Primo (lighter portion), 1 serving	24
Pecan-Smoked Pork Loin, 1 serving	1
Penne Pasta & Meatballs, 1 serving	42
Penne Pasta & Meatballs (lighter portion), 1 serving	27
Pollo Mexicano (lighter portion), 1 serving	28
Pollo Mexicano Potato, 1 serving	43
Pot Roast, 1 serving	4
Zucchini Garden Pasta (lighter portion), 1 serving	24

Soup

	SmartPoints® value
Broccoli Cheese Soup, 1 bowl	19
Broccoli Cheese Soup, 1 cup	14
Chicken Noodle Soup, 1 bowl	7
Chicken Noodle Soup, 1 cup	5
Chicken Pot Pie Soup, 1 bowl	19
Chicken Pot Pie Soup, 1 cup	10
Chili Soup, 1 bowl	15
Chili Soup, 1 cup	11
Fire Roasted Tortilla Soup, 1 bowl	7
Fire Roasted Tortilla Soup, 1 cup	5
French Onion Soup, 1 bowl	8
French Onion Soup, 1 cup	7
Organic Vegetable Soup, 1 bowl	5
Organic Vegetable Soup, 1 cup	4
Potato Soup, 1 bowl	22
Potato Soup, 1 cup	15
Southwest Chicken Chili Soup, 1 bowl	8
Southwest Chicken Chili Soup, 1 cup	6
Spicy Seafood Gumbo Soup, 1 bowl	8
Spicy Seafood Gumbo Soup, 1 cup	6
Tomato Basil Soup, 1 bowl	18
Tomato Basil Soup, 1 cup	15

Extras

	SmartPoints® value
Artichoke Hearts, 1 serving	0
Aujus Sauce, 1 serving	1
Bacon Bits, 1 serving	3
Baked Lays, 1	3
Balsamic Vinaigrette Dressing, 1 serving	1
Basil Pesto, 1 serving	4
Bleu Cheese Dressing, 1 serving	3
Cashew Butter, 1 serving	4
Chipotle Aioli, 1 serving	4
Cornbread Muffin, 1	3
Cottage Cheese, 1 serving	1
Cranberry Relish, 1 serving	9
Cream Cheese, 1 serving	10
Creamy Ceasar Dressing, 1 serving	1
Creamy Fruit Dip, 1 serving	8
Croutons, 1 serving	4
Cucumber Slice, 1 serving	0
House Chips (Ruffles), 1 bag	5
Kettle Chips, 1 bag	5
Marinara Sauce, 1 serving	1
Mayonnaise, 1 serving	6
Organic Blue Chips, 1 bag	7
Pickle Spear, 1	0
Pico De Gallo, 1 serving	0
Sauerkraut, 1 serving	0
Stone Ground Mustard, 1 serving	0
Yellow Mustard, 1 serving	1

	SmartPoints® value

Bread

Focaccia Bread, 2 slices	7
French Bread, 1	6
Garlic Toast, 2 pieces	1
Gingerbread Muffin, 1	4
Gluten-Free Bread, 2 slices	8
Olive Oil Blend - Bread, 1 serving	4
White Bread, 2 slices	8
Whole Grain Wheat Bread, 2 slices	6

Kids Menu

Hot Dog, 1	11
Hot Dog Bun, 1	5
Hot Dog with Chili, 1	16
Kid's Baked Potato, 1 serving	17
Mac & Cheese, 1 serving	15
Pepperoni Pizza, 1	16

Desserts

Banana Pudding, 1 serving	7
Carrot Cake, 1 slice	23
Chocolate Caramel Bite, ⅛ bar	5
Chocolate Chip Cookie, 1	13
Chocolate Coffee Cake, 1 slice	16
Chocolate Ice Cream, 1 serving	11
Chocolate Mousse, 1 serving	9
Chocolate Syrup, 1 serving	6
Cranberry Walnut Cookie, 1	12
Cranberry Walnut Mix, 1 serving	5
Cream Cheese Pecan Bite, ⅛ bar	7
Fudge Nut Brownie, 1	20
Ice Cream Cone, 1	1
Mixed Berry Granola, 1 serving	5
Mixed Fruit and Yogurt, 1 serving	4
Peanut Butter Cookie, 1	15
Plain Cheesecake, 1 slice	26

	SmartPoints® value
Pumpkin Coffee Cake, 1 slice	18
Strawberry Shortcake, 1 slice	31
Strawberry-Topped Cheesecake, 1 slice	27
Vanilla Ice Cream, 1 serving	11
Whipped Topping, 1 serving	6
White Chocolate Macadamia Nut, 1	15
White Chocolate Raspberry Bite, ⅛ bar	5

Beverages

Citrus Sweet Leaf Green Tea, 1 serving	9
Jason's Deli Bottled Black Cherry, 1 serving	10
Jason's Deli Bottled Cream Soda, 1 serving	10
Jason's Deli Bottled Ginger Ale, 1 serving	9
Jason's Deli Bottled Root Beer, 1 serving	10
Jason's Deli Pomegranate Blueberry Sports Drink, 1 serving	6
Kids Tree Top Apple Juice, 1 serving	6
Peach Sweet Leaf Tea, 1 serving	9
Raspberry Sweet Leaf Tea, 1 serving	9
Sweet Tea, 1 serving	9

"We Like This!" item

8" Sub Sandwiches – French Bread

	SmartPoints® value
BIG JOHN Sandwich on French Bread, 1 sub	10
BOOTLEGGER CLUB Sandwich on French Bread, 1 sandwich	14
CLUB TUNA Sandwich on French Bread, 1 sandwich	30
CLUB TUNA Sandwich on French Bread (without provolone), 1 sandwich	23
J.J.B.L.T Sandwich on French Bread, 1 sub	14
PEPE Sandwich on French Bread, 1 sub	13
PEPE Sandwich on French Bread (without provolone), 1 sub	9
TOTALLY TUNA Sandwich on French Bread, 1 sub	20
TURKEY TOM Sandwich on French Bread, 1 sub	11
ULTIMATE PORKER™ Sandwich on French Bread, 1 sandwich	17
VEGETARIAN Sandwich on French Bread, 1 sub	16
VEGETARIAN Sandwich on French Bread (without provolone), 1 sub	9
VITO Sandwich on French Bread, 1 sub	20
VITO Sandwich on French Bread (without provolone), 1 sub	16

8" Sub Sandwiches – Wheat Bread

	SmartPoints® value
BIG JOHN Sandwich on Wheat Bread, 1 sandwich	12
HUNTERS CLUB Sandwich on Wheat Bread, 1 sandwich	17
J.J.B.L.T Sandwich on Wheat Bread, 1 sandwich	16
PEPE Sandwich on Wheat Bread, 1 sandwich	15
PEPE Sandwich on Wheat Bread (without provolone), 1 sandwich	12
TOTALLY TUNA Sandwich on Wheat Bread, 1 sandwich	22
TURKEY TOM Sandwich on Wheat Bread, 1 sandwich	13
VEGETARIAN Sandwich on Wheat Bread, 1 sandwich	19
VEGETARIAN Sandwich on Wheat Bread (without provolone), 1 sandwich	11
VITO Sandwich on Wheat Bread, 1 sandwich	19

Giant Club Sandwiches – French Bread

	SmartPoints® value
BEACH CLUB Sandwich on French Bread, 1 sandwich	20
BEACH CLUB Sandwich on French Bread (without provolone), 1 sandwich	13
BILLY CLUB Sandwich on French Bread, 1 sandwich	17
BILLY CLUB Sandwich on French Bread (without provolone), 1 sandwich	14
CLUB LULU Sandwich on French Bread, 1 sandwich	17
COUNTRY CLUB Sandwich on French Bread, 1 sandwich	17
COUNTRY CLUB Sandwich on French Bread (without provolone), 1 sandwich	14
GOURMET SMOKED HAM CLUB On French Bread, 1 sandwich	17
GOURMET SMOKED HAM CLUB On French Bread (without p rovolone), 1 sandwich	13
GOURMET VEGGIE CLUB Sandwich on French Bread, 1 sandwich	26
GOURMET VEGGIE CLUB Sandwich on French Bread (without provolone), 1 sandwich	12

Giant Club Sandwiches – French Bread (cont'd)

	SmartPoints® value
HUNTER'S CLUB Sandwich on French Bread, 1 sandwich	17
HUNTER'S CLUB Sandwich on French Bread (without provolone), 1 sandwich	14
ITALIAN NIGHT CLUB Sandwich on French Bread, 1 sandwich	24
ITALIAN NIGHT CLUB Sandwich on French Bread (without provolone), 1 sandwich	20

Giant Club Sandwiches – Wheat Bread

	SmartPoints® value
BEACH CLUB Sandwich on Wheat Bread, 1 sandwich	20
BEACH CLUB Sandwich on Wheat Bread (without provolone), 1 sandwich	12
BILLY CLUB Sandwich on Wheat Bread, 1 sandwich	17
BILLY CLUB Sandwich on Wheat Bread (without provolone), 1 sandwich	14
Bootlegger Club Sandwich, 1 sandwich	14
Club Lulu Sandwich, 1 sandwich	17
COUNTRY CLUB Sandwich on Wheat Bread, 1 sandwich	17
COUNTRY CLUB Sandwich on Wheat Bread (without provolone), 1 sandwich	14
GOURMET SMOKED HAM CLUB Sandwich on Wheat Bread, 1 sandwich	17
GOURMET SMOKED HAM CLUB Sandwich on Wheat Bread (without provolone), 1 sandwich	13
Gourmet Veggie Club Sandwich, 1 sandwich	26
Gourmet Veggie Club Sandwich (without provolone), 1 sandwich	11
HUNTERS CLUB Sandwich on Wheat Bread (without provolone), 1 sandwich	13
ITALIAN NIGHT CLUB Sandwich on Wheat Bread, 1 sandwich	24
ITALIAN NIGHT CLUB Sandwich on Wheat Bread (without provolone), 1 sandwich	20
Tuna Club Sandwich, 1 sandwich	30
Tuna Club Sandwich (without provolone), 1 sandwich	22
Ultimate Poker Sandwich, 1 sandwich	17

Plain Slims – French Bread

	SmartPoints® value
Slim 1 Ham, 1 sandwich	10
Slim 1 Ham & cheese, 1 sandwich	14
Slim 2 Roast Beef, 1 sandwich	11
Slim 3 Tuna Salad, 1 sandwich	21
Slim 4 Turkey Breast, 1 sandwich	10
Slim 5 Salami & Capicola, 1 sandwich	14
Slim 5 Salami, Capicola & Cheese, 1 sandwich	18
Slim 6 Double Provolone, 1 sandwich	16

Low Fat/Low Carb Options

	SmartPoints® value
Beach Club Lettuce Wrap, 1 wrap	10
Beach Club Lettuce Wrap (without provolone), 1 serving	2
BIG JOHN Low Carb Lettuce Wrap, 1 wrap	2
Billy Club Lettuce Wrap, 1 wrap	7
Billy Club Lettuce Wrap (without provolone), 1 wrap	3
Bootlegger Club Lettuce Wrap, 1 wrap	4
Club Lulu Lettuce Wrap, 1 wrap	7
Club Tuna Lettuce Wrap, 1 wrap	19
Club Tuna Lettuce Wrap (without provolone), 1 wrap	12
Country Club Lettuce Wrap, 1 wrap	7

"We Like This!" item

	SmartPoints® value
Country Club Lettuce Wrap (without provolone), 1 wrap	3
Gourmet Smoked Ham Club Lettuce Wrap, 1 wrap	6
Gourmet Smoked Ham Club Lettuce Wrap (without provolone), 1 wrap	3
Gourmet Veggie Club Lettuce Wrap, 1 wrap	15
Gourmet Veggie Club Lettuce Wrap (without provolone), 1 serving	1
Hunter's Club Lettuce Wrap, 1 wrap	7
Hunter's Club Lettuce Wrap (without provolone), 1 serving	3
Italian Night Club Lettuce Wrap, 1 wrap	13
Italian Night Club Lettuce Wrap (without provolone), 1 wrap	10
J.J.B.L.T Low Carb Lettuce Wrap, 1 wrap	5
PEPE Low Carb Lettuce Wrap, 1 wrap	5
PEPE Low Carb Lettuce Wrap (without provolone), 1 wrap	2
Slim 1 Ham & Cheese Lettuce Wrap, 1 sandwich	5
Slim 1 Ham Lettuce Wrap, 1 wrap	1
Slim 2 Roast Beef Lettuce Wrap, 1 wrap	1
Slim 3 Tuna Salad Lettuce Wrap, 1 wrap	12
Slim 4 Turkey Breast Lettuce Wrap, 1 wrap	2
Slim 5 Salami & Capicola Lettuce Wrap, 1 wrap	5
Slim 5 Salami, Capicola & Cheese Lettuce Wrap, 1 wrap	9
Slim 6 Double Provolone Lettuce Wrap, 1 wrap	7
TOTALLY TUNA Low Carb Lettuce Wrap, 1 wrap	12
TURKEY TOM Low Carb Lettuce Wrap, 1 wrap	3
Ultimate Porker Lettuce Wrap, 1 wrap	6
VEGETARIAN Low Carb Lettuce Wrap, 1 wrap	8
VEGETARIAN Low Carb Lettuce Wrap (without provolone), 1 wrap	1
VITO Low Carb Lettuce Wrap, 1 wrap	9

Plain Slims – Wheat Bread

Slim 1 Ham, 1 sandwich	11
Slim 1 Ham & Cheese, 1 sandwich	15
Slim 2 Roast Beef, 1 sandwich	12
Slim 3 Tuna Salad, 1 sandwich	22
Slim 4 Turkey Breast, 1 sandwich	12
Slim 5 Salami & Capicola, 1 sandwich	15
Slim 5 Salami, Capicola & Cheese, 1 sandwich	19
Slim 6 Double Provolone, 1 sandwich	17

Sides

Avocado Spread, 1 serving	0
BBQ Potato Chips, 1 oz	5
Giant Chocolate Chip Cookie, 1 cookie	19
Giant Oatmeal Raisin Cookie, 1 cookie	16
Hot Peppers, 11 pieces	0
Jalapeño Potato Chips, 1 oz	5
Jumbo Kosher Dill Pickle, 1 serving	1
Reduced Fat Potato Chips, 1 oz	4
Regular Potato Chips, 1 oz	5
Salt & Vinegar Potato Chips, 1 oz	5
Sprouts, 1 serving	0

Burgers & Sandwiches

	SmartPoints® value
Artisan Grilled Chicken Sandwich, 1 serving	9
Bacon and Cheese Sirloin Third Pound Burger, 1 serving	26
Bacon Buffalo Ranch McChicken, 1	13
Bacon Cheddar McChicken, 1	15
Bacon Clubhouse Burger, 1	24
Bacon Clubhouse Crispy Chicken Sandwich, 1	24
Bacon Clubhouse Grilled Chicken Sandwich, 1	17
Bacon McDouble, 1	14
BBQ Ranch Burger, 1	11
Big Mac, 1	17
Buffalo Ranch McChicken, 1	11
Buttermilk Crispy Chicken Deluxe Sandwich, 1 serving	17
Cheeseburger, 1	10
Daily Double, 1	14
Double Cheeseburger, 1	14
Double Quarter Pounder with Cheese, 1	25
Hamburger, 1	8
Lettuce and Tomato Sirloin Third Pound Burger, 1 serving	25
McDouble, 1	13
McRib, 1	17
Premium Crispy Chicken Deluxe Sandwich, 1 serving	16
Premium McWrap Chicken & Bacon (crispy), 1	19
Premium McWrap Chicken & Bacon (grilled), 1	14
Premium McWrap Chicken & Ranch (crispy), 1	19
Premium McWrap Chicken & Ranch (grilled), 1	13
Premium McWrap Chicken Sweet Chili (crispy), 1	17
Premium McWrap Chicken Sweet Chili (grilled), 1	11
Quarter Pounder Deluxe, 1	20
Quarter Pounder with Cheese, 1	18
Ranch Snack Wrap (crispy), 1	11
Ranch Snack Wrap (grilled), 1	8
Steakhouse Sirloin Third Pound Burger, 1 serving	24

Chicken & Fish

	SmartPoints® value
Chicken McNuggets, 10 pieces	13
Chicken McNuggets, 20 pieces	27
Chicken McNuggets, 4 pieces	5
Chicken McNuggets, 40 pieces	54
Chicken McNuggets, 6 pieces	8
Chicken Selects, 3 pieces	10
Filet O Fish, 1	12
McChicken, 1	11
Southern Style Buttermilk Crispy Chicken Sandwich, 1	13
Southern Style Chicken Biscuit (large size biscuit), 1	16
Southern Style Chicken Biscuit (regular size biscuit), 1	13

Salads

	SmartPoints® value
Premium Asian Salad (without chicken), 1 serving	5
Premium Asian Salad with Crispy Chicken, 1 serving	12
Premium Asian Salad with Grilled Chicken, 1 serving	7
Premium Bacon Ranch Salad (without chicken), 1 serving	6
Premium Bacon Ranch Salad with Crispy Chicken, 1 serving	12
Premium Bacon Ranch Salad with Grilled Chicken (no dressing), 1 serving	8
Premium Southwest Salad (without chicken), 1 serving	5
Premium Southwest Salad with Crispy Chicken, 1 serving	14
Premium Southwest Salad with Grilled Chicken, 1 serving	9
Side Salad (no dressing), 1 serving	0

"We Like This!" item

Snacks & Sides

	SmartPoints® value
Apple Slices, 1 serving	0
Baked Hot Apple Pie, 1	11
Baked Mozzarella Sticks, 3 pieces	6
Chocolate Chip Cookie, 1	7
French Fries, 1 large	16
French Fries, 1 medium	11
French Fries, 1 small	7
French Fries (kids), 1 serving	4
Fried Cherry Pie, 1 serving	10
Fruit 'n Yogurt Parfait, 1	7
Grilled Onion Cheddar, 1	10
Hash Browns, 1	5
Mac Snack Wrap, 1	11
Oatmeal Raisin Cookie, 1	7

Breakfast

	SmartPoints® value
Bacon, Egg, & Cheese Bagel, 1	20
Bacon, Egg, & Cheese Bagel with Egg Whites, 1 serving	18
Bacon, Egg, & Cheese Biscuit (large size biscuit), 1	18
Bacon, Egg, & Cheese Biscuit (regular size biscuit), 1	16
Bacon, Egg, & Cheese Biscuit with Egg Whites (large size biscuit), 1 serving	16
Bacon, Egg, & Cheese Biscuit with Egg Whites (regular size biscuit), 1 serving	14
Bacon, Egg, & Cheese McGriddles, 1	16
Bacon, Egg, & Cheese McGriddles with Egg Whites, 1 serving	14
Big Breakfast (large size biscuit), 1	27
Big Breakfast (regular size biscuit), 1	25
Big Breakfast with Egg Whites (large size biscuit), 1 serving	23
Big Breakfast with Egg Whites (regular size biscuit), 1 serving	21
Big Breakfast with Hotcakes (large size biscuit), 1 serving	39
Big Breakfast with Hotcakes (regular size biscuit), 1 serving	37
Big Breakfast with Hotcakes and Egg Whites (large size biscuit), 1 serving	35
Big Breakfast with Hotcakes and Egg Whites (regular size biscuit), 1 serving	33
Egg McMuffin, 1	9
Egg White Delight, 1 serving	7
Fruit & Maple Oatmeal, 1 serving	13
Fruit & Maple Oatmeal without Brown Sugar, 1 serving	10
Hotcake Syrup, 1 packet	9
Hotcakes, 1	12
Hotcakes and Sausage, 1 serving	18
Sausage Biscuit (large size biscuit), 1	17
Sausage Biscuit (regular size biscuit), 1	15
Sausage Biscuit with Egg (large size biscuit), 1	20
Sausage Biscuit with Egg (regular Size biscuit), 1	18
Sausage Biscuit with Egg Whites (large size biscuit), 1 serving	18
Sausage Biscuit with Egg Whites (regular size biscuit), 1 serving	16
Sausage Burrito, 1 serving	10
Sausage McGriddles, 1 serving	16
Sausage McMuffin, 1	12
Sausage McMuffin with Egg, 1	15
Sausage McMuffin with Egg Whites, 1 serving	13
Sausage, Egg, & Cheese McGriddles, 1 serving	20
Sausage, Egg, & Cheese McGriddles with Egg Whites, 1 serving	18
Steak & Egg Biscuit (regular size biscuit), 1 serving	19
Steak & Egg McMuffin, 1 serving	13
Steak, Egg, & Cheese Bagel, 1 serving	22

Condiments

	SmartPoints® value
Creamy Ranch Sauce, 1 packet	4
Grape Jam, 1 serving	2
Honey, 1 packet	3
Honey Mustard Sauce, 1 packet	3
Hot Habanero Sauce, 1 packet	3
Jalapeño Double, 1	14
Ketchup, 1 packet	1
Marinara Sauce, 1 package	1
Salt Packet, 1 packet	0
Spicy Buffalo Sauce, 1 packet	1
Strawberry Preserves, 1 serving	2
Sugar, 1 packet	1
Sweet 'N Sour Sauce, 1 packet	3
Tangy Barbeque Sauce, 1 packet	3
Tartar Sauce, 1 packet	5
Whipped Margarine, 1 pat	2

Desserts & Shakes

	SmartPoints® value
Cinnamon Melts, 1	20
Hot Caramel Sundae, 1 serving	16
Hot Fudge Sundae, 1 serving	17
Kiddie Cone (includes ice cream), 1	2
McFlurry with M&M'S Candies, 12 fl oz cup	33
McFlurry with OREO Cookies, 12 fl oz cup	25
Oreo Frappe, 1 small	27
Peanuts (for sundaes), 1 serving	1
Pumpkin and Creme Pie, 1 serving	12
Shamrock McCafe Shake, 12 fl oz	27
Snack Size McFlurry with M&M'S Candies, 1 serving	22
Snack Size McFlurry with OREO Cookies, 1 serving	16
Strawberry and Creme Pie, 1 serving	13
Strawberry McCafe Shake, 12 fl oz	28
Strawberry Sundae, 1 serving	14
Sweet Potato and Creme Pie, 1 serving	13
Vanilla McCafe Shake, 12 fl oz	25
Vanilla Reduced Fat Ice Cream Cone, 1	8

Beverages

	SmartPoints® value
Blueberry Pomegranate Smoothie, 12 fl oz	12
Caramel Latte, 12 fl oz	13
Chocolate McCafe Shake, 12 fl oz	28
Coffee Cream, 1	1
Frappe Caramel, 12 fl oz	23
Frappe Chocolate Chip, 12 fl oz	27
Frappe Mocha, 12 fl oz	23
French Vanilla Latte, 12 fl oz	13
Frozen Classic Lemonade, 1 small	9
Frozen Strawberry Lemonade, 1 small	11
Hazelnut Latte, 12 fl oz	13
Hot Chocolate with Nonfat Milk, 12 fl oz	13
Iced Classic Lemonade, 1 small	6
Iced Coffee Caramel, 16 fl oz	7
Iced Coffee French Vanilla, 16 fl oz	7
Iced Coffee Hazelnut, 16 fl oz	7
Iced Coffee Regular, 16 fl oz	8
Iced Coffee with Sugar Free French Vanilla Syrup, 16 fl oz	3
Iced Mocha with Nonfat Milk, 12 fl oz	11
Iced Nonfat Caramel Mocha, 12 fl oz	11
Iced Strawberry Lemonade, 1 small	7

"We Like This!" item

	SmartPoints® value
Iced Tea, 12 fl oz	0
Latte with Sugar Free French Vanilla Syrup, 12 fl oz	8
Mango Pineapple Smoothie, 12 fl oz	12
McCafe Caramel Mocha, 12 fl oz	15
McCafe Hot Chocolate, 12 fl oz	17
McCafe Iced Caramel Mocha, 12 fl oz	13
McCafe Iced Mocha, 12 fl oz	14
McCafe Latte, 12 fl oz	7
McCafe Latte with Nonfat Milk, 12 fl oz	4
McCafe Mocha, 12 fl oz	16
McCafe White Chocolate Mocha, 12 fl oz	15
McCafe White Hot Chocolate, 1 small	17
Mocha with Nonfat Milk, 12 fl oz	13
Nonfat Caramel Latte, 12 fl oz	10
Nonfat Caramel Mocha, 12 fl oz	12
Nonfat French Vanilla Latte, 12 fl oz	9
Nonfat Hazelnut Latte, 12 fl oz	10

	SmartPoints® value
Nonfat Latte with Sugar Free French Vanilla Syrup, 12 fl oz	5
Nonfat White Hot Chocolate, 1 small	13
Premium Roast Iced Coffee, 16 fl oz	8
Southern Style Frozen Lemonade, 1 small	14
Southern Style Frozen Strawberry Lemonade, 1 small	16
Southern Style Iced Lemonade, 1 small	8
Southern Style Iced Strawberry Lemonade, 1 small	10
Strawberry Banana Smoothie, 12 fl oz	11
Sweet Tea, 12 fl oz	7

Appetizers

	SmartPoints® value
Antipasti Italian Meats & Cheese Topper, 1 serving	12
Artichoke Fritti, 1 serving	15
Breadstick (with garlic butter spread), 1 serving	4
Bruschetta Caprese, 1 serving	21
Calamari (create a sampler portion), 1 serving	10
Chicken Fingers (create a sampler portion), 1 serving	5
Classic Calamari, 1 serving	19
Classic Shrimp Scampi Fritta, 1 serving	19
Crispy Chicken Fritta, 1 serving	6
Crispy Risotto Bites, 1 serving	11
Fried Mozzarella (create a sampler portion), 1 serving	11
Fried Zucchini (create a sampler portion), 1 serving	12
Lasagna Fritta, 1 serving	37
Smoked Mozzarella Fonduta, 1 serving	32
Stuffed Mushrooms (create a sampler portion), 1 serving	13
Toasted Beef & Pork Ravioli (create a sampler portion), 1 serving	10

Dinner Entrées

	SmartPoints® value
Asiago Garlic Alfredo, 1 serving	43
Baked Parmesan Shrimp, 1 serving	31
Baked Tilapia with Shrimp, 1 serving	8
Braised Beef & Tortelloni, 1 serving	41
Cavatappi, 1 serving	13
Cheese Ravioli with Marinara Sauce, 1 serving	26
Cheese Ravioli with Meat Sauce, 1 serving	29
Chicken & Shrimp Carbonara, 1 serving	59
Chicken Alfredo, 1 serving	56
Chicken Marsala, 1 serving	28
Chicken Meatballs, 2	5
Chicken Parmigiana, 1 serving	31
Chicken Picata Mediterranean Fresh Lighter Fare, 1 serving	14
Chicken Scampi, 1 serving	27
Citrus Chicken Sorrento, 1 serving	15
Creamy Chicken Firenze, 1 serving	46
Eggplant Parmigiana, 1 serving	34
Fettuccine Alfredo, 1 serving	42
Five Cheese Marinara, 1 serving	20
Five Cheese Ziti Al Forno, 1 serving	45
Florentine Rollatini, 1 serving	28
Florentine Rollatini with Chicken, 1 serving	34
Garlic Rosemary Chicken, 1 serving	13
Grilled Chicken (add on), 1 serving	2
Grilled Shrimp (add on), 1 serving	1
Herb Grilled Salmon (gluten free), 1 serving	12
Italian Sausage, 2 links	16
Lasagna Classico, 1 serving	34
Meatballs, 3	13
Pappardelle Pescatore, 1 serving	28
Pappardelle Portobello Alfredo, 1 serving	54
Pecorino Parmesan Ravioli with Shrimp, 1 serving	35
Ravioli Di Portobello, 1 serving	30
Rigatoni, 1 serving	13
Rotini (gluten free), 1 serving	12
Rotini Primavera (dinner), 1 serving	33
Rotini with Marinara (dinner), 1 serving	16

"We Like This!" item

	SmartPoints® value
Rotini with Meat Sauce (dinner), 1 serving	20
Sausage Stuffed Giant Rigatoni, 1 serving	34
Seafood Alfredo, 1 serving	45
Shrimp Alfredo, 1 serving	43
Shrimp Fresco, 1 serving	6
Spaghetti, 1 serving	8
Spaghetti with Chicken Meatballs, 1 serving	27
Spaghetti with Italian Sausage, 1 serving	38
Spaghetti with Meatballs, 1 serving	35
Spicy Calamari, 1 serving	25
Spicy Shrimp Scampi Fritta, 1 serving	17
Steak Gorgonzola Alfredo, 1 serving	50
Steak Toscano, 1 serving	25
Steak Toscano (gluten free), 1 serving	20
Stuffed Chicken Marsala, 1 serving	30
Tortellini Al Forno, 1 serving	16
Tour Of Italy, 1 serving	54
Tri Colored Vegetable Penne, 1 serving	10
Tuscan Three Meat Fettuccine, 1 serving	28
Whole Wheat Linguine, 1 serving	12

Lunch Entrées

	SmartPoints® value
Breadstick Bun Chicken Parmigiana, 1 serving	17
Breadstick Bun Italian Meatball, 1 serving	21
Cheese Ravioli with Marinara Sauce, 1 serving	20
Cheese Ravioli with Meat Sauce, 1 serving	22
Chicken Alfredo, 1 serving	39
Chicken Parmigiana, 1 serving	20
Chicken Scampi, 1 serving	30
Citrus Chicken Sorrento, 1 serving	13
Eggplant Parmigiana, 1 serving	22
Fettuccine Alfredo, 1 serving	27
Fettuccine Alfredo Pasta Bowl, 1 serving	20
Five Cheese Ziti Al Forno, 1 serving	25
Garden Primavera, 1 serving	18
Garlic Rosemary Chicken, 1 serving	11
Grilled Chicken Caesar Salad, 1 serving	11
Italian Mac & Cheese Pasta Bowl, 1 serving	19
Lasagna Classico, 1 serving	22
Parmesan Garlic Fries, 1 serving	8
Ravioli Di Portobello, 1 serving	21
Risotto Bites, 1 serving	11
Rotini Primavera, 1 serving	20
Rotini with Marinara, 1 serving	11
Rotini with Meat Sauce, 1 serving	14
Seafood Alfredo, 1 serving	29
Shrimp Fresco, 1 serving	4
Spaghetti with Chicken Meatballs, 1 serving	19
Spaghetti with Italian Sausage, 1 serving	31
Spaghetti with Meat Sauce, 1 serving	15
Spaghetti with Meat Sauce - Tuscan Duos/Trios, 1 serving	8
Spaghetti with Meatballs, 1 serving	24
Tortellini Al Forno Mini Pasta Bowl, 1 serving	16
Tri Colored Penne with Basil Garlic Bowl, 1 serving	10

Flatbreads

	SmartPoints® value
Grilled Chicken Flatbread, 1 serving	25
Grilled Chicken Flatbread (lunch), 1 serving	25
Mediterranean Flatbread, 1 serving	23
Mediterranean Flatbread (lunch), 1 serving	23
Pizzaiola Flatbread, 1 serving	23

Soups & Salads

	SmartPoints® value
Chicken & Gnocchi Soup, 1 serving	8
Famous House Salad & Dressing without Croutons, 1 serving	4
Famous House Salad (with dressing), 1 serving	5
Famous House Salad (with low fat dressing), 1 serving	3
Famous House Salad (without dressing), 1 serving	2
Grilled Chicken Caesar Salad, 1 serving	11
Grilled Chicken Salad Topper, 1 serving	2
Minestrone Soup, 1 serving	3
Pasta e Fagioli Soup, 1 serving	6
Zuppa Toscana, 1 serving	8

Sauces

	SmartPoints® value
Alfredo Dipping Sauce, 1 serving	20
Alfredo Sauce (kids create your own pasta), 1 serving	15
Citrus Aioli Sauce, 1 serving	11
Five Cheese Marinara Dipping Sauce, 1 serving	9
Fresco Sauce, 1 serving	6
Garlic White Wine Sauce, 1 serving	20
Marinara Dipping Sauce, 1 serving	3
Marinara Sauce, 1 serving	2
Meat Sauce (kids create your own pasta), 1 serving	4
Parmesan Peppercorn Sauce, 1 serving	11
Primavera Sauce (gluten free), 1 serving	21
Tomato Sauce, 1 serving	2
Tomato Sauce (kids create your own pasta), 1 serving	3
Traditional Meat Sauce, 1 serving	11

Kids' Selections

	SmartPoints® value
Apple Juice, 1 serving	2
Cavatappi, 1 serving	6
Cheese Pizza, 1 serving	13
Cheese Ravioli, 1 serving	12
Cheese Tortelloni, 1 serving	10
Chicken Fingers & Pasta, 1 serving	11
Cranberry Juice, 1 serving	4
Fettuccine, 1 serving	5
Grapes, 1 serving	0
Grilled Chicken, 1 serving	12
Herb Grilled Salmon, 1 serving	12
Italian Sausage, 1 serving	8
Macaroni & Cheese, 1 serving	11
Meatball, 1 serving	4
Orange Juice, 1 serving	4
Peach Mango Smoothie (kids), 1 serving	10
Pepperoni, 1 serving	3
Raspberry Lemonade, 1 serving	6
Rotini with Marinara, 1 serving	9
Rotini with Meat Sauce, 1 serving	12
Shrimp, 1 serving	0
Small Shells, 1 serving	6
Spaghetti, 1 serving	4
Steamed Broccoli, 1 serving	0
Strawberry Smoothie, 1 serving	11
Sundae, 1 serving	7
Whole Wheat Linguine, 1 serving	7

"We Like This!" item

Desserts

	SmartPoints® value
Amaretto Tiramisu, 1 serving	10
Black Tie Mousse Cake, 1 serving	38
Chocolate Mousse Cake, 1 serving	17
Chocolate Mousse Mini Dessert, 1 serving	11
Dark Chocolate Caramel Cream, 1 serving	12
Lemon Cream Cake, 1 serving	26
Limoncello Mousse, 1 serving	14
Strawberry & White Chocolate Cake, 1 serving	9
Tiramisu, 1 serving	22
Vanilla Panna Cotta with Fresh Blueberries, 1 serving	24
White Chocolate Raspberry Cheesecake, 1 serving	36
Zeppoli, 1 serving	27

Dessert Sauces

	SmartPoints® value
Chocolate Sauce, 1 serving	12
Raspberry Sauce, 1 serving	11

Beverage Selections

	SmartPoints® value
Apple Juice, 1 serving	5
Bellini Peach Raspberry Iced Tea, 1 serving	6
Berry Bianco Spritzer, 1 serving	5
Berry Sangria Glass, 1 serving	7
Berry Sangria Pitcher, 1 serving	29
Caffe Latte, 1 serving	6
Caffe Mocha, 1 serving	20
Cappuccino, 1 serving	4
Cappuccino with Whipped Cream, 1 serving	7
Caramel Hazelnut Macchiato, 1 serving	10
Chocolate Almond Amore, 1 serving	21
Cranberry Juice, 1 serving	10
Fresh Brewed Iced Tea, 1 serving	0
Frozen Cappuccino, 1 serving	18
Hot Chocolate, 1 serving	18
Italian Margarita, 1 serving	8
Kiwi Melon Frozen Limonata, 1 serving	5
Kiwi Melon Limonata, 1 serving	10
Lavazza Espresso, 1 serving	2
Long Island Limoncello, 1 serving	10
Mango Martini, 1 serving	6
Moscato Citrus Berry Cocktail, 1 serving	13
Orange Juice, 1 serving	8
Peach Bellini, 1 serving	12
Peach Mango Smoothie, 1 serving	16
Peach Sangria Glass, 1 serving	8
Peach Sangria Pitcher, 1 serving	32
Pineapple Juice, 1 serving	13
Raspberry Lemonade, 1 serving	10
Sangarita, 1 serving	9
Strawberry Frozen Margarita, 1 serving	11
Strawberry Mango Frozen Margarita, 1 serving	11
Strawberry Passion Fruit Frozen Limonata, 1 serving	4
Strawberry Passion Fruit Limonata, 1 serving	10
Strawberry Smoothie, 1 serving	18
Traditional Margarita, 1 serving	11

Appetizers

Item	SmartPoints® value
Alice Springs Chicken Quesadillas (Aussie-tizer to share), 1 serving	53
Aussie Cheese Fries Aussie-tizer, 1 small	42
Aussie Cheese Fries Aussie-tizer (regular), 1 serving	63
Bloomin Onion (serves 6), 1 serving	75
Chicken Artichoke Flatbread, 1 serving	8
Coconut Shrimp Aussi-tizers to Share (serves 2), 1 serving	25
Crab and Avocado Stack Aussi-tizers to Share, 1 serving	21
Crab Stack, 1 serving	12
Spinach Artichoke Dip, 1 serving	9
Tomato Mozzarella Caprese, 1 serving	21
Wings Aussie-tizer to Share, 1 serving	39
Wings with Hot Sauce, 1 serving	16
Wings with Medium Sauce, 1 serving	17
Wings with Mild Sauce, 1 serving	16

Under 600 Calories

Item	SmartPoints® value
4 oz Lobster Tails (2 steamed) and Light Balsamic Vinaigrett House Salad, 1 serving	16
4 oz Lobster Tails (2 Steamed) and Tangy Tomato House Salad, 1 serving	15
Asian Sesame Salad with Chicken, 1 serving	15
California Chicken Salad with Light Balsamic Vinaigrette, 1 serving	19
Chicken Artichoke Flatbread, 1 serving	16
Crab and Avocado Stack, 1 serving	18
Crab Stuffed Mushroom, 1 serving	16
Grilled Chicken on the Barbie with Fresh Seasonal Mixed Veggies, 1 serving	10
Grilled Shrimp on the Barbie, 1 serving	5
Norwegian Salmon, 1 serving	13
Outback Special (6 oz) with Mixed Veggies And Tangy Tomato House Salad, 1 serving	16
Outback Special (6 oz) with Mixed Veggies and Light Balsamic Vinaigrette House Salad, 1 serving	17
Perfectly Grilled Salmon, 1 serving	13
Seared Ahi Tuna (regular under 600 calories), 1 serving	14
Simply Grilled Mahi with Mixed Vegetables, 1 serving	9
Simply Grilled Mahi without Sides, 1 serving	3
Victoria's Filet (6 oz) with Mixed Veggies And Light Balsamic Vinaigrette House Salad, 1 serving	16
Victoria's Filet (6 oz) with Mixed Veggies And Tangy Tomato House Salad, 1 serving	15

Steaks

Item	SmartPoints® value
10 oz New York Strip, 1 serving	15
10 oz Ribeye Steak (no sides), 1 serving	15
12 oz Outback Sirloin (no sides), 1 serving	11
12 oz Sirloin and Coconut Shrimp (no sides), 1 serving	26
12 oz Sirloin and Grilled Shrimp on the Barbie (no sides), 1 serving	14
12 oz Slow Roasted Prime Rib (no sides), 1 serving	45
14 oz New York Strip (no sides), 1 serving	12
16 oz Slow Roasted Prime Rib (no sides), 1 serving	61
6 oz Outback Sirloin (no sides), 1 serving	5

"We Like This!" item

	SmartPoints® value
6 oz Sirloin and Coconut Shrimp, 1 serving	16
6 oz Sirloin and Coconut Shrimp (no sides), 1 serving	19
6 oz Sirloin and Grilled Shrimp (no sides), 1 serving	10
6 oz Sirloin with Grilled Shrimp on the Barbie (no sides), 1 serving	10
8 oz Slow Roasted Prime Rib (no sides), 1 serving	30
9 oz Outback Sirloin (no sides), 1 serving	8
9 oz Sirloin and Coconut Shrimp (no sides), 1 serving	23
9 oz Sirloin and Grilled Shrimp on the Barbie (no sides), 1 serving	10
9 oz Sirloin with Grilled Shrimp on the Barbie (no sides), 1 serving	10
Filet (6 oz) and Lobster Tail (4 oz), 1 serving	20
Filet and Grilled Shrimp On The Barbie, 1 serving	11
Filet with Wild Mushroom Sauce, 1 serving	8
Herb Roasted Prime Rib, 1 serving	24
Outback flat Iron Steak (no sides), 1 serving	12
Outback Special, 12 oz	11
Outback Special, 6 oz	5
Outback Special, 9 oz	8
Porterhouse, 22 oz	34
Prime Rib with Aujus, 12 oz	12
Prime Rib with Aujus, 16 oz	16
Prime Rib with Aujus, 8 oz	8
Ribeye Grilled Steak, 10 oz	15
Ribeye Grilled Steak, 14 oz	22
Ribeye Skewer, 1 serving	29
Ribeye Steak, 14 oz	21
Sirloin Diablo, 1 serving	10
Sirloin with Wild Mushroom Sauce, 1 serving	7
Teriyaki Filet Medallions (no sides), 1 serving	8
The Bloomin' Sirloin, 1 serving	9
Victoria's Filet, 6 oz	4

	SmartPoints® value
Victoria's Filet, 8 oz	4
Woodfire grilled Prime Rib with Aujus, 12 oz	13
Woodfire grilled Prime Rib with Aujus, 16 oz	17
Woodfire grilled Prime Rib with Aujus, 8 oz	9
WoodFire Herb Roasted Prime Rib, 12 oz	37
WoodFire Herb Roasted Prime Rib, 16 oz	49

Straight From the Sea

2 Lobster Tails, 5 oz	13
7 oz Perfectly Grilled Salmon (no sides), 1 serving	9
Coconut Shrimp, 4	10
Coconut Shrimp (add ons), 1 serving	15
Grilled Scallops, 4	13
Grilled Scallops (add on), 1 serving	6
Grilled Shrimp, 4	8
Grilled Shrimp, 8	12
Grilled Shrimp (add on), 1 serving	6
Grilled Shrimp on the Barbie Aussi-tizers to Share, 1 serving	18
Hearts of Gold Mahi, 1 serving	19
Hearts of Gold Mahi (no sides), 1 serving	10
Lobster, 5 oz	12
Lobster Tails, 4 oz	13
Royal Port Tilapia, 1 serving	25
Seafood Mixed Grill, 1 serving	21
Snow Crab, ½ lb	11
Tilapia with Pure Lump Crab Meat (no sides), 1 serving	11
WoodFire Grilled Ahi Tuna, 1 serving	14

Chicken, Ribs, Chops, & More

Alice Springs Chicken (lunch), 5 oz	14
Alice Springs Chicken (no sides), 1 serving	21

Chicken, Ribs, Chops, & More (cont'd)

	SmartPoints® value
Baby Back Ribs (no sides), ½ order	19
Baby Back Ribs (no sides), full order	27
Braized Short Ribs, 1 serving	31
Chicken on the Barbie (regular), 1 serving	5
Chicken Tender Platter (no sides), 1 serving	35
Grilled Chicken, 5 oz	11
Grilled Chicken on the Barbie (no sides), 1 serving	5
Hand-Breaded Chicken Tenders Buffalo Style, 1 serving	27
New Zealand Rack Of Lamb (no sides), 1 serving	18
Parmesan Herb Crusted Chicken (no sides), 1 serving	13
Pork Porterhouse (no sides), 1 serving	12
Rack of Lamb, 12 oz	19
Ribs and Chicken On The Barbie (no sides), 1 serving	13
Sweet Glazed Pork Tenderloin, 1 serving	6
WoodFire Grilled Pork Chop, 1 pork chop	10

Burgers and Sandwiches

	SmartPoints® value
Aged Cheddar Bacon Burger, 1 serving	34
Bloomin Burger (no sides), 1 serving	38
Classic Cheeseburger with American Cheese, 1 serving	27
Classic Cheeseburger with Cheddar, 1 serving	29
Classic Cheeseburger with Provolone, 1 serving	30
Classic Cheeseburger with Swiss Cheese, 1 serving	29
Crispy Chicken Sandwich (no sides), 1 serving	25
Double Burger (no sides), 1 serving	32
Filet Focaccia Sandwich, 1 serving	21
Grilled Chicken and Swiss Sandwich, 1 serving	21
Prime Burger, 1 serving	31
Prime Rib Dip Sandwich, 1 serving	29
Ribeye Melt Steak Sandwich (no sides), 1 serving	30
Steak Flatbread Sandwich, 1 serving	29
The Outbacker Burger (no cheese no sides), 1 serving	21
The Outbacker Burger with American, 1 serving	27
The Outbacker Burger with Swiss, 1 serving	29
Wood Grilled California Chicken Sandwich (no sides), 1 serving	16
Woodfire Grilled Chicken Flatbread Sandwich, 1 serving	31

Joey Menu

	SmartPoints® value
Joey Boomerang Cheese Burger, 1 serving	16
Joey Chicken Fingers, 1 serving	16
Joey Grilled Cheese-A-Roo, 1 serving	9
Joey Grilled Chicken on the Barbie, 1 serving	1
Joey Junior Ribs, 1 serving	9
Joey Mac-A-Roo 'N Cheese, 1 serving	17
Joey Sirloin, 1 serving	5
Joey Sirloin Medallions, 1 serving	5
Joey Sirloin Medallions with Apple Juice, 1 serving	5
Kids Live Well Grilled Chicken with Apple Juice, 1 serving	8
Kids Live Well Grilled Chicken with Orange Juice, 1 serving	7
Kids Live Well Sirloin Medalliions with Apple Juice, 1 serving	10
Kids Live Well Sirloin Medalliions with Orange Juice, 1 serving	9

"We Like This!" item

Soups and Salads

Item	SmartPoints® value
Aussie Chicken Cobb Salad Crispy, 1 serving	28
Aussie Chicken Cobb Salad Fried (dressing not included), 1 serving	30
Aussie Chicken Cobb Salad Grilled, 1 serving	14
Blue Cheese Pecan Chopped Salad, 1 serving	12
Caesar Salad, 1 serving	3
Caesar Salad (dressing included), 1 serving	12
Caesar Salad Chicken, 1 serving	17
Caesar Salad Shrimp, 1 serving	16
California Chicken Salad (dressing included), 1 serving	24
Chicken Caesar Salad (dressing included), 1 serving	18
Chicken Tortilla Soup, 1 bowl	10
Chicken Tortilla Soup, 1 cup	6
Clam Chowder, 1 bowl	26
Clam Chowder, 1 cup	13
Classic Blue Cheese Wedge Salad, 1 serving	4
Classic Blue Cheese Wedge Salad (dressing included), 1 serving	16
Filet Wedge Salad, 1 serving	20
French Onion Soup, 1 serving	16
House Salad with Blue Cheese Dressing, 1 serving	12
House Salad with Honey Mustard Dressing, 1 serving	12
House Salad with Mustard Vinaigrette Dressing, 1 serving	13
House Salad with Ranch Dressing, 1 serving	12
House Salad with Tangy Tomato Dressing, 1 serving	7
House Salad with Thousand Island Dressing, 1 serving	12
House Salad without Dressing, 1 serving	4
Potato Soup, 1 bowl	18
Potato Soup, 1 cup	10
Sesame Salad with Ahi Tuna, 1 serving	6
Sesame Salad with Grilled Chicken, 1 serving	5
Sesame Salad with Salmon, 1 serving	13
Shrimp Caesar Salad (dressing included), 1 serving	18
Shrimp Caesar Salad (under 600 calories), 1 serving	16
Steakhouse Salad, 1 serving	30

Dressings, Sauces, & Toppings

Item	SmartPoints® value
Au Jus (add on), 1½ oz	0
Barbeque Sauce, 1½ oz	3
Bloomin Onion Sauce, 1½ oz	8
Blue Cheese Dressing, 1½ oz	8
Blue Cheese Vinaigrette Dressing, 1½ oz	10
Butter, 1 serving	6
Butter and Sour Cream, 1 serving	4
Cabernet Wine Sauce, 1½ oz	3
Caesar Dressing, 3 oz	12
Honey Butter, 1 serving	5
Honey Mustard Dressing, 1½ oz	9
Honey Salsa Vinaigrette Dressing, 1½ oz	6
Horseradish Crumb Crust, 1 serving	13
Horseradish Crumb Topping, 1 serving	10
Hot Sauce, 1 serving	8
Light Balsamic, 1½ oz	3
Medium Sauce, 1 serving	9
Mild Sauce, 1 serving	4
Mustard Vinaigrette Dressing, 1½ oz	9
Mustard Vinaigrette Dressing, 3 oz	17
Orange Marmalade, 1½ oz	6
Ranch Dressing, 1½ oz	7
Ranch Dressing, 3 oz	15
Raspberry Sauce, 1 oz	4
Remoulade Sauce, 1½ oz	7
Sour Cream, 1 serving	2

	SmartPoints® value
Soy Dressing, 1½ oz	7
Tangy Tomato Dressing, 1½ oz	2
Thousand Island Dressing, 1½ oz	8
Wasabi Vinaigrette Dressing, 1½ oz	6
Wild Mushroom Sauce, 1 serving	3

Sides

Aussie Fries (sides), 1 serving	11
Baked Potato Everything, 1 serving	12
Bread and Butter, 1 serving	5
Broccoli and Cheese, 1 serving	15
Bushman Shrooms, 1 serving	27
Dressed Baked Potato, 1 serving	7
Dressed Baked Potato with Butter, 1 serving	13
Dressed Baked Potato with Butter And Sour Cream, 1 serving	11
Dressed Baked Potato with Sour Cream, 1 serving	9
Fresh Seasonal Mixed Veggies, 1 serving	6
Fresh Steamed Broccoli, 1 serving	5
Fresh Steamed French Green Beans, 1 serving	2
Garlic Mashed Potatoes, 1 serving	10
Green Beans, 1 serving	2
Grilled Asparagus (premium sides), 1 serving	2
Loaded Mashed Potatoes, 1 serving	12
Sauteed Mushrooms, 1 serving	5
Seasoned Rice, 1 serving	11
Steakhouse Mac and Cheese, 1 serving	30
Sweet Potato (everything), 1 serving	16
Sweet Potato (plain), 1 serving	10
Sweet Potato Fries, 1 serving	18
Sweet Potato with Brown Sugar, 1 serving	14
Sweet Potato with Honey Butter, 1 serving	16

Extras

Bacon, 1 serving	1
Blue Cheese Crumbles, 1 serving	4
Brown Sugar, 1 serving	3
Cheese, 1 serving	1
Chives, 1 serving	0

Desserts

Carrotcake Lollipop (under 600 calories), 1 serving	11
Cheesecake (under 600 calories), 1 serving	16
Cheesecake Lollipop (under 600 calories), 1 serving	8
Chocolate Sauce, 1 oz	8
Chocolate Thunder From Down Under, 1 serving	76
Classic Key Lime Mini Dessert Parfait, 1 serving	28
Double Chocolate Mini Dessert Parfait, 1 serving	31
Ice Cream Scoop, 1 serving	6
NY Style Cheese Cake, 1 serving	68
Oreo Crumbs, 1 serving	6
Sampler Carrot Cake, 1 serving	35
Sampler Chocolate Thunder From Down Under, 1 serving	32
Spotted Dog Sundae, 1 serving	6
Sweet Adventure Sampler Trio, 1 serving	20
Sydney's Sinful Sundae, 1 serving	49
Triple Layer Carrot Cake, 1 serving	58

Milkshakes

Chocolate Mini Milkshake, 1 serving	30
Oreo Mini Milkshake, 1 serving	28
Strawberry Mini Milkshake, 1 serving	21
Vanilla Mini Milkshake, 1 serving	23

"We Like This!" item

Outback Steakhouse

	SmartPoints® value

Appetizers

Chicken Egg Roll, 1	7
Chicken Potsticker, 3	7
Cream Cheese Rangoon, 3	7
Crispy Shrimp, 6	8
Veggie Spring Roll, 2	5

Chicken

Black Pepper Chicken, 1 serving	6
Grilled Teriyaki Chicken, 1 serving	8
Kung Pao Chicken, 1 serving	7
Mandarin Chicken, 1 serving	8
Mushroom Chicken, 1 serving	5
Mushroom Chicken (kids), 1 serving	4
Orange Chicken, 1 serving	15
Orange Chicken (kids), 1 serving	10
Potato Chicken, 1 serving	6
Potato Chicken (kids), 1 serving	5
String Bean Chicken Breast, 1 serving	4
String Bean Chicken Breast (kids), 1 serving	3
Sweet & Sour Chicken Breast, 1 serving	14
Sweet & Sour Chicken Breast (kids), 1 serving	11
SweetFire Chicken Breast (kids), 1 serving	12
Teriyaki Chicken, 1 serving	8
Teriyaki Chicken (kids), 1 serving	5

Beef

Beijing Beef, 1 serving	24
Beijing Beef (kids), 1 serving	18
Broccoli Beef, 1 serving	3
Broccoli Beef (kids), 1 serving	3
Shanghai Angus Steak, 1 serving	7
Shanghai Angus Steak (kids), 1 serving	5

	SmartPoints® value

Seafood

Golden Treasure Shrimp, 1 serving	13
Golden Treasure Shrimp (kids), 1 serving	8
Honey Walnut Shrimp, 1 serving	12
Honey Walnut Shrimp (kids), 1 serving	6
Peppercorn Shrimp, 1 serving	6

Soup

Hot & Sour Soup, 1 serving	3

Sides

Brown Steamed Rice (kids), 1 serving	9
Chow Mein, 1 serving	16
Chow Mein (kids), 1 serving	9
Fried Rice, 1 serving	16
Fried Rice (kids), 1 serving	11
Steamed Brown Rice, 1 serving	12
Steamed White Rice, 1 serving	11
White Steamed Rice (kids), 1 serving	7

Vegetables

Eggplant & Tofu, 1 serving	11
Eggplant & Tofu (kids), 1 serving	9
Mixed Veggies, 1 serving	0
Mixed Veggies (kids), 1 serving	0

Sauces & Cookies

Chili Sauce, 1 packet	1
Fortune Cookies, 1	1
Hot Mustard, 1 packet	0
Mandarin Sauce, 1 serving	10
Plum Sauce, 1 packet	1
Potsticker Sauce, 1 packet	1
Sweet & Sour Sauce, 1 serving	5

Bagels

	SmartPoints® value
Asiago Cheese Bagel, 1	10
Blueberry Bagel, 1	11
Chocolate Chip Bagel, 1	13
Cinnamon Crunch Bagel, 1	17
Cinnamon Swirl & Raisin Bagel, 1	10
Everything Bagel, 1	9
French Toast Bagel, 1	12
Plain Bagel, 1	8
Sesame Bagel, 1	9
Sprouted Grain Bagel Flat, 1	7
Whole Grain Bagel, 1	10

Muffins

	SmartPoints® value
Apple Crunch Muffin, 1	20
Blueberry Muffin with Fresh Blueberries, 1	19
Chocolate Chip Muffie, 1	14
Pumpkin Muffin, 1	25

Scones

	SmartPoints® value
Cinnamon Crunch Scone, 1	25
Orange Mini Scone, 1	8
Orange Scone, 1	24
Triple Berry Mini Scone, 1	7
Triple Berry Scone, 1	19
Wild Blueberry Mini Scone, 1	7
Wild Blueberry Scone, 1	20

Freshly Baked Breads

	SmartPoints® value
All Natural White Loaf, 1	4
All Natural White Miche, 1	4
Asiago Cheese Focaccia Loaf, 1 serving	4
Asiago Cheese Loaf, 1	5
Ciabatta Loaf, 1	4
Cinnamon Raisin Swirl Loaf, 1	8
Country Loaf, 1	4
Country Miche, 1	4
Focaccia, 1	5
French Baguette, 1 (2½ oz)	4
Grain Baguette, 1	5
Honey Wheat Loaf, 1	5
Rye Loaf, 1 serving	4
Rye Miche, 1	4
Sesame Semolina Loaf, 1	4
Sesame Semolina Miche, 1	4
Sourdough Bread Bowl, 1	18
Sourdough Loaf, 1	4
Sourdough XL Loaf, 1	4
Three Cheese Demi, 1	5
Three Cheese Loaf, 1	4
Three Cheese Miche, 1	4
Three Seed Demi, 1	4
Tomato Basil XL Loaf, 1	4
Whole Grain Baguette, 1	4
Whole Grain Loaf, 1	4
Whole Grain Miche, 1	4

"We Like This!" item

Panini & Sandwiches

	SmartPoints® value
Bacon Turkey Bravo on Tomato Basil Panini Sandwich, 1 whole	26
Bacon Turkey Bravo on Tomato Basil Sandwich, 1 half	12
Classic Grilled Cheese on All Natural White Miche, 1 half	10
Classic Grilled Cheese on All Natural White Miche, 1 whole	20
Classic Grilled Cheese on White Bread, 1 whole	20
Frontega Chicken Panini on Focaccia, 1 half	10
Frontega Chicken Panini on Focaccia, 1 whole	21
Italian Combo Sandwich on Ciabatta, 1 half	16
Italian Combo Sandwich on Ciabatta, 1 whole	32
Kids Peanut Butter and Jelly on All Natural White Bread, 1 whole	14
Kids Smoked Ham Sandwich on All Natural White Bread, 1 whole	10
Mediterranean Veggie Sandwich on Tomato Basil Sandwich, 1 whole	17

	SmartPoints® value
Mediterranean Veggie Sandwich on Tomato Basil Sandwich (half), 1 serving	9
Napa Almond Chicken Salad on Sesame Semolina Sandwich, 1 half	11
Napa Almond Chicken Salad on Sesame Semolina Sandwich, 1 whole	22
Roasted Turkey and Avocado BLT on Sourdough Sandwich, 1	7
Roasted Turkey and Avocado BLT on Sourdough Sandwich, 1 whole	15
Sierra Turkey Sandwich on Asiago Cheese Focaccia Sandwich, 1 half	10
Sierra Turkey Sandwich on Asiago Cheese Focaccia Sandwich, 1 whole	21
Smoked Ham and Swiss Sandwich on Rye, 1 half	9
Smoked Ham and Swiss Sandwich on Rye, 1 whole	19
Smoked Turkey Breast Sandwich on Country, 1 half	5
Smoked Turkey Breast Sandwich on Country, 1 whole	11
Smokehouse Turkey Panini on Three Cheese, 1 half	10
Southwestern Chicken Flatbread Sandwich, 1	13
Steak and Arugula on Sourdough, 1 serving	16
Steak and Arugula on Sourdough (half sandwich), 1 serving	8
Tomato & Mozzarella Panini on Ciabatta, 1 half	12
Tomato & Mozzarella Panini on Ciabatta, 1 whole	23
Tuna Salad Sandwich on Honey Wheat, 1 half	8
Tuna Salad Sandwich on Honey Wheat, 1 whole	16

Pastas

Lentil Quinoa Bowl with Cage Free Egg Broth Bowl, 1 serving	10
Lentil Quinoa Bowl with Chicken Broth Bowl, 1 serving	11
Ricotta Sacchettini Pasta with Chicken Broth Bowl, 1 serving	14

	SmartPoints® value
Signature Mac & Cheese, 1 large	35
Signature Mac & Cheese, 1 small	17

Soufflés

Four Cheese Soufflé, 1	18
Roasted Tomato & Feta Soufflé, 1	19
Spinach & Bacon Soufflé, 1	21

Salads

Asian Sesame Chicken Salad, 1 half with dressing	6
Asian Sesame Chicken Salad, 1 whole with dressing	11
Caesar Salad, 1 half with dressing	6
Caesar Salad, 1 whole with dressing	11
Chicken Caesar Salad, 1 half with dressing	6
Chicken Caesar Salad, 1 whole with dressing	12
Chicken Cobb with Avocado Salad, 1 half with dressing	10
Chicken Cobb with Avocado Salad, 1 whole with dressing	20
Chicken Soba Noodle Salad with Peanut Sauce, 1 half	7
Chicken Soba Noodle Salad with Peanut Sauce, 1 whole	14
Classic Salad, 1 half with dressing	3
Classic Salad, 1 whole with dressing	7
Classic with Chicken Salad, 1 half with dressing	4
Classic with Chicken Salad, 1 whole with dressing	9
Fuji Apple with Chicken Salad, 1 half with dressing	9
Fuji Apple with Chicken Salad, 1 whole with dressing	18
Greek Salad, 1 half with dressing	7
Greek Salad, 1 whole with dressing	13
Greek with Chicken Salad, 1 half with dressing	8
Greek with Chicken Salad, 1 whole with dressing	15
Mediterranean & Quinoa Salad with Almonds, 1 half with dressing	7

	SmartPoints® value
Mediterranean & Quinoa Salad with Almonds, 1 whole with dressing	14
Power Kale Caesar Salad with Chicken, 1 half with dressing	9
Power Kale Caesar Salad with Chicken, 1 whole with dressing	18
Power Mediterranean Roasted Turkey, 1	7
Strawberry Poppyseed & Chicken, 1 whole with dressing	11
Strawberry Poppyseed & Chicken, 1 half with dressing	5
Thai Chicken Salad, 1 half with dressing	7
Thai Chicken Salad, 1 whole with dressing	13

Dressings and Spreads

Asian Sesame Vinaigrette, 1½ Tbsp	2
Asian Sesame Vinaigrette, 3 Tbsp	3
Caesar Dressing, 1½ Tbsp	3
Greek Dressing/Herb Vinaigrette, 1½ Tbsp	4
Low Fat Thai Chili Vinaigrette, 1½ Tbsp	1
Plain Cream Cheese Spread, 2 oz	9
Reduced Fat Balsamic Vinaigrette, 1½ Tbsp	3
Reduced Fat Chive & Onion Cream Cheese Spread, 2 oz	6
Reduced Fat Hazelnut Cream Cheese Spread, 2 oz	6
Reduced Fat Honey Walnut Cream Cheese Spread, 2 oz	7
Reduced Fat Plain Cream Cheese Spread, 2 oz	5
Reduced Fat Roasted Vegetable Medley Cream Cheese Spread, 2 oz	5
Reduced Fat Wild Blueberry Cream Cheese Spread, 2 oz	7
Tortellini Alfredo Sauce2 cups	25
White Balsamic Apple Vinaigrette, 1½ Tbsp	3

"We Like This!" item

Soups

	SmartPoints® value
All Natural Low Fat Chicken Noodle Soup, 1 bowl	5
All Natural Low Fat Chicken Noodle Soup, 1 cup	3
All Natural Turkey Chili, 1 bowl	9
All Natural Turkey Chili, 1 cup	6
All Natural Turkey Chili (bread bowl), 1 serving	26
Baked Potato Soup, 1 bowl	14
Baked Potato Soup, 1 cup	9
Bistro French Onion Soup, 1 bowl	13
Bistro French Onion Soup, 1 cup	8
Broccoli Cheddar Soup, 1 bowl	14
Broccoli Cheddar Soup, 1 cup	9
Broccoli Cheddar Soup (bread bowl), 1 serving	27
Cream of Chicken and Wild Rice Soup, 1 bowl	11
Cream of Chicken and Wild Rice Soup, 1 cup	7
Low Fat Garden Vegetable with Pesto Soup, 1 cup	3
Low Fat Vegetarian Black Bean Soup, 1 bowl	6
Low Fat Vegetarian Black Bean Soup, 1 cup	4
Low Fat Vegetarian Garden Vegetable Soup with Pesto, 1 bowl	4
New England Clam Chowder, 1 bowl	23
New England Clam Chowder, 1 cup	15
Thai Garden Chicken Wonton Broth, 1 bowl	8
Vegetarian Creamy Tomato Soup, 1 bowl	13
Vegetarian Creamy Tomato Soup, 1 cup	9
Vegetarian Summer Corn Chowder, 1 cup	9

Sides

Panera Baked Crisps, 1	4
Panera Potato Chips, 1	4
Pickle Spear, 1	0

Breakfast Favorites	SmartPoints® value
Seasonal Fruit Cup, 1	0
Steel Cut Oatmeal with Strawberries & Pecans, 1 serving	12
Steel Cut Oatmeal with Summer Blueberries & Granola, 1 serving	13
Strawberry Granola Parfait, 1	7

Breakfast Sandwiches

Avocado Egg White and Spinach Breakfast Power Sandwich, 1	13
Bacon, Egg, and Cheese on Asiago Cheese Bagel, 1	21
Egg & Cheese on Ciabatta, 1	13
Ham, Egg, and Cheese Breakfast Power Sandwich, 1 sandwich	11
Mediterranean Egg White on Ciabatta, 1	13
Sausage, Egg, and Cheese on Ciabatta Sandwich, 1	18
Steak and Egg on Everything Bagel, 1	17
Turkey, Sausage, Egg White, and Spinach Breakfast Power Sandwich, 1 sandwich	12

Sweet Rolls

Cinnamon Roll, 1	26
Cobblestone, 1	25
Pecan Roll, 1	31

Cookies

Candy Cookie, 1	19
Chocolate Chipper Cookie, 1	21
Chocolate Chipper Petites Cookie, 1	5
Flip Flop Shaped Shortbread Cookie, 1	20
Gluten Conscious Triple Chocolate Cookie with Walnuts, 1	17
Oatmeal Raisin Cookie, 1	18
Shortbread Cookie, 1	16
White Chocolate Macadamia Nut Cookie, 1	18

Cakes	SmartPoints® value
Carrot Cake with Walnuts, 1	29
Cinnamon Coffee Crumb Cake, 1 slice	20
Strawberry Rhubarb Mini Cake, 1	11
Vanilla Cupcake, 1	21

Pastries

Bear Claw, 1	24
Cherry Pastry, 1	18
French Croissant, 1	12
Pastry Ring, 1 slice	10

Smoothies

Low Fat Mango Smoothie, 16 fl oz	14
Low Fat Strawberry Smoothie, 16 fl oz	15

Espresso & Coffee

Caffe Latte, 16 fl oz	5
Caffe Mocha, 16 fl oz	17
Cappuccino, 16 fl oz	5
Caramel Latte, 16 fl oz	19
Coffee, 12 fl oz	0
Decaf Coffee, 12 fl oz	0
Frozen Caramel Drink, 16 fl oz	29
Skinny Caffe Mocha, 16 fl oz	11
Vanilla Latte, 16 fl oz	11
Vanilla Latte with Sugar Free Vanilla Syrup, 16 fl oz	4

Teas

Brewed Tea Black, 20 fl oz	0
Chai Tea Latte, 16 fl oz	12
Iced Chai Tea Latte, 16 fl oz	10
Iced Infused Green Tea with Passionfruit & Papaya, 20 fl oz	8

Drinks

Kid's Organic Apple Juice, 8 fl oz	7
Lemonade, 16 fl oz	6
Organic Chocolate Milk, 8 fl oz	7
Signature Hot Chocolate, 16 fl oz	24

Pizzas

	SmartPoints® value
BBQ Chicken Bacon Pizza (original crust extra large), 1 slice	12
BBQ Chicken Bacon Pizza (original crust for one), 1 slice	8
BBQ Chicken Bacon Pizza (original crust large), 1 slice	11
BBQ Chicken Bacon Pizza (original crust medium), 1 slice	8
BBQ Chicken Bacon Pizza (original crust small), 1 slice	8
BBQ Chicken Bacon Pizza (thin crust large), 1 slice	9
Buffalo Chicken Pizza (original crust extra large), 1 slice	13
Buffalo Chicken Pizza (original crust for one), 1 slice	8
Buffalo Chicken Pizza (original crust large), 1 slice	12
Buffalo Chicken Pizza (original crust medium), 1 slice	8
Buffalo Chicken Pizza (original crust small), 1 slice	8
Buffalo Chicken Pizza (thin crust large), 1 slice	10
Cheese Pizza (original crust extra large), 1 slice	10
Cheese Pizza (original crust for one), 1 slice	7
Cheese Pizza (original crust large), 1 slice	10
Cheese Pizza (original crust medium), 1 slice	7
Cheese Pizza (original crust small), 1 slice	6
Cheese Pizza (thin crust large), 1 slice	7
Chicken and Veggie Pizza (original crust extra large), 1 slice	10
Chicken and Veggie Pizza (original crust for one), 1 slice	6

	SmartPoints® value
Chicken and Veggie Pizza (original crust large), 1 slice	9
Chicken and Veggie Pizza (original crust medium), 1 slice	6
Chicken and Veggie Pizza (original crust small), 1 slice	6
Chicken and Veggie Pizza (thin crust large), 1 slice	7
Chicken Cordon Blue Pizza (original crust extra large), 1 slice	12
Chicken Cordon Blue Pizza (original crust large), 1 slice	12
Chicken Cordon Blue Pizza (original crust medium), 1 slice	8
Chicken Cordon Blue Pizza (original crust small), 1 slice	8
Chicken Cordon Blue Pizza (thin crust large), 1 slice	9
Double Bacon Six Cheese Pizza (original crust extra large), 1 slice	12
Double Bacon Six Cheese Pizza (original crust large), 1 slice	11
Double Bacon Six Cheese Pizza (original crust medium), 1 slice	8
Double Bacon Six Cheese Pizza (original crust small), 1 slice	8
Double Bacon Six Cheese Pizza (thin crust large), 1 slice	9
Garden Fresh Pizza (original crust extra large), 1 slice	10
Garden Fresh Pizza (original crust for one), 1 slice	7
Garden Fresh Pizza (original crust large), 1 slice	10
Garden Fresh Pizza (original crust medium), 1 slice	7
Garden Fresh Pizza (original crust small), 1 slice	6
Garden Fresh Pizza (thin crust large), 1 slice	8
Greek Pizza (original crust extra large), 1 slice	13

"We Like This!" item

	SmartPoints® value
Greek Pizza (original crust for one), 1 slice	8
Greek Pizza (original crust large), 1 slice	12
Greek Pizza (original crust medium), 1 slice	8
Greek Pizza (original crust small), 1 slice	8
Greek Pizza (thin crust large), 1 slice	10
Grilled Chicken and Canadian Bacon Pizza (original crust extra large), 1 slice	9
Grilled Chicken and Canadian Bacon Pizza (original crust for one), 1 slice	6
Grilled Chicken and Canadian Bacon Pizza (original crust large), 1 slice	8
Grilled Chicken and Canadian Bacon Pizza (original crust medium), 1 slice	6
Grilled Chicken and Canadian Bacon Pizza (original crust small), 1 slice	5
Grilled Chicken and Canadian Bacon Pizza (thin crust large), 1 slice	6
Hawaiian BBQ Chicken Pizza (original crust extra large), 1 slice	13
Hawaiian BBQ Chicken Pizza (original crust for one), 1 slice	8
Hawaiian BBQ Chicken Pizza (original crust large), 1 slice	12
Hawaiian BBQ Chicken Pizza (original crust medium), 1 slice	9
Hawaiian BBQ Chicken Pizza (original crust small), 1 slice	8
Hawaiian BBQ Chicken Pizza (thin crust large), 1 slice	10
Hawaiian Chicken Pizza (original crust extra large), 1 slice	9

	SmartPoints® value
Hawaiian Chicken Pizza (original crust for one), 1 slice	6
Hawaiian Chicken Pizza (original crust large), 1 slice	8
Hawaiian Chicken Pizza (original crust medium), 1 slice	6
Hawaiian Chicken Pizza (original crust small), 1 slice	6
Hawaiian Chicken Pizza (thin crust large), 1 slice	6
Johns Favorite Pizza (original crust extra large), 1 slice	14
Johns Favorite Pizza (original crust for one), 1 slice	9
Johns Favorite Pizza (original crust large), 1 slice	13
Johns Favorite Pizza (original crust medium), 1 slice	9
Johns Favorite Pizza (original crust small), 1 slice	9
Johns Favorite Pizza (thin crust large), 1 slice	11
Mediterranean Veggie Pizza (original crust extra large), 1 slice	10
Mediterranean Veggie Pizza (original crust for one), 1 slice	6
Mediterranean Veggie Pizza (original crust large), 1 slice	9
Mediterranean Veggie Pizza (original crust medium), 1 slice	6
Mediterranean Veggie Pizza (original crust small), 1 slice	6
Mediterranean Veggie Pizza (thin crust large), 1 slice	7
Pepperoni Pizza (original crust extra large), 1 slice	11
Pepperoni Pizza (original crust for one), 1 slice	7
Pepperoni Pizza (original crust large), 1 slice	11
Pepperoni Pizza (original crust medium), 1 slice	7

	SmartPoints® value
Pepperoni Pizza (original crust small), 1 slice	7
Pepperoni Pizza (thin crust large), 1 slice	8
Philly Cheesesteak Pizza (original crust extra large), 1 slice	13
Philly Cheesesteak Pizza (original crust for one), 1 slice	9
Philly Cheesesteak Pizza (original crust large), 1 slice	12
Philly Cheesesteak Pizza (original crust medium), 1 slice	8
Philly Cheesesteak Pizza (original crust small), 1 slice	8
Philly Cheesesteak Pizza (thin crust large), 1 slice	10
Sausage Pizza (original crust extra large), 1 slice	11
Sausage Pizza (original crust for one), 1 slice	8
Sausage Pizza (original crust large), 1 slice	11
Sausage Pizza (original crust medium), 1 slice	8
Sausage Pizza (original crust small), 1 slice	7
Sausage Pizza (thin crust large), 1 slice	9
Spicy Italian Pizza (original crust extra large), 1 slice	13
Spicy Italian Pizza (original crust for one), 1 slice	9
Spicy Italian Pizza (original crust large), 1 slice	13
Spicy Italian Pizza (original crust medium), 1 slice	9
Spicy Italian Pizza (original crust small), 1 slice	8
Spicy Italian Pizza (thin crust large), 1 slice	10
Spinach Alfredo Pizza (original crust extra large), 1 slice	10

	SmartPoints® value
Spinach Alfredo Pizza (original crust for one), 1 slice	7
Spinach Alfredo Pizza (original crust large), 1 slice	9
Spinach Alfredo Pizza (original crust medium), 1 slice	7
Spinach Alfredo Pizza (original crust small), 1 slice	6
Spinach Alfredo Pizza (thin crust large), 1 slice	7
The Meats Pizza (original crust extra large), 1 slice	13
The Meats Pizza (original crust for one), 1 slice	9
The Meats Pizza (original crust large), 1 slice	13
The Meats Pizza (original crust medium), 1 slice	8
The Meats Pizza (original crust small), 1 slice	8
The Meats Pizza (thin crust large), 1 slice	10
The Works Pizza (original crust extra large), 1 slice	13
The Works Pizza (original crust for one), 1 slice	8
The Works Pizza (original crust large), 1 slice	12
The Works Pizza (original crust medium), 1 slice	8
The Works Pizza (original crust small), 1 slice	8
The Works Pizza (thin crust large), 1 slice	10
Tropical Luau Pizza (original crust extra large), 1 slice	9
Tropical Luau Pizza (original crust for one), 1 slice	6
Tropical Luau Pizza (original crust large), 1 slice	8
Tropical Luau Pizza (original crust medium), 1 slice	6

"We Like This!" item

	SmartPoints® value
Tropical Luau Pizza (original crust small), 1 slice	5
Tropical Luau Pizza (thin crust large), 1 slice	6
Tuscan Six Cheese Pizza (original crust extra large), 1 slice	11
Tuscan Six Cheese Pizza (original crust for one), 1 slice	7
Tuscan Six Cheese Pizza (original crust large), 1 slice	10
Tuscan Six Cheese Pizza (original crust medium), 1 slice	8
Tuscan Six Cheese Pizza (original crust small), 1 slice	7
Tuscan Six Cheese Pizza (thin crust large), 1 slice	8

Sides

BBQ Wings, 2	6
Breadsticks, 2 sticks	9
Bruschetta Cheesesticks (10"), 4 sticks	14
Bruschetta Cheesesticks (12"), 4 sticks	17
Cheesesticks, 4 sticks	15
Chicken Poppers, 5	5
Garlic Knots, 2 sticks	7
Garlic Parmesan Breadsticks, 2 sticks	11
Honey Chipotle Wings, 2	7
Spicy Buffalo Wings, 2	6
Unsauced Roasted Wings, 2	5

Sauces

	SmartPoints® value
BBQ Sauce, 1 oz	3
Blue Cheese Sauce, 1 oz	6
Buffalo Sauce, 1 oz	1
Cheese Sauce, 1 oz	2
Honey Mustard Sauce, 1 oz	6
Pizza Sauce, 1 oz	1
Ranch Sauce, 1 oz	3
Special Garlic Sauce, 1 oz	5

Extras

Crushed Red Pepper, 1 packet	0
Parmesan Cheese, 1 packet	1
Pepperoncinis, 1	0
Special Seasonings, 1 packet	0

Desserts

Brookie, 1 slice	9
Chocolate Chip Cookie, 1 slice	9
Cinnamon Knots, 2	15
Cinnapie, 4 sticks	23
Double Chocolate Chip Brownie, 1 square	11

Appetizers/Sides

	SmartPoints® value
Baked Boneless Wings, 2 pieces	2
Baked Hot Wings, 2 pieces	3
Baked Mild Wings, 2 pieces	3
Breadsticks, 1	4
Cheese Sticks, 1	5
Fiery Red Pepper Flavor Sticks, 1	4
Honey Sriracha Flavor Sticks, 1	4
Hut Favorite Flavor Sticks, 1	4
Toasted Asiago Flavor Sticks, 1	4
Toasted Cheddar Flavor Sticks, 1	4
Toasted Parmesan Flavor Sticks, 1	4
Waffle Fries (side order), 1 serving	21

12″ Medium Hand Tossed Pizza (serves 8)

7-Alarm Fire™, 1 slice	7
BBQ Bacon Cheeseburger, 1 slice	8
BBQ Lover's, 1 slice	8
Buffalo State of Mind™, 1 slice	6
Cheese, 1 slice	7
Cherry Pepper Bombshell, 1 slice	7
Cock-A-Doodle Bacon, 1 slice	7
Garden Party, 1 slice	6
Giddy-Up BBQ Chicken™, 1 slice	7
Hot and Twisted™, 1 slice	6
Meat Lover's®, 1 slice	9
Old Fashioned Meatbrawl™, 1 slice	7
Pepperoni, 1 slice	7
Pepperoni Lover's®, 1 slice	9
Pretzel Piggy, 1 slice	7
Supreme, 1 slice	8
Sweet Sriracha Dynamite, 1 slice	7
Ultimate Cheese Lover's®, 1 slice	7
Veggie Lover's®, 1 slice	6

12″ Medium Pan Pizza (serves 8)

	SmartPoints® value
7-Alarm Fire™, 1 slice	8
BBQ Bacon Cheeseburger, 1 slice	9
BBQ Lover's, 1 slice	10
Buffalo State of Mind™, 1 slice	8
Cheese, 1 slice	8
Cherry Pepper Bombshell, 1 slice	8
Cock-A-Doodle Bacon, 1 slice	7
Garden Party, 1 slice	7
Giddy-Up BBQ Chicken™, 1 slice	9
Hot and Twisted™, 1 slice	8
Meat Lover's®, 1 slice	10
Old Fashioned Meatbrawl™, 1 slice	8
Pepperoni, 1 slice	8
Pepperoni Lover's®, 1 slice	10
Pretzel Piggy, 1 slice	8
Supreme, 1 slice	9
Sweet Sriracha Dynamite, 1 slice	8
Ultimate Cheese Lover's®, 1 slice	9
Veggie Lover's®, 1 slice	7

12″ Medium Thin 'N Crispy Pizza (serves 8)

7-Alarm Fire™, 1 slice	7
BBQ Bacon Cheeseburger, 1 slice	9
BBQ Lover's, 1 slice	9
Buffalo State of Mind™, 1 slice	7
Cheese, 1 slice	7
Cherry Pepper Bombshell, 1 slice	7
Cock-A-Doodle Bacon, 1 slice	8
Garden Party, 1 slice	7
Giddy-Up BBQ Chicken™, 1 slice	8
Hot and Twisted™, 1 slice	7
Meat Lover's®, 1 slice	9
Old Fashioned Meatbrawl™, 1 slice	7
Pepperoni, 1 slice	7
Pepperoni Lover's®, 1 slice	9
Pretzel Piggy, 1 slice	7

"We Like This!" item

	SmartPoints® value
Supreme, 1 slice	8
Sweet Sriracha Dynamite, 1 slice	7
Ultimate Cheese Lover's®, 1 slice	8
Veggie Lover's®, 1 slice	6

14" Large Original Stuffed Crust Pizza (serves 8)

7-Alarm Fire™, 1 slice	11
BBQ Bacon Cheeseburger, 1 slice	13
BBQ Lover's, 1 slice	13
Buffalo State of Mind™, 1 slice	10
Cheese, 1 slice	10
Cherry Pepper Bombshell, 1 slice	11
Cock-A-Doodle Bacon, 1 slice	11
Garden Party, 1 slice	10
Giddy-Up BBQ Chicken™, 1 slice	12
Hot and Twisted™, 1 slice	10
Meat Lover's®, 1 slice	14
Old Fashioned Meatbrawl™, 1 slice	11
Pepperoni, 1 slice	11
Pepperoni Lover's®, 1 slice	13
Pretzel Piggy, 1 slice	11
Supreme, 1 slice	12
Sweet Sriracha Dynamite, 1 slice	11
Ultimate Cheese Lover's®, 1 slice	11
Veggie Lover's®, 1 slice	10

14" Large Hand Tossed Pizza (serves 8)

	SmartPoints® value
7-Alarm Fire™, 1 slice	9
BBQ Bacon Cheeseburger, 1 slice	11
BBQ Lover's, 1 slice	11
Buffalo State of Mind™, 1 slice	9
Cheese, 1 slice	9
Cherry Pepper Bombshell, 1 slice	9
Cock-A-Doodle Bacon, 1 slice	10
Garden Party, 1 slice	9
Giddy-Up BBQ Chicken™, 1 slice	10
Hot and Twisted™, 1 slice	9
Meat Lover's®, 1 slice	13
Old Fashioned Meatbrawl™, 1 slice	10
Pepperoni, 1 slice	10
Pepperoni Lover's®, 1 slice	12
Pretzel Piggy, 1 slice	10
Supreme, 1 slice	11
Sweet Sriracha Dynamite, 1 slice	9
Ultimate Cheese Lover's®, 1 slice	10
Veggie Lover's®, 1 slice	8

14" Large Hot Dog Bites Pizza (serves 8)

Cheese, 1 slice	11
Meat Lover's® (maximum calories), 1 slice	14
Pepperoni, 1 slice	11
Spinach, 1 slice	10

14" Large Pan Pizza (serves 8)

7-Alarm Fire™, 1 slice	12
BBQ Bacon Cheeseburger, 1 slice	14
BBQ Lover's, 1 slice	14
Buffalo State of Mind™, 1 slice	11
Cheese, 1 slice	11
Cherry Pepper Bombshell, 1 slice	12
Cock-A-Doodle Bacon, 1 slice	12
Garden Party, 1 slice	10
Giddy-Up BBQ Chicken™, 1 slice	12
Hot and Twisted™, 1 slice	11
Meat Lover's®, 1 slice	15
Old Fashioned Meatbrawl™, 1 slice	12
Pepperoni, 1 slice	12
Pepperoni Lover's®, 1 slice	14
Pretzel Piggy, 1 slice	12
Supreme, 1 slice	13
Sweet Sriracha Dynamite, 1 slice	11
Ultimate Cheese Lover's®, 1 slice	12
Veggie Lover's®, 1 slice	10

14″ Large Skinny Slice Pizza (serves 8)

	SmartPoints® value
Skinny Beach, 1 slice	6
Skinny Club™, 1 slice	7
Skinny Italy, 1 slice	7
Skinny Luau™, 1 slice	6
Skinny with a Kick™, 1 slice	8

14″ Large Thin 'N Crispy Pizza (serves 8)

	SmartPoints® value
7-Alarm Fire™, 1 slice	9
BBQ Bacon Cheeseburger, 1 slice	12
BBQ Lover's, 1 slice	12
Buffalo State of Mind™, 1 slice	9
Cheese, 1 slice	9
Cherry Pepper Bombshell, 1 slice	9
Cock-A-Doodle Bacon, 1 slice	10
Garden Party, 1 slice	9
Giddy-Up BBQ Chicken™, 1 slice	10
Hot and Twisted™, 1 slice	9
Meat Lover's®, 1 slice	13
Old Fashioned Meatbrawl™, 1 slice	10
Pepperoni, 1 slice	10
Pepperoni Lover's®, 1 slice	12
Pretzel Piggy, 1 slice	10
Supreme, 1 slice	10
Sweet Sriracha Dynamite, 1 slice	9
Ultimate Cheese Lover's®, 1 slice	10
Veggie Lover's®, 1 slice	8

6″ Personal Pan Pizza

	SmartPoints® value
7-Alarm Fire™, 1 whole pizza	20
BBQ Bacon Cheeseburger, 1 whole pizza	25
BBQ Lover's, 1 whole pizza	25
Buffalo State of Mind™ (whole pizza), 1 whole pizza	20
Cheese, 1 whole pizza	20
Cherry Pepper Bombshell, 1 whole pizza	20
Cock-A-Doodle Bacon, 1 whole pizza	22
Garden Party, 1 whole pizza	20
Giddy-Up BBQ Chicken™, 1 whole pizza	22
Hot and Twisted™, 1 whole pizza	19
Meat Lover's®, 1 whole pizza	28
Old Fashioned Meatbrawl™, 1 whole pizza	23
Pepperoni, 1 whole pizza	20
Pepperoni Lover's®, 1 whole pizza	24
Pretzel Piggy, 1 whole pizza	21
Supreme, 1 whole pizza	23
Sweet Sriracha Dynamite, 1 whole pizza	19
Ultimate Cheese Lover's®, 1 whole pizza	22
Veggie Lover's®, 1 whole pizza	18

Rectangular/Dinner Box Pizza (serves 8)

	SmartPoints® value
7-Alarm Fire™, 1 piece	8
BBQ Bacon Cheeseburger, 1 piece	10
BBQ Lover's, 1 piece	10
Buffalo State of Mind™, 1 piece	8
Cheese, 1 piece	8
Cherry Pepper Bombshell, 1 piece	8
Cock-A-Doodle Bacon, 1 piece	11
Garden Party, 1 piece	8
Giddy-Up BBQ Chicken™, 1 piece	9
Hot and Twisted™, 1 piece	7
Meat Lover's®, 1 piece	10
Old Fashioned Meatbrawl™, 1 piece	8
Pepperoni, 1 piece	8
Pepperoni Lover's®, 1 piece	10
Pretzel Piggy, 1 piece	8

"We Like This!" item

	SmartPoints® value
Supreme, 1 piece	9
Sweet Sriracha Dynamite, 1 piece	8
Ultimate Cheese Lover's®, 1 piece	9
Veggie Lover's®, 1 piece	7

10" Gluten-Free Pizza (serves 6)

Cheese, 1 slice	5
Pepperoni, 1 slice	6

Tuscani Pasta

Creamy Chicken Alfredo, 1 serving	16
Meaty Marinara, 1 serving	15

WingStreet Traditional Wings

Buffalo Burnin' Hot, 1 serving	4
Buffalo Medium, 1 serving	4
Buffalo Mild, 1 serving	4
Garlic Parmesan, 1 serving	6
Honey BBQ, 1 serving	6
Honey Sriracha, 1 serving	4
Naked, 1 serving	2
Spicy BBQ, 1 serving	5
Sweet Chili, 1 serving	5

WingStreet Bone-Out Wings

Buffalo Burnin' Hot, 1 serving	6
Buffalo Medium, 1 serving	6
Buffalo Mild, 1 serving	6
Garlic Parmesan, 1 serving	8
Honey BBQ, 1 serving	8
Honey Sriracha, 1 serving	6
Naked, 1 serving	4
Spicy BBQ, 1 serving	7
Sweet Chili, 1 serving	8

SmartPoints® value

WingStreet Breaded Bone-In Wings

Buffalo Burnin' Hot, 1 serving	7
Buffalo Medium, 1 serving	7
Buffalo Mild, 1 serving	7
Garlic Parmesan, 1 serving	9
Honey BBQ, 1 serving	9
Honey Sriracha, 1 serving	6
Naked, 1 serving	5
Spicy BBQ, 1 serving	8
Sweet Chili, 1 serving	9

Condiments/Dipping Sauces

BBQ Wing Sauce for Baked Boneless Wings, 3 oz	9
Blue Cheese Dipping Sauce, 1½ oz	8
Buffalo Wing Sauce for Baked Boneless Wings, 3 oz	1
Marinara Dipping Sauce, 3 oz	2
Ranch Dipping Sauce, 1½ oz	8

Desserts

Cinnamon Sticks, 2 pieces	6
HERSHEY'S® Chocolate Dipping Sauce, 1½ oz	6
HERSHEY'S® Chocolate Dunkers®, 2 pieces	7
The Ultimate HERSHEY'S® Chocolate Chip Cookie, 1 serving	8
White Icing Dipping Sauce, 2 oz	10

Appetizers

	SmartPoints® value
Buffalo Chicken Wings with Blue Cheese Dressing, 1 serving	28
Chicken Breast Strips (create your own app), 1 serving	16
Chilled Jumbo Shrimp Cocktail, 1 serving	1
Clam Strips (create your own app), 1 serving	18
Crispy Calamari and Vegetables, 1 serving	58
Crispy Calamari and Vegetables (create your own app), 1 serving	33
Crispy Shrimp Lettuce Wraps, 1 serving	22
Fried Green Beans (create your own app), 1 serving	13
Fried Oysters (create your own app), 1 serving	18
Fried Oysters with French Fries and Sauces, 1 serving	32
Langostino Lobster Artichoke and Seafood Dip, 1 serving	34
Lobster Artichoke and Seafood Dip, 1 serving	34
Mozzarella Cheesesticks, 1 serving	26
Mozzarella Cheesesticks (create your own app), 1 serving	14
Parrot Isle Jumbo Coconut Shrimp Appetizer, 1 serving	23
Parrot Isle Shrimp (add five more), 1 serving	15
Raw Oysters on the Half Shell, 1 dozen	8
Raw Oysters on the Half Shell, ½ dozen	6
Seaside Sampler, 1 serving	30
Shrimp Nachos, 1 serving	39
Shrimp Your Way - Coconut Bites, 1 serving	15
Signature Shrimp Cocktail, 1 serving	3
Steamed Clams, 1 serving	21
Steamed Oysters on the Half Shell, 1 dozen	21
Steamed Oysters on the Half Shell, ½ dozen	20
Stuffed Mushrooms (create your own app), 1 serving	10
Sweet Chili Shrimp, 1 serving	40
Tomato Mozzarella Caprese, 1 serving	5
White Wine and Roasted-Garlic Mussels, 1 serving	21

Lobster & Signature Combos

	SmartPoints® value
Bar Harbor Lobster Bake, 1 serving	55
Coastal Lobster and Shrimp, 1 serving	43
Grilled Lobster and Red Shrimp, 1 serving	23
Langostino Lobster and Shrimp Caprese Pasta, 1 serving	56
Lighthouse Rock Lobster Tail, 1 serving	9
Live Maine Lobster (1¼ lb steamed includes fixed sides and sauces), 1 serving	17
Lobster and Langostino Pizza, 1 serving	22
Lobster and Shrimp Overboard, 1 serving	66
Lobster Scampi Linguini, 1 serving	25
Lobster, Crab and Seafood Stuffed Mushrooms, 1 serving	15
NY Strip and Rock Lobster Tail, 1 serving	35

"We Like This!" item

	SmartPoints® value
Roasted Maine Lobster Bake, 1 serving	21
Roasted Maine Lobster Tail with Melted Butter Add-On, 1 serving	16
Rock Lobster Tail with Melted Butter, 1 serving	22
Seaport Lobster and Shrimp, 1 serving	30
Ultimate Feast (includes fixed sides and sauces), 1 serving	38
Wood-Grilled Lobster Tacos, 1 serving	19
Wood-Grilled Lobster, Shrimp and Salmon, 1 serving	27

Shrimp & Classic Combos

Admiral's Feast, 1 serving	41
Garlic Shrimp Scampi (create your own), 1 serving	7
Garlic-Grilled Shrimp (4-course feast), 1 serving	9
Garlic-Grilled Shrimp (create your own), 1 serving	6
Jumbo Coconut Shrimp (4-course feast), 1 serving	29
Lighthouse Garlic Grilled Shrimp, 1 serving	10
Parrot Isle Jumbo Coconut Shrimp (create your own), 1 serving	29
Parrot Isle Jumbo Coconut Shrimp (dinner entrée), 1 serving	34
Seaside Shrimp Trio, 1 serving	38
Shrimp Linguini Alfredo (create your own), 1 serving	20
Shrimp Linguini Alfredo (full), 1 serving	40
Shrimp Linguini Alfredo (half), 1 serving	20
Shrimp Your Way - Fried, 1 serving	8
Shrimp Your Way - Popcorn, 1 serving	13
Shrimp Your Way - Scampi, 1 serving	7
Walt's Favorite Shrimp, 1 serving	19
Walt's Favorite Shrimp (add a half dozen more), 1 serving	11
Walt's Favorite Shrimp (create your own), 1 serving	13
Wood-Grilled Shrimp Skewers, 1 serving	8
Wood-Grilled Tacos with Grilled Shrimp, 1 serving	16

Crab Entrées & Seafood Bakes

Crab Linguini Alfredo (full), 1 serving	64
Crab Linguini Alfredo (half/lunch), 1 serving	32
Jumbo Lump Crab Cakes, 1 serving	9
Lighthouse Snow Crab Legs, 1 serving	17
North Pacific King Crab Legs, 1½ pounds	19
Portofino Seafood Bake, 1 serving	35
Snow Crab Legs (includes fixed sides and dipping sauces), 1 pound	16
Steamed Snow Crab Legs with Fixed Sides and Dipping Sauces (create your own), 1 serving	16

Fish

Arctic Char (lunch/dinner), 1 serving	8
Baked Flounder Dinner (with crab-and-seafood stuffing), 1 serving	12
Batterfried Canadian Walleye, 1 serving	30
Batterfried Crawfish, 1 serving	44

Fish (cont'd)

	SmartPoints® value
Batterfried Crawfish (create your own), 1 serving	30
Blackened Canadian Walleye, 1 serving	6
Broiled Canadian Walleye, 1 serving	5
Canadian Walleye-Fried, 1 serving	6
Cod (lunch/dinner), 1 serving	2
Crunch-Fried Fish Sandwich, 1 serving	46
Flounder (lunch/dinner), 1 serving	3
Golden Fried Canadian Walleye, 1 serving	12
Golden Fried Catfish, 1 serving	12
Golden Fried Flounder/Sole, 1 serving	20
Grouper (lunch/dinner), 1 serving	2
Gulf Snapper (lunch/dinner), 1 serving	3
Haddock (lunch/dinner), 1 serving	2
Halibut (lunch/dinner), 1 serving	3
Hand-Battered Fish and Chips, 1 serving	29
Lake Whitefish (lunch/dinner), 1 serving	6
Ono/Wahoo (lunch/dinner), 1 serving	7
Oven Broiled Flounder/Sole, 1 serving	6
Pacific Snapper (lunch/dinner), 1 serving	2
Parmesan Crusted Tilapia (dinner), 1 serving	18
Perch (lunch/dinner), 1 serving	2
Rainbow Trout (dinner), 1 serving	10
Red Rockfish (lunch/dinner), 1 serving	2
Salmon (dinner), 1 serving	15
Salmon New Orleans (full), 1 serving	28
Salmon New Orleans (half), 1 serving	23
Seafood Stuffed Flounder (create your own), 1 serving	6
Sole (lunch/dinner), 1 serving	3
Soy Ginger Salmon (4-course feast), 1 serving	9
Tilapia (dinner), 1 serving	6
Tilapia with Roasted Vegetables, 1 serving	15
Tuna (lunch/dinner), 1 serving	3
Wood-Grilled Fresh Salmon (create your own), 1 serving	7
Wood-Grilled Fresh Tilapia (create your own), 1 serving	3
Wood-Grilled Tacos with Grilled Fresh Tilapia, 1 serving	21

Land & Sea

Bacon Cheddar Chicken Club, 1 serving	32
Cajun Chicken Linguini Alfredo (4-course feast), 1 serving	23
Center-Cut NY Strip Steak, 1 serving	18
Garlic Grilled Sea Scallops, 1 serving	2
Garlic Grilled Sea Scallops (create your own), 1 serving	2
Lighthouse Maple Glazed Chicken, 1 serving	11
Lighthouse Wood-Grilled Peppercorn Sirloin and Shrimp, 1 serving	12
Maple-Glazed Chicken Dinner, 1 serving	11
Peppercorn-Grilled Sirloin (create your own), 1 serving	5
Shrimp and Wood-Grilled Chicken (hand-breaded shrimp), 1 serving	11
Shrimp and Wood-Grilled Chicken (shrimp scampi), 1 serving	9
Shrimp and Wood-Grilled Chicken (shrimp skewer), 1 serving	7

"We Like This!" item

	SmartPoints® value
Wood-Grilled Burger, 1 serving	38
Wood-Grilled Cheeseburger, 1 serving	42
Wood-Grilled Chicken Sandwich, 1 serving	28
Wood-Grilled Peppercorn Sirloin, 1 serving	12
Wood-Grilled Peppercorn Sirloin and Shrimp, 1 serving	14
Wood-Grilled Tacos with Chicken, 1 serving	17

Soup & Salad Combos

Grilled Shrimp Salad and Creamy Potato Bacon Soup (lunch), 1 serving	14
Grilled Shrimp Salad and Lobster and Langostino Bisque (lunch), 1 serving	16
Grilled Shrimp Salad and Manhattan Clam Chowder (lunch), 1 serving	7
Grilled Shrimp Salad and New England Clam Chowder (lunch), 1 serving	12
Grilled Shrimp Salad and Seafood Gumbo (lunch), 1 serving	9
Lobster and Langostino Bisque and Grilled Shrimp Salad, 1 serving	28
Manhattan Clam Chowder and Grilled Shrimp Salad, 1 serving	11

Soups, Salads & More

	SmartPoints® value
Caesar Salad, 1 serving	10
Classic Caesar Salad, 1 serving	18
Classic Caesar Salad with Chicken, 1 serving	19
Classic Caesar Salad with Salmon, 1 serving	25
Classic Caesar Salad with Shrimp, 1 serving	18
Creamy Potato Bacon Soup, 1 bowl	22
Creamy Potato Bacon Soup, 1 cup	11
Creamy Potato Bacon Soup and Grilled Shrimp Salad, 1 serving	25
Garden Salad (without dressing), 1 serving	2
Grilled Zucchini and Squash, 1 serving	6
Lobster Bisque, 1 bowl	25
Lobster Bisque, 1 cup	12
Manhattan Clam Chowder, 1 bowl	7
Manhattan Clam Chowder, 1 cup	4
New England Chowder and Grilled Shrimp Salad, 1 serving	20
New England Clam Chowder, 1 bowl	17
New England Clam Chowder, 1 cup	8
Seafood Gumbo, 1 bowl	10
Seafood Gumbo, 1 cup	5
Seafood Gumbo and Grilled Shrimp Salad, 1 serving	14

Dressings and Sauces

Blue Cheese Dressing, 1 serving	8
Blueberry Balsamic Dressing, 1 serving	4
Butter (for baked potato), 1 serving	4
Caesar Dressing, 1 serving	11
Champagne Vinaigrette Dressing, 1 serving	3
Cocktail Sauce, 1 serving	2
French Dressing, 1 serving	7
Honey Mustard Dressing, 1 serving	7
Honey-Mustard Dipping Sauce, 1 serving	7
Marinara Sauce, 1 serving	1
Pico de Gallo, 1 serving	0
Piña Colada Sauce, 1 serving	5
Pineapple Salsa, 1 serving	2

	SmartPoints® value
Pure Melted Butter, 1 serving	15
Ranch Dressing, 1 serving	5
Red Wine Vinaigrette, 1 serving	3
Sriracha Aioli, 1 serving	8
Tartar Sauce, 1 serving	8
Thousand Island Dressing, 1 serving	8

Lunch Classics

	SmartPoints® value
Batterfried Canadian Walleye, 1 serving	15
Batterfried Crawfish, 1 serving	16
Blackened Canadian Walleye, 1 serving	3
Broiled Bay Scallops, 1 serving	2
Broiled Canadian Walleye, 1 serving	3
Cajun Chicken Linguini Alfredo (full), 1 serving	33
Cajun Chicken Linguini Alfredo (half), 1 serving	23
Crunchy Popcorn Shrimp, 1 serving	13
Fried Bay Scallops, 1 serving	5
Fried Farm-Raised Catfish, 1 serving	4
Fried Flounder, 1 serving	15
Garlic Shrimp Scampi (create your own portion), 1 serving	4
Garlic Shrimp Scampi (no sides), 1 serving	7
Garlic-Grilled Shrimp Skewer, 1 serving	5
Hand Breaded Shrimp, 1 serving	6
Hand-Breaded Shrimp, 1 serving	9
Lunch Crunch-Fried Fish, 1 serving	18
Maple-Glazed Chicken, 1 serving	10
Opah, 1 serving	2
Oven Broiled Flounder, 1 serving	2
Rainbow Trout, 1 serving	5
Sailor's Platter, 1 serving	11
Salmon, 1 serving	7
Seafood-Stuffed Flounder, 1 serving	6
Tilapia, 1 serving	3

Add-Ons

	SmartPoints® value
Garlic-Grilled Shrimp Skewer, 1 serving	2
Grilled Main Lobster Tail, 1 serving	16
Lemon Garlic Beurre Blanc Topping, 1 serving	7
Petite Shrimp (for salad), 1 serving	1
Sour Cream (for baked potato), 1 serving	1

Sides

	SmartPoints® value
Asparagus, 1 serving	2
Baked Potato, 1 potato	6
Broccoli, 1 serving	1
Cheddar Bay Biscuit, 1	5
Coleslaw, 1 serving	10
Creamy Lobster Baked Potato, 1 serving	11
Creamy Lobster Mashed Potatoes, 1 serving	12
French Fries, 1 serving	14
Mashed Potatoes, 1 serving	7
Petite Green Beans, 1 serving	4
Wild Rice Pilaf, 1 serving	4

Kid's Menu

	SmartPoints® value
Broiled Fish, 1 serving	2
Chicken Fingers, 1 serving	9
Frozen Strawberry Lemonade Casco Bay Cooler, 1 serving	22
Garlic-Grilled Shrimp Skewer, 1 serving	2
Grilled Chicken, 1 serving	1
Macaroni and Cheese, 1 serving	10

"We Like This!" item

	SmartPoints® value
Peachy Breezy Smoothie Casco Bay Cooler, 1 serving	14
Popcorn Shrimp, 1 serving	5
Raspberry Bay Smoothie Casco Bay Cooler, 1 serving	10
Snow Crab Legs, 1 serving	1
Sunset Strawberry Casco Bay Cooler, 1 serving	10

Desserts

Brownie Overboard, 1 serving	32
Carrot Cake, 1 serving	26
Chocolate Wave, 1 serving	48
Homemade Berry Shore Cake, 1 serving	31
Key Lime Pie, 1 serving	19
New York Cheesecake with Strawberries, 1 serving	29
Surf's Up Sundae, 1 serving	7
Triple-Chocolate Brownie à la Mode, 1 serving	19
Warm Apple Crostada, 1 serving	27
Warm Chocolate Chip Lava Cookie, 1 serving	41

Drinks

	SmartPoints® value
Berry Bootlegger Cocktail, 1 serving	5
Boston Iced Tea, Classic Cranberry, 1 serving	5
Boston Iced Tea, Peach, 1 serving	7
Boston Iced Tea, Raspberry, 1 serving	6
Cherry Wave Slushy, 1 serving	9
Chocolate Martini, 1 serving	16
Classic Lemonade, 1 serving	9
Classic Margarita (on the rocks), 1 serving	5
Cosmopolitan, 1 serving	7
Fruit Smoothie, Peach, 1 serving	25
Fruit Smoothie, Raspberry, 1 serving	24
Fruit Smoothie, Strawberry, 1 serving	24
Handcrafted Flavored Lemonade, Peach, 1 serving	16
Handcrafted Flavored Lemonade, Strawberry, 1 serving	15
Martini (gin), 1 serving	5
Martini (vodka), 1 serving	6
Raspberry Lobsterita, 1 serving	24
Sail Away Sangria, 1 serving	9
Skinny Margarita (on the rocks), 1 serving	6
Strawberry Lobsterita, 1 serving	24
Traditional Lobsterita, 1 serving	20

Appetizers

	SmartPoints® value
Ahi Tuna Tartare, 1 serving	13
Asian Glazed Grilled Chicken Skewers, 1 serving	8
Blistered Shishito Peppers, 1 serving	9
Duck Wing Lollipops, 1 serving	13
Fresh Summer Truffle Risotto, 1 serving	10
Hummus Duo with Crisp Hawaiian Sea Salt Lavosh, 1 serving	12
Lump Crab Cake, 1 serving	10
Lump Crab Roasted Shrimp and Spinach Stuffed Mushrooms, 1 serving	5
Roasted Prosciutto Wrapped Figs, 1 serving	11
Shrimp Scampi Skillet with Bomba Rice, 1 serving	15
Sweet Corn & Ricotta Ravioli, 1 serving	10
Toasted Meyer Lemon and Ricotta Ravioli, 1 serving	11
Wood-Grilled Artichokes, 1 serving	12
Wood-Grilled Artichokes, 1 serving	12

Poultry & Meat

	SmartPoints® value
Boneless Beef Short Rib, 1 serving	24
Grilled Chipotle Chicken Skewers, 1 serving	8
Honey and Herb Roasted Half Chicken, 1 serving	11
Wood-Grilled Filet Mignon, 1 serving	12
Wood-Grilled Flat Iron Steak Entrée, 1 serving	11
Wood-Grilled NY Strip Steak, 1 serving	18
Wood-Grilled Pork Tenderloin, 1 serving	16
Wood-Grilled Rack of Lamb, 1 serving	13

Fish & Seafood

	SmartPoints® value
Ahi Tuna Tartare, 1 serving	13
Asian Glazed Chilean Sea Bass, 1 serving	17
Caramelized Grilled Sea Scallops Dinner, 1 serving	15
Cedar Plank Roasted Salmon, 1 serving	12
Grilled Boneless Rainbow Trout, 1 serving	11
Halibut, 1 serving	12
Lobster Pappardelle, 1 serving	23
Shrimp Scampi Skillet with Bomba Rice Entrée, 1 serving	15
Southern Style Shrimp and Grits, 1 serving	26
Wild Alaskan Copper River Salmon, 1 serving	15

Flatbreads

	SmartPoints® value
All Natural Pepperoni Flatbread, 1 flatbread	18
All Natural Pepperoni Flatbread, ½ flatbread	9
Artichoke and Laura Chenel Goat Cheese Flatbread, 1 flatbread	13
Artichoke Flatbread, ½ flatbread	6
Blackened Steak and Blue Cheese Flatbread, 1 flatbread	15
Crispy Prosciutto and Camembert Flatbread, 1 flatbread	16
Fig & Bacon Flatbread, 1 flatbread	15

"We Like This!" item

	SmartPoints® value
Garlic Pesto Chicken Flatbread, 1 flatbread	13
Garlic Pesto Chicken Flatbread, ½ flatbread	7
Lobster and Fresh Mozzarella Flatbread, 1 flatbread	12
Plum Tomato Flatbread, ½ flatbread	6
Roasted Roma Tomato Flatbread, 1 flatbread	13
Steak & Mushroom Flatbread, ½ flatbread	8

Handhelds

Blackened Mahi Mahi Tacos, 1 serving	11
Braised Beef Tacos, 1 serving	13
Crispy Braised Short Rib Sandwich, 1 serving	15
Grilled Chicken Caprese Sandwich, 1 serving	18
Lobster BLT Lettuce Wraps, 1 serving	5
Lump Crab Cake Sandwich, 1 serving	14
Signature Burger, 1 serving	16

Soups

Asparagus Soup, 1 bowl	7
Asparagus Soup, 1 cup	6
Chicken and White Bean Chili, 1 bowl	13
Chicken and White Bean Chili, 1 cup	11
Chicken Chili, 1 bowl	13
Corn Soup, 1 cup	13
Potato Leek Soup, 1 bowl	9
Potato Leek Soup, 1 cup	8

	SmartPoints® value
Roasted Tomato Soup, 1 bowl	10
Roasted Tomato Soup, 1 cup	9
Summer Corn Soup, 1 bowl	13
Summer Corn Soup, 1 cup	10
Tomato Soup, 1 bowl	10

Salads

Baby Spinach and Strawberries Salad, 1 small salad	8
BBQ Chicken Salad, 1 entrée salad	13
Crisp Romaine and Baby Kale Caesar, 1 small salad	10
Field Greens Salad, 1 serving	6
Grilled Flat Iron Steak Salad, 1 entrée salad	14
Heirloom Tomato & Haas Avocado, 1 small salad	14
Kalymnos Greek Salad, 1 small salad	8
Lump Crab Wedge Salad, 1 entrée salad	10
Maui Tuna Crunch, 1 entrée salad	12
Maui Tuna Crunch, 1 entrée salad	12
Organic Field Greens, 1 small salad	6
Quinoa and Citrus Salad, 1 serving	9
Sesame Grilled Salmon Salad, 1 entrée salad	13
Shaved Kale Salad, 1 small salad	16
Spring Vegetarian Tasting, 1 entrée salad	13
Summer Vegetarian Tasting, 1 entrée salad	15
Warm Heirloom Tomato Caprese, 1 small salad	16
Watermelon & Heirloom Tomato Salad, 1 small salad	8
Wood-Grilled Flat Iron Steak Salad, 1 serving	14

Sides

	SmartPoints® value
Charcoal Roasted Vegetables, 1 serving	5
Farro Quinoa Citrus, 1 serving	9
French Green Bean Salad, 1 serving	3
Grilled Asparagus with Sriracha Hollandaise, 1 serving	4
Housemade Pickles, 1 serving	1
Mac 'n' Cheese en Brodo, 1 serving	15
Roasted Summer Corn Skillet, 1 serving	15
Shaved Kale Salad, 1 serving	11
Snow Peas with Mushrooms, 1 serving	8
Sweet Corn & Black Bean Salad, 1 serving	5
Warm California Golden Beets, 1 serving	8
Wood-Grilled Potato Salad, 1 serving	6

Add-Ons

Caramelized Sea Scallops, 1 serving	12
Lobster Tail, 1 serving	5
Shrimp Scampi Skillet with Bomba Rice, 1 serving	15

Happy Hour

	SmartPoints® value
Caramelized Grilled Scallops, 1 serving	6
Chicken Yakitori Skewers, 1 serving	10
Duck Lollipops, 1 serving	8
Kona Crusted Lamb Chop, 1 serving	4
Shishito Peppers, 1 serving	7
Shrimp Scampi Skillet, 1 serving	7
Tuna Tataki, 1 serving	2
Wood-Grilled Meatballs, 1 serving	10

Kid's Menu

Cheese Flatbread, 1 serving	8
Chicken Tenders, 1 serving	6
Pasta with Sauce, 1 serving	10
Signature Burger, 1 serving	17

Desserts

Carrot Cake Mini, 1 serving	11
Fresh Fruit Mini, 1 serving	2
Key Lime with Pecan Crust Mini, 1 serving	15
Mocha Macchiato Mini, 1 serving	14
Peanut Butter and Chocolate Mousse Mini, 1 serving	14
Pecan Pie Mini, 1 serving	17
Raspberry Chocolate Cannoli Mini, 1 serving	10
S'more Mini, 1 serving	14
Toasted Almond Amaretto Mini, 1 serving	13
Traverse City Cherry Crème Brulee Mini, 1 serving	16

"We Like This!" item

	SmartPoints® value

Brewed Coffee

Bold Pick of the Day Tall, 1 serving	0
Clover Brewed Coffee Tall, 1 serving	0
Decaf Pike Place Roast Tall, 1 serving	0
Pike Place Roast Tall, 1 serving	0

Espresso Beverages

Caffe Latte Short with Nonfat Milk, 1 serving	3
Caffe Latte Tall with Nonfat Milk, 1 serving	4
Caffe Mocha Short with 2% Milk No Whipped Cream, 1 serving	6
Caffe Mocha Short with 2% Milk Whipped Cream, 1 serving	8
Caffe Mocha Short with Nonfat Milk No Whipped Cream, 1 serving	5
Caffe Mocha Short with Nonfat Milk Whipped Cream, 1 serving	7
Caffe Mocha Short with Soy Milk No Whipped Cream, 1 serving	6
Caffe Mocha Short with Soy Milk Whipped Cream, 1 serving	8
Caffe Mocha Short with Whole Milk No Whipped Cream, 1 serving	7
Caffe Mocha Short with Whole Milk Whipped Cream, 1 serving	9
Caffe Mocha Tall with 2% Milk No Whipped Cream, 1 serving	9
Caffe Mocha Tall with 2% Milk Whipped Cream, 1 serving	12
Caffe Mocha Tall with Nonfat Milk No Whipped Cream, 1 serving	8
Caffe Mocha Tall with Nonfat Milk Whipped Cream, 1 serving	11
Caffe Mocha Tall with Soy Milk No Whipped Cream, 1 serving	9
Caffe Mocha Tall with Soy Milk Whipped Cream, 1 serving	12
Caffe Mocha Tall with Whole Milk No Whipped Cream, 1 serving	11
Caffe Mocha Tall with Whole Milk Whipped Cream, 1 serving	14
Cappuccino Short with 2% Milk, 1 serving	3
Cappuccino Short with Coconut Milk, 1 serving	4
Cappuccino Short with Nonfat Milk, 1 serving	2
Cappuccino Short with Soy Milk, 1 serving	2
Cappuccino Short with Whole Milk, 1 serving	4
Cappuccino Tall with 2% Milk, 1 serving	4
Cappuccino Tall with Coconut Milk, 1 serving	6
Cappuccino Tall with Nonfat Milk, 1 serving	2
Cappuccino Tall with Soy Milk, 1 serving	4
Cappuccino Tall with Whole Milk, 1 serving	5
Caramel Macchiato Short with Nonfat Milk, 1 serving	4
Caramel Macchiato Tall with Nonfat Milk, 1 serving	6
Cinnamon Dolce Latte Short with 2% Milk No Whipped Cream, 1 serving	6
Cinnamon Dolce Latte Short with 2% Milk Whipped Cream, 1 serving	9
Cinnamon Dolce Latte Short with Nonfat Milk No Whipped Cream, 1 serving	5
Cinnamon Dolce Latte Short with Nonfat Milk Whipped Cream, 1 serving	8
Cinnamon Dolce Latte Short with Soy Milk No Whipped Cream, 1 serving	6
Cinnamon Dolce Latte Short with Soy Milk Whipped Cream, 1 serving	8

"We Like This!" item

	SmartPoints® value
Cinnamon Dolce Latte Short with Whole Milk No Whipped Cream, 1 serving	7
Cinnamon Dolce Latte Short with Whole Milk Whipped Cream, 1 serving	10
Cinnamon Dolce Latte Tall with 2% Milk No Whipped Cream, 1 serving	9
Cinnamon Dolce Latte Tall with 2% Milk Whipped Cream, 1 serving	13
Cinnamon Dolce Latte Tall with Nonfat Milk No Whipped Cream, 1 serving	8
Cinnamon Dolce Latte Tall with Nonfat Milk Whipped Cream, 1 serving	11
Cinnamon Dolce Latte Tall with Soy Milk No Whipped Cream, 1 serving	9
Cinnamon Dolce Latte Tall with Soy Milk Whipped Cream, 1 serving	12
Cinnamon Dolce Latte Tall with Whole Milk No Whipped Cream, 1 serving	11
Cinnamon Dolce Latte Tall with Whole Milk Whipped Cream, 1 serving	14
Espresso Con Panna Doppio No Milk, 1 serving	1
Espresso Con Panna Solo, 1 serving	1
Espresso Con Panna Solo No Milk, 1 serving	1
Espresso Macchiato Doppio with 2% Milk, 1 serving	0
Espresso Macchiato Doppio with Nonfat Milk, 1 serving	0
Espresso Macchiato Doppio with Soy Milk, 1 serving	0
Espresso Macchiato Doppio with Whole Milk, 1 serving	0
Espresso Macchiato Solo with 2% Milk, 1 serving	0

	SmartPoints® value
Espresso Macchiato Solo with Nonfat Milk, 1 serving	0
Espresso Macchiato Solo with Soy Milk, 1 serving	0
Espresso Macchiato Solo with Whole Milk, 1 serving	0
Espresso Short, 1 serving	0
Espresso Tall, 1 serving	0
Flavored Latte Short with 2% Milk, 1 serving	6
Flavored Latte Short with Nonfat Milk, 1 serving	5
Flavored Latte Short with Soy Milk, 1 serving	6
Flavored Latte Short with Whole Milk, 1 serving	7
Flavored Latte Tall with Nonfat Milk, 1 serving	7
Flavored Latte Tall with Soy Milk, 1 serving	8
Hazelnut Macchiato Short with 2% Milk, 1 serving	5
Hazelnut Macchiato Short with Nonfat Milk, 1 serving	4
Hazelnut Macchiato Short with Soy Milk, 1 serving	5
Hazelnut Macchiato Short with Whole Milk, 1 serving	6
Hazelnut Macchiato Tall with 2% Milk, 1 serving	8
Hazelnut Macchiato Tall with Nonfat Milk, 1 serving	6
Hazelnut Macchiato Tall with Soy Milk, 1 serving	8
Hazelnut Macchiato Tall with Whole Milk, 1 serving	9
Pumpkin Spice Latte Tall with 2% Milk No Whipped Cream, 1 serving	11
Pumpkin Spice Latte Tall with 2% Milk Whipped Cream, 1 serving	15
Pumpkin Spice Latte Tall with Nonfat Milk No Whipped Cream, 1 serving	9

	SmartPoints® value
Pumpkin Spice Latte Tall with Nonfat Milk Whipped Cream, 1 serving	13
Pumpkin Spice Latte Tall with Soy Milk No Whipped Cream, 1 serving	11
Pumpkin Spice Latte Tall with Soy Milk Whipped Cream, 1 serving	14
Pumpkin Spice Latte Tall with Whole Milk No Whipped Cream, 1 serving	13
Pumpkin Spice Latte Tall with Whole Milk Whipped Cream, 1 serving	16
Salted Caramel Mocha Tall with 2% Milk No Whipped Cream, 1 serving	12
Salted Caramel Mocha Tall with 2% Milk Whipped Cream, 1 serving	16
Salted Caramel Mocha Tall with Nonfat Milk No Whipped Cream, 1 serving	11
Salted Caramel Mocha Tall with Nonfat Milk Whipped Cream, 1 serving	15
Salted Caramel Mocha Tall with Soy Milk No Whipped Cream, 1 serving	12
Salted Caramel Mocha Tall with Soy Milk Whipped Cream, 1 serving	16
Salted Caramel Mocha Tall with Whole Milk No Whipped Cream, 1 serving	14
Salted Caramel Mocha Tall with Whole Milk Whipped Cream, 1 serving	18
Short Flat White (2% milk), 1 serving	4
Short Flat White (coconut milk), 1 serving	3
Short Flat White (soy milk), 1 serving	3

	SmartPoints® value
Short Flat White (whole milk), 1 serving	5
Sugar-free Short Flat White (nonfat milk), 1 serving	2
Sugar-free Tall Flat White (nonfat milk), 1 serving	4
Tall Flat White (2% milk), 1 serving	6
Tall Flat White (coconut milk), 1 serving	6
Tall Flat White (soy milk), 1 serving	5
Tall Flat White (whole milk), 1 serving	7
Vanilla Latte Short with 2% Milk, 1 serving	6
Vanilla Latte Short with Nonfat Milk, 1 serving	5
Vanilla Latte Short with Whole Milk, 1 serving	7
Vanilla Latte Tall with 2% Milk, 1 serving	9
Vanilla Latte Tall with Nonfat Milk, 1 serving	7
Vanilla Latte Tall with Whole Milk, 1 serving	10
White Chocolate Mocha Short with 2% Milk No Whipped Cream, 1 serving	10
White Chocolate Mocha Short with 2% Milk Whipped Cream, 1 serving	12
White Chocolate Mocha Short with Nonfat Milk No Whipped Cream, 1 serving	9
White Chocolate Mocha Short with Nonfat Milk Whipped Cream, 1 serving	11
White Chocolate Mocha Short with Soy Milk No Whipped Cream, 1 serving	10
White Chocolate Mocha Short with Soy Milk Whipped Cream, 1 serving	12
White Chocolate Mocha Short with Whole Milk No Whipped Cream, 1 serving	11

"We Like This!" item

Item	SmartPoints® value
White Chocolate Mocha Short with Whole Milk Whipped Cream, 1 serving	13
White Chocolate Mocha Tall with 2% Milk No Whipped Cream, 1 serving	15
White Chocolate Mocha Tall with 2% Milk Whipped Cream, 1 serving	18
White Chocolate Mocha Tall with Nonfat Milk No Whipped Cream, 1 serving	13
White Chocolate Mocha Tall with Nonfat Milk Whipped Cream, 1 serving	16
White Chocolate Mocha Tall with Soy Milk No Whipped Cream, 1 serving	15
White Chocolate Mocha Tall with Soy Milk Whipped Cream, 1 serving	18
White Chocolate Mocha Tall with Whole Milk No Whipped Cream, 1 serving	16
White Chocolate Mocha Tall with Whole Milk Whipped Cream, 1 serving	19

Frappuccinos

Item	SmartPoints® value
Bottled Caramel Frappuccino Coffee Drink, 1 serving	10
Caffe Vanilla Frappuccino Grande with Whole Milk No Whipped Cream, 1 serving	18
Caffe Vanilla Frappuccino Grande with Whole Milk Whipped Cream, 1 serving	23
Caffe Vanilla Frappuccino Light Grande, 1 serving	10
Caffe Vanilla Frappuccino Light Venti with Nonfat Milk, 1 serving	14
Caffe Vanilla Frappuccino Tall with 2% Milk No Whipped Cream, 1 serving	12
Caffe Vanilla Frappuccino Tall with 2% Milk Whipped Cream, 1 serving	16
Caffe Vanilla Frappuccino Tall with Nonfat Milk No Whipped Cream, 1 serving	11
Caffe Vanilla Frappuccino Tall with Nonfat Milk Whipped Cream, 1 serving	15
Caffe Vanilla Frappuccino Tall with Soy Milk No Whipped Cream, 1 serving	12
Caffe Vanilla Frappuccino Tall with Soy Milk Whipped Cream, 1 serving	16
Caffe Vanilla Frappuccino Tall with Whole Milk No Whipped Cream, 1 serving	12
Caffe Vanilla Frappuccino Tall with Whole Milk Whipped Cream, 1 serving	16
Caramel Frappuccino Light Grande, 1 serving	7
Caramel Frappuccino Light Grande with Nonfat Milk, 1 serving	7
Caramel Frappuccino Light Tall with Nonfat Milk, 1 serving	5
Caramel Frappuccino Light Venti with Nonfat Milk, 1 serving	10
Caramel Frappuccino Tall with 2% Milk No Whipped Cream, 1 serving	12
Caramel Frappuccino Tall with 2% Milk Whipped Cream, 1 serving	16
Caramel Frappuccino Tall with Nonfat Milk No Whipped Cream, 1 serving	11
Caramel Frappuccino Tall with Nonfat Milk Whipped Cream, 1 serving	15
Caramel Frappuccino Tall with Soy Milk No Whipped Cream, 1 serving	11
Caramel Frappuccino Tall with Soy Milk Whipped Cream, 1 serving	16

	SmartPoints® value
Caramel Frappuccino Tall with Whole Milk No Whipped Cream, 1 serving	11
Caramel Frappuccino Tall with Whole Milk Whipped Cream, 1 serving	16
Caramel Ribbon Crunch Creme Frappuccino Tall with 2% Milk No Whipped Cream, 1 serving	15
Caramel Ribbon Crunch Creme Frappuccino Tall with 2% Milk Whipped Cream, 1 serving	21
Caramel Ribbon Crunch Creme Frappuccino Tall with Nonfat Milk No Whipped Cream, 1 serving	15
Caramel Ribbon Crunch Creme Frappuccino Tall with Nonfat Milk Whipped Cream, 1 serving	20
Caramel Ribbon Crunch Frappuccino Tall with 2% Milk No Whipped Cream, 1 serving	16
Caramel Ribbon Crunch Frappuccino Tall with 2% Milk Whipped Cream, 1 serving	22
Caramel Ribbon Crunch Frappuccino Tall with Nonfat Milk No Whipped Cream, 1 serving	16
Caramel Ribbon Crunch Frappuccino Tall with Nonfat Milk Whipped Cream, 1 serving	21
Chocolate Cookie Crumble Frappuccino Tall with 2% Milk No Whipped Cream, 1 serving	11
Chocolate Cookie Crumble Frappuccino Tall with 2% Milk Whipped Cream, 1 serving	16
Chocolate Cookie Crumble Frappuccino Tall with Nonfat Milk No Whipped Cream, 1 serving	11
Chocolate Cookie Crumble Frappuccino Tall with Nonfat Milk Whipped Cream, 1 serving	15
Cinnamon Dolce Creme Frappuccino Tall with 2% Milk No Whipped Cream, 1 serving	9

	SmartPoints® value
Cinnamon Dolce Creme Frappuccino Tall with 2% Milk Whipped Cream, 1 serving	13
Cinnamon Dolce Creme Frappuccino Tall with Nonfat Milk No Whipped Cream, 1 serving	8
Cinnamon Dolce Creme Frappuccino Tall with Nonfat Milk Whipped Cream, 1 serving	12
Cinnamon Dolce Creme Frappuccino Tall with Soy Milk No Whipped Cream, 1 serving	8
Cinnamon Dolce Creme Frappuccino Tall with Soy Milk Whipped Cream, 1 serving	12
Cinnamon Dolce Creme Frappuccino Tall with Whole Milk No Whipped Cream, 1 serving	9
Cinnamon Dolce Creme Frappuccino Tall with Whole Milk Whipped Cream, 1 serving	13
Cinnamon Dolce Frappuccino Light Grande with Nonfat Milk, 1 serving	6
Cinnamon Dolce Frappuccino Light Tall with Nonfat Milk, 1 serving	5
Cinnamon Dolce Frappuccino Light Venti with Nonfat Milk, 1 serving	9
Cinnamon Dolce Frappuccino Tall with 2% Milk No Whipped Cream, 1 serving	10
Cinnamon Dolce Frappuccino Tall with 2% Milk Whipped Cream, 1 serving	15
Cinnamon Dolce Frappuccino Tall with Nonfat Milk No Whipped Cream, 1 serving	10
Cinnamon Dolce Frappuccino Tall with Nonfat Milk Whipped Cream, 1 serving	14
Cinnamon Dolce Frappuccino Tall with Soy Milk No Whipped Cream, 1 serving	10
Cinnamon Dolce Frappuccino Tall with Soy Milk Whipped Cream, 1 serving	14

"We Like This!" item

	SmartPoints® value
Cinnamon Dolce Frappuccino Tall with Whole Milk No Whipped Cream, 1 serving	11
Cinnamon Dolce Frappuccino Tall with Whole Milk Whipped Cream, 1 serving	15
Coffee Frappuccino Light Grande, 1 serving	6
Coffee Frappuccino Light Grande with Nonfat Milk, 1 serving	6
Coffee Frappuccino Light Tall with Nonfat Milk, 1 serving	5
Coffee Frappuccino Light Venti with Nonfat Milk, 1 serving	8
Coffee Frappuccino Tall with 2% Milk, 1 serving	10
Coffee Frappuccino Tall with Nonfat Milk, 1 serving	9
Coffee Frappuccino Tall with Soy Milk, 1 serving	9
Coffee Frappuccino Tall with Whole Milk, 1 serving	10
Double Chocolaty Chip Frappuccino Tall with 2% Milk No Whipped Cream, 1 serving	11
Double Chocolaty Chip Frappuccino Tall with 2% Milk Whipped Cream, 1 serving	15
Double Chocolaty Chip Frappuccino Tall with Nonfat Milk No Whipped Cream, 1 serving	10
Double Chocolaty Chip Frappuccino Tall with Nonfat Milk Whipped Cream, 1 serving	15
Double Chocolaty Chip Frappuccino Tall with Soy Milk No Whipped Cream, 1 serving	11
Double Chocolaty Chip Frappuccino Tall with Soy Milk Whipped Cream, 1 serving	15
Double Chocolaty Chip Frappuccino Tall with Whole Milk No Whipped Cream, 1 serving	12
Double Chocolaty Chip Frappuccino Tall with Whole Milk Whipped Cream, 1 serving	16

	SmartPoints® value
Espresso Frappuccino Tall with 2% Milk, 1 serving	8
Espresso Frappuccino Tall with Nonfat Milk, 1 serving	8
Espresso Frappuccino Tall with Soy Milk, 1 serving	8
Espresso Frappuccino Tall with Whole Milk, 1 serving	9
Hazelnut Frappuccino Tall with 2% Milk No Whipped Cream, 1 serving	10
Hazelnut Frappuccino Tall with 2% Milk Whipped Cream, 1 serving	15
Hazelnut Frappuccino Tall with Nonfat Milk No Whipped Cream, 1 serving	10
Hazelnut Frappuccino Tall with Nonfat Milk Whipped Cream, 1 serving	14
Hazelnut Frappuccino Tall with Soy Milk No Whipped Cream, 1 serving	10
Hazelnut Frappuccino Tall with Soy Milk Whipped Cream, 1 serving	15
Hazelnut Frappuccino Tall with Whole Milk No Whipped Cream, 1 serving	11
Hazelnut Frappuccino Tall with Whole Milk Whipped Cream, 1 serving	15
Java Chip Frappuccino Light Grande, 1 serving	11
Java Chip Frappuccino Light Grande with Nonfat Milk, 1 serving	11
Java Chip Frappuccino Light Tall with Nonfat Milk, 1 serving	8
Java Chip Frappuccino Light Venti with Nonfat Milk, 1 serving	14
Java Chip Frappuccino Tall with 2% Milk No Whipped Cream, 1 serving	13
Java Chip Frappuccino Tall with 2% Milk Whipped Cream, 1 serving	17

	SmartPoints® value
Java Chip Frappuccino Tall with Nonfat Milk No Whipped Cream, 1 serving	13
Java Chip Frappuccino Tall with Nonfat Milk Whipped Cream, 1 serving	16
Java Chip Frappuccino Tall with Soy Milk No Whipped Cream, 1 serving	13
Java Chip Frappuccino Tall with Soy Milk Whipped Cream, 1 serving	17
Java Chip Frappuccino Tall with Whole Milk No Whipped Cream, 1 serving	13
Java Chip Frappuccino Tall with Whole Milk Whipped Cream, 1 serving	18
Mocha Cookie Crumble Frappuccino Tall with 2% Milk No Whipped Cream, 1 serving	13
Mocha Cookie Crumble Frappuccino Tall with 2% Milk Whipped Cream, 1 serving	18
Mocha Cookie Crumble Frappuccino Tall with Nonfat Milk No Whipped Cream, 1 serving	12
Mocha Cookie Crumble Frappuccino Tall with Nonfat Milk Whipped Cream, 1 serving	17
Mocha Frappuccino Light Grande with Nonfat Milk, 1 serving	7
Mocha Frappuccino Light Tall with Nonfat Milk, 1 serving	6
Mocha Frappuccino Light Venti with Nonfat Milk, 1 serving	10
Mocha Frappuccino Tall with 2% Milk No Whipped Cream, 1 serving	11
Mocha Frappuccino Tall with 2% Milk Whipped Cream, 1 serving	14
Mocha Frappuccino Tall with Nonfat Milk No Whipped Cream, 1 serving	10

	SmartPoints® value
Mocha Frappuccino Tall with Nonfat Milk Whipped Cream, 1 serving	14
Mocha Frappuccino Tall with Soy Milk No Whipped Cream, 1 serving	10
Mocha Frappuccino Tall with Soy Milk Whipped Cream, 1 serving	15
Mocha Frappuccino Tall with Whole Milk No Whipped Cream, 1 serving	11
Mocha Frappuccino Tall with Whole Milk Whipped Cream, 1 serving	15
Salted Caramel Mocha Frappuccino Tall with 2% Milk No Whipped Cream, 1 serving	12
Salted Caramel Mocha Frappuccino Tall with 2% Milk Whipped Cream, 1 serving	17
Salted Caramel Mocha Frappuccino Tall with Skimmed Milk No Whipped Cream, 1 serving	11
Salted Caramel Mocha Frappuccino Tall with Skimmed Milk Whipped Cream, 1 serving	16
Salted Caramel Mocha Frappuccino Tall with Soy Milk No Whipped Cream, 1 serving	12
Salted Caramel Mocha Frappuccino Tall with Soy Milk Whipped Cream, 1 serving	17
Salted Caramel Mocha Frappuccino Tall with Whole Milk No Whipped Cream, 1 serving	13
Salted Caramel Mocha Frappuccino Tall with Whole Milk Whipped Cream, 1 serving	18
Strawberries and Creme Frappuccino Tall with 2% Milk No Whipped Cream, 1 serving	10
Strawberries and Creme Frappuccino Tall with 2% Milk Whipped Cream, 1 serving	14

"We Like This!" item

	SmartPoints® value
Strawberries and Creme Frappuccino Tall with 2% Milk Whipped Cream Unsweetened, 1 serving	14
Strawberries and Creme Frappuccino Tall with Nonfat Milk No Whipped Cream, 1 serving	9
Strawberries and Creme Frappuccino Tall with Nonfat Milk Whipped Cream, 1 serving	13
Strawberries and Creme Frappuccino Tall with Nonfat Milk Whipped Cream Unsweetened, 1 serving	13
Strawberries and Creme Frappuccino Tall with Soy Milk No Whipped Cream, 1 serving	10
Strawberries and Creme Frappuccino Tall with Soy Milk Whipped Cream, 1 serving	14
Strawberries and Creme Frappuccino Tall with Whole Milk No Whipped Cream, 1 serving	10
Strawberries and Creme Frappuccino Tall with Whole Milk Whipped Cream, 1 serving	15
Tall Teavana® Oprah Cinnamon Chai Crème Frappucino with 2% Milk (no whipped cream), 1 serving	8
Tall Teavana® Oprah Cinnamon Chai Crème Frappucino with 2% Milk (with whipped cream), 1 serving	12
Tall Teavana® Oprah Cinnamon Chai Crème Frappucino with Coconut Milk (no whipped cream), 1 serving	8
Tall Teavana® Oprah Cinnamon Chai Crème Frappucino with Coconut Milk (with whipped cream), 1 serving	12
Tall Teavana® Oprah Cinnamon Chai Crème Frappucino with Nonfat Milk (no whipped cream), 1 serving	8

	SmartPoints® value
Tall Teavana® Oprah Cinnamon Chai Crème Frappucino with Nonfat Milk (with whipped cream), 1 serving	12
Tall Teavana® Oprah Cinnamon Chai Crème Frappucino with Soy Milk (no whipped cream), 1 serving	8
Tall Teavana® Oprah Cinnamon Chai Crème Frappucino with Soy Milk (with whipped cream), 1 serving	12
Tall Teavana® Oprah Cinnamon Chai Crème Frappucino with Whole Milk (no whipped cream), 1 serving	8
Tall Teavana® Oprah Cinnamon Chai Crème Frappucino with Whole Milk (with whipped cream), 1 serving	13
Tazo Chai Frappuccino Tall with 2% Milk No Whipped Cream, 1 serving	9
Tazo Chai Frappuccino Tall with 2% Milk Whipped Cream, 1 serving	13
Tazo Chai Frappuccino Tall with Nonfat Milk No Whipped Cream, 1 serving	8
Tazo Chai Frappuccino Tall with Nonfat Milk Whipped Cream, 1 serving	12
Tazo Chai Frappuccino Tall with Soy Milk No Whipped Cream, 1 serving	8
Tazo Chai Frappuccino Tall with Soy Milk Whipped Cream, 1 serving	12
Tazo Chai Frappuccino Tall with Whole Milk No Whipped Cream, 1 serving	9
Tazo Chai Frappuccino Tall with Whole Milk Whipped Cream, 1 serving	13
Tazo Green Tea Frappuccino Grande with 2% Milk No Whipped Cream Unsweetened, 1 serving	17

	SmartPoints® value
Tazo Green Tea Frappuccino Tall with 2% Milk No Whipped Cream Unsweetened, 1 serving	13
Tazo Green Tea Frappuccino Tall with 2% Milk Whipped Cream Unsweetened, 1 serving	16
Tazo Green Tea Frappuccino Tall with Nonfat Milk No Whipped Cream Unsweetened, 1 serving	12
Tazo Green Tea Frappuccino Tall with Nonfat Milk Whipped Cream Unsweetened, 1 serving	16
Tazo Green Tea Frappuccino Tall with Soy Milk No Whipped Cream Unsweetened, 1 serving	12
Tazo Green Tea Frappuccino Tall with Soy Milk Whipped Cream Unsweetened, 1 serving	16
Tazo Green Tea Frappuccino Tall with Whole Milk No Whipped Cream Unsweetened, 1 serving	13
Tazo Green Tea Frappuccino Tall with Whole Milk Whipped Cream Unsweetened, 1 serving	17
Vanilla Bean Creme Frappuccino Tall with 2% Milk No Whipped Cream, 1 serving	10
Vanilla Bean Creme Frappuccino Tall with 2% Milk Whipped Cream, 1 serving	14
Vanilla Bean Creme Frappuccino Tall with Nonfat Milk No Whipped Cream, 1 serving	9
Vanilla Bean Creme Frappuccino Tall with Nonfat Milk Whipped Cream, 1 serving	13
Vanilla Bean Creme Frappuccino Tall with Soy Milk No Whipped Cream, 1 serving	10
Vanilla Bean Creme Frappuccino Tall with Soy Milk Whipped Cream, 1 serving	14
Vanilla Bean Creme Frappuccino Tall with Whole Milk No Whipped Cream, 1 serving	11

	SmartPoints® value
Vanilla Bean Creme Frappuccino Tall with Whole Milk Whipped Cream, 1 serving	15
White Chocolate Creme Frappuccino Tall with 2% Milk No Whipped Cream, 1 serving	10
White Chocolate Creme Frappuccino Tall with 2% Milk Whipped Cream, 1 serving	14
White Chocolate Creme Frappuccino Tall with Nonfat Milk No Whipped Cream, 1 serving	10
White Chocolate Creme Frappuccino Tall with Nonfat Milk Whipped Cream, 1 serving	14
White Chocolate Creme Frappuccino Tall with Soy Milk No Whipped Cream, 1 serving	10
White Chocolate Creme Frappuccino Tall with Soy Milk Whipped Cream, 1 serving	14
White Chocolate Creme Frappuccino Tall with Whole Milk No Whipped Cream, 1 serving	11
White Chocolate Creme Frappuccino Tall with Whole Milk Whipped Cream, 1 serving	15
White Chocolate Mocha Frappuccino Tall with 2% Milk No Whipped Cream, 1 serving	13
White Chocolate Mocha Frappuccino Tall with 2% Milk Whipped Cream, 1 serving	17
White Chocolate Mocha Frappuccino Tall with Nonfat No Whipped Cream, 1 serving	12
White Chocolate Mocha Frappuccino Tall with Nonfat Whipped Cream, 1 serving	16
White Chocolate Mocha Frappuccino Tall with Soy Milk No Whipped Cream, 1 serving	13
White Chocolate Mocha Frappuccino Tall with Soy Milk Whipped Cream, 1 serving	17

"We Like This!" item

	SmartPoints® value
White Chocolate Mocha Frappuccino Tall with Whole Milk No Whipped Cream, 1 serving	13
White Chocolate Mocha Frappuccino Tall with Whole Milk Whipped Cream, 1 serving	17

Americano

Caffe Americano, 1 serving	0
Caffe Americano Short, 1 serving	0
Caffe Americano Short No Milk, 1 serving	0
Caffe Americano Tall, 1 serving	0
Caffe Americano Tall No Milk, 1 serving	0
Iced Caffe Americano Tall, 1 serving	0

Hot Chocolate

	SmartPoints® value
Hot Chocolate Short with 2% Milk No Whipped Cream, 1 serving	7
Hot Chocolate Short with 2% Milk Whipped Cream, 1 serving	10
Hot Chocolate Short with Nonfat Milk No Whipped Cream, 1 serving	6
Hot Chocolate Short with Nonfat Milk Whipped Cream, 1 serving	9
Hot Chocolate Short with Soy Milk No Whipped Cream, 1 serving	7
Hot Chocolate Short with Soy Milk Whipped Cream, 1 serving	10
Hot Chocolate Short with Whole Milk No Whipped Cream, 1 serving	8
Hot Chocolate Short with Whole Milk Whipped Cream, 1 serving	11
Hot Chocolate Tall with 2% Milk No Whipped Cream, 1 serving	14
Hot Chocolate Tall with 2% Milk Whipped Cream, 1 serving	14
Hot Chocolate Tall with Nonfat Milk No Whipped Cream, 1 serving	9
Hot Chocolate Tall with Nonfat Milk Whipped Cream, 1 serving	12
Hot Chocolate Tall with Soy Milk No Whipped Cream, 1 serving	10
Hot Chocolate Tall with Soy Milk Whipped Cream, 1 serving	13
Hot Chocolate Tall with Whole Milk No Whipped Cream, 1 serving	12
Hot Chocolate Tall with Whole Milk Whipped Cream, 1 serving	16
Peppermint Hot Chocolate Short with 2% Milk No Whipped Cream, 1 serving	10
Peppermint Hot Chocolate Short with 2% Milk Whipped Cream, 1 serving	13
Peppermint Hot Chocolate Short with Nonfat Milk No Whipped Cream, 1 serving	8
Peppermint Hot Chocolate Short with Nonfat Milk Whipped Cream, 1 serving	11
Peppermint Hot Chocolate Short with Soy Milk No Whipped Cream, 1 serving	9
Peppermint Hot Chocolate Short with Soy Milk Whipped Cream, 1 serving	12
Peppermint Hot Chocolate Short with Whole Milk No Whipped Cream, 1 serving	10
Peppermint Hot Chocolate Short with Whole Milk Whipped Cream, 1 serving	13
Peppermint Hot Chocolate Tall with 2% Milk No Whipped Cream, 1 serving	14
Peppermint Hot Chocolate Tall with 2% Milk Whipped Cream, 1 serving	18
Peppermint Hot Chocolate Tall with Nonfat Milk No Whipped Cream, 1 serving	12
Peppermint Hot Chocolate Tall with Nonfat Milk Whipped Cream, 1 serving	16
Peppermint Hot Chocolate Tall with Soy Milk No Whipped Cream, 1 serving	14

	SmartPoints® value
Peppermint Hot Chocolate Tall with Soy Milk Whipped Cream, 1 serving	17
Peppermint Hot Chocolate Tall with Whole Milk No Whipped Cream, 1 serving	15
Peppermint Hot Chocolate Tall with Whole Milk Whipped Cream, 1 serving	19
White Hot Chocolate Short with 2% Milk No Whipped Cream, 1 serving	10
White Hot Chocolate Short with 2% Milk Whipped Cream, 1 serving	13
White Hot Chocolate Short with Nonfat Milk No Whipped Cream, 1 serving	9
White Hot Chocolate Short with Nonfat Milk Whipped Cream, 1 serving	11
White Hot Chocolate Short with Soy Milk No Whipped Cream, 1 serving	10
White Hot Chocolate Short with Soy Milk Whipped Cream, 1 serving	13
White Hot Chocolate Short with Whole Milk No Whipped Cream, 1 serving	11
White Hot Chocolate Short with Whole Milk Whipped Cream, 1 serving	14

Iced Brewed Coffee

	SmartPoints® value
Caramel Iced Coffee, 1 serving	6
Iced Coffee and Milk, 1 serving	6
Iced Coffee Grande Unsweetened, 1 serving	0
Iced Coffee Tall Sweetened, 1 serving	4
Iced Coffee with Milk Tall with 2% Milk Sweetened, 1 serving	5
Iced Coffee with Milk Tall with 2% Milk Unsweetened, 1 serving	1
Iced Coffee with Milk Tall with Nonfat Milk Sweetened, 1 serving	4
Iced Coffee with Milk Tall with Nonfat Milk Unsweetened, 1 serving	1
Iced Coffee with Milk Tall with Soy Milk Sweetened, 1 serving	5
Iced Coffee with Milk Tall with Soy Milk Unsweetened, 1 serving	1
Iced Coffee with Milk Tall with Whole Milk Sweetened, 1 serving	5
Iced Coffee with Milk Tall with Whole Milk Unsweetened, 1 serving	1
Orange Spice Iced Coffee Tall Sweetened, 1 serving	4

"We Like This!" item

Iced Espresso Beverages

	SmartPoints® value
Iced Caffe Mocha Tall with 2% Milk No Whipped Cream, 1 serving	7
Iced Caffe Mocha Tall with 2% Milk Whipped Cream, 1 serving	11
Iced Caffe Mocha Tall with Nonfat Milk No Whipped Cream, 1 serving	6
Iced Caffe Mocha Tall with Nonfat Milk Whipped Cream, 1 serving	10
Iced Caffe Mocha Tall with Soy Milk No Whipped Cream, 1 serving	7
Iced Caffe Mocha Tall with Soy Milk Whipped Cream, 1 serving	11
Iced Caffe Mocha Tall with Whole Milk No Whipped Cream, 1 serving	8
Iced Caffe Mocha Tall with Whole Milk Whipped Cream, 1 serving	12
Iced Caramel Macchiato Tall with Nonfat Milk, 1 serving	7
Iced Cinnamon Dolce Latte Tall with 2% Milk No Whipped Cream, 1 serving	7
Iced Cinnamon Dolce Latte Tall with 2% Milk Whipped Cream, 1 serving	12
Iced Cinnamon Dolce Latte Tall with Nonfat Milk No Whipped Cream, 1 serving	6

	SmartPoints® value
Iced Cinnamon Dolce Latte Tall with Nonfat Milk Whipped Cream, 1 serving	10
Iced Cinnamon Dolce Latte Tall with Soy Milk No Whipped Cream, 1 serving	7
Iced Cinnamon Dolce Latte Tall with Soy Milk Whipped Cream, 1 serving	11
Iced Cinnamon Dolce Latte Tall with Whole Milk No Whipped Cream, 1 serving	9
Iced Cinnamon Dolce Latte Tall with Whole Milk Whipped Cream, 1 serving	12
Iced Flavored Latte Tall with Nonfat Milk, 1 serving	6
Iced Hazelnut Macchiato Tall with 2% Milk, 1 serving	8
Iced Hazelnut Macchiato Tall with Nonfat Milk, 1 serving	6
Iced Hazelnut Macchiato Tall with Soy Milk, 1 serving	7
Iced Hazelnut Macchiato Tall with Whole Milk, 1 serving	9
Iced Skinny Flavored Latte Tall with Nonfat Milk, 1 serving	2
Iced Skinny Mocha Tall with Nonfat Milk, 1 serving	3
Iced Vanilla Latte Tall with 2% Milk, 1 serving	7
Iced Vanilla Latte Tall with Nonfat Milk, 1 serving	6
Iced Vanilla Latte Tall with Whole Milk, 1 serving	8
Iced Vanilla Spice Latte Tall with 2% Milk No Whipped Cream, 1 serving	7
Iced Vanilla Spice Latte Tall with 2% Milk Whipped Cream, 1 serving	11
Iced Vanilla Spice Latte Tall with Nonfat Milk No Whipped Cream, 1 serving	6
Iced Vanilla Spice Latte Tall with Nonfat Milk Whipped Cream, 1 serving	10

	SmartPoints® value
Iced Vanilla Spice Latte Tall with Soy Milk No Whipped Cream, 1 serving	7
Iced Vanilla Spice Latte Tall with Soy Milk Whipped Cream, 1 serving	11
Iced Vanilla Spice Latte Tall with Whole Milk No Whipped Cream, 1 serving	8
Iced Vanilla Spice Latte Tall with Whole Milk Whipped Cream, 1 serving	12
Iced White Chocolate Mocha Tall with 2% Milk No Whipped Cream, 1 serving	13
Iced White Chocolate Mocha Tall with 2% Milk Whipped Cream, 1 serving	17
Iced White Chocolate Mocha Tall with Nonfat Milk No Whipped Cream, 1 serving	12
Iced White Chocolate Mocha Tall with Nonfat Milk Whipped Cream, 1 serving	16
Iced White Chocolate Mocha Tall with Soy Milk No Whipped Cream, 1 serving	13
Iced White Chocolate Mocha Tall with Soy Milk Whipped Cream, 1 serving	17
Iced White Chocolate Mocha Tall with Whole Milk No Whipped Cream, 1 serving	14
Iced White Chocolate Mocha Tall with Whole Milk Whipped Cream, 1 serving	18

Teas

Chai Tea Latte Short with 2% Milk, 1 serving	6
Chai Tea Latte Short with Nonfat Milk, 1 serving	5
Chai Tea Latte Short with Soy Milk, 1 serving	6
Chai Tea Latte Short with Whole Milk, 1 serving	7

Teas (cont'd)

	SmartPoints® value
Chai Tea Latte Tall with 2% Milk, 1 serving	9
Chai Tea Latte Tall with Nonfat Milk, 1 serving	8
Chai Tea Latte Tall with Soy Milk, 1 serving	9
Chai Tea Latte Tall with Whole Milk, 1 serving	10
Chocolate Chai Tea Latte Tall with 2% Milk, 1 serving	10
Chocolate Chai Tea Latte Tall with Nonfat Milk, 1 serving	8
Chocolate Chai Tea Latte Tall with Soy Milk, 1 serving	9
Chocolate Chai Tea Latte Tall with Whole Milk, 1 serving	10
Earl Grey Tea Latte Short with 2% Milk, 1 serving	5
Earl Grey Tea Latte Short with Nonfat Milk, 1 serving	4
Earl Grey Tea Latte Short with Soy Milk, 1 serving	4
Earl Grey Tea Latte Short with Whole Milk, 1 serving	5
Earl Grey Tea Latte Tall with 2% Milk, 1 serving	7
Earl Grey Tea Latte Tall with Nonfat Milk, 1 serving	6
Earl Grey Tea Latte Tall with Soy Milk, 1 serving	7
Earl Grey Tea Latte Tall with Whole Milk, 1 serving	8
Grande Teavana® Oprah Chai Herbal Blend Brewed Tea, 1 serving	0
Grande Teavana® Oprah Cinnamon Chai Brewed Tea, 1 serving	0
Green Tea Latte Short with 2% Milk, 1 serving	5
Green Tea Latte Short with Nonfat Milk, 1 serving	4

	SmartPoints® value
Green Tea Latte Short with Soy Milk, 1 serving	5
Green Tea Latte Short with Whole Milk, 1 serving	6
Green Tea Latte Tall with 2% Milk, 1 serving	9
Green Tea Latte Tall with Nonfat Milk, 1 serving	6
Green Tea Latte Tall with Soy Milk, 1 serving	8
Green Tea Latte Tall with Whole Milk, 1 serving	10
Short Teavana® Oprah Chai Herbal Blend Brewed Tea, 1 serving	0
Short Teavana® Oprah Cinnamon Chai Brewed Tea, 1 serving	0
Short Teavana® Oprah Cinnamon Chai Tea Latte with 2% Milk, 1 serving	5
Short Teavana® Oprah Cinnamon Chai Tea Latte with Coconut Milk, 1 serving	5
Short Teavana® Oprah Cinnamon Chai Tea Latte with Nonfat Milk, 1 serving	4
Short Teavana® Oprah Cinnamon Chai Tea Latte with Soy Milk, 1 serving	5
Short Teavana® Oprah Cinnamon Chai Tea Latte with Whole Milk, 1 serving	5
Tall Teavana® Oprah Chai Herbal Blend Brewed Tea, 1 serving	0
Tall Teavana® Oprah Cinnamon Chai Brewed Tea, 1 serving	0
Tall Teavana® Oprah Cinnamon Chai Tea Latte with 2% Milk, 1 serving	7
Tall Teavana® Oprah Cinnamon Chai Tea Latte with Coconut Milk, 1 serving	7
Tall Teavana® Oprah Cinnamon Chai Tea Latte with Nonfat Milk, 1 serving	6

"We Like This!" item

	SmartPoints® value
Tall Teavana® Oprah Cinnamon Chai Tea Latte with Soy Milk, 1 serving	7
Tall Teavana® Oprah Cinnamon Chai Tea Latte with Whole Milk, 1 serving	8
Vanilla Rooibos Tea Latte Short with 2% Milk, 1 serving	5
Vanilla Rooibos Tea Latte Short with Nonfat Milk, 1 serving	4
Vanilla Rooibos Tea Latte Short with Soy Milk, 1 serving	5
Vanilla Rooibos Tea Latte Short with Whole Milk, 1 serving	5
Vanilla Rooibos Tea Latte Tall with 2% Milk, 1 serving	7
Vanilla Rooibos Tea Latte Tall with Nonfat Milk, 1 serving	6
Vanilla Rooibos Tea Latte Tall with Soy Milk, 1 serving	7
Vanilla Rooibos Tea Latte Tall with Whole Milk, 1 serving	8
Venti Teavana® Oprah Chai Herbal Blend Brewed Tea, 1 serving	0
Venti Teavana® Oprah Cinnamon Chai Brewed Tea, 1 serving	0

Iced Tea

Iced Chai Tea Latte Tall with Nonfat Milk, 1 serving	8
Iced Chai Tea Latte Tall with 2% Milk, 1 serving	9
Iced Chai Tea Latte Tall with Soy Milk, 1 serving	9
Iced Chai Tea Latte Tall with Whole Milk, 1 serving	10
Iced Chocolate Chai Tea Latte Tall with 2% Milk, 1 serving	7
Iced Chocolate Chai Tea Latte Tall with Nonfat Milk, 1 serving	6
Iced Chocolate Chai Tea Latte Tall with Soy Milk, 1 serving	7
Iced Chocolate Chai Tea Latte Tall with Whole Milk, 1 serving	8

	SmartPoints® value
Iced Green Tea Latte Tall with 2% Milk, 1 serving	7
Iced Green Tea Latte Tall with Nonfat Milk, 1 serving	5
Iced Green Tea Latte Tall with Soy Milk, 1 serving	7
Iced Green Tea Latte Tall with Whole Milk, 1 serving	8
Shaken Iced Passion Tea Tall Iced Sweetened, 1 serving	4
Shaken Sweet Tea Lemonade Tall, 1 serving	7
Shaken Sweet Tea Tall, 1 serving	5
Tall Teavana® Iced Oprah Cinnamon Chai Tea Latte with 2% Milk, 1 serving	7
Tall Teavana® Iced Oprah Cinnamon Chai Tea Latte with Coconut Milk, 1 serving	7
Tall Teavana® Iced Oprah Cinnamon Chai Tea Latte with Nonfat Milk, 1 serving	6
Tall Teavana® Iced Oprah Cinnamon Chai Tea Latte with Soy Milk, 1 serving	7
Tall Teavana® Iced Oprah Cinnamon Chai Tea Latte with Whole Milk, 1 serving	8

Bottled Beverages

Coffee Frappuccino Coffee Drink, 1 serving	10
Dark Chocolate Mocha Frappuccino Coffee Drink, 1 serving	14
Discoveries Caffe Mocha, 1 serving	6
Discoveries Caramel Macchiato, 1 serving	6
Discoveries-Vanilla Latte, 1 serving	6
Doubleshot Energy Mocha Drink, 1 serving	8
Doubleshot Energy Vanilla Drink, 1 serving	9

	SmartPoints® value
Doubleshot Energy Vanilla Light Drink, 1 serving	5
Doubleshot Energy White Chocolate Drink, 1 serving	9
Doubleshot Light Espresso Drink, 1 serving	3
Mocha Frappuccino Coffee Drink, 1 serving	9
Mocha Light Frappuccino Coffee Drink, 1 serving	4
Tazo Berry Blossom White, 1 serving	4
Tazo Black Mango, 1 serving	9
Tazo Black with Lemon, 1 serving	8
Tazo Brambleberry, 1 serving	8
Tazo Giant Peach, 1 serving	9
Tazo Iced Passion, 1 serving	4
Tazo Lemon Ginger, 1 serving	7
Tazo Organic Black Lemonade, 1 serving	8
Tazo Organic Golden Amber, 1 serving	3
Tazo Organic Himalayan, 1 serving	3
Tazo Organic Iced Black Tea, 1 serving	4
Tazo Organic Iced Green Tea, 1 serving	7
Tazo Organic Jasmine Green, 1 serving	3
Tazo Plum Pomegranate, 1 serving	8
Tazo Tazoberry, 1 serving	9
Tazo White Cranberry, 1 serving	8
Vanilla Frappuccino Coffee Drink, 1 serving	10
Vanilla Light Frappuccino Coffee Drink, 1 serving	4

Smoothies

	SmartPoints® value
Chocolate Smoothie with 2% Milk, 1 serving	12
Chocolate Smoothie with Nonfat Milk, 1 serving	11
Chocolate Smoothie with Soy Milk, 1 serving	12
Orange Mango Smoothie with 2% Milk, 1 serving	11
Orange Mango Smoothie with Nonfat Milk, 1 serving	11
Orange Mango Smoothie with Soy Milk, 1 serving	11
Strawberry Smoothie with 2% Milk, 1 serving	13
Strawberry Smoothie with Nonfat Milk, 1 serving	12
Strawberry Smoothie with Soy Milk, 1 serving	13

Starbucks Refreshers

Cool Lime Refreshers Beverage Tall, 1 serving	2
Valencia Orange Refreshers Beverage Tall, 1 serving	4
Very Berry Hibiscus Refreshers Beverage Tall, 1 serving	3

Sandwiches, Paninis, & Salads

Chicken and Greens Caesar Salad Bowl, 1 serving	10
Chicken and Hummus, 1 serving	6
Chicken Santa Fe Panini, 1	12
Egg Salad Sandwich, 1	15
Ham and NY Cheddar Sandwich, 1	14
Ham and Swiss Panini, 1	9
Hearty Veggie and Brown Rice Salad Bowl, 1 serving	14
Roasted Tomato and Mozzarella Panini, 1	12

"We Like This!" item

	SmartPoints® value
Roasted Vegetable Panini, 1	11
Tomato and Cheese Croissant, 1	10
Turkey and Havarti Sandwich, 1	13
Turkey Rustico Panini, 1	15
Wheat Spinach Croissant, 1	13

Bakery

8 Grain Roll, 1 serving	14
Almond Cookie, 1 serving	9
Apple Fritter, 1	18
Asiago and Cheddar Bavarian Style Pretzel, 1 serving	11
Banana Chocolate Swirl, 1 serving	14
Banana Pecan Walnut Loaf Cake, 1 serving	16
Banana Walnut Bread, 1 serving	20
Birthday Cake Pop, 1	9
Blueberry Oat Bar, 1	15
Blueberry Scone with Buttermilk and Lemon, 1	16
Blueberry Scone with Sugar Crystals, 1	19
Blueberry Yogurt Muffin with Honey, 1	13
Bountiful Blueberry Muffin, 1	15
Butter Croissant, 1	12
Carrot Cake Muffin with Pecans, 1	14
Cheese Danish from La Boulange, 1	13
Cheese Danish with Cream Cheese Filling, 1	18
Cheesecake Brownie, 1	14
Chewy Chocolate Meringue Cookie, 1 serving	8
Chocolate Cake Pop, 1	6
Chocolate Chip Cookie, 1 serving	9
Chocolate Chunk Cookie, 1 serving	18
Chocolate Croissant, 1	13
Chocolate Croissant from La Boulange, 1	14
Chocolate Marble Loaf Cake, 1 serving	17
Chocolate Molten Cake, 1 serving	15
Chocolate Old Fashioned Doughnut, 1	19
Chonga Bagel, 1	9
Cinnamon Chip Scone, 1	21
Cinnamon Roll, 1	18
Classic Coffee Cake, 1 serving	18
Cranberry Orange Scone, 1	21
Double Chocolate Brownie, 1 serving	17
Everything with Cheese Bagel, 1 serving	8
Ginger Molasses Cookie, 1 serving	16
Iced Lemon Pound Cake, 1 serving	24
Mallorca Sweet Bread, 1 serving	17
Maple Oat Pecan Scone, 1	18
Marble Pound Cake, 1 serving	16
Marshmallow Dream Bar, 1	9
Morning Bun from La Boulange, 1	16
Multigrain Bagel, 1	8
Oatmeal Cookie, 1 serving	10
Old Fashioned Glazed Doughnut, 1	21
Outrageous Oatmeal Cookie, 1 serving	16
Peaches and Cream Muffin, 1	16
Petite Vanilla Bean Scone, 1	5
Plain Bagel, 1	8
Pumpkin Bread, 1 serving	17
Pumpkin Scone, 1	22
Raspberry Blueberry Doughnut, 1	13
Raspberry Passion Fruit Loaf Cake, 1 serving	19
Raspberry Scone, 1	20
Raspberry Swirl Pound Cake, 1 serving	21

	SmartPoints® value
Reduced Fat Banana Chocolate Chip Coffee Cake, 1 serving	19
Reduced Fat Berry Coffee Cake with Lemon Crumble, 1 serving	14
Reduced Fat Cinnamon Swirl Coffee Cake, 1 serving	16
Reduced Fat Lemon Loaf Cake, 1 serving	16
Reduced Fat Pumpkin Cream Cheese Loaf Cake, 1 serving	14
Reduced Fat Very Berry Coffee Cake, 1 serving	15
Salted Caramel Cake Pop, 1	9
Stoneground Dijon Bavarian Style Pretzel, 1	10
Summer Berry Croissant, 1	12
Sweet Lemon Cake Pop, 1	7
Zucchini Walnut Muffin, 1	18

Breakfast Sandwiches

Bacon and Gouda Artisan Breakfast Sandwich, 1	11
Chicken Sausage Breakfast Wrap, 1	9
Egg and Cheddar Breakfast Sandwich, 1	9
Ham and Cheddar Artisan Breakfast Sandwich, 1	10
Ham and Cheese Croissant, 1	11
Reduced Fat Turkey Bacon and White Cheddar Classic Breakfast Sandwich, 1	7
Sausage and Cheddar Classic Breakfast Sandwich, 1	16
Spinach and Feta Breakfast Wrap, 1	8
Veggie and Monterey Jack Artisan Breakfast Sandwich, 1 serving	11

Kid's Drinks and More

	SmartPoints® value
Caramel Apple Spice Short with No Whipped Cream, 1 serving	8
Caramel Apple Spice Short with Whipped Cream, 1 serving	11
Caramel Apple Spice Tall with No Whipped Cream, 1 serving	12
Caramel Apple Spice Tall with Whipped Cream, 1 serving	16
Cold Apple Juice Tall, 1 serving	11
Flavored Steamed Milk Short with 2% Milk No Whipped Cream, 1 serving	4
Flavored Steamed Milk Short with 2% Milk Whipped Cream, 1 serving	9
Flavored Steamed Milk Short with Nonfat Milk No Whipped Cream, 1 serving	3
Flavored Steamed Milk Short with Nonfat Milk Whipped Cream, 1 serving	7
Flavored Steamed Milk Short with Soy Milk No Whipped Cream, 1 serving	8
Flavored Steamed Milk Short with Soy Milk Whipped Cream, 1 serving	8
Flavored Steamed Milk Short with Whole Milk No Whipped Cream, 1 serving	5
Flavored Steamed Milk Short with Whole Milk Whipped Cream, 1 serving	10
Flavored Steamed Milk Tall with 2% Milk No Whipped Cream, 1 serving	6
Flavored Steamed Milk Tall with 2% Milk Whipped Cream, 1 serving	12
Flavored Steamed Milk Tall with Nonfat Milk No Whipped Cream, 1 serving	4

"We Like This!" item

	SmartPoints® value
Flavored Steamed Milk Tall with Nonfat Milk Whipped Cream, 1 serving	10
Flavored Steamed Milk Tall with Soy Milk No Whipped Cream, 1 serving	5
Flavored Steamed Milk Tall with Soy Milk Whipped Cream, 1 serving	12
Flavored Steamed Milk Tall with Whole Milk No Whipped Cream, 1 serving	8
Flavored Steamed Milk Tall with Whole Milk Whipped Cream, 1 serving	14
Kids Milk Tall with 2% Milk, 1 serving	8
Kids Milk Tall with Soy Milk, 1 serving	8
Kids Milk Tall with Whole Milk, 1 serving	10
Steamed Apple Juice Short, 1 serving	7
Steamed Apple Juice Tall, 1 serving	10

Yogurt and Fruit

	SmartPoints® value
Cheese and Fruit, 1 serving	18
Greek Yogurt with Honey Parfait, 1 serving	14
Peach Raspberry Yogurt Parfait, 1 serving	12
Seasonal Harvest Fruit Blend, 1 serving	0
Strawberry Blueberry Yogurt Parfait, 1 serving	12

Sandwiches

	SmartPoints® value
6″ B.L.T., 1 serving	12
6″ Barbecue Rib Patty Sub, 1 serving	14
6″ Big Hot Pastrami Melt Sub, 1 serving	19
6″ Big Philly Cheesesteak on Sub, 1 serving	15
6″ Black Forest Ham Sandwich (low fat), 1 serving	8
6″ Buffalo Chicken Sub with Regular Ranch Dressing, 1 serving	12
6″ Chicken and Bacon Ranch Sandwich, 1 serving	19
6″ Chicken Pizziola Melt Sub, 1 serving	14
6″ Cold Cut Combo Sandwich, 1 serving	11
6″ Italian B.M.T. Sandwich, 1 serving	13
6″ Meatball Marinara Sandwich, 1 serving	16
6″ Oven Roasted Chicken Sandwich (low fat), 1 serving	9
6″ Roast Beef Sandwich (low fat), 1 serving	9
6″ Spicy Italian Sandwich, 1 serving	16
6″ Steak and Cheese Sandwich, 1 serving	11
6″ Subway Club Sandwich (low fat), 1 serving	8
6″ Subway Melt Sub, 1 serving	12
6″ Sweet Onion Chicken Teriyaki Sandwich (low fat), 1 serving	11
6″ Tuna Sandwich, 1 serving	15
6″ Turkey and Bacon Avocado Sub, 1 serving	12
6″ Turkey Breast Sandwich (low fat), 1 serving	8
6″ Veggie Delite Sandwich (low fat), 1 serving	7
6″ Veggie Patty Sub, 1 serving	11
Footlong B.L.T., 1 serving	23
Footlong Barbecue Rib Patty, 1 serving	28
Footlong Big Hot Pastrami Melt, 1 serving	38
Footlong Big Philly Cheesesteak, 1 serving	30
Footlong Black Forest Ham, 1 serving	17
Footlong Cold Cut Combo, 1 serving	22
Footlong Italian B.M.T. Sandwich, 1 serving	26
Footlong Meatball Marinara, 1 serving	32
Footlong Oven Roasted Chicken, 1 serving	17
Footlong Roast Beef, 1 serving	17
Footlong Spicy Italian, 1 serving	32
Footlong Steak and Cheese, 1 serving	23
Footlong Sweet Onion Chicken Teriyaki, 1 serving	22
Footlong Tuna, 1 serving	29
Footlong Turkey and Bacon Avocado, 1 serving	25
Footlong Turkey Breast, 1 serving	16
Footlong Veggie Delite, 1 serving	14
Footlong Veggie Patty, 1 serving	22

Pizza

	SmartPoints® value
8″ Cheese and Veggies Pizza, 1 serving	23
8″ Cheese Pizza, 1 serving	21
8″ Pepperoni Pizza, 1 serving	25
8″ Sausage Pizza, 1 serving	26
Spicy Italian Flatizza, 1 serving	16

"We Like This!" item

Salads	SmartPoints® value
Black Forest Ham Chopped Salad (without dressing), 1 serving	3
Chicken and Bacon Ranch Melt Chopped Salad (includes ranch dressing), 1 serving	17
Club Chopped Salad (without dressing), 1 serving	3
Cold Cut Combo Chopped Salad (without dressing), 1 serving	6
Double Chicken Chopped Salad (without dressing), 1 serving	4
Italian B.M.T. Chopped Salad (without dressing), 1 serving	8
Meatball Marinara Chopped Salad (without dressing), 1 serving	11
Oven Roasted Chicken Breast Chopped Salad (without dressing), 1 serving	3
Roast Beef Chopped Salad (without dressing), 1 serving	3
Spicy Italian Chopped Salad (without dressing), 1 serving	11
Steak and Cheese Chopped Salad (without dressing), 1 serving	6
Sweet Onion Chicken Teriyaki Chopped Salad (includes sweet onion dressing), 1 serving	8
Tuna Chopped Salad, 1 serving	10
Turkey Breast Chopped Salad (without dressing), 1 serving	3
Veggie Delite Chopped Salad (without dressing), 1 serving	2

Salad Dressings (amount mixed into chopped salad)

Chipotle Southwest Salad Dressing, 1 serving	7
Fat Free Red Wine Vinaigrette, 1 serving	1
Honey Mustard Salad Dressing, 1 serving	3
Low Fat Balsamic Vinaigrette Dressing, 1 serving	1
Oil and Vinegar Salad Dressings, 1 serving	6
Ranch Dressing, 1 serving	4
Ranch Salad Dressings, 1 serving	8

Soup

Beef Chili, 1 serving	13
Chicken and Dumpling Soup, 1 serving	5
Chicken Noodle Soup, 1 serving	3
Clam Chowder, 1 serving	8
Creamy Broccoli and Cheese Soup, 1 serving	6
Creamy Wild and Brown Rice Soup, 1 serving	6
Green Chili and Tomato Soup, 1 serving	3
Loaded Baked Potato Soup, 1 serving	8
Minestrone Soup, 1 serving	3
Poblano Corn Chowder, 1 serving	6
Vegetable Beef Soup, 1 serving	3

Breakfast

6″ Bacon Egg White and Cheese on Flatbread, 1 serving	12
6″ Bacon Egg White and Cheese Sandwich, 1 serving	12
6″ Bacon, Egg, and Cheese on Flatbread, 1 serving	14
6″ Bacon, Egg, and Cheese Sandwich, 1 serving	14
6″ Egg and Cheese Ham Sandwich, 1 serving	12
6″ Egg and Cheese on Flatbread, 1 serving	11
6″ Egg and Cheese Sandwich, 1 serving	11
6″ Egg and Cheese with ham on Flatbread, 1 serving	12

	SmartPoints® value
6″ Egg White and Cheese on Flatbread, 1 serving	10
6″ Egg White and Cheese Sandwich, 1 serving	9
6″ Egg White and Cheese with ham on Flatbread, 1 serving	12
6″ Egg White and Cheese with Ham Sandwich, 1 serving	10
6″ Mega Melt Egg White on Flatbread, 1 serving	15
6″ Mega Melt Omelet Sandwich with Egg White, 1 serving	15
6″ Mega Melt Omelet Sandwich with Regular Egg, 1 serving	18
6″ Mega Melt Regular Egg on Flatbread, 1 serving	18
6″ Sausage Egg White and Cheese on Flatbread, 1 serving	12
6″ Sausage Egg White and Cheese Sandwich, 1 serving	12
6″ Sausage, Egg, and Cheese on Flatbread, 1 serving	16
6″ Sausage, Egg, and Cheese Sandwich, 1 serving	16
6″ Steak Egg and Cheese on Flatbread, 1 serving	13
6″ Steak Egg and Cheese Sandwich, 1 serving	13
6″ Steak Egg White and Cheese on Flatbread, 1 serving	11
6″ Steak Egg White and Cheese Sandwich, 1 serving	11

Breakfast Side

	SmartPoints® value
Hash Browns, 1 serving	7

Kids Meal Sandwiches

	SmartPoints® value
Black Forest Ham Kids Meal Sandwiches, 1 serving	5
Roast Beef Kids Meal Sandwiches, 1 serving	6
Turkey Breast Kids Meal Sandwiches, 1 serving	5
Veggie Delite Kids Meal Sandwich, 1 serving	4

Desserts

	SmartPoints® value
Apple Slices, 1 serving	2
Chocolate Chip Cookie, 1	9
Chocolate Chunk Cookie, 1	10
Double Chocolate Chip Cookie, 1	10
Gingerbread, 1 serving	8
M & M Cookie, 1	10
Oatmeal Raisin Cookie, 1	9
Peanut Butter Cookie, 1	10
Raspberry Cheesecake, 1 serving	9
White Chip Macadamia Nut Cookie, 1	10

Beverages

	SmartPoints® value
Diet Unsweetened Tea, 16 oz	0
Juice Box, 1	6
Reduced Fat Chocolate Milk, 1 serving	10
Reduced Fat Strawberry Milk, 1 serving	14
Sweetened Tea, 16 oz	15

"We Like This!" item

Tacos

	SmartPoints® value
Beef Soft Taco, 1	6
Beef Soft Taco Supreme, 1	7
Cheesy Gordita Crunch, 1 serving	16
Cool Ranch Doritos Cheesy Gordita Crunch, 1 serving	17
Cool Ranch Doritos Double Decker Taco, 1 serving	10
Cool Ranch Doritos Locos Taco, 1 serving	5
Cool Ranch Doritos Locos Taco Supreme, 1 serving	6
Crunchy Taco, 1 serving	5
Crunchy Taco Supreme, 1 serving	6
Double Decker Taco, 1 serving	10
Double Decker Taco Supreme, 1 serving	11
Express Fiesta Taco Salad, 1 serving	18
Fiery Doritos Cheesy Gordita Crunch, 1 serving	16
Fiery Doritos Double Decker Taco, 1 serving	10
Fiery Doritos Locos Taco, 1 serving	5
Fiery Doritos Locos Taco Supreme, 1 serving	6
Fresco Crunchy Taco with Beef, 1 serving	4
Fresco Soft Taco with Beef, 1 serving	5
Fresco Soft Taco with Shredded Chicken, 1 serving	4
Fresco Soft Taco with Steak, 1 serving	4
Gordita Supreme with Beef, 1 serving	9
Gordita Supreme with Chicken, 1 serving	8
Gordita Supreme with Steak, 1 serving	8
Grilled Steak Soft Taco, 1 serving	6
Nacho Cheese Doritos Cheesy Gordita Crunch, 1 serving	16
Nacho Cheese Doritos Double Decker Taco, 1 serving	10
Nacho Cheese Doritos Locos Taco, 1 serving	5
Nacho Cheese Doritos Locos Taco Supreme, 1 serving	6
Soft Taco Supreme with Beef, 1 serving	7
Soft Taco with Beef, 1 serving	6
Soft Taco with Chicken, 1 serving	4
Spicy Potato Soft Taco, 1 serving	7

Burritos

7-Layer Burrito, 1 serving	14
Bean Burrito, 1 serving	11
Beef Burrito Supreme, 1 serving	13
Beefy 5-Layer Burrito, 1 serving	16
Beefy Crunch Burrito, 1 serving	15
Beefy Fritos Burrito, 1 serving	13
Black Bean Burrito, 1 serving	12
Burrito Supreme with Chicken, 1 serving	11
Burrito Supreme with Steak, 1 serving	12
Cantina Power Burrito with Chicken, 1 serving	14
Cantina Power Burrito with Steak, 1 serving	14
Cantina Power Burrito with Veggie, 1 serving	14
Cheesy Bean and Rice Burrito, 1 serving	13
Cheesy Burrito Bacon Fresco Style, 1 serving	12
Cheesy Burrito Fiesta Potato, 1 serving	17
Cheesy Burrito Fiesta Potato Fresco Style, 1 serving	13
Cheesy Burrito Sausage Fresco Style, 1 serving	12
Cheesy Burrito Steak and Egg, 1 serving	15
Cheesy Burrito Steak and Egg Fresco Style, 1 serving	11
Cheesy Burrito with Bacon, 1 serving	16

	SmartPoints® value
Cheesy Burrito with Sausage, 1 serving	16
Cheesy Double Beef Burrito, 1 serving	13
Cheesy Potato Burrito, 1 serving	15
Chicken Burrito Supreme, 1	11
Chili Cheese Burrito, 1 serving	12
Combo Burrito, 1 serving	14
Fresco Bean Burrito, 1 serving	11
Fresco Burrito Supreme with Chicken, 1 serving	10
Fresco Burrito Supreme with Steak, 1 serving	10
Grilled Chicken Stuft Burrito, 1 serving	19
Loaded Potato Griller, 1 serving	13
Shredded Chicken Burrito, 1 serving	12
Smothered Burrito with Beef, 1 serving	22
Smothered Burrito with Shredded Chicken, 1 serving	19
Smothered Burrito with Steak, 1 serving	20
Steak Burrito Supreme, 1 serving	12
Steak Quesarito, 1 serving	20
XXL Grilled Stuft Burrito with Beef, 1 serving	28
XXL Grilled Stuft Burrito with Shredded Chicken, 1 serving	25
XXL Grilled Stuft Burrito with Steak, 1 serving	25

Quesadillas

	SmartPoints® value
Beefy Mini Quesadilla, 1 serving	7
Cheese Quesadilla, 1 serving	15
Chicken Quesadilla, 1 serving	16
Chicken Quesarito, 1 serving	20
Crunchwrap Supreme, 1 serving	17
DoubleDilla Chicken, 1 serving	20
DoubleDilla Chicken with Chips and Salsa, 1 serving	28
DoubleDilla Steak, 1 serving	21
DoubleDilla Steak with Chips and Salsa, 1 serving	29
MexiMelt®, 1	8
Sausage Flatbread Quesadilla, 1 serving	11
Shredded Chicken Mini Quesadilla, 1 serving	5
Steak Quesadilla, 1 serving	16

Specialties

	SmartPoints® value
Beef Chalupa Supreme, 1	12
Beefy Nacho Loaded Griller, 1 serving	12
Cantina Power Bowl with Chicken, 1 serving	14
Cantina Power Bowl with Steak, 1 serving	15
Cantina Power Bowl with Veggie, 1 serving	14
Chalupa Supreme with Beef, 1 serving	12
Chalupa Supreme with Chicken, 1 serving	10
Chalupa Supreme with Steak, 1 serving	10
Cheese Roll Up, 1 serving	6
Chicken Chalupa Supreme, 1	10
Chipotle Chicken Loaded Griller, 1 serving	11
Double Tostada, 1 serving	8
Mexican Pizza, 1 serving	17
Nachos BellGrande, 1 serving	23
Nachos Supreme, 1 serving	14
Quesalupa with Beef, 1 serving	15
Quesalupa with Chicken, 1 serving	11
Quesalupa with Steak, 1 serving	12
Spicy Tostada, 1 serving	7
Steak Chalupa Supreme, 1	10
Steak Enchirito, 1	10
Triple Layer Nachos, 1 serving	10

"We Like This!" item

	SmartPoints® value
Salads	
Chicken Cantina Bowl, 1 serving	15
Fiesta Taco Salad with Beef, 1 serving	24
Fiesta Taco Salad with Chicken, 1 serving	21
Fiesta Taco Salad with Steak, 1 serving	22
Sauces	
Diablo Sauce, 1 serving	0
Fire Border Sauce, ¼ oz	0
Hot Border Sauce, ¼ oz	0
Mild Border Sauce, ¼ oz	0
Salsa Del Sol, 1 serving	0
Salsa Verde Border Sauce, 1 serving	0
Sides and Extras	
Black Beans, 1 serving	2
Black Beans and Rice, 1 serving	5
Cheesy Fiesta Potatoes, 1 serving	7
Chips and Guacamole, 1 serving	10
Chips and Nacho Cheese Sauce, 1 serving	9
Chips and Pico de Gallo, 1 serving	7
Chips and Salsa, 1 serving	8
Nacho Cheese Doritos Chips, 1 serving	4
Pintos 'n Cheese, 1 serving	6
Premium Latin Rice, 1 serving	3
Quesarito Beef, 1 serving	21
Breakfast	
A.M. Grilled Taco with Egg and Cheese, 1 serving	5
Breakfast Crunchwrap California, 1 serving	20
Breakfast Crunchwrap with Sausage, 1	23
Breakfast Crunchwrap with Steak, 1 serving	21
Breakfast Grilled Taco with Bacon, 1 serving	8

	SmartPoints® value
Breakfast Grilled Taco with Egg and Cheese, 1 serving	5
Breakfast Grilled Taco with Sausage, 1 serving	8
Breakfast Quesalupa with Bacon, 1 serving	19
Breakfast Quesalupa with Sausage, 1 serving	20
Grande Scrambler Burrito with Bacon, 1 serving	21
Grande Scrambler Burrito with Sausage, 1 serving	20
Grande Scrambler Burrito with Steak, 1 serving	19
Grilled Breakfast Burrito Fiesta Potato, 1 serving	11
Grilled Breakfast Burrito with Bacon, 1 serving	11
Grilled Breakfast Burrito with Sausage, 1 serving	11
Hashbrown, 1 serving	5
Mini Skillet Bowl, 1 serving	6
Desserts	
Caramel Apple Empanada, 1 serving	11
Cinnabon Delights (2-pack), 1 serving	6
Cinnamon Twists, 1 serving	7
Drinks	
Crush Orange Vanilla Float Freeze, 16 oz	12
Diet Mountain Dew Baja Blast, 16 oz	0
Iced Coffee (mocha), 1 serving	11
Mountain Dew Baja Blast, 16 oz	14
Mountain Dew Baja Blast Freeze, 16 oz	14
Mountain Dew Kickstart Orange Citrus, 16 oz	5
Mountain Dew Sangrita Blast, 16 oz	14
Rainforest Coffee, 1 serving	0
Rainforest Coffee with Nestle Coffee Mate Original Creamer, 1 serving	1
Starburst Strawberry Freeze, 16 oz	13

Wendy's

	SmartPoints® value
Burgers	
¼ lb Hamburger Patty, 1	7
¼ lb. Single with Cheese, 1	19
½ lb. Double with Cheese, 1	27
¾ lb. Triple with Cheese, 1	36
Bacon Portabella Melt on Brioche, 1 serving	20
Baconator, 1	30
Cheeseburger, 1	10
Double Stack, 1	12
Hamburger, 1	8
Jr. Cheeseburger, 1	9
Jr. Cheeseburger Deluxe, 1	11
Jr. Hamburger, 1	7
Jr. Hamburger Patty, 1	7
Jr. Single Sunny Side Burger, 1	16
Pretzel Bacon Cheeseburger, 1	22
Pulled Pork Cheeseburger with Smoky BBQ, 1	20
Pulled Pork Cheeseburger with Spicy BBQ, 1	22
Pulled Pork Cheeseburger with Sweet BBQ, 1	21
Son of Baconator, 1	21
Chicken, Wraps, & More	
Asiago Ranch Club with Homestyle Chicken, 1	20
Asiago Ranch Club with Spicy Chicken, 1	20
Asiago Ranch Club with Ultimate Chicken Grill, 1 serving	15
Chicken Nuggets, 10 pieces	18
Chicken Nuggets, 4 pieces	5
Chicken Nuggets, 6 pieces	10

	SmartPoints® value
Cod Fillet, 1 serving	5
Crispy Chicken Caesar Wrap, 1	13
Crispy Chicken Patty, 1	5
Crispy Chicken Sandwich, 1	10
Grilled Chicken Go Wrap, 1	7
Grilled Chicken Wrap, 1	8
Homestyle Chicken Fillet, 1	7
Homestyle Chicken Go Wrap, 1	10
Homestyle Chicken Sandwich, 1	15
Honey Butter Chicken Biscuit, 1	18
Jalapeño Fresco Spicy Chicken Sandwich, 1 serving	18
Premium Cod Sandwich, 1	15
Pretzel Pub Sandwich with Homestyle Chicken, 1	20
Pretzel Pub Sandwich with Spicy Chicken, 1	20
Pretzel Pub Sandwich with Ultimate Chicken Grill, 1	15
Pulled Pork Sandwich with Smoky BBQ, 1	14
Pulled Pork Sandwich with Spicy BBQ, 1	16
Pulled Pork Sandwich with Sweet BBQ, 1	15
Spicy Chicken Fillet, 1	7
Spicy Chicken Go Wrap, 1	10
Spicy Chicken Nuggets, 10 pieces	22
Spicy Chicken Nuggets, 4 pieces	6
Spicy Chicken Nuggets, 6 pieces	8
Spicy Chicken Sandwich, 1	15
Ultimate Chicken Grill Fillet (without roll), 1	4
Ultimate Chicken Grill Sandwich, 1	8

"We Like This!" item

Fries & Sides

	SmartPoints® value
Bacon and Cheese Baked Potato, 1 serving	16
Broccoli and Cheese Baked Potato, 1 serving	14
Ghost Pepper Fries, 1 serving	18
Natural Cut Fries, 1 large	17
Natural Cut Fries, 1 medium	13
Natural Cut Fries, 1 small	10
Natural Cut Fries (value size), 1 serving	7
Oatmeal Bar, 1	12
Plain Baked Potato, 10 oz	8
Pulled Pork Cheese Fries with Smoky BBQ, 1	16
Pulled Pork Cheese Fries with Spicy BBQ, 1 serving	17
Pulled Pork Cheese Fries with Sweet BBQ, 1 serving	17
Rich and Meaty Chili, 1 large	7
Rich and Meaty Chili, 1 small	5
Seasoned Homestyle Potatoes, 1 serving	7
Sour Cream and Chive Baked Potato, 1 serving	10

Salads

	SmartPoints® value
Apple Pecan Chicken Salad (full size), 1 serving	22
Apple Pecan Chicken Salad (half size), 1 serving	13
Asian Cashew Chicken Salad (full size), 1 serving	11
Asian Cashew Chicken Salad (half size), 1 serving	7
BBQ Ranch Chicken (half size), 1 serving	11
BBQ Ranch Chicken Salad (full size), 1 serving	20
Caesar Side Salad with Lemon Garlic Caesar dressing, 1 serving	8
Garden Side Salad (no croutons no dressing), 1 serving	0
Garden Side Salad (with croutons and ranch dressing), 1 serving	7
Spicy Chicken Caesar Salad (full size), 1 serving	25
Spicy Chicken Caesar Salad (half size), 1 serving	14
Strawberry Fields Chicken Salad, 1 serving	10
Strawberry Fields Chicken Salad (half size), 1 serving	5

Salad Dressings

	SmartPoints® value
Apple Balsamic Vinaigrette, 1 serving	4
BBQ Ranch Dressing, 1 serving	4
Italian Vinaigrette, 1 serving	2
Lemon Garlic Caesar Dressing, 1 packet	8
Light Honey French Dressing, 1 packet	2
Light Ranch Dressing, 1 packet	2
Light Spicy Asian Chili Vinaigrette, 1 packet	4
Pomegranate Vinaigrette, 1 serving	6
Ranch Dressing, 1 packet	4
Thousand Island Dressing, 1 packet	5

Condiments

	SmartPoints® value
Barbecue Dipping Sauce, 1 serving	2
Brown Sugar, 1 serving	2
Buttermilk Ranch Dipping Sauce, 1 serving	4
Buttery Best Spread, 1 serving	2
Spicy BBQ Side Sauce, 1 serving	4

Extras

	SmartPoints® value
American Cheese, 1 serving	2
Applewood Smoked Bacon, 1 serving	2
Asiago Cheese, 1 serving	2
Cheddar Cheese Sauce, 1 serving	5
Cheddar Cheese Slice, 1 serving	3
Crinkle Cut Pickles, 3 slices	0
Gourmet Croutons, 1 serving	3
Honey Mustard Dipping Sauce, 1 serving	3
Honey Roasted Sunflower Seeds, 1 serving	2
Hot Chili Seasoning Packet, 1 serving	0
Hot Sauce, 1 serving	0
Ketchup, 1 packet	1
Muenster Cheese Slice, 1 serving	3
Premium Bun Toasted, 1	6
Pretzel Bun Toasted, 1	7
Ranch Sauce, 1 packet	4
Roasted Pecans, 1 packet	4
Saltine Crackers, 1 packet	1
Sandwich Bun, 1	4
Shredded Cheddar Cheese, 1 serving	3
Smoky BBQ Side Sauce, 1 serving	2
Smoky Honey Mustard, 1	2
Spicy Roasted Cashews, 1 serving	3
Sweet and Sour Dipping Sauce, 1 serving	2
Sweet BBQ Side Sauce, 1 serving	3
Tartar Sauce, 1 packet	4
Tortilla, 1	4

Breakfast

	SmartPoints® value
Artisan Egg Sandwich with All Natural Sausage, 1	17
Artisan Egg Sandwich with Applewood Smoked Bacon, 1	12
Artisan Sandwich with Egg and Cheese, 1	9
Fresh Baked Biscuit with All Natural Sausage, 1	21
Fresh Baked Biscuit with Applewood Smoked Bacon, 1	15
Fresh Baked Biscuit with Egg and Cheese, 1	13
Mornin' Melt Panini with All Natural Sausage, 1	23
Mornin' Melt Panini with Applewood Smoked Bacon, 1 serving	18
Mornin' Melt Panini with Egg and Cheese, 1	16
Plain Steel Cut Oatmeal, 1 serving	5
Plain Toasted Bagel, 1	8
Sausage and Egg Burrito, 1	9
Sausage Biscuit, 1	17
Sausage Gravy and Biscuit, 1 serving	17
Steel Cut Oatmeal with Apples and Caramel, 1 serving	9
Steel Cut Oatmeal with Cranberries and Pecans, 1 serving	14

"We Like This!" item

	SmartPoints® value
Steel Cut Oatmeal with Summer Berries, 1 serving	7
Toasted Bagel Sandwich with All Natural Sausage, 1	20
Toasted Bagel Sandwich with Applewood Smoked Bacon, 1	14
Toasted Bagel Sandwich with Egg and Cheddar, 1	12

Frosty

Chocolate Frosty, 1 junior	10
Chocolate Frosty, 1 small	17
Chocolate Frosty Waffle Cone, 1 serving	14
Strawberry Frosty Shake, 1 large	39
Strawberry Frosty Shake, 1 small	27
Vanilla Frosty, 1 junior	9
Vanilla Frosty, 1 small	16
Vanilla Frosty Waffle Cone, 1 serving	13

Fresh Baked Favorites

Chocolate Chunk Cookie, 1 serving	18
Double Chocolate Chip Cookie, 1 serving	16
Espresso Chip Bar, 1 serving	12
Sugar Cookie, 1 serving	17

	SmartPoints® value

Desserts & Shakes

Apple Slices, 1 serving	0
Caramel Frosty Shake, 1 large	44
Caramel Frosty Shake, 1 small	29

Beverages

All Natural Lemonade, 1 large	23
All Natural Lemonade, 1 small	11
Brewed Unsweetened Iced Tea, 1 large	0
Brewed Unsweetened Iced Tea, 1 small	0
Caramel Iced Coffee, 1 small	9
Mocha Iced Coffee, 1 small	9
Orange Juice, 1 small	7
Original Redhead Hot Coffee Decaffeinated, 1 small	0
Original Regular Redhead Hot Coffee, 1 small	0
Skinny Vanilla Iced Coffee, 1 small	3
Strawberry Lemonade, 1 small	14
Strawberry Tea, 1 small	3
Vanilla Iced Coffee, 1 small	9

table of contents

Printed in U.S.A.

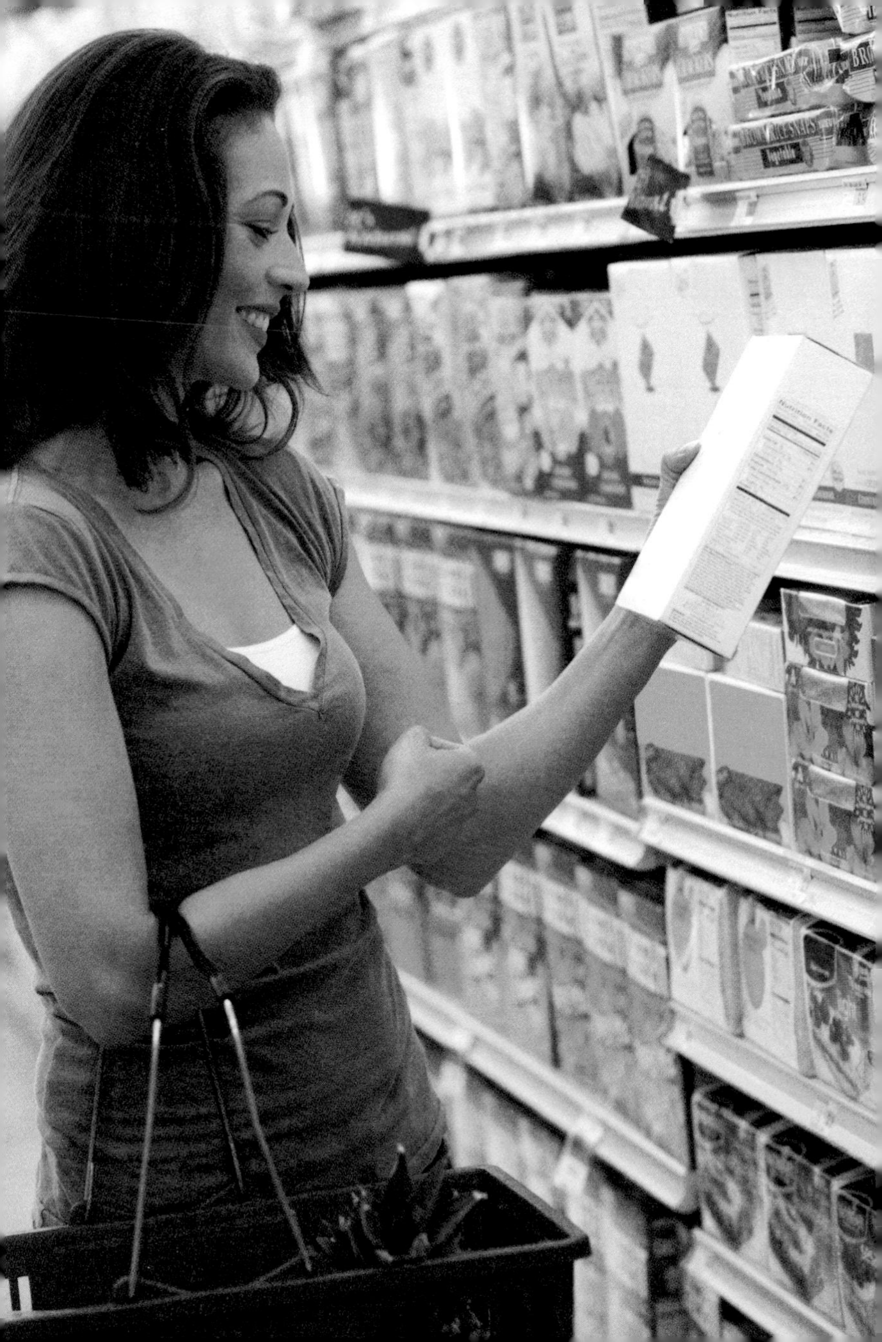

supermarket shopping

where do you begin?

You walk into the grocery, and what do you see? Thousands of items. How do you decide what to buy? Looking for a way to narrow down the search? You've got it in your hands!

We've identified the foods most searched for on our website and have included only those items in our listings here. No longer will you have to wade through a countless number of products only a handful of folks have been interested in checking out. We've even noted some as **"We Like This!" items.**

So go ahead, take a look. Plan a menu. Make a list. And head for the store. Shopping just got easier!

in this book
you will find:

- **SmartPoints® values** for each and every food item listed.
- Our indispensable **A-Z Food List,** a comprehensive general list of foods, updated to focus on those tracked most on our website. For those following the **Simply Filling technique,** we've marked no-count foods with an icon (◉) to make finding them easy. And for the first time ever, our A-Z Food List includes...
- **"We Like This!" items:** 👍 Some extra support for after you leave your meeting! Not sure what to choose? Just browse the A-Z Food List for those items shaded in gray. Think of us as a menu planning companion, giving you ideas to help you stay the course.
- The latest **Brand Name Food List,** filled with thousands of the products most searched for on our website! Check out what others are checking out—the popular ones are right here! This extensive list includes SmartPoints values for each and every product. And to help you find what you're looking for fast, each section begins with a shopping guide.
- The most current list of **Weight Watchers Food Products** available in grocery stores, and at participating meeting room locations.
- A user-friendly **Index,** with all the categories of our brand-name listings alphabetized, along with their page numbers, to make finding what you're looking for a cinch.

What makes something a "We Like This!" item?

Looking though a *l-o-n-g* list of foods could be onerous. So we've made the first cut for you. **Our "We Like This!" items are:**

- Those that, in general, have a lower SmartPoints value per serving than others in that category. Keep in mind that SmartPoints reflect the serving size, so the SmartPoints listed could change if a different serving size is taken.
- Those lower in fat (e.g., lean or trimmed) than others with the same SmartPoints value in the category.
- Those that might bring new ideas to your menu planning.
- Those that might satisfy with just a few bites.

You might decide on something else, and that's fine. **"We Like This! items** are a way to make it easier to focus on these lower SmartPoints choices first.

A note about branded foods:

In order to help make finding what you're looking for and comparison shopping easier, products in the **Brand Name Food List** are grouped by category. However, for many products there are numerous categories into which a product could be placed. Therefore, if you can't find the product you're looking for in a specific category, try another category. The **Index** at the end of the book is a great resource for finding categories, and the pages where they begin.

Inclusion of the products in this book does not imply endorsement or sponsorship of such products by Weight Watchers International, Inc. Endorsed products are specifically marked as such on the products' labels.

A note about the SmartPoints value for each listing:

The SmartPoints values for the foods in this book were calculated by Weight Watchers International, Inc. using the most current nutrition information supplied by manufacturers and available from the USDA at the time of the book's publication. However, since product formulations may change during the year, it's a good idea to continue to use the nutrition labels on products to confirm SmartPoints values.

One more thing to keep in mind:

Note that the alcohol content of certain foods, especially alcoholic beverages, can impact their total SmartPoints values. Because alcohol is not typically included on nutrition labels, you might notice discrepancies with the values of alcoholic beverages you see in these lists and that you calculate with nutrition information. For beverages that contain alcohol, as with all the products in this book, you can feel confident using the SmartPoints values listed here.

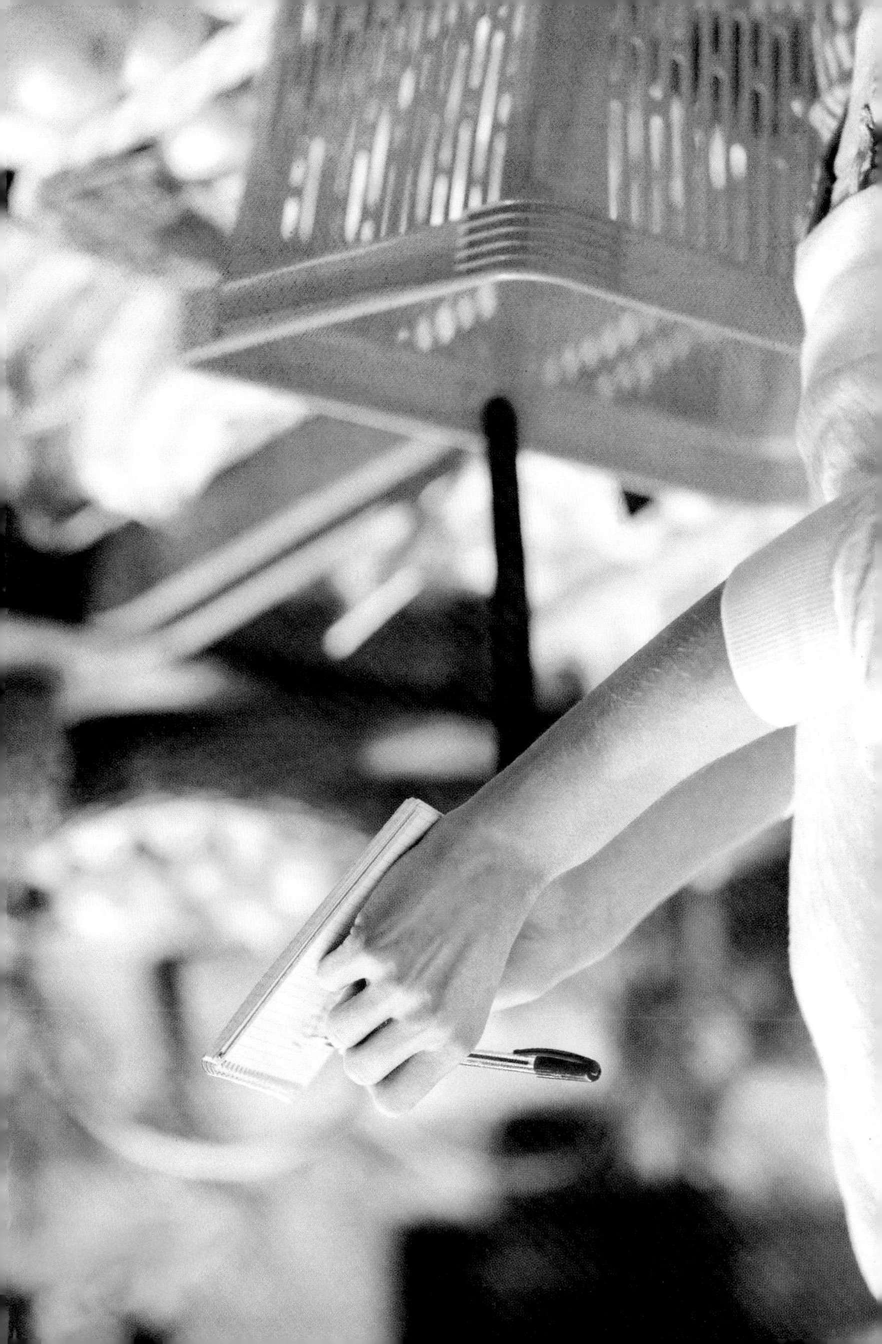

a-z
food list

A

Food (○ No Count)	SmartPoints® value
Alcoholic beverages	
bourbon, 1½ fl oz	4
brandy, 1½ fl oz	3
cognac, 1½ fl oz	4
crème de menthe, 1½ fl oz	9
gin, 1½ fl oz	3
Irish cream, 1½ fl oz	8
liqueur, any type, 1½ fl oz	9
mirin, 1 fl oz	1
rum, 1½ fl oz	3
sake, 1 fl oz	1
schnapps, any flavor, 1½ fl oz	13
scotch, 1½ fl oz	3
tequila, 1½ fl oz	3
vodka, 1½ fl oz	3
vodka, raspberry-flavored, 1½ fl oz	3
whiskey, 1½ fl oz	3
Alcoholic mixed drinks	
bay breeze, 5½ fl oz	7
bellini, 6 fl oz	6
black Russian, 3 fl oz	11
bloody Mary, 5 fl oz	5
brandy Alexander, 3 fl oz	13
chocolate martini, 2½ fl oz	7
citrus vodka and soda, 5 fl oz	3
cosmopolitan, 3½ fl oz	7
daiquiri, 3 fl oz	7
gin and diet tonic, 5 fl oz	4
gin and tonic, 5 fl oz	6
gin gimlet, 2½ fl oz	5
highball, 5 fl oz	6
Jack and cola, 5 fl oz	6
Jack and diet cola, 5 fl oz	4
kamikazi, 4½ fl oz	15
Long Island iced tea, 8 fl oz	18
mai tai, 3½ fl oz	11
Manhattan, 4 fl oz	10

"We Like This!" item

Food (○ No Count)	SmartPoints® value
Margarita, 6 fl oz	17
martini, 2 fl oz	6
mimosa, 6 fl oz	4
mojito, 12 fl oz	8
old-fashioned, 4 fl oz	12
piña colada, 6 fl oz	16
Rob Roy, 4 fl oz	10
rum and cola, 5 fl oz	6
rum and diet cola, 5 fl oz	3
sakatini, 3 fl oz	6
sangria, 5 fl oz	5
screwdriver, 6 fl oz	7
sex on the beach, 6 fl oz	8
Singapore sling, 6 fl oz	8
sour apple martini, 3 fl oz	10
strawberry daiquiri, frozen, 7 fl oz	11
tequila sunrise, canned, 3 fl oz	3
Tom Collins, 6 fl oz	4
vanilla vodka and soda, 5 fl oz	4
vodka and cranberry juice, 5 fl oz	7
vodka and diet soda, 5 fl oz	3
vodka and tonic, 5 fl oz	6
vodka gimlet, 3 fl oz	5
whiskey sour, 4 fl oz	7
white Russian, 3 fl oz	10
Almond butter	
2 Tbsp	6
Almond meal	
1 tsp	0
Almond milk	
plain, unsweetened, 8 fl oz	1
vanilla, unsweetened, 8 fl oz	1
Almond paste	
firmly packed, 1 Tbsp	3
Almonds	
¼ cup	4
blanched, ¼ cup	6
chopped, ¼ cup	5
dry-roasted, ¼ cup	6

⭘ No Count	SmartPoints® value
honey roasted, 1 oz	5
sliced, ¼ cup	4
slivered, ¼ cup	5
smoked, 23 pieces (1 oz)	5
Aloo gobi	
1 cup	3
Aloo palak	
8 oz	4
Amaranth	
⭘ cooked, 1 cup	7
⭘ uncooked, ¼ cup	5
Ambrosia	
½ cup	1
Anchovy paste	
1 Tbsp	1
Apple	
baked, with nuts, butter, and sugar, 1 medium (4 ¾ oz)	9
candied, 1 medium (6 oz)	13
canned, with sugar, sliced, drained, ½ cup	4
caramel, 1 medium (5 ½ oz)	11
dried, ¼ cup	3
dried, stewed, without sugar, ¼ cup	2
Apple brown Betty	
4 ¾ oz	10
Apple butter	
1 Tbsp	2
Apple crisp	
5 oz	10
Apple streusel	
3 ½ oz	6
Applesauce	
canned, with sugar, ½ cup	5
⭘ unsweetened	0
Apricots	
canned halves, heavy syrup pack, with skin, 1 (1 ½ oz)	2
canned or frozen, with sugar, ½ cup	7

⭘ No Count	SmartPoints® value
canned, heavy syrup pack, without skin, 1 cup	12
canned, heavy syrup, drained, 1 cup	9
halves, canned, extra light syrup pack, 1 cup	7
halves, canned, heavy syrup, drained, 1 cup	9
halves, canned, juice pack, with skin, 1 (1 ⅓ oz)	1
halves, canned, light syrup packed, with skin, 1 (1 ½ oz)	1
halves, dried, ¼ cup	4
halves, dried, stewed, with sugar, ½ cup	9
⭘ halves, stewed, without sugar, ¼ cup	3
Arroz con leche (Mexican rice pudding)	
restaurant-type, 10 oz	18
Arroz con pollo	
11 ⅓ oz	16
Artichoke	
marinated, 1 cup	6
stuffed, 8 oz	16
Avocado	
California (hass), raw, ¼ (1 ¼ oz)	2
California (hass), raw, pureed, ¼ cup	3
Florida, raw, ¼ (2 ¾ oz)	3
Florida, raw, pureed, ¼ cup	2

B

Baba ghanoush	
1 ¼ oz	3
Bacon	
cooked, crisp, 3 slices (1 ¼ oz)	5
imitation, cooked, 3 slices (½ oz)	1
reduced/low-sodium, uncooked, 3 slices (2 ¾ oz)	11
turkey, cooked, 3 slices (¾ oz)	3
turkey, uncooked, 3 slices (1 ¾ oz)	3

A-Z Food List

Bacon (cont'd)

○ No Count		SmartPoints® value
	uncooked, 3 slices (3 oz)	13
	vegetarian, uncooked, ½ oz	2
	Bacon bits	
	imitation, ¼ oz	1
	Bacon fat	
	1 Tbsp	5
	Bacon, Canadian	
○	cooked, 3 slices (1½ oz)	1
○	uncooked, 2 slices (2 oz)	1
	Bagel	
	any type other than those listed here, 1 large (4½ oz)	12
	any type, store-bought, 1 (3½ oz)	8
	blueberry, restaurant-type, 1 (4 oz)	10
	cinnamon-raisin, store-bought, 1 (3½ oz)	9
	egg, small, 1 (2½ oz)	5
	multi-grain, restaurant-type, 1 (4½ oz)	9
	oat bran, small, 1 (2½ oz)	5
	onion, restaurant-type, 1 (4 oz)	9
	poppyseed, restaurant-type, 1 (4 oz)	9
	pumpernickel, restaurant-type, 1 (4 oz)	8
	salt, restaurant-type, 1 (4 oz)	8
	store-bought (plain, onion, poppy seed, or sesame), small, 1 (2½ oz)	5
	wheat, store-bought, 1 (3½ oz)	7
	Bagel with cream cheese and lox	
	6½ oz	17
	Baklava	
	1 (2½ oz)	14
	Banana	
	dehydrated, or freeze-dried, ¼ cup	4
	Banana bread	
	with nuts, 1 piece (2½ oz)	9
	without nuts, 1 piece (2 oz)	8

○ No Count		SmartPoints® value
	Barley	
○	cooked, 1 cup	6
	hulled (groats), 2 oz	5
○	quick-cooking, prepared, 1 cup	6
○	uncooked, 2 oz	6
	Beans	
○	adzuki, cooked, ½ cup	4
○	adzuki, dried, ¼ cup	4
○	black, canned, ½ cup	3
○	black, canned, low-sodium, ½ cup	3
○	black, cooked, ½ cup	3
○	black, dry, ¼ cup	4
○	butter beans, canned, ½ cup	2
○	cannellini, canned, ½ cup	4
○	cranberry (Roman), cooked, ½ cup	3
○	fava, canned (broadbeans), ½ cup	2
○	fava, dried, not in pod (broadbeans), ¼ cup	3
○	garbanzo (chickpeas), bengal gram, raw, ¼ cup	5
○	garbanzo (chickpeas), canned, drained, ½ cup	3
○	garbanzo (chickpeas), cooked, ½ cup	3
○	garbanzo (chickpeas), dry, 1 cup	22
○	great northern, canned, ½ cup	4
○	great northern, canned, low-sodium, 1 cup	8
○	great northern, cooked, ½ cup	2
○	great northern, dry, ¼ cup	4
○	kidney, canned, all types, ¼ cup	1
○	kidney, cooked, ½ cup	3
○	kidney, dry, ¼ cup	4
○	lima, canned, ½ cup	2
○	lima, cooked, ½ cup	3
○	lima, dry, ¼ cup	4
○	lupini (lupin) beans, cooked, 1 cup	4
○	mung, cooked, ½ cup	2
○	mung, dry (mungo), ¼ cup	5

"We Like This!" item

⭘ No Count	SmartPoints® value
⭘ navy, canned, ½ cup	4
⭘ navy, cooked, ½ cup	3
⭘ navy, dry, ¼ cup	4
⭘ pink, cooked, ½ cup	3
⭘ pink, dry, ¼ cup	5
⭘ pinto, canned, ½ cup	3
⭘ pinto, cooked, ½ cup	3
⭘ pinto, dry, 1 cup	17
⭘ red kidney, canned, low-sodium, 1 cup	6
⭘ small white, cooked, ½ cup	3
⭘ small white, dry, ¼ cup	4
⭘ soy, cooked, ½ cup	4
⭘ soy, dry, ¼ cup	5
⭘ soy, green, cooked, ½ cup	3
⭘ soy, green, raw, ¼ cup	2
⭘ white, canned, ½ cup	4
⭘ white, cooked, ½ cup	3
⭘ white, dry, ¼ cup	4
Beans, baked	
½ cup	7
canned, ½ cup	5
canned, vegetarian, ½ cup	4
canned, with beef, ½ cup	5
canned, with franks, ½ cup	7
canned, with pork, ½ cup	4
canned, with pork and sweet sauce, ½ cup	5
deli, ½ cup	7
fast food, 6⅓ oz	9
Beans, black, and rice	
5¼ oz	6
Beans, chili, barbecue	
ranch style, cooked, ½ cup	4
Beans, red, and rice	
6¼ oz	7
Beans, refried	
½ cup	6
black, canned, ½ cup	3
canned, ½ cup	3

⭘ No Count	SmartPoints® value
⭘ canned, fat-free, ½ cup	2
⭘ canned, reduced-sodium, ½ cup	3
red, canned, ¼ cup	2
restaurant-type, 1 cup	7
with sausage, canned, ½ cup	7
Bear claw	
restaurant-type, 1 (4 oz)	17
Beef	
back rib, lean and fat, cooked, 3 oz	10
back rib, lean and fat, raw, 3 oz	10
back rib, lean and trimmed, cooked, 3 oz	7
back rib, barbecued, 3 oz	7
blade roast, lean, trimmed, cooked, 3 oz	5
bottom round, trimmed, raw, 4 oz	6
⭘ bottom sirloin (tri-tip), lean, trimmed, raw, 4 oz	3
⭘ bottom sirloin (tri-tip), trimmed, cooked, 3 oz	3
brisket, barbecued, 3 oz	9
brisket, cooked, 3 oz	11
brisket, lean, trimmed, cooked, 3 oz	4
brisket, lean, trimmed, raw, 4 oz	4
brisket, trimmed, raw, 4 oz	9
chuck, arm pot roast, cooked, 3 oz	7
chuck, arm pot roast, lean only, trimmed, cooked, 3 oz	3
chuck, blade roast, cooked, 3 oz	9
chuck, blade roast, trimmed, cooked, 3 oz	5
chuck, boneless, lean and trimmed, raw, 4 oz	3
cube steak, cooked, 3 oz	3
⭘ cube steak, trimmed, cooked, 3 oz	2
cured, thin-sliced beef, 3 oz	3
⭘ eye round, lean, trimmed, raw, 4 oz	2

Beef (cont'd)

No Count		SmartPoints® value
○	eye round, steak or roast, trimmed, cooked, 3 oz	2
	filet mignon, cooked, 3 oz	6
○	filet mignon, lean only, trimmed, cooked, 3 oz	3
○	filet mignon, trimmed, raw, 4 oz	3
○	flank steak, raw, 4 oz	3
○	flank, lean, raw, 4 oz	3
○	flank, lean, trimmed, cooked, 3 oz	3
	flanken, cooked, 3 oz	7
	KC strip, cooked, 3 oz	5
○	KC strip, lean and trimmed, cooked, 3 oz	3
○	KC strip, lean, trimmed, raw, 4 oz	3
	New York steak, cooked, 3 oz	5
○	New York steak, lean, trimmed, cooked, 3 oz	3
	New York steak, raw, 4 oz	7
	oxtails, raw, 4 oz	8
	porterhouse steak, cooked, 3 oz	9
	porterhouse steak, trimmed, cooked, 3 oz	7
	rib eye roast, boneless lean, cooked, 3 oz	4
	rib eye roast, boneless lean, raw, 3 oz	3
	rib eye, trimmed, cooked, 3 oz	5
	rib, large end, cooked, 3 oz	9
	rib, large end, trimmed, cooked, 3 oz	9
	rib, small end, trimmed, cooked, 3 oz	5
	rib, whole (ribs 6-12), lean and fat, cooked, 3 oz	10
	rib, whole (ribs 6-12), lean and fat, raw, 4 oz	12
	rib, whole (ribs 6-12), lean only, cooked, 3 oz	5
	rib, whole (ribs 6-12), lean only, raw, 4 oz	4
	round, lean and fat, raw, 4 oz	6
○	round, lean and trimmed, cooked, 3 oz	2
○	round, lean only, raw, 4 oz	3
	round, steak or roast, cooked, 3 oz	5
○	rump roast, lean, trimmed, cooked, 3 oz	3
○	shanks, lean, trimmed, raw, 4 oz	2
	shortribs, cooked, barbecued, 3 oz	16
	shortribs, lean and fat, cooked, 3 oz	14
	shortribs, lean and fat, raw, 4 oz	17
	shortribs, trimmed, cooked, 3 oz	8
	shortribs, trimmed, raw, 4 oz	9
	sirloin, cooked, 3 oz	6
○	sirloin, lean and trimmed, cooked, 3 oz	3
○	sirloin lean, trimmed, raw, 4 oz	2
	sirloin, trimmed, cooked, 3 oz	4
	skirt steak, cooked, 3 oz	5
	steak, flat iron, cooked, 3 oz	5
	steak, flat iron, raw, 4 oz	5
○	steak, lean, cooked (round or loin cuts with all visible fat trimmed), 3 oz	3
	steak, regular, cooked, 3 oz	8
	steak, sirloin, family-style, restaurant-type, 6 oz	7
	steak, skirt, lean and fat, trimmed, cooked, 3 oz	5
	strip sirloin, cooked, 3 oz	6
○	strip sirloin, lean, trimmed, cooked, 3 oz	3
○	strip sirloin, lean, trimmed, raw, 4 oz	3
	t-bone steak, cooked, 3 oz	8
	t-bone steak, lean, trimmed, cooked, 3 oz	6
	t-bone steak, lean, trimmed, raw, 3 oz	6
	tenderloin, cooked, 3 oz	6

"We Like This!" item

○ No Count	SmartPoints® value
○ tenderloin, lean only, trimmed, cooked, 3 oz	3
tenderloin, lean, raw, 4 oz	3
○ tenderloin, lean, trimmed, raw, 4 oz	3
tongue, cooked, 3 oz	8
top round, trimmed, raw, 4 oz	4
Beef and broccoli	
6 ½ oz	4
frozen, 7 oz	9
Beef balls	
Vietnamese (thit bo vien), 6 (1 ¼ oz)	2
Beef Bourguignon	
7 ½ oz	13
Beef heart	
○ cooked, 3 oz	2
Beef jerky or stick	
1 oz	4
Beef macaroni, with tomato sauce	
frozen, reduced-fat, 9 ⅔ oz	9
Beef patty	
country-fried, 3 oz	8
country-fried, store-bought, 3 oz	8
frozen, cooked, 3 oz	8
Beef sandwich steak	
processed, raw, 3 oz	9
Beef sticks	
smoked, 1 (¾ oz)	4
Beef stroganoff	
with noodles, 15 oz	21
Beef Wellington	
5 oz	15
Beef, chopped	
smoked, 3 oz	2
Beef, corned	
canned, 3 oz	6
cooked, 3 oz	6
cooked, lean, 3 oz	6
loaf, jellied, 2 oz	2
raw, 4 oz	7

○ No Count	SmartPoints® value
Beef, dried	
3 oz	2
Beef, ground	
75% lean/25% fat (regular), cooked, 3 oz	6
75% lean/25% fat (regular), raw, 4 oz	11
80% lean/20% fat, cooked, 3 oz	6
80% lean/20% fat, raw, 4 oz	9
85% lean/15% fat, cooked, 3 oz	6
85% lean/15% fat, raw, 4 oz	7
90% lean/10% fat, cooked, 3 oz	4
90% lean/10% fat, raw, 4 oz	5
90% lean/10% fat, sirloin, cooked, 3 oz	4
○ 93% lean/7% fat, cooked, 3 oz	3
○ 93% lean/7% fat, raw, 4 oz	3
○ 95% lean/5% fat, cooked, 3 oz	3
○ 95% lean/5% fat, raw, 4 oz	3
lean, raw, 4 oz	5
sirloin, cooked, 3 oz	4
sirloin, raw, 4 oz	5
Beefalo	
○ cooked, 3 oz	3
○ uncooked, 4 oz	3
Beer	
ginger, 12 fl oz	11
light, 12 fl oz	3
malt, 8 fl oz	5
non-alcoholic, 12 fl oz	7
regular, 12 fl oz	5
Beets	
pickled, ½ cup	3
Beignet	
¾ oz	3
from mix, prepared, 1 (¾ oz)	4
Bhuna gosht	
9 oz	8
Bialy	
1 (3 oz)	8

○ No Count	SmartPoints® value
Biryani	
chicken, 10 oz	12
lamb, 10 oz	19
Biscotti	
chocolate, 1 (1 oz)	6
fat-free, 1 (1 oz)	5
plain, 1 (1 oz)	6
Biscuit	
2″ square, fast food, 1 (2 oz)	11
cheese, 1 (1 ¾ oz)	8
commercially baked, 1 (1 ¼ oz)	4
small, 1 (1 ½ oz)	4
small, refrigerated, baked, 1 (1 oz)	3
with egg and bacon, fast food, 5 ⅓ oz	15
with egg and ham, fast food, 6 ½ oz	13
with egg and sausage, fast food, 6 ½ oz	19
with sausage, fast food, 4 oz	14
with steak, fast food, 5 oz	15
Biscuit dough	
mixed grain, refrigerated, 1 (1 ½ oz)	3
refrigerated, 1 (1 ½ oz)	4
Biscuit mix	
⅓ cup	6
buttermilk, reduced-fat, ⅓ cup	6
prepared, 1 (2 oz)	6
Bison (buffalo)	
○ lean, all visible fat trimmed, cooked, 3 oz	2
○ lean, all visible fat trimmed, raw, 4 oz	2
○ ribeye, lean and trimmed, raw, 4 oz	2
○ top sirloin steak, cooked, 3 oz	3
○ top sirloin steak, raw, 4 oz	2
Bison (buffalo), ground	
cooked, 3 oz	4
grass-fed, 3 oz	3
raw, 4 oz	8

"We Like This!" item

○ No Count	SmartPoints® value
Bistec de palomilla (Cuban fried steak)	
3 oz	6
Blackberries	
canned, heavy syrup, ½ cup	6
Blackened chicken	
3 oz	10
Blackened fish	
6 oz	14
Blackened steak	
3 oz	9
Blanquette of veal	
5 ¼ oz	5
Blintz	
cheese, 1 (4 ¾ oz)	8
cheese, frozen, 1 (2 ¼ oz)	3
fruit, frozen, 1 (2 ¼ oz)	3
potato, frozen, 1 (2 ¼ oz)	3
Blueberries	
canned, heavy syrup, ½ cup	7
dried, sweetened, ¼ cup	7
frozen, sweetened, 1 cup	11
in light syrup, canned, drained, ½ cup	6
Bologna	
beef and pork, low-fat, 2 oz	4
beef and pork, low-fat, 1″ cubes, 2 oz	4
beef, low-fat, 2 oz	4
beef, reduced-sodium, 2 oz	6
chicken and pork, 2 oz	7
chicken, pork, and beef, 2 oz	5
chicken, turkey, and pork, 2 oz	6
Lebanon, beef, 2 oz	2
pork and turkey, light, 2 oz	4
turkey, 2 oz	4
Borscht	
1 cup	6
low-calorie, store-bought, 1 cup	1
store-bought, 1 cup	5

○ No Count	SmartPoints® value
Boston brown bread	
1 slice (1 ½ oz)	3
Bouillon	
canned, 1 cup	0
cube, 1	0
granules, 1 tsp	0
Bran	
oat, uncooked, ⅓ cup	4
wheat, uncooked, ¼ cup	1
Brazil nuts	
¼ cup	7
Bread	
any type (white, wheat, rye, Italian, French, pumpernickel), 1 slice (1 oz)	2
challah, 1 slice (1 ½ oz)	3
cinnamon-raisin swirl, 1 slice (1 ¼ oz)	4
French baguette, 1 piece (2 ¼ oz)	5
high fiber (3 g or more dietary fiber per slice), 1 slice (1 oz)	2
pan Cubano, 1 (4 ½ oz)	12
potato, 1 slice (1 oz)	3
protein-enriched (includes gluten), 1 slice (⅔ oz)	1
○ reduced-calorie, 1 slice (¾ oz)	1
○ reduced-calorie, any type, 2 slices (1 ⅔ oz)	3
○ sandwich thin, 1 (1 ½ oz)	3
sourdough, 1 slice (1 ¼ oz)	3
wheat germ, 1 slice (1 oz)	2
Bread pudding	
½ cup	12
Bread, cheese	
1 slice (1 ¾ oz)	6
Bread, garlic	
1 slice (1 ½ oz)	8
frozen, 1 slice (1 ½ oz)	5
Breadcrumbs	
dried, plain, ¼ cup	3
dried, seasoned, ¼ cup	3

○ No Count	SmartPoints® value
fresh, ¼ cup	1
panko, white, ¼ cup	3
panko, whole-wheat, ¼ cup	3
whole-wheat, ¼ cup	2
Breadfruit	
○ uncooked, ½ cup	5
Breadstick dough	
refrigerated, 1 (1 oz)	2
Breadsticks	
any type, 1 (⅓ oz)	1
soft, 1 (1 ⅓ oz)	3
Breakfast powder	
instant, 1 Tbsp	1
Brioche	
1 (1 oz)	5
Broccoli-rice casserole	
5 ¼ oz	6
Broth	
any type other than those listed here, 1 cup	0
○ beef, reduced-sodium, 1 cup	0
○ beef, with tomato juice, 1 cup	3
chicken, canned, 1 cup	1
chicken, canned, condensed, ½ cup	1
○ chicken, canned, low-sodium, 1 cup	1
chicken, canned, reduced-sodium, 1 cup	0
○ chicken, gluten-free, fat-free, reduced-sodium, 1 cup	0
consomme, dehydrated, prepared with water, 1 cup	0
fish, 1 cup	1
vegetable, 1 cup	1
○ vegetable, reduced-sodium, 1 cup	1
Brownie	
fat-free, store-bought, 1 (1 ½ oz)	6
low-fat, store-bought, 1 (1 ½ oz)	8
prepared, 1 (2 ½ oz)	15

No Count	SmartPoints® value
Brownie mix	
special dietary, prepared, 1 (¾ oz)	3
Bruschetta	
3 ¼ oz	4
Bubble and squeak	
8 oz	5
Bubble tea (milk tea)	
8 fl oz	4
Buckwheat	
(No Count) 2 oz	5
Buffalo wings	
1 (1 ½ oz)	4
frozen, prepared without fat, 1 (1 oz)	2
Bulgogi (beef stir-fry)	
4 ⅓ oz	4
Bulgur	
(No Count) cooked, 1 cup	4
(No Count) uncooked, 2 oz	5
Bunuelos (fried yeast bread)	
restaurant-type, 1 slice (2 ½ oz)	12
Burger, vegetable or soy	
unprepared, 3 oz	4
Burrito	
bean, 1 (7 ½ oz)	8
bean and cheese, reduced-fat, store-bought, 1 (5 ½ oz)	7
bean and cheese, store-bought, 1 (5 oz)	10
bean, fast food, 7 ¾ oz	14
beef and cheese, large, 1 (6 oz)	11
beef and cheese, small, 1 (3 ⅔ oz)	7
beef or chicken and cheese, reduced-fat, store-bought, 1 (4 oz)	7
chicken and cheese, large, 1 (6 oz)	9
chicken and cheese, small, 1 (3 ⅔ oz)	6
chicken, store-bought, 1 (5 oz)	8
vegetable, large, 11 oz	14
vegetable, small, 5 ½ oz	6
with beans and cheese, fast food, 6 ¾ oz	12
with beans and chili peppers, fast food, 7 ⅓ oz	14
with beans and meat, fast food, 8 ¼ oz	13
with beans, cheese, and beef, fast food, 8 ⅔ oz	14
with beans, cheese, and chili peppers, fast food, 12 oz	20
with beef and chili peppers, fast food, 7 oz	13
with beef, cheese, and chili peppers, fast food, 10 ¾ oz	18
with beef, fast food, 7 ¾ oz	16
with fruit, fast food, 2 ⅔ oz	10
Burrito, breakfast	
egg, cheese and bacon, ham, or sausage, store-bought, 1 (3 ½ oz)	8
ham and cheese, frozen, 1 package (3 ½ oz)	6
Butter	
1 Tbsp	5
light, 1 Tbsp	3
whipped, 1 Tbsp	3
Butter chicken	
10 ¾ oz	9
Butternuts	
dried, ¼ cup	5

C

No Count	SmartPoints® value
Cabbage	
Japanese style, fresh, pickled, ¼ cup	0
stuffed, 11 oz	8
Cacao nibs	
1 oz	6
Café mocha	
made with fat-free milk, without whipped cream, 8 fl oz	7

"We Like This!" item

No Count	SmartPoints® value
Cake	
angel food, 1 piece (2 oz)	4
apple, 1 slice (3 oz)	10
Boston cream pie, commercially prepared, 1 piece (3 ¼ oz)	11
cherry fudge, with chocolate frosting, 1 piece (2 ½ oz)	9
corn, sweet, 4 oz	16
fat-free, store-bought, 1 piece (3 ½ oz)	9
fruit, 1 piece (2 oz)	9
gingerbread, 1 piece (2 ⅔ oz)	10
honey, 1 piece (4 oz)	14
Passover sponge, 1 piece (2 ½ oz)	6
petit fours, 1 (1 oz)	5
pineapple upside-down (⅑ of 8″ square), 1 piece (4 oz)	16
pound, 1 piece (3 oz)	15
pound, butter, store-bought, 1 piece (1 ¾ oz)	8
pound, store-bought, 1 piece (2 ½ oz)	13
sachertorte, 1 piece (2 ¾ oz)	15
shortcake, store-bought, 1 piece (1 oz)	4
shortcake, strawberry, 1 piece (4 ⅓ oz)	11
sponge, commercially prepared, 1 piece (1 ⅓ oz)	5
sugar-free, store-bought, 1 piece (2 ½ oz)	7
with icing, store-bought, 1 piece (3 oz)	13
yellow, with chocolate frosting, store-bought, 1 piece (5 oz)	25
yellow, with vanilla frosting, store-bought, 1 piece (2 ⅓ oz)	12
Cake mix	
angel food, 1 oz	5
angel food, prepared, 1 piece (1 ¾ oz)	5
banana, ⅛ package (2 ⅓ oz)	12

No Count	SmartPoints® value
banana, unprepared, ⅛ package (2 ⅓ oz)	12
carrot, pudding-type, ⅛ package (2 ¼ oz)	8
chocolate, pudding-type, ⅛ package (2 ⅓ oz)	11
chocolate, regular, 1 oz	5
coffee cake, cinnamon with crumb topping, 1 oz	5
coffee cake, cinnamon with crumb topping, prepared, 1 piece (2 oz)	7
devil's food, 1 oz	5
German chocolate, ¼ package (4 ⅔ oz)	20
gingerbread, 1 oz	5
marble, pudding-type, ⅛ package (2 ⅓ oz)	11
vanilla, unprepared, ⅛ package (2 ⅓ oz)	13
white, pudding-type, enriched, 1 oz	5
white, regular, 1 oz	5
white, unprepared, ⅛ package (2 ⅓ oz)	13
yellow, regular, enriched, 1 oz	5
yellow, unprepared, ⅛ package (2 ⅓ oz)	12
Cake, coffee	
1 piece (3 ¼ oz)	14
cheese, 1 piece (2 ¾ oz)	11
cinnamon, store-bought, 1 piece (2 oz)	10
crème-filled with chocolate frosting, 1 (3 oz)	12
fat-free, store-bought, 1 piece (2 oz)	6
fruit, 1 piece (1 ¾ oz)	7
Cake, snack	
crème-filled, chocolate with frosting, 1 (1 ¾ oz)	9
crème-filled, sponge, 1 (1 ½ oz)	7
crème-filled, store-bought, 1 (1 oz)	5

◯ No Count	SmartPoints® value
Calamari	
fried, 3 ½ oz	13
◯ grilled, 3 oz	2
Candy, chocolate	
any type other than those listed here, 1 (1 ½ oz)	12
caramels, chocolate-flavor roll, 6 (1 ½ oz)	7
chocolate toffee bar, 1 (1 ⅓ oz)	10
dark 60-69%, 1 oz	8
dark 70-85%, 1 oz	8
fun-size bar, 1 (⅔ oz)	4
milk chocolate, with almonds, 1 (1 ½ oz)	11
milk chocolate, with rice cereal, 1 (1 ⅔ oz)	11
milk chocolate-covered coffee beans, 1 oz	8
mint, chocolate-covered, 1 (1 ¼ oz)	8
sweet chocolate-coated fondant, 1 (1 ½ oz)	9
Candy, non-chocolate	
butterscotch, 3 (½ oz)	4
candy bits, yogurt-covered, 1 oz	6
candy cane, any type, 1 (½ oz)	3
candy corn, 1 oz	6
caramels, 1 oz	6
cotton candy, 1 oz	6
gum drops, 1 small	1
gum drops, low-calorie, 1	1
hard, 1 (¼ oz)	1
hard, low-calorie, 1	1
jelly beans, 10 (⅓ oz)	2
licorice, 1 (1 oz)	4
licorice rope, 1 (⅔ oz)	3
lollipop, 1 (1 oz)	6
nougat, with almonds, 1 piece (½ oz)	2
peanut bar, 1 (1 ⅔ oz)	9
peanut brittle, store-bought, 1 oz	6

◯ No Count	SmartPoints® value
praline, 1 (1 ⅓ oz)	8
rolls, yogurt-covered, fruit-flavored, 1 (¾ oz)	4
sesame, 1 (¾ oz)	5
sesame crunch, 20 (1 ¼ oz)	7
Cannelloni	
cheese, with tomato sauce, frozen, 7 oz	9
spinach and cheese, with tomato sauce, 12 oz	14
Cannoli	
1 (3 ⅓ oz)	13
Capers	
1 Tbsp	0
Capon	
cooked, with skin, without bone, 3 oz	4
Caponata (eggplant appetizer)	
6 ½ oz	5
store-bought, ½ cup	5
Cappuccino	
◯ made with fat-free milk, 8 fl oz	2
made with reduced-fat (2%) milk, 8 fl oz	3
made with whole milk, 8 fl oz	3
ready-made, from machine, any flavor, 8 fl oz	4
Cappuccino mix	
any flavor, 1 Tbsp	3
Carne asada	
5 oz	12
Carnitas	
5 ½ oz	8
Cashew butter	
2 Tbsp	6
Cashew chicken	
6 ⅓ oz	7
Cashews	
¼ cup	6
dry-roasted, ¼ cup	7
oil-roasted, ¼ cup	6

"We Like This!" item

No Count		SmartPoints® value
	Catfish	
	channel, breaded and fried, 3 oz	5
	Cavatelli with sausage and broccoli	
	5 oz	8
	Caviar	
	any type, 1 Tbsp	1
	Cereal bar/snack bar	
	crisped rice bar, chocolate chip, 1 (1 oz)	4
	crispy rice and marshmallow treat, store-bought, 1 (¾ oz)	4
	fat-free, 1 (1½ oz)	6
	mixed berry, 1 bar (1⅓ oz)	6
	regular, 1 (1¼ oz)	4
	rice and wheat, 1 bar (¾ oz)	3
	Cereal, hot	
●	cream of rice, cooked, 1 cup	4
●	cream of wheat, cooked, 1 cup	4
●	farina, cooked, 1 cup	4
	farina, uncooked, 1 oz	3
●	oatmeal, cooked, 1 cup	5
	oatmeal, flavored, cooked, 1 cup	8
	oatmeal, instant, with cinnamon and spice, uncooked, 1 packet (1⅔ oz)	6
	oatmeal, instant, with raisins and spice, uncooked, 1 packet (1½ oz)	6
	oatmeal, uncooked, ½ cup	4
●	whole-wheat , cooked, 1 cup	4
	Cereal, ready-to-eat	
	amaranth flakes, 1 cup	4
	any type, with sugar substitute, 1 cup	3
	bran flakes, ¾ cup	3
	corn flakes, 1 cup	3
	crisp rice, 1 cup	3
	frosted, 1 cup	7
	granola, low-fat, 1 cup	13
	granola, store-bought, 1 cup	19

No Count		SmartPoints® value
	museli, with dried fruit and nuts, 1 cup	11
	nuggets, 1 cup	12
	oat, corn and wheat squares, sweetened, maple flavor, 1 cup	5
	puffed millet, 1 cup	2
	puffed rice, 1 cup	2
	puffed wheat, 1 cup	1
	raisin bran, 1 cup	8
●	shredded wheat, bite-size, 1 oz	3
	whole-grain, fortified, 1 cup	4
	Ceviche	
	4¾ oz	2
	Chai tea latte	
	made with fat-free milk, 8 fl oz	4
	made with reduced-fat (2%) milk, 8 fl oz	6
	Chalupa (pork and bean dish)	
	5⅓ oz	8
	Champagne	
	5 fl oz	4
	Chana dal	
	9 oz	6
	Char shiu bao (roast pork bun)	
	char shiu bao (roast pork bun), 1 (2½ oz)	6
	Cheese	
	American, 1 slice (1 oz)	4
●	American, fat-free, 1 oz	1
	American, low-fat , single, 1 slice (¾ oz)	1
	American, spread, 1 oz	3
	asiago, 1 oz	5
	blue, 1 oz	4
	blue, crumbled, reduced-fat, ¼ cup	3
	brick, 1 oz	4
	brie, 1 oz	4
	camembert, 1 oz	3
	cheddar or colby, 1 oz	4

Cheese (cont'd)

No Count		SmartPoints® value
	cheddar or colby, low-fat, 1 oz	1
	cheddar or colby, low-sodium, 1 oz	4
●	cheddar, fat-free, 2 slices (1½ oz)	1
●	cheddar, fat-free, shredded, ¼ cup	1
	cheddar, reduced-fat, 1 oz	3
	cheddar, shredded, ¼ cup	4
	cheddar, shredded, low-fat, ¼ cup	1
●	cottage, fat-free, 1 cup	3
	cottage, low-fat (1%), 1 cup	3
	cottage, low-fat (1%), with vegetables, 1 cup	3
	cottage, reduced-fat (2%), 1 cup	5
	cottage, regular (4%), 1 cup	6
	cottage, regular, with fruit, 1 cup	6
	cottage, with vegetables, 1 cup	6
	cream, ⅓ less fat, 1 Tbsp	2
●	cream, fat-free, ¼ cup	2
	cream, light, 1 Tbsp	1
	cream, regular, 1 Tbsp	2
	cream, soy, 1 oz	3
	cream, whipped, 1 Tbsp	2
	edam, 1 oz	4
	farmer, 1 oz	3
	feta, 1 oz	3
●	feta, fat-free, 2 oz	1
	feta, reduced-fat, 1 oz	2
	fontina, 1 oz	4
	gjetost, 1 oz	5
	goat, hard-type, 1 oz	5
	goat, reduced-fat, 1 oz	2
	goat, semisoft-type, 1 oz	4
	goat, soft-type, 1 oz	3
	gorgonzola, 1 oz	4
	gouda, 1 oz	4
	gruyère, 1 oz	4
	halloumi, 1 oz	3
●	hard or semisoft, fat-free, 1 oz	1
	hard or semisoft, low-fat, 1 oz	2

"We Like This!" item

No Count		SmartPoints® value
	hard or semisoft, regular, 1 oz	4
	havarti, 1 oz	4
	manchego, 1 oz	4
	mascarpone, 1 oz	6
	Mexican, reduced-fat, shredded, ¼ cup	3
	Monterey, 1 oz	4
	Monterey Jack, shredded, reduced-fat, 1 oz	3
●	mozzarella, fat-free, shredded, 2 oz	1
	mozzarella, fresh, 1 oz	3
	mozzarella, low-sodium, 1 oz	3
	mozzarella, low-sodium, diced, 1 oz	3
	mozzarella, part-skim, 1 oz	2
	mozzarella, whole milk, 1 oz	3
	mozzarella, whole milk, low moisture, 1 oz	3
	muenster, 1 oz	4
	muenster, low-fat, 1 oz	3
	neufchâtel (reduced-fat cream cheese), 1 oz	3
	Parmesan, 1 oz	4
	Parmesan, fat-free, 2 Tbsp	1
	Parmesan, low-sodium, grated, 1 oz	4
	Parmesan, reduced-fat, 1 oz	3
	Parmesan, shredded, ¼ cup	3
	Parmigiano Reggiano, shredded, ¼ cup	3
	pasteurized process, Swiss, 1 oz	3
	Pecorino Romano, grated, ¼ cup	3
	Pecorino, grated, 1 Tbsp	1
	pepper Jack, 1 oz	4
	port de salut, 1 oz	4
	pot, 1 cup	2
	provolone, 1 oz	4
	provolone, reduced-fat, 1 oz	3
	queso anejo, 1 oz	4
	queso asadero, 1 oz	4

No Count	Food	SmartPoints® value
	queso chihuahua, 1 oz	4
	queso cotija, 1 oz	4
	queso fresco, 1 oz	3
	ricotta salata, 1 oz	3
O	ricotta, fat-free, ½ cup	2
	ricotta, part-skim, ½ cup	5
	ricotta, whole milk, ½ cup	8
	Romano, 1 oz	4
	Roquefort, 1 oz	4
	Roquefort, crumbled, ¼ cup	4
O	soy, Parmesan-flavored, 1 oz	3
	soybean, curd, 1 oz	1
	Swiss, 1 oz	4
O	Swiss, fat-free, 2 oz	1
O	Swiss, fat-free, shredded, ¼ cup	1
	Swiss, low-fat, 1 oz	1
	Swiss, low-fat, shredded, ¼ cup	1
	white, dry, queso seco, grated, 1 oz	3
	white, queso blanco, crumbled, 1 oz	3
	Cheese ball	
	store-bought, 1 oz	3
	Cheese food	
	cold pack, American, 1 oz	3
	pasteurized process, Swiss, 1 oz	3
	Cheese product	
	American, yellow loaf, 1 oz	5
	Cheese puffs	
	hot, 1 oz	3
	Cheese squares	
	mini, regular, 1 oz	4
	Cheese sticks	
	breaded, prepared without fat, store-bought, 1 (½ oz)	2
	Cheese straws	
	2 (2 oz)	3
	Cheese substitute	
	mozzarella, 1 oz	3

No Count	Food	SmartPoints® value
	Cheese twists or balls	
	1 oz	5
	Cheeseburger	
	double, fast food, 5 ⅓ oz	15
	double, regular patty and bun, with condiments, fast food, 5 ½ oz	15
	large, with condiments and vegetables, fast food, 1 (8 ⅓ oz)	16
	microwave, 4 ¾ oz	14
	on bun, plain, without mayonnaise, lettuce, and tomato, 6 ¾ oz	14
	single patty, with condiments, fast food, 4 ½ oz	12
	single, large patty, with condiments, fast food, 7 oz	18
	small, fast food, 1 (3 ¼ oz)	9
	small, with condiments and vegetables, fast food, 4 oz	10
	with bacon, microwave, 5 oz	15
	Cheesecake	
	any type, fast food, 1 piece (2 ¾ oz)	12
	frozen, 1 piece (4 oz)	17
	plain, 1 piece (4 ½ oz)	18
	prepared from mix, no-bake type, 1 piece (3 ½ oz)	12
	with fruit topping, 1 piece (5 ¾ oz)	19
	Cherries	
	dried, ¼ cup	8
	sour, red, canned, light syrup pack, ½ cup	5
	sweet, canned, heavy syrup pack, ½ cup	6
	sweet, canned, juice pack, ½ cup	4
	sweet, canned, light syrup pack, ½ cup	5
	sweet, frozen, sweetened, 1 cup	13
	Cherries, chocolate-covered	
	chocolate-covered, 1 (½ oz)	3

No Count	Food	SmartPoints® value
	Chestnuts	
	Chinese, boiled and steamed, ¼ cup	1
	European, boiled and steamed, 1 oz	1
	Chicken adobo	
	4 oz	6
	Chicken and broccoli	
	6 ½ oz	3
	Chicken and dumplings	
	canned, 8 ½ oz	6
	cooked, with skin, 5 oz	9
	cooked, without skin, 5 oz	8
	frozen, 8 ½ oz	6
	Chicken and meatball fricassee	
	14 ½ oz	8
	Chicken and rice	
	restaurant-type, 5 oz	6
	Chicken asopao	
	10 ¾ oz	10
	Chicken breast	
	barbecued, with skin and bone, 4 ½ oz	8
●	boneless, skinless, raw, 4 oz	2
	cooked, with skin, without bone, 1 oz	1
●	cooked, without bone, without skin, 3 oz	2
	deli-style, sliced, 4 slices (1 ¾ oz)	1
	fat-free, mequite flavor, sliced, 3 slices (2 ¼ oz)	1
	fillet, breaded, frozen, prepared without fat, 3 oz	4
●	fillet, grilled, without skin and bone, 3 oz	2
	five-spice, 4 ½ oz	7
	fried, with skin and bone, 4 ½ oz	11
	fried, with skin, without bone, 3 oz	5
	oven roasted, fat-free, sliced, 3 oz	1

No Count	Food	SmartPoints® value
	patty, breaded, fat-free, prepared without fat, 3 oz	2
●	raw, without skin, without bone, 4 oz	2
●	roasted, without skin and bone, 1 oz	1
	rotisserie, barbecue, with skin, 3 oz	3
	rotisserie, barbecue, without skin, 3 oz	2
●	rotisserie, without skin, 3 oz	1
	tenders, breaded, cooked, 3 oz	6
	Chicken breast, ground	
●	raw, 4 oz	1
	Chicken broilers and fryers	
	dark meat, with skin, cooked, 3 oz	5
	dark meat, without skin, cooked, 3 oz	4
	dark meat, without skin, raw, 4 oz	2
	Chicken cacciatore	
	6 ½ oz	10
	Chicken cordon bleu	
	6 ¾ oz	13
	frozen, 4 ⅓ oz	12
	Chicken cutlet	
	pan-fried, 3 oz	4
	Chicken drumstick	
	cooked, skinless, with bone, 1 drumstick (4 ⅓ oz)	2
	cooked, with skin, without bone, 1 (3 ¾ oz)	4
	cooked, without skin and bone, 1 (3 ½ oz)	4
	fried, with skin and bone, 1 (1 ½ oz)	6
	raw, skinless, boneless, 4 oz	4
	raw, with skin and bone, 4 oz	3
	rotisserie, barbecue, with skin, 1 (2 ½ oz)	3
	rotisserie, barbecue, without skin, 1 (2 ½ oz)	2

"We Like This!" item

● No Count	SmartPoints® value
Chicken feet	
boiled, 1 oz	2
Chicken fingers	
family-style, restaurant-type, 4 oz	10
Chicken giblets	
cooked, 2 ½ oz	2
Chicken gizzard	
● cooked, 3 oz	2
Chicken heart	
cooked, 5 oz	5
Chicken hekka	
8 oz	8
Chicken jalfrezi	
6 oz	6
Chicken Kiev	
6 ½ oz	21
frozen, 6 oz	11
Chicken leg	
drumstick and thigh, roasted, with skin and bone, 1 (9 oz)	10
five-spice, 6 oz	9
Chicken long rice	
7 oz	4
Chicken mole	
7 oz	7
Chicken neck	
simmered, without skin and bone, 1 (⅔ oz)	1
Chicken nuggets	
fried, 2 ½ oz	8
fried, fast food, 6 (3 ¾ oz)	9
frozen, 3 oz	7
Chicken paprika	
10 oz	8
Chicken parmigiana	
patty, store-bought, 5 oz	8
without sauce, 5 ½ oz	10

● No Count	SmartPoints® value
Chicken patty	
fried, frozen, 3 oz	6
frozen, cooked, 3 oz	7
frozen, uncooked, 4 oz	10
with sauce, 13 ¾ oz	13
Chicken pilaf (kotta pilafi)	
13 ⅔ oz	12
Chicken roaster	
raw, with skin and bone, 4 oz	7
Chicken tenders	
breaded, frozen, prepared, 3 oz	6
family-style, restaurant-type, 7 oz	16
fast food, 3 oz	6
restaurant-type, 3 oz	4
Chicken thigh	
barbecued, with skin and bone, 3 oz	6
boneless, skinless, raw, 4 oz	2
cooked, with skin, 5 oz	8
cooked, without skin, 3 oz	5
fried, with skin and bone, 3 oz	8
rotisserie, barbecue, with skin, 1 (3 ⅓ oz)	5
rotisserie, barbecue, without skin, 1 (3 ⅓ oz)	4
skinless, boneless, raw, 3 oz	2
skinless, with bone, raw, 1 oz	1
with skin, meat only, roasted, 4 oz	4
Chicken tikka	
4 ½ oz	5
Chicken wing	
cooked, with skin, with bone, 1 (3 oz)	6
glazed, barbecue flavor, frozen, 1 (1 oz)	2
glazed, barbecue flavor, frozen, conventional oven heated, 3 ½ oz	6
glazed, barbecue flavor, frozen, microwave heated, 2 ⅔ oz	5
raw, with skin, with bone, 4 oz	6

Chicken wing (cont'd)

○ No Count	SmartPoints® value
raw, without skin, 4 oz	2
rotisserie, barbecue, with skin, 1 (1 ¾ oz)	3
rotisserie, barbecue, without skin, 1 (1 ¾ oz)	2
Chicken with cashews	
7 oz	11
Chicken, breaded and fried	
light meat (from breast or wing), fast food, 3 oz	7
Chicken, canned	
with broth, 3 oz	3
without broth, 3 oz	3
Chicken, dark meat	
cooked, 2 oz	2
Chicken, fried	
breast, with skin, breaded, fast food, 3 oz	5
breast, without skin and breading, fast food, 3 oz	2
drumstick, with skin and breading, fast food, 3 oz	6
drumstick, without skin and breading, fast food, 3 oz	3
thigh, with skin, fast food, 3 oz	7
thigh, without skin and breading, fast food, 3 oz	3
wing, with skin, fast food, 3 oz	7
wing, without skin and breading, fast food, 3 oz	4
Chicken, ground	
93% lean/7% fat, cooked, 3 oz	3
93% lean/7% fat, raw, 4 oz	4
cooked, 3 oz	4
Chicken, light meat	
cooked, 1 slice (2 oz)	2
Chicken, meat only	
roasted, 5 oz	5
stewed, 5 oz	5

○ No Count	SmartPoints® value
Chili cheese dog	
restaurant-type, 5 oz	12
Chili con carne	
fast food, 1 cup	7
with beans, 1 cup	8
with beans, family-style, restaurant-type, 6 ½ oz	9
without beans, 1 cup	8
Chili con queso	
store-bought, 1 cup	9
Chili dog on roll	
8 ½ oz	12
fast food, 4 oz	9
Chili mac	
canned, 1 cup	8
Chili with beans	
canned, 1 cup	8
in a cup, 1 container (2 oz)	5
microwavable bowl, 1 cup	7
turkey, canned, 1 cup	6
Chili without beans	
canned, 1 cup	8
frozen, 1 cup	16
turkey, canned, 1 cup	4
Chili, low-fat	
canned, 1 cup	7
Chili, vegetarian	
low-fat or fat-free, canned, 1 cup	5
Chimichanga	
beef, 1 (8 ⅓ oz)	13
beef or chicken, with beans, frozen, 1 (6 ½ oz)	10
chicken, 1 (8 ⅓ oz)	11
with beef, fast food, 1 (6 ¼ oz)	13
Chinese lemon chicken	
restaurant-type, 2 ⅔ oz	6
Chinese orange chicken	
restaurant-type, 2 ¼ oz	6

"We Like This!" item

No Count	SmartPoints® value
Chinese roast pork	
5 oz	5
Chinese vegetables	
with beef, 5 ¾ oz	6
with chicken, 5 ¾ oz	5
with pork, 5 ¾ oz	8
with shrimp, restaurant-type, 1 order (21 ½ oz)	13
with tofu, 5 ¾ oz	4
Chips, bagel	
1 oz	4
fat-free, 1 oz	4
Chips, banana	
¼ cup	16
Chips, brown rice	
1 (⅓ oz)	1
Chips, corn	
10 (1 oz)	5
barbecue-flavor, 1 oz	5
Chips, pita	
1 oz	4
whole-wheat, 1 oz	3
Chips, plantain	
1 oz	5
Chips, potato	
baked, 1 oz	3
barbecue-flavor, 1 oz	5
cheese-flavor, 1 oz	5
fat-free, 1 oz	2
light, 1 oz	5
lightly salted, 1 oz	5
plain, unsalted, 1 oz	5
reduced-calorie, 1 oz	4
reduced-fat, 1 oz	4
regular, 1 oz	5
sour-cream-and-onion-flavor, 1 oz	5
Chips, soy	
1 oz	3

No Count	SmartPoints® value
Chips, sweet potato	
1 oz	5
Chips, taro	
1 oz	5
Chips, tortilla	
12 chips (1 oz)	4
baked, low-fat, 12 (1 oz)	3
blue corn, baked, 10 chips (1 oz)	3
light, 1 oz	4
low-fat, 1 oz	3
nacho cheese, 1 oz	5
nacho cheese, low-fat, made with olestra, 1 oz	3
nacho-flavor, 1 oz	4
nacho-flavor, light, 1 oz	4
ranch-flavor, 1 oz	4
reduced-fat, 12 (1 oz)	4
taco-flavor, 1 oz	4
white corn, plain, 1 oz	4
yellow corn, plain, 1 oz	4
Chips, vegetable	
1 oz	4
Chips, yucca (cassava)	
1 oz	5
Chitterlings	
cooked, 3 oz	7
Chocolate and candy, baking	
bittersweet chocolate, 1 piece (½ oz)	3
bittersweet chocolate, shavings, 1 Tbsp	2
carob, without sugar, ¼ cup	4
Mexican, squares, 1 piece (¾ oz)	5
milk chocolate chips, 1 Tbsp	3
milk chocolate, shavings, 1 Tbsp	2
mini chocolate chips, 1 Tbsp	3
peanut butter chips, 1 Tbsp	4
semisweet chocolate chips, 1 Tbsp	3

Chocolate and candy, baking (cont'd)

No Count	SmartPoints® value
semisweet chocolate chips, made with butter, 1 Tbsp	3
toffee baking bits, 1 Tbsp	3
unsweetened chocolate, grated, 1 Tbsp	2
unsweetened, liquid, 1 Tbsp	3
unsweetened, squares, 1 piece (1 oz)	8
white chocolate chips, 1 Tbsp	3
white chocolate, shavings, 1 Tbsp	2
Chocolate drink	
8 fl oz	7
Chocolate milk	
fat-free, 1 cup	7
low-fat (1%), 1 cup	8
reduced-fat (2%), 1 cup	8
whole, 1 cup	10
Chocolate mousse	
½ cup	22
sugar-free, prepared, 1 container (2 oz)	2
Cholent	
4 oz	5
Chop suey	
beef, 7 oz	5
chicken, 7 oz	3
pork, 7 oz	4
vegetable, 11 oz	3
Chorizo	
3 oz	13
chicken, 1 oz	1
Chow fun	
beef, 5 oz	10
chicken, 5 oz	10
pork, 5 oz	10
shrimp, 5 oz	10
Chow mein	
beef, 8 oz	4
chicken, 8 ¼ oz	4
chicken, restaurant-type, 21 ½ oz	14

No Count	SmartPoints® value
chow mein, beef, chicken, or pork, canned, 8 ¾ oz	2
pork, 8 ½ oz	4
subgum chicken, 8 ¼ oz	3
vegetable, without meat or noodles, restaurant-type, 27 ¾ oz	12
Chow mein noodles	
packaged, 2 oz	9
Chuleta	
1 (6 oz)	13
Chutney	
2 Tbsp	3
Cider	
apple, ½ cup	2
Cinnamon bun or roll	
frosted, 1 (2 ⅓ oz)	13
homemade, 1 (4 oz)	11
mini, fast food, 1 (1 oz)	4
Clam juice	
canned, 2 Tbsp	0
clam-tomato, 8 fl oz	4
Clams, baked	
2 ½ oz	11
Clams, fried	
6 ⅔ oz	12
breaded, 3 oz	5
frozen, prepared without fat, 3 oz	9
Clams, stuffed	
frozen, prepared without fat, 3 oz	3
Cobbler	
fruit, 7 ¾ oz	21
fruit, frozen, 4 ½ oz	12
Cocktail mix	
daiquiri, 3 fl oz	4
Margarita, 3 fl oz	6
piña colada, 3 fl oz	5
tonic water, 8 fl oz	5
whiskey sour, 3 fl oz	5
Cocoa powder, unsweetened	
1 Tbsp	0

"We Like This!" item

No Count	SmartPoints® value
Cocoa, hot, instant	
fat-free, prepared, 8 fl oz	2
no sugar added, prepared, 8 fl oz	4
regular, prepared, 8 fl oz	4
sugar-free, fat-free, 1 Tbsp	1
Coconut cream	
canned, 2 Tbsp	8
raw, 2 Tbsp	5
Coconut flakes	
sweetened, 2 Tbsp	4
unsweetened, 1 tsp	0
Coconut juice	
8 fl oz	6
Coconut meat	
dried, without sugar, 2 Tbsp	10
raw, ¼ cup	4
sweetened, shredded, 2 Tbsp	3
Coconut milk	
fresh, canned, 8 fl oz	25
light, store-bought, 8 fl oz	7
Coconut rice	
Indian, 4 ⅓ oz	8
Thai, 10 ⅓ oz	16
Coconut water	
8 fl oz	2
Coffee drink	
Jamaican, store-bought, 8 fl oz	5
with milk, canned, 8 fl oz	8
Coffee mix	
flavored, sugar-free, prepared, 8 fl oz	1
flavored, sugar-free, unprepared, 1 Tbsp	1
flavored, with sugar, prepared, 8 fl oz	3
Coffee powder, instant	
with sugar, French flavor, 1 Tbsp	2
with sugar, mocha flavor, 1 Tbsp	1

No Count	SmartPoints® value
Coffee substitute or cereal beverage powder	
1 Tbsp	1
Coffee, Irish	
7 fl oz	7
Coffee, Mexican	
6 fl oz	6
Coffee, regular or decaffeinated	
black, without sugar, 8 fl oz	0
Colcannon	
9 oz	12
Coleslaw	
family-style, restaurant-type, 3 ¾ oz	7
fast food, 6 ¾ oz	12
homemade, 3 ½ oz	5
Conch fritters	
1 ¾ oz	3
Conch, cracked	
4 oz	9
Cookie dough, refrigerated	
baked, 2 (1 oz)	6
chocolate chip, ¼ cup	11
oatmeal, 1 (½ oz)	3
peanut butter, 1 (½ oz)	3
sugar, 1 (⅔ oz)	3
Cookie mix	
chocolate chip, 1 oz	6
oatmeal, 1 oz	6
Cookies	
amaretti, 1 (1 oz)	4
animal crackers, 13 (1 oz)	4
animal crackers, fast food, 1 oz	4
bar, 1 (1 ¼ oz)	5
butter, commercially prepared, 1 (¼ oz)	1
buttercrunch toffee, 1 (2 oz)	12
Chinese almond, 1 (½ oz)	3
chocolate chip, commercially prepared, higher fat, 1 (⅓ oz)	2

Cookies (cont'd)

No Count	SmartPoints® value
chocolate chip, commercially prepared, soft-type, 1 (½ oz)	2
chocolate chip, commercially prepared, special dietary, 1 (¼ oz)	1
chocolate chip, fast food, 1 package (2 oz)	8
chocolate sandwich, with crème filling, 1 (⅓ oz)	2
chocolate sandwich, with crème filling, chocolate-coated, 1 (⅔ oz)	4
chocolate sandwich, with crème filling, special dietary, 1 (⅓ oz)	2
chocolate sandwich, with extra crème filling, 1 (½ oz)	3
chocolate wafers, 2 (½ oz)	2
chruscik, 1 (¼ oz)	1
fig bar, 1 (½ oz)	3
fortune, 1 (¼ oz)	1
fruit bar, 1 (½ oz)	3
fudge, cake-type, 1 (¾ oz)	3
gingerbread, 1 (¾ oz)	4
gingersnaps, 1 (¼ oz)	1
homemade, chocolate chip, oatmeal, sugar, or similar type, 1 (½ oz)	3
kolache (fruit filled), 1 (2 oz)	7
kolache (without filling), 1 (2 oz)	6
kringla, 1 (¾ oz)	3
lace, 1 (¼ oz)	2
ladyfinger, 1 (⅓ oz)	2
ladyfingers, store-bought, 1 (½ oz)	2
macaroon, 1 (⅔ oz)	3
mandelbrot, 1 (2 oz)	8
marshmallow, chocolate-coated, 1 (½ oz)	2
Mexican wedding, 2 (½ oz)	3
molasses, 1 (½ oz)	2
oatmeal, chocolate chip, sugar, or similar type, packaged, 1 (½ oz)	3
oatmeal, commercially prepared, 1 (⅔ oz)	3

No Count	SmartPoints® value
oatmeal, commercially prepared, fat-free, 1 oz	4
oatmeal, commercially prepared, special dietary, 1 (¼ oz)	1
peanut butter sandwich, regular, 1 (½ oz)	3
peanut butter sandwich, special dietary, 1 (⅓ oz)	2
peanut butter, commercially prepared, 1 (1 oz)	5
rainbow, 1 (⅔ oz)	3
raisin, soft, 1 (½ oz)	3
reduced-calorie, store-bought, 1 (½ oz)	2
rugalach, 1 (1 oz)	6
sesame seed, 2 (1 oz)	5
shortbread, commercially prepared, 1 (½ oz)	2
shortbread, commercially prepared, pecan, 1 (½ oz)	3
social tea biscuit, 1	1
sugar wafers with crème filling, 1 (⅓ oz)	2
sugar wafers with crème filling, special dietary, 2 (⅓ oz)	1
sugar, commercially prepared, 1 (⅔ oz)	3
sugar, commercially prepared, special dietary, 1 (¼ oz)	1
sugar-free, store-bought, 1 (½ oz)	2
vanilla sandwich with crème filling, 1 (½ oz)	3
vanilla wafers, 1 (⅓ oz)	2
vanilla wafers, reduced-fat, 1 (¼ oz)	1
Viennese wafers, chocolate cream, store-bought, 1 (1 oz)	6
white macadamia, restaurant-type, 1 (1 ¾ oz)	11

Cooking spray

5 sprays	0
butter-flavored, 1 spray	0
olive oil, 1 spray	0

"We Like This!" item

No Count	Food	SmartPoints® value
	Coquilles St. Jacques	
	13 ¾ oz	10
	Corn	
	breaded, prepared without fat, 6 (3 oz)	7
○	canned, with red and green peppers, ½ cup	2
	cream-style, ½ cup	3
○	dried, 1 oz	3
○	frozen, kernels cut off cob, cooked, ½ cup	3
○	frozen, kernels cut off cob, unprepared, ½ cup	2
○	frozen, kernels on cob, cooked, ½ cup	2
○	frozen, kernels on cob, unprepared, ½ cup	3
○	kernels, cooked, ½ cup	2
	on the cob, with butter, fast food, 5 ¼ oz	5
	on the grill, with butter, 1 (4 oz)	8
○	white, canned, ½ cup	2
	white, canned, cream-style, ½ cup	3
○	white, kernels on cob, cooked, ½ cup	3
○	white, kernels on cob, raw, ½ cup	3
○	white, raw, ½ cup	2
○	yellow, canned (vacuum-packed), ½ cup	3
○	yellow, frozen, cooked, ½ cup	2
○	yellow, kernels, cooked, ½ cup	2
○	yellow, on the cob, 1 medium (3 ⅔ oz)	3
○	yellow, raw, ½ cup	2
	Corn cakes	
	corn, 1 (⅓ oz)	1
	popcorn, mini, 3 (⅓ oz)	1
	popcorn, other than plain or butter-flavored, 1 (½ oz)	2
	popcorn, plain or butter-flavored, 1 (⅓ oz)	1

No Count	Food	SmartPoints® value
	Corn casserole	
	6 ¼ oz	14
	Corn dog	
	1 (2 ¾ oz)	6
	fast food, 6 ¼ oz	15
	frozen, prepared, 1 (2 ¾ oz)	7
	mini, frozen, prepared, 1 (⅔ oz)	2
	Corn flake crumbs	
	¼ cup	2
	Corn nuts	
	1 oz	4
	barbecue-flavor, 1 oz	4
	chile picante, ⅓ cup	4
	nacho-flavor, 1 oz	4
	Corn pudding	
	home prepared, ½ cup	6
	Cornbread	
	made with fat-free milk, 1 piece (1 ¾ oz)	4
	Mexican, 1 piece (3 ⅔ oz)	12
	Cornbread and muffin mix	
	1 ½ oz	6
	Cornbread dressing	
	6 ⅓ oz	11
	Cornbread mix	
	¼ package (2 oz)	9
	prepared, 1 slice (2 oz)	7
	Cornish hen	
	cooked, with skin, 3 oz	6
○	cooked, without skin, 3 oz	2
	with skin, raw, 4 oz	6
○	without skin, raw, 4 oz	2
	Cornmeal	
○	blue, ¼ cup	3
○	cooked, ¼ cup	1
	self-rising, white, ¼ cup	3
	white, enriched, raw, ¼ cup	4
	white, unenriched, raw, ¼ cup	4
○	whole-grain, white, ¼ cup	3
○	yellow, ¼ cup	4

Cornmeal (cont'd)

○ No Count	SmartPoints® value
yellow, degermed, self-rising, ¼ cup	3
○ yellow, enriched, raw, ¼ cup	4
○ yellow, whole-grain, ¼ cup	3
Cornmeal mix	
self-rising, ¼ cup	4
Cornstarch	
1 Tbsp	1
Couscous	
cooked, 1 cup	5
in a cup, unprepared, 2 oz	6
Israeli, raw, 2 oz	6
○ Israeli, whole-wheat, raw, 2 oz	5
uncooked, 2 oz	6
○ whole-wheat, cooked, 1 cup	6
○ whole-wheat, raw, 2 oz	6
Cowpeas	
○ common (blackeyes, crowder, southern), canned, ½ cup	2
○ common (blackeyes, crowder, southern), cooked, ½ cup	3
○ common (blackeyes, crowder, southern), dry, ¼ cup	4
common (blackeyes, crowder, southern), with pork, canned, ½ cup	3
○ young pods with seeds, raw, 1 cup	2
Crab cakes	
5 oz	4
blue crab, 2 oz	2
fast food, 2 oz	5
Crab puffs	
2 oz	6
Crab rangoon	
1 (2 ¼ oz)	7
frozen, 5 ⅓ oz	12
Crab, stuffed	
frozen, 3 oz	3
Cracker meal	
¼ cup	3

○ No Count	SmartPoints® value
Crackers	
arare, 50 (1 oz)	3
cheese squares, mini, reduced-fat, 1 oz	4
cheese, sandwich-type with peanut butter filling, 1 oz	4
cheese, sandwich-type, with cheese filling, 1 oz	5
cheese, whole-grain, 1 oz	3
fat-free, 1 oz	3
graham, 2 squares (½ oz)	2
graham, chocolate, 2 squares (½ oz)	2
graham, chocolate-coated, 1 piece (⅓ oz)	2
graham, cinnamon, reduced-fat, 2 squares (½ oz)	2
graham, cinnamon-honey, reduced-fat, 2 squares (½ oz)	2
graham, low-fat, 1 whole (⅔ oz)	3
graham, mini, any variety, 1 oz	5
graham, reduced-fat, 2 squares (½ oz)	2
milk, 1 oz	4
multi-grain, 1 oz	5
oyster, 5 (¼ oz)	1
rice, 8 (½ oz)	2
rusk toast, 1 oz	3
rye, sandwich-type with cheese filling, 2 (½ oz)	2
rye, wafers, plain, 1 oz	3
rye, wafers, seasoned, 1 oz	3
saltines, 1 oz	4
saltines, fat-free, low-sodium, 6 (1 oz)	3
saltines, whole-wheat, 1 oz	3
snack, 1 oz	5
snack, with filling (cheese, wheat, rye, toast, or wafer crackers with cheese, peanut butter, or cream cheese filling), 6 (1 ½ oz)	7

"We Like This!" item

○ No Count	SmartPoints® value
standard snack-type, sandwich, with peanut butter filling, 2 (½ oz)	2
wheat, regular, 16 thin (1¼ oz)	5
wheat, sandwich, with cheese filling, 2 (½ oz)	2
wheat, sandwich, with peanut butter filling, 2 (½ oz)	2
whole-wheat, 1 oz	4
whole-wheat, reduced-fat, 1 oz	3
Cranberries	
dried, ¼ cup	7
Cranberry sauce	
canned, ¼ cup	6
Cream	
clotted, 2 Tbsp	7
fat-free, 2 Tbsp	1
half and half, 2 Tbsp	2
heavy, unwhipped, 2 Tbsp	5
light, 2 Tbsp	3
whipping, heavy, 2 Tbsp	5
whipping, light, 2 Tbsp	4
Cream puff	
homemade, 1 (2 oz)	13
Cream substitute	
flavored, liquid, 1 Tbsp	2
flavored, powder, 1 tsp	1
light, powder, 1 tsp	0
liquid, light, 1 Tbsp	1
Cream, sour	
○ fat-free, 2 Tbsp	1
imitation, cultured, 2 Tbsp	3
light, 1 tsp	0
reduced-fat, 2 Tbsp	2
regular, 2 Tbsp	3
soy, 2 Tbsp	1
Cream, whipped	
aerosol, 2 Tbsp	1
chocolate, aerosol, 2 Tbsp	1
dairy or nondairy, frozen, 2 Tbsp	1

○ No Count	SmartPoints® value
Creamer	
fat-free, 2 Tbsp	1
fat-free, liquid, flavored, 2 Tbsp	2
nondairy, liquid, 2 Tbsp	2
nondairy, powder, 2 Tbsp	3
Crème brûlée	
½ cup	13
Crème caramel	
½ cup	7
Crème fraiche	
2 Tbsp	5
Creole, chicken	
without rice, 9⅓ oz	6
Creole, shrimp	
store-bought, 9⅔ oz	5
without rice, 9⅓ oz	5
Crêpe	
6″ diameter, 1 (1⅓ oz)	3
Crêpes Suzette	
4¾ oz	19
Crispbread	
5 (¾ oz)	2
rye, crushed, 1 oz	3
rye, wafer, 1 oz	3
wafer, thin, 1 oz	3
Croissant	
apple, 1 (2 oz)	6
butter, 1 (2 oz)	9
cheese, 1 (2 oz)	9
chocolate-filled, 1 (3¾ oz)	10
plain, 1 (1¾ oz)	9
Croquette	
beef, 5 oz	11
chicken, 5 oz	10
Croutons	
homemade, 7 (1 oz)	4
packaged, fat-free, 7 (¼ oz)	1
packaged, regular, 7 (1 oz)	4
plain, 7 (1 oz)	3
seasoned, 1 cup	6

No Count	SmartPoints® value
Cruller	
2 oz	9
French, glazed, 1 (1 ½ oz)	7
glazed, 1 (2 ⅓ oz)	10
Crumpet	
2 ¼ oz	5
Cuban rice	
8 oz	6
Cupcake	
any type, homemade, prepared from mix, with 2 Tbsp frosting, 1 (2 ¾ oz)	14
chocolate, with frosting, low-fat, 1 (1 ½ oz)	6
crème-filled, store-bought, 1 (1 ¾ oz)	8
extra-large, with frosting, store-bought, any type, 1 (4 ½ oz)	23
large, with frosting, store-bought, any type, 1 (3 oz)	15
mini, with frosting, store-bought, any type, 1 (1 oz)	5
with frosting, store-bought, any type, 1 (2 oz)	9
Currants (zante)	
dried, ¼ cup	6
Curry	
African, fish, 4 ¼ oz	9
African, shrimp, 4 ¼ oz	10
beef, 7 ⅔ oz	13
Bengali fish, 13 ¾ oz	7
chicken, 7 ⅔ oz	12
egg, 7 ½ oz	4
goat, 9 oz	5
green chicken (gaeng kheow wan gai), 7 ⅓ oz	13
lamb, 7 ⅔ oz	15
Vietnamese chicken, 8 oz	11
Curry paste	
green, 1 Tbsp	0
panang, 1 Tbsp	1

"We Like This!" item

No Count	SmartPoints® value
Custard	
½ cup	7
Custard mix	
dessert, egg, ¾ oz	3
dessert, egg, prepared with whole milk, ½ cup	6

D

Dairy drink/shake mix	
reduced-calorie, 1 packet (¾ oz)	3
Danish pastry	
cheese, 1 (2 ½ oz)	9
cheese, fast food, 1 (3 ¼ oz)	15
cinnamon, 1 (2 ⅓ oz)	10
cinnamon, fast food, 1 (3 oz)	14
fast food, 1 (3 ¼ oz)	15
fruit, 1 (2 ½ oz)	11
fruit, fast food, 1 (3 ⅓ oz)	13
nut, 1 (2 ⅓ oz)	11
store-bought, 1 (2 ⅓ oz)	10
Date-nut bread	
1 slice (2 ½ oz)	11
Dates	
dried, ¼ cup	7
Deviled crab	
4 oz	6
Deviled egg	
2 oz	5
Dim sum	
bean curd roll with shrimp and vegetables, 1 (3 ½ oz)	2
bean curd roll with vegetables, 1 (2 ½ oz)	2
sesame seed balls, 1 (2 oz)	9
Dip	
artichoke, baked, 2 Tbsp	4
bean, fat-free, ¼ cup	1
black bean, fat-free, 2 Tbsp	1
Mexican 7-layer, 2 Tbsp	1

No Count	SmartPoints® value
spinach, 2 Tbsp	4
spinach-artichoke, restaurant-type, 2 oz	5
strawberry-yogurt, 2 Tbsp	3
Dirty rice	
12 oz	12
Dirty rice mix	
prepared without fat, 8 ½ oz	4
Dolma	
4 (3 ½ oz)	6
store-bought, 3 ½ oz	5
Donair	
9 oz	21
Doro wat	
6 ¾ oz	8
Dosa mix	
instant, 2 Tbsp	4
ready-to-cook, 1 ½ oz	2
Doughnut	
cake-type, sugared or glazed, 1 (2 oz)	9
cake-type, wheat, sugared or glazed, 1 (2 oz)	8
cake-type, with icing, 1 (2 oz)	11
malasadas (Portuguese doughnuts), 1 (1 ¼ oz)	4
mini, chocolate-covered, store-bought, 1 (2 oz)	12
mini, powdered, sugar-covered, store-bought, 1 (2 oz)	10
with crème filling, 1 (3 oz)	12
yeast, glazed, 1 (2 oz)	10
yeast, with jelly filling, 1 (3 oz)	12
Doughnut holes	
yeast, glazed, 1 (½ oz)	2
Dressing, salad	
bacon and tomato, 2 Tbsp	3
balsamic vinaigrette, fat-free, 2 Tbsp	1
balsamic vinaigrette, light, gluten-free, 2 Tbsp	2

No Count	SmartPoints® value
balsamic, vinaigrette, low-fat, 1 Tbsp	1
blue cheese, fat-free, 2 Tbsp	1
blue cheese, light, 2 Tbsp	3
blue cheese, regular, 2 Tbsp	5
blue or roquefort cheese, light, 2 Tbsp	1
buttermilk, light, 2 Tbsp	2
Caesar, fat-free, 2 Tbsp	2
Caesar, low-calorie, 2 Tbsp	2
Caesar, regular, 2 Tbsp	6
coleslaw, 2 Tbsp	5
coleslaw, reduced-fat, 2 Tbsp	5
creamy, fat-free, 2 Tbsp	1
creamy, reduced-calorie, 2 Tbsp	3
French, 2 Tbsp	6
French, diet, 2 Tbsp	3
French, fat-free, 2 Tbsp	2
French, reduced-calorie, 1 Tbsp	2
French, reduced-fat, 2 Tbsp	3
French, regular, 2 Tbsp	5
ginger, 2 Tbsp	3
green goddess, 2 Tbsp	5
honey-mustard, fat-free, 1 Tbsp	2
honey-mustard, light, 2 Tbsp	5
honey-mustard, regular, 2 Tbsp	5
Italian, commerically prepared, reduced-fat, 2 Tbsp	1
Italian-tyle, regular, 2 Tbsp	3
Italian-type, diet, 2 Tbsp	1
Italian-type, fat-free, 2 Tbsp	1
Italian-type, reduced-calorie, 2 Tbsp	2
mayonnaise and mayonnaise-type, low-calorie, 2 Tbsp	3
mayonnaise, imitation, low-calorie, 2 Tbsp	1
mayonnaise, light, 2 Tbsp	3
mayonnaise-type, 2 Tbsp	3
peppercorn, commercially prepared, 2 Tbsp	5

Dressing, salad (cont'd)

● No Count	SmartPoints® value
poppy seed, creamy, 2 Tbsp	5
ranch, commercially prepared, 2 Tbsp	5
ranch, creamy, regular, 2 Tbsp	5
ranch, fat-free, 2 Tbsp	1
ranch, reduced-fat, 2 Tbsp	2
raspberry vinaigrette, 2 Tbsp	2
raspberry vinaigrette, fat-free, 2 Tbsp	2
red wine vinaigrette, fat-free, 2 Tbsp	1
red wine vinaigrette, low-fat, 2 Tbsp	2
Russian, low-calorie, 2 Tbsp	2
Russian, regular, 2 Tbsp	4
sesame ginger, light, 1 Tbsp	1
sesame seed, 2 Tbsp	5
sweet and sour, ¼ cup	1
Thousand Island, 2 Tbsp	5
Thousand Island, diet (10 calories per tsp), 2 Tbsp	2
Thousand Island, fat-free, 2 Tbsp	2
vinaigrette, fat-free, 1 Tbsp	0
vinaigrette, low-fat, 2 Tbsp	1
vinaigrette, regular, 2 Tbsp	5
Drunken noodles	
7 ⅓ oz	6
Duck	
domestic, cooked, with skin, ¼ (5 oz)	15
domestic, cooked, without skin, 3 oz	4
tea smoked, 2 oz	3
uncooked, without skin, 4 oz	4
Duck a l'orange	
17 ¾ oz	17
Dumpling	
beef or pork, fried, 1 (1 ⅔ oz)	2
beef or pork, steamed, 1 (1 ½ oz)	2
chicken, fried, 1 (1 ⅔ oz)	1
chicken, steamed, 1 (1 ½ oz)	1

"We Like This!" item

● No Count	SmartPoints® value
kroppkakor (potato dumpling), boiled, 1 (2 oz)	5
kroppkakor (potato dumpling), fried, 1 (2 oz)	5
potato, 5 ¾ oz	4
shrimp, fried, 1 (1 ⅔ oz)	1
shrimp, steamed, 1 (1 ½ oz)	1
vegetarian, fried, 1 (¾ oz)	1

E

Eclair	
1 (5 ⅓ oz)	16
Edamame	
● in pods, 1 cup	3
● shelled, ½ cup	3
Egg	
fried, 1	3
● hard-boiled, 1	2
scrambled, fast food (2 eggs), 3 ½ oz	7
scrambled, with butter and milk, 2 large eggs	6
● whole, 1	2
Egg foo yung	
beef, 1 (3 oz)	5
chicken, 1 (2 ¾ oz)	5
pork, 1 (3 oz)	5
shrimp, 1 (2 ¾ oz)	4
Egg roll snack	
pork or shrimp, store-bought, 3 oz	5
vegetable, store-bought, 3 oz	5
Egg roll, Chinese	
beef, 1 (2 ½ oz)	7
chicken, 1 (2 ½ oz)	5
chicken, store-bought, 1 (3 oz)	5
pork, 1 (2 ½ oz)	6
pork, store-bought, 1 (3 oz)	5
shrimp, 1 (2 ½ oz)	5
shrimp, store-bought, 1 (3 oz)	6
vegetable, store-bought, 1 (3 oz)	5

● No Count	SmartPoints® value
Egg substitute	
● fat-free, ½ cup	1
● regular, liquid, ½ cup	1
Egg white	
● 3	1
Egg yolk	
1	2
Eggnog	
1 cup	15
homemade, with liquor, 4 fl oz	8
homemade, without liquor, 1 cup	15
reduced-calorie, store-bought, without liquor, 1 cup	14
Eggnog mix	
powder, 1 Tbsp	9
Eggplant	
breaded and baked, without oil, 1½ oz	1
breaded and fried, 2⅔ oz	3
pickled, ¼ cup	1
Eggplant Parmesan	
frozen, 5 oz	6
Eggplant parmigiana	
with sauce, 13¼ oz	16
without sauce, 6¾ oz	12
Empanadas	
2 (1¾ oz)	7
restaurant-type, 3 oz	10
Enchilada	
beef, cheese, or chicken, 4⅓ oz	8
sour cream, 1 (5½ oz)	12
Enchilada de camarones	
7 oz	5
Energy drink	
regular, 8 fl oz	8
sugar-free, 8 fl oz	0
English muffin	
cinnamon-raisin, 1 (2 oz)	5
● light, 1 (2 oz)	2

● No Count	SmartPoints® value
● light, whole-wheat, 1 (2 oz)	3
plain, 1 (2 oz)	4
English muffin breakfast	
egg and cheese with meat, frozen, 4½ oz	9
egg, cheese, and Canadian bacon, 5 oz	9
with butter, fast food, 1 (2¼ oz)	6
with cheese and sausage, fast food, 4 oz	13
with egg, cheese, and Canadian bacon, fast food, 4½ oz	9
with egg, cheese, and sausage, fast food, 6 oz	16
Escargots	
3 oz	14
Étouffée	
crawfish or shrimp, store-bought, 9 oz	8
Extract	
almond, 1 Tbsp	2
coconut, imitation, 1 tsp	0
lemon, 1 Tbsp	2
mint, 1 Tbsp	1
orange, with alcohol, 1 Tbsp	2
rum, 1 Tbsp	1
vanilla, 1 Tbsp	1
vanilla, imitation, with alcohol, 1 Tbsp	1
vanilla, imitation, without alcohol, 1 Tbsp	0

F

Fadge (Irish potato bread)	
1 slice (3⅓ oz)	3
Fajita	
beef, 9 oz	15
chicken, 2 (8¾ oz)	9
shrimp, 9¼ oz	9
vegetarian, 5½ oz	7

No Count		SmartPoints® value
	Falafel	
	in pita, 6 ¾ oz	15
	Falafel patty	
	4 (4 ⅔ oz)	10
	prepared, 2 ⅓ oz	6
	Faro	
O	cooked, 1 cup	6
O	hulled, 2 oz	5
O	uncooked, ¼ cup	4
	Fattoush	
	8 oz	7
	Fettucine Alfredo	
	with broccoli and chicken, frozen, 8 oz	13
	Fig	
	canned, heavy syrup pack, ½ cup	7
	canned, light syrup pack, ½ cup	5
	dried, ¼ cup	5
	dried, stewed, ¼ cup	4
	Filberts	
	¼ cup	7
	dry-roasted, ¼ cup	6
	Fillo (phyllo) dough	
	1 sheet (⅔ oz)	2
	wheat, 1 sheet (⅔ oz)	2
	Fillo (phyllo) shells	
	mini, 4 (½ oz)	2
	Fish	
	anchovy, canned in oil, drained, 1	0
O	arctic char, cooked, 3 oz	2
O	bass, fresh water, cooked, 1 fillet (2 ¼ oz)	1
O	bass, striped, cooked, 3 oz	1
O	bluefish, cooked, 3 oz	2
O	butterfish, cooked, 3 oz	3
O	carp, cooked, 3 oz	3
O	catfish, farm-raised, cooked, 3 oz	3
O	catfish, wild, cooked, 3 oz	1
O	cod, Atlantic, canned, solids and liquid, 3 oz	1

"We Like This!" item

No Count		SmartPoints® value
O	cod, Atlantic, cooked, 3 oz	1
	cod, Atlantic, dried and salted, 3 oz	2
O	cod, Pacific, cooked, 3 oz	1
	dried, 3 oz	2
O	drum, cooked, 3 oz	2
	eel, cooked, 3 oz	5
	eel, raw, 4 oz	5
O	flounder, cooked, 3 oz	1
O	grouper, cooked, 3 oz	1
O	haddock, cooked, 3 oz	1
	haddock, smoked, 3 oz	1
O	halibut, cooked, 3 oz	1
	herring, cooked, 3 oz	4
	lox, 3 oz	2
	mackerel, Atlantic, cooked, 3 oz	6
O	mackerel, canned, 3 oz	3
	mackerel, cooked, 3 oz	4
O	mackerel, Spanish, cooked, 3 oz	3
O	mahimahi (dolphinfish), cooked, 3 oz	1
O	monkfish, cooked, 3 oz	1
O	mullet, striped, cooked, 3 oz	2
O	orange roughy, cooked, 3 oz	1
O	orange roughy, farm-raised, cooked, 6 oz	2
O	perch, cooked, 3 oz	1
O	pollack, cooked, 3 oz	1
	pompano, cooked, 3 oz	4
O	rockfish, cooked, 3 oz	1
	sable, cooked, 3 oz	6
	sable, smoked, 3 oz	6
	salmon, Atlantic, farmed, cooked, 3 oz	4
O	salmon, canned, drained, 3 oz	2
	salmon, chinook, cooked, 3 oz	5
	salmon, chinook, smoked, 3 oz	2
O	salmon, chum, canned, 3 oz	2
O	salmon, chum, cooked, 3 oz	2

No Count	Food	SmartPoints® value
	salmon, patty, 3 oz	3
○	salmon, pink, canned, 3 oz	2
○	salmon, pink, cooked, 3 oz	2
	salmon, raw, 4 oz	5
	salmon, smoked, 3 oz	2
○	salmon, sockeye, canned, 3 oz	3
○	salmon, sockeye, canned, with bone, drained, 3 oz	3
○	salmon, sockeye, cooked, 3 oz	2
○	salmon, sockeye, raw, 4 oz	2
○	salmon, wild, cooked, 3 oz	3
○	salmon, wild, pink canned, ¼ cup	2
	sardines, canned in oil, drained, 2 oz	3
	sardines, canned in tomato sauce, 3 oz	4
○	sea bass, cooked, 3 oz	1
○	sheepshead, cooked, 3 oz	1
○	smelt, cooked, 3 oz	1
○	snapper, cooked, 3 oz	1
○	sole, cooked, 3 oz	1
○	sturgeon, cooked, 3 oz	2
○	sturgeon, raw, 4 oz	2
	sturgeon, smoked, 3 oz	2
○	sucker, white, cooked, 3 oz	1
○	swordfish, cooked, 3 oz	3
○	tilapia, cooked, 3 oz	1
○	tilefish, cooked, 3 oz	2
○	trout, cooked, 3 oz	3
○	trout, rainbow, farmed, cooked (steelhead), 1 fillet (2 ½ oz)	2
○	trout, rainbow, wild, cooked (steelhead), 3 oz	2
○	tuna, bluefin, cooked, 3 oz	3
	tuna, canned in oil, drained, 3 oz	3
○	tuna, canned in water, drained, 3 oz	1
○	tuna, canned, chunk light tuna in water, ½ cup	1
○	tuna, canned, chunk white tuna in water, 3 oz	2

No Count	Food	SmartPoints® value
○	tuna, cooked, 3 oz	1
○	tuna, raw, 4 oz	1
○	turbot, European, cooked, 3 oz	2
○	whitefish, cooked, 3 oz	3
	whitefish, smoked, 2 oz	1
○	yellowtail, cooked, 3 oz	3
	Fish and chips	
	11 ½ oz	17
	Fish fillet	
	battered or breaded, fried, family-style, restaurant-type, 8 oz	13
	battered or breaded, fried, fast food, 3 ¼ oz	6
	battered, prepared without fat, 3 oz	6
	breaded, prepared without fat, 3 ¾ oz	7
	grilled, with garlic butter, 3 ¾ oz	2
○	grilled, with lemon-pepper, 3 ¾ oz	2
	light, breaded, prepared without fat, 3 ¾ oz	4
	Fish roe	
	cooked, 3 oz	3
	raw, 2 Tbsp	1
	Fish sticks	
	breaded, 2 ½ oz	5
	frozen, prepared (4" x 1" x ½"), 1 (1 oz)	2
	frozen, prepared (4" x 2" x ½"), 1 (2 oz)	5
	Fish, baked, stuffed	
	6 ¾ oz	11
	Fish, fried	
	without flour, 6 oz	13
	Fish, imitation (surimi)	
○	3 oz	1
	Fish, stuffed	
	frozen, 5 oz	5
	Flan	
	½ cup	11

No Count	SmartPoints® value
Flan mix	
caramel custard, ¾ oz	5
caramel custard, prepared with whole milk, ½ cup	5
Flatbread	
1 (¾ oz)	2
chapati, 1 piece (¾ oz)	3
Indian (navajo) fry, 1 piece (5 ½ oz)	17
injera, 1 (1 ⅔ oz)	2
lavash, 1 (2 ¼ oz)	8
lefse, 1 (4 ½ oz)	8
naan, 1 (3 oz)	6
paratha, 1 (1 ¼ oz)	5
puris, 1 (1 ½ oz)	4
Flauta	
beef, 4 oz	14
chicken, 4 oz	13
pork, 4 oz	13
Flax seed meal	
ground, ¼ cup	3
Flour	
bread, ¼ cup	3
cake, ¼ cup	4
chickpea (besan), ¼ cup	3
corn, masa, enriched, white, ¼ cup	3
masa harina, ¼ cup	3
millet, ¼ cup	3
peanut, low-fat, ¼ cup	2
rice, brown, ¼ cup	4
rice, white, ¼ cup	4
rye, ¼ cup	4
tortilla mix, enriched, ¼ cup	3
wheat, white, self-rising, ¼ cup	3
wheat, whole-grain, ¼ cup	3
white, ¼ cup	3
whole-wheat, ¼ cup	3
whole-wheat, pastry, ¼ cup	3
whole-wheat, white, ¼ cup	3

No Count	SmartPoints® value
Focaccia bread	
1 slice (2 oz)	4
Frankfurter	
beef, 1 (1 ¾ oz)	6
beef or pork, fat-free, 1 (1 ¾ oz)	1
beef or pork, light, 1 (1 ¾ oz)	3
beef or pork, regular, 1 (2 oz)	6
beef, low-fat, 1 (2 oz)	5
chicken, 1 (2 oz)	4
turkey, 1 (2 oz)	4
turkey, fat-free, 1 (1 ½ oz)	1
turkey, light, 1 (2 oz)	4
Frankfurter on roll	
plain, 3 ½ oz	10
Frankfurter roll or bun	
1 (2 oz)	5
○ light, 1 (1 ½ oz)	2
Franks (pigs) in blankets	
1 oz	9
frozen, 1 (½ oz)	2
Freekeh	
○ uncooked, ¼ cup	4
French fries	
20 (5 ⅔ oz)	13
crinkle cut, frozen, cooked, 10 (2 ½ oz)	4
crinkle cut, frozen, uncooked, 10 (3 oz)	4
cross cut, frozen, uncooked, 3 oz	5
family-style, restaurant-type, 6 oz	16
fast food, 4 oz	11
frozen, prepared without fat, 3 oz	4
shoestring, frozen, cooked, 10 (¾ oz)	1
shoestring, frozen, uncooked, 10 (1 oz)	2
small, 2 ½ oz	7
steak fries, frozen, cooked, 10 (4 ¾ oz)	6

"We Like This!" item

● No Count	SmartPoints® value
steak fries, frozen, uncooked, 10 (5 ½ oz)	6
wedges, frozen, uncooked, 3 oz	5
French toast	
2 slices (4 ⅔ oz)	11
frozen, 2 slices (4 ¼ oz)	8
with butter, fast food, 2 slices (4 ¾ oz)	13
French toast sticks	
fast food, 1 (1 oz)	3
frozen, 3 (2 ½ oz)	8
Fried rice	
beef, 8 ½ oz	11
chicken, 8 ½ oz	11
chicken or pork, frozen, 2 ½ oz	4
kho-phat, 6 oz	10
plain, homemade, 8 ¾ oz	11
pork, 8 ½ oz	10
shrimp, 8 ¼ oz	10
without meat, restaurant-type, 5 oz	7
Frijoles	
with cheese, fast food, 6 oz	7
Fritters	
apple, restaurant-type, 1 (4 oz)	16
corn, 4 oz	7
vegetable, 7 oz	13
Frog legs	
fried, 1 oz	4
Frosting/icing	
chocolate, creamy, ready-to-eat, 1 Tbsp	4
coconut-nut, ready-to-eat, 2 Tbsp	7
cream cheese-flavor, ready-to-eat, 1 Tbsp	7
decorating icing, 1 Tbsp	4
store-bought, regular, 1 Tbsp	3
vanilla, creamy, ready-to-eat, 1 Tbsp	3

● No Count	SmartPoints® value
Frosting/icing mix	
chocolate, creamy, 1 oz	3
chocolate, creamy, prepared with butter, 2 Tbsp	7
chocolate, creamy, prepared with margarine, 1 Tbsp	2
vanilla, creamy, 1 oz	4
vanilla, creamy, prepared with butter, 1 Tbsp	10
vanilla, creamy, prepared with margarine, 1 Tbsp	2
white, fluffy, prepared with water, 1 Tbsp	3
Frozen yogurt	
chocolate, ½ cup	6
chocolate, fat-free, ½ cup	5
chocolate, fat-free, reduced-sugar, 1 cup	8
chocolate, soft-serve, ½ cup	6
coffee-flavored, low-fat, ½ cup	6
fat-free, no sugar added, ½ cup	3
fat-free, sweetened with sugar, ½ cup	5
low-fat, ½ cup	5
vanilla, fat-free, ½ cup	5
vanilla, fat-free, reduced-sugar, ½ cup	3
Frozen yogurt bar	
chocolate-covered, frozen, 1 (2 ¾ oz)	6
Fruit	
● all individual or mixed fruits: canned or jarred in its own or another juice, without added sugar, drained	0
● all individual or mixed fruits: fresh, frozen, or canned or jarred in water, without added sugar	0
Fruit butter	
1 Tbsp	2

A-Z Food List

No Count		SmartPoints® value
	Fruit cocktail	
	canned, extra heavy syrup, ½ cup	7
	canned, heavy syrup, ½ cup	5
	canned, light syrup, ½ cup	4
●	mixed fruits without added sugar	0
	Fruit compote	
	½ cup	8
	Fruit juice bar	
	frozen, 1 (2 ¾ oz)	4
	frozen, without sugar, 1 (1 ¾ oz)	0
	Fruit juice cup	
	frozen, 1 (6 ½ oz)	10
	Fruit juices and drinks	
	apple and grape juice, 8 fl oz	7
	apple juice, 8 fl oz	7
	apple juice, unsweetened, 8 fl oz	7
	blackberry juice, canned, 8 fl oz	5
	citrus juice drink, frozen concentrate, prepared with water, 8 fl oz	6
	cranberry juice cocktail, frozen concentrate, 2 fl oz	8
	cranberry juice cocktail, low-calorie, 8 fl oz	3
	cranberry juice cocktail, regular, 8 fl oz	8
	cranberry juice, unsweetened, 8 fl oz	7
	cranberry-apple drink, 8 fl oz	9
	cranberry-apple juice, low-calorie, 8 fl oz	3
	cranberry-apple juice, store-bought, 8 fl oz	9
	cranberry-grape drink, 8 fl oz	8
	fruit drink mix, powdered, prepared, 8 fl oz	5
	fruit juice (combined), 8 fl oz	6
	fruit juice, low-calorie, 8 fl oz	0
	fruit punch drink, 8 fl oz	7
	fruit punch drink, concentrate, prepared with water, 8 fl oz	6
	fruit punch drink, powder, 1 Tbsp	3

"We Like This!" item

No Count		SmartPoints® value
	grape drink, 8 fl oz	9
	grape drink, canned, 8 fl oz	9
	grape juice, 8 fl oz	9
	grapefruit juice, 8 fl oz	5
	grapefruit juice, canned, sweetened, 8 fl oz	7
	grapefruit juice, pink, raw, 8 fl oz	3
	grapefruit juice, white, raw, 8 fl oz	6
	grapefruit juice, white, sweetened, canned, 8 fl oz	7
	grapefruit-mango juice, 8 fl oz	6
	lemon juice, canned or bottled, 8 fl oz	2
	lemon juice, fresh, 1 Tbsp	0
	lime juice, canned or bottled, unsweetened, 8 fl oz	2
	lime juice, fresh, 1 Tbsp	0
	mango juice, 8 fl oz	8
	orange and apricot juice drink, 8 fl oz	7
	orange juice, canned, unsweetened, 8 fl oz	6
	orange juice, fresh, 8 fl oz	6
	orange juice, frozen concentrate, unsweetened, undiluted, 8 fl oz	19
	orange-flavor drink, breakfast type, powder, 1 Tbsp	3
	orange-flavor drink, breakfast-type, frozen concentrate, prepared with water, 8 fl oz	7
	orange-flavor drink, breakfast-type, powder, prepared with water, 8 fl oz	8
	orange-grapefruit juice, 8 fl oz	6
	passionfruit juice, purple, 8 fl oz	8
	passionfruit juice, yellow, 8 fl oz	9
	pineapple and grapefruit drink, 8 fl oz	7
	pineapple and orange drink, 8 fl oz	7
	pineapple juice, 8 fl oz	7
	pineapple juice, canned, without sugar and ascorbic acid, 8 fl oz	7

◎ No Count	SmartPoints® value
pomegranate juice, 8 fl oz	9
prune juice, 8 fl oz	10
tangerine juice, 8 fl oz	6
tangerine juice, canned, sweetened, 8 fl oz	5
vegetable and fruit juice blend (100% juice), 8 fl oz	6
vegetable and fruit juice drink, reduced-calorie, 8 fl oz	0
vegetable and fruit juice, cold-pressed, detox-type, 8 fl oz	4
Fruit leather	
pieces, 1 oz	5
roll, 2 oz	10
snack bars, 1 (¾ oz)	4
snack bars, with cream, 1 (¾ oz)	4
Fruit tart	
with custard, individual, 1 (7½ oz)	24
Fruit, candied	
¼ cup	8
Fruit, dried	
mixed, ¼ cup	6
Fruit, mixed	
peach, cherry, sweet and sour, raspberry, grape, and boysenberry, frozen, sweetened, ½ cup	4
peach, pear, and pineapple, canned, heavy syrup, ½ cup	6
Fudge	
1 piece (1 oz)	6

G

Gefilte fish	
3 oz	2
Gelatin	
unflavored, 1 Tbsp	0
Gelatin dessert	
fruit-flavored, ½ cup	5
fruit-flavored, sugar-free, prepared, ½ cup	0

◎ No Count	SmartPoints® value
Gelatin-fruit mold	
½ cup	4
Gelato	
½ cup	7
General Tso's chicken	
restaurant-type, 2 oz	5
Ghee	
ghee, 1 tsp	2
Ginger	
crystalized, 7 pieces (1 oz)	6
pickled, 1 Tbsp	1
Ginger chicken	
7¾ oz	6
Ginger fish	
7⅓ oz	9
Glaze, balsamic	
1 Tbsp	1
Glaze, strawberry	
2 Tbsp	3
Gnocchi	
any type, frozen, 5½ oz	10
cheese, 6½ oz	17
potato, 4 oz	7
potato, refrigerated, 5 oz	8
spinach, 7¼ oz	19
Goat	
◎ cooked, 3 oz	2
Goose	
cooked, with skin, without bone, 3 oz	7
cooked, without skin and bone, 3 oz	4
Gordita	
beef, 4¼ oz	14
Goulash	
beef, 7⅔ oz	10
Hungarian, 1 cup	9
Graham cracker crumbs	
¼ cup	4
low-fat, 1 Tbsp	1

○ No Count	SmartPoints® value
Granola	
homemade, 1 cup	21
Granola bar	
chewy, reduced-sugar, all flavors, 1 (¾ oz)	4
chocolate-coated, 1 (1 oz)	7
chocolate-coated, with coconut, 1 (1 oz)	7
hard, chocolate chip, 1 bar (¾ oz)	4
hard, peanut butter, 1 (¾ oz)	4
hard, plain, 1 bar (1 oz)	4
hard, with almonds, 1 bar (¾ oz)	4
reduced-calorie, 1 (1 oz)	4
soft, chocolate chip, 1 bar (1½ oz)	7
soft, chocolate chip, graham, and marshmallow, 1 bar (1 oz)	4
soft, nut and raisin, uncoated, 1 bar (1 oz)	4
soft, peanut butter, milk chocolate-coated, 1 (1 oz)	6
soft, peanut butter, uncoated, 1 bar (1 oz)	4
soft, raisin, uncoated, 1 bar (1½ oz)	7
soft, uncoated, 1 (1 oz)	5
Granola bites	
mixed flavors, 1 package (¾ oz)	4
Grapefruit	
canned, light syrup pack, ½ cup	5
sections, juice pack, ½ cup	3
Gravy	
au jus, canned, 2 Tbsp	0
au jus, dry, 2 Tbsp	2
beef, canned, 2 Tbsp	0
brown, 2 Tbsp	2
brown, dry, 2 Tbsp	1
chicken, canned, 2 Tbsp	0
chicken, dry, 2 Tbsp	2
cream, 2 Tbsp	3
fat-free, canned, 2 Tbsp	0
giblet, 2 Tbsp	1

○ No Count	SmartPoints® value
meat or poultry, low-sodium, prepared, 1 Tbsp	0
mushroom, canned, 2 Tbsp	0
mushroom, dehydrated, dry, 2 Tbsp	0
onion, dehydrated, dry, 1 cup	2
pork, dry, 2 Tbsp	6
sausage, 2 Tbsp	3
sausage, canned, 2 Tbsp	2
turkey, canned, 2 Tbsp	0
turkey, dry, 2 Tbsp	5
Green bean casserole	
8 oz	8
Green rice	
10¾ oz	8
Greens	
seasoned with bacon or salt pork, 1 cup	5
Grits	
○ white, cooked, 1 cup	5
white, uncooked, ¼ cup	4
○ yellow, quick, cooked, 1 cup	4
Guacamole	
homemade or restaurant-type, 2 Tbsp	1
store-bought, 2 Tbsp	2
Guine hen	
○ cooked, 4 oz	1
Gum, chewing	
sugarless, 1 piece	0
with sugar, 1 piece	1
Gumbo	
chicken, 8¾ oz	6
seafood, 1 cup	5
seafood, with rice, store-bought, 1 cup	5
Gyoza	
1 (⅔ oz)	1
Gyro	
11½ oz	19

"We Like This!" item

H

No Count	Food	SmartPoints® value
	Halvah	
	store-bought, 1½ oz	8
	Ham	
○	boneless, extra-lean, low-sodium, cooked, 1 oz	1
	chopped, canned, 3 oz	6
	chopped, not canned, 3 oz	4
	cooked, lean, 3 oz	2
	cooked, regular, 3 oz	3
	extra-lean (approximately 4% fat), canned, 3 oz	2
	extra-lean (approximately 4% fat), canned, roasted, 3 oz	2
	extra-lean (approximately 5% fat), 3 oz	2
	glazed, with pineapple, 6½ oz	7
○	honey, smoked, 2 oz	1
	minced, 3 oz	7
	roasted, lean only, 3 oz	2
	serrano, 1 oz	2
○	slice, bone-in, lean, pan-broil, 3 oz	2
○	slice, bone-in, lean, uncooked, 3 oz	2
	slice, country-style, lean, raw, 1 oz	1
○	spiral slice, lean, roasted, 3 oz	2
	steak, extra-lean, unheated, 3 oz	2
	Ham hocks	
	smoked, 4 oz	6
	Hamantaschen	
	1 (1⅓ oz)	4
	Hamburger	
	dinner in a box, prepared, 7 oz	10
	double patty, plain, fast food, 1 (4¼ oz)	11
	double, large patty, with condiments and vegetables, fast food, 8 oz	16
	large, fast food with condiments, 1 (6 oz)	14
	large, plain, fast food, 1 (5 oz)	13
	microwave, 1½ oz	4

No Count	Food	SmartPoints® value
	on bun, plain (without mayonnaise, lettuce, and tomato), 4½ oz	11
	single, large patty, with condiments and vegetables, fast food, 7¾ oz	16
	single, with condiments, fast food, 3½ oz	8
	small, fast food, 2¾ oz	7
	small, with condiments and vegetables, fast food, 4 oz	9
	Hamburger roll or bun	
	1 (1½ oz)	4
○	light, 1 (1½ oz)	2
	Harissa paste	
	1 tsp	0
	Haroset	
	1 Tbsp	0
	Hash	
	corned beef, canned, 3 oz	4
	pork, 6 oz	7
	roast beef, canned, 3 oz	5
	Hash browns	
	family-style, restaurant-type, 4⅓ oz	8
	fast food, 1 patty (2 oz)	5
○	frozen, uncooked, 3¾ oz	2
	frozen, with butter sauce, cooked, 3½ oz	6
	frozen, with butter sauce, unprepared, 6 oz	8
	homemade, 1 cup	13
	patty, frozen, prepared without fat, 1 oz	2
	refrigerated, pan-fried in canola oil, 1 cup	10
	refrigerated, uncooked, 1 cup	4
	Haupia (coconut pudding)	
	½ cup	3
	Hazelnuts	
	¼ cup	7
	dry-roasted, ¼ cup	6

○ No Count	SmartPoints® value
Herbs	
fresh or dried, 1 tsp	0
Herring fillets	
chopped, 3 oz	5
in cream sauce, store-bought, 2 oz	5
in wine sauce, store-bought, 2 oz	3
kippered, 3 oz	4
pickled, 3 oz	7
store-bought, 3 oz	4
Hibachi chicken	
6 ½ oz	6
Hibachi shrimp	
6 ½ oz	4
Hibachi steak	
6 ½ oz	9
Hibachi vegetables	
6 ⅔ oz	4
Hominy	
○ canned, ½ cup	2
○ canned, yellow, ½ cup	2
○ whole, cooked, 1 cup	4
Honey	
1 Tbsp	4
Honeybun	
glazed, 1 (2 ⅓ oz)	10
Horseradish	
prepared, 1 Tbsp	0
Hot chocolate	
homemade, with whipped topping, 8 fl oz	14
homemade, without whipped topping, 8 fl oz	13
Hot cross buns	
1 (2 ⅓ oz)	9
Hot fudge	
fat-free, 2 Tbsp	5
Huevos rancheros	
10 oz	18

○ No Count	SmartPoints® value
Huli huli chicken	
breast, with skin and bone, 7 ⅓ oz	13
drumstick, with skin and bone, 2 oz	3
thigh, with skin and bone, 3 oz	6
Hummus	
2 Tbsp	2
Hunan beef	
9 oz	11
Hush puppies	
1 ½ oz	5
fast food, 1 (¾ oz)	2
frozen, prepared without fat, 2 oz	4
Hush puppy mix	
⅓ cup	4

I

Ice cream	
chocolate, ½ cup	7
chocolate, light, ½ cup	6
chocolate, light, no sugar added, ½ cup	5
chocolate, light, soft-serve, ½ cup	6
chocolate, regular, low-carbohydrate, ½ cup	6
chocolate, rich, ½ cup	9
chocolate, soft-serve, ½ cup	9
fat-free, no sugar added, ½ cup	3
French vanilla, soft-serve, ½ cup	9
fried, ½ cup	17
green tea, ½ cup	6
light, any flavor, no sugar added, ½ cup	5
premium, ½ cup	13
strawberry, ½ cup	7
vanilla, ½ cup	7
vanilla, fat-free, ½ cup	3
vanilla, light, ½ cup	6

"We Like This!" item

No Count	SmartPoints® value
vanilla, light, soft-serve, ½ cup	5
vanilla, regular, low-carbohydrate, ½ cup	6
vanilla, rich, ½ cup	13
Ice cream bar	
chocolate- or caramel-covered, with nuts, 1 bar (2 oz)	9
chocolate-covered, 1 (1 ¾ oz)	8
chocolate-covered, with crisp rice, 1 (2 oz)	9
chocolate-covered, with crisp rice, no sugar added, 1 (1 ½ oz)	5
Ice cream cone only	
cake or wafer, 1 (1 oz)	4
plain or sugar, 1 (⅓ oz)	1
Ice cream in cone	
light, vanilla, soft-serve, fast food, 4 ¼ oz	9
sundae cone, 1 (3 ½ oz)	15
Ice cream sandwich	
1 (2 ½ oz)	7
cookie-type, 1 (3 oz)	8
light, vanilla, 1 (2 ½ oz)	5
light, vanilla, no sugar added, 1 (2 ½ oz)	5
Ice cream soda	
8 fl oz	15
Ice cream sundae	
caramel, fast food, 5 ½ oz	15
hot fudge, fast food, 5 ⅔ oz	15
strawberry, fast food, 5 ½ oz	13
Ice pop	
fruit-flavored, 1 (1 ¾ oz)	2
fruit-flavored, artificially sweetened, 1 (2 oz)	0
Ices	
fruit, ½ cup	8
Italian, restaurant-type, ½ cup	3
water, pineapple-coconut, 4 fl oz	6

No Count	SmartPoints® value
Idli mix	
1 ½ oz	2
rava, 1 Tbsp	2
rice, 3 Tbsp	4
Imperial roll	
2 oz	5
Indian pudding	
½ cup	7
Irish soda bread	
1 slice (3 ½ oz)	12
Italian toast snack	
store-bought, 4 (1 oz)	4

J

Jackfruit	
canned, syrup pack, ½ cup	4
Jalapeño bread	
1 slice (1 ½ oz)	4
Jalapeño poppers	
1 (1 ⅔ oz)	5
Jalapeños, stuffed	
prepared without fat, store-bought, 2 oz	7
Jam	
all-fruit, 1 Tbsp	3
any type, 1 Tbsp	3
reduced-sugar, 1 Tbsp	1
Jamaican akee (ackee)	
canned, drained, 3 ½ oz	4
Jambalaya	
chicken, with rice, 12 ½ oz	12
fish, with rice, 12 ¾ oz	12
Jambalaya mix	
1 ½ oz	4
Japchae	
beef, 4 oz	8
chicken, 4 oz	9
pork, 4 oz	10

○ No Count	SmartPoints® value
Jelly	
any type, 1 Tbsp	3
Jerk chicken breast	
6 oz	3
Jerusalem artichokes (sunchokes)	
○ 1 cup	5
Juice, carrot	
canned, 8 fl oz	4
Juice, tomato	
8 fl oz	2
Juice, vegetable	
cold-pressed, 8 fl oz	4
low-sodium, canned, 8 fl oz	2
mixed, 8 fl oz	2

K

○ No Count	SmartPoints® value
Kabobs	
beef, 3 oz	5
chicken, 4 ¾ oz	4
fish, 4 ¾ oz	4
lamb, 4 ¾ oz	9
Kahlua pig	
3 oz	3
Kasha (buckwheat groats)	
○ cooked, 1 cup	4
○ dry, 2 oz	5
Kasha varnishkes	
7 ¾ oz	7
Kashmiri (lamb meatballs)	
3 ¾ oz	13
Kataifi	
1 (2 oz)	11
Katsu (4 ½" x 1 ½" x ¾" thick)	
ahi, 4 ⅓ oz	5
chicken, 4 ⅓ oz	5
pork, 4 ⅓ oz	7
Ketchup	
1 Tbsp	1
Khal bi	
4 oz	9

"We Like This!" item

○ No Count	SmartPoints® value
Kibbe	
baked, 1 piece (⅓ oz)	1
uncooked, 3 oz	6
Kielbasa	
grilled or pan-fried, 3 oz	10
Polish, turkey and beef, smoked, 3 oz	6
turkey, uncooked, 1 oz	1
Kim chee	
4 oz	1
King ranch chicken casserole	
8 oz	9
Kishke	
¾ oz	3
Knish	
potato, 4 oz	9
potato, store-bought, 4 ½ oz	15
Knockwurst	
boiled, 3 oz	9
Kofta (vegetable balls without sauce)	
3 oz	8
Korean barbecue beef	
4 oz	7
Korean barbecue chicken thighs	
5 oz	14
Korean barbecue short ribs	
4 oz	9
Korma	
vegetable, 14 ¾ oz	12
Kreplach	
boiled, 2 ¾ oz	8
fried, 3 oz	9
Kugel	
lukschen, with fruit, 6 ⅔ oz	12
lukschen, without fruit, 5 ⅔ oz	7
noodle, store-bought, 4 oz	7
potato, 6 ¼ oz	6
potato, store-bought, 3 ½ oz	6
Kung pao beef	
11 oz	11

No Count	Food	SmartPoints® value
	Kung pao chicken	
	9 ¼ oz	8
	Kung pao pork	
	10 ½ oz	10
	Kung pao shrimp	
	10 ½ oz	9

L

No Count	Food	SmartPoints® value
	Lamb	
●	chop, baby, cooked, 3 oz	3
●	chop, baby, raw, 4 oz	3
●	chop, cooked, 3 oz	4
●	chop, raw, 4 oz	4
	leg, cooked, 3 oz	6
●	leg, cooked, lean, trimmed, 3 oz	3
●	leg, lean, trimmed, raw, 4 oz	2
	loin, cooked, 3 oz	8
	loin, cooked, trimmed, 3 oz	4
	rib, cooked, 3 oz	10
	rib, lean and fat, raw, 4 oz	14
	shoulder, cooked, 3 oz	9
	shoulder, raw, 4 oz	9
	Lamb, ground	
	cooked, 3 oz	7
	raw, 4 oz	11
	Lasagna	
	chicken, 7 oz	8
	meat, 7 ⅔ oz	9
	vegetable, 7 ½ oz	10
	vegetarian, with cheese and spinach, 10 ½ oz	13
	with meat sauce, 7 ½ oz	8
	Latkes, potato	
	6 ½ oz	8
	Latte	
●	made with fat-free milk, 8 fl oz	3
	made with low-fat (1%) milk, 8 fl oz	4
	made with low-fat (1%) milk, 12 fl oz	6

No Count	Food	SmartPoints® value
	made with reduced-fat (2%) milk, 12 fl oz	6
	made with whole milk, 8 fl oz	5
	Lau Lau (pork and fish in taro or spinach leaves)	
	7 ⅔ oz	8
	Lechon asado (roast pork)	
	3 oz	4
	Lemon curd	
	1 Tbsp	3
	Lemon grass chicken	
	8 ¾ oz	9
	Lemonade	
	8 fl oz	6
	frozen concentrate, pink, prepared, 8 fl oz	6
	frozen concentrate, white, prepared, 8 fl oz	6
	prepared with water, 8 fl oz	6
	Lemonade mix	
	1 Tbsp	3
	low-calorie, prepared with water, 8 fl oz	0
	Lentils	
●	cooked, ½ cup	3
●	dry, ¼ cup	4
●	sprouted, raw, ½ cup	1
	Limeade	
	8 fl oz	8
	frozen concentrate, 2 fl oz	6
	Linguine	
	with red clam sauce, 6 ¾ oz	9
	with white clam sauce, 7 ½ oz	11
	Liver	
●	beef, cooked, 3 oz	3
	chicken, cooked, 1 ½ oz	1
	chopped, 3 oz	5
●	veal, cooked, 3 oz	3
	veal, pan-fried, 3 oz	3
	Liver with onions	
	3 oz	3

○ No Count	SmartPoints® value
Lo mein	
beef, 8 ½ oz	11
chicken, 9 oz	10
pork, 8 ¾ oz	10
shrimp, 8 ¾ oz	10
vegetable, 8 oz	9
Lobster Cantonese	
7 ¾ oz	9
Lomi lomi salmon	
3 ¾ oz	2
Luncheon meat	
3 g fat or less per oz (lean), 2 oz	1
4 g fat or more per oz (regular), 2 oz	7
barbecue loaf, pork or beef, 1 slice (¾ oz)	1
beef, jellied, 2 oz	1
beef, thin sliced, 2 oz	1
bratwurst, 2 oz	6
braunschweiger, 2 oz	7
chicken roll, 2 oz	1
Dutch loaf, pork or beef, 2 oz	5
○ fat-free, 3 oz	1
ham and cheese, loaf or roll, 2 oz	4
ham, 11% fat, sliced, regular, 2 oz	2
ham, 96% fat-free, prepackaged, water added, 2 oz	1
ham, honey, lean, deli-sliced, 2 oz	2
light, canned, 3 oz	5
liver cheese (leberkase), 2 oz	6
liverwurst, 2 oz	6
mother's loaf, pork, 2 oz	5
olive loaf, 2 oz	4
peppered loaf, 2 oz	2
pickle and pimiento loaf, 2 oz	5
picnic loaf, 2 oz	4
pork, canned, 2 oz	7
roast beef, deli-style, 2 oz	2
roast beef, deli-style, prepackaged, sliced, 1 piece (⅓ oz)	0

"We Like This!" item

○ No Count	SmartPoints® value
turkey breast, 2 oz	1
○ turkey breast, low-sodium, deli-type, 2 oz	1
turkey ham, 2 oz	2

M

Macadamia nuts	
dry-roasted, ¼ cup	8
shelled, ¼ cup	8
Macaroni and cheese	
9 ¾ oz	14
Bahamian, 9 ¾ oz	13
family-style, restaurant-type, 7 ½ oz	11
frozen, 7 ½ oz	12
in a cup, 2 oz	8
Macaroni and cheese mix	
prepared, 6 ¼ oz	13
Macchiato	
caramel, made with fat-free milk, 8 fl oz	6
caramel, made with reduced-fat (2% milk), 8 fl oz	7
Malai kofta (vegetable balls in cream sauce)	
7 oz	12
Malanga	
○ cooked, ½ cup	3
Malted milk-flavor mix	
chocolate, added nutrients, powder, 2 Tbsp	8
chocolate, added nutrients, powder, prepared with whole milk, 8 fl oz	11
natural, added nutrients, powder, 2 Tbsp	2
Manapua with char shiu filling	
1 (3 ¼ oz)	6
Mandarin orange	
○ canned, in juice, drained, 1 cup	4
canned, in light syrup, ½ cup	5

No Count	SmartPoints® value
Mango	
dried, ¼ cup	5
Manicotti	
cheese, with tomato sauce, frozen, 10 oz	14
cheese, without sauce, frozen, 5 ½ oz	9
with tomato sauce, 12 oz	15
Margarine	
fat-free, 1 Tbsp	0
reduced-calorie, 1 Tbsp	3
regular, 1 Tbsp	4
soft, 1 Tbsp	4
Margarine-butter blend	
1 Tbsp	4
Marmalade	
orange, 1 Tbsp	3
orange, low-sugar, 1 Tbsp	1
Marsala, chicken	
10 ¾ oz	20
Marsala, veal	
10 ½ oz	25
Marshmallow	
1 (¼ oz)	1
mini, 10 (¼ oz)	1
Marshmallow crème	
store-bought, 1 Tbsp	1
Marzipan	
1 Tbsp	3
Masala	
beef, 12 ⅓ oz	9
chana, 8 oz	10
goat, 8 ½ oz	4
lamb, 8 ½ oz	5
Masala dosa	
with filling, 8 oz	16
without filling, 1 (5 ⅓ oz)	14
Matzo	
1 board (1 oz)	3
egg, 1 oz	3

No Count	SmartPoints® value
egg and onion, 1 oz	3
plain, 1 oz	3
whole-wheat, 1 oz	3
Matzo brei	
3 oz	7
Matzo cake meal	
¼ cup	3
Matzo farfel	
store-bought, ½ oz	2
Matzo meal	
¼ cup	3
Mayonnaise	
fat-free, 1 Tbsp	1
light, 1 Tbsp	2
regular, 1 Tbsp	3
Meal replacement/supplement bar for weight loss	
1 (1 oz)	6
Meal replacement/supplement drink	
8 fl oz	10
Meal replacement/supplement drink for weight loss	
prepared from powder using fat-free milk, or canned, 8 fl oz	8
Meat loaf	
4 oz	8
vegetarian, 3 oz	4
Meatballs	
with sauce, 10 oz	15
without sauce, 1 (1 ¾ oz)	6
without sauce, frozen, 3 oz	8
Meatballs, Swedish	
4 oz	12
with noodles, frozen, 6 ½ oz	10
Melba toast	
plain, 1 oz	3
rye or pumpernickel, 1 oz	3
wheat, 1 oz	3
Menudo	
10 oz	7

○ No Count	SmartPoints® value
Milk	
○ buttermilk, fat-free, 8 fl oz	3
buttermilk, low-fat (1%), 8 fl oz	4
buttermilk, reduced-fat (2%), 8 fl oz	6
buttermilk, whole, 8 fl oz	7
dry, nonfat, instant, ¼ cup	2
dry, nonfat, instant, 1 cup	9
evaporated, fat-free, 8 fl oz	8
evaporated, low-fat, 8 fl oz	9
evaporated, whole, 8 fl oz	15
○ fat-free, 8 fl oz	3
flavored, reduced-fat, ready-to-drink, 8 fl oz	9
goat, 1 8 fl oz	7
low-fat or light (1%), 8 fl oz	4
oat, any flavor, 8 fl oz	6
reduced-fat (2%), 8 fl oz	5
whole, 8 fl oz	7
Milk shake	
chocolate, thick, 8 fl oz	14
vanilla, thick, 8 fl oz	13
Milk, sweetened condensed	
2 Tbsp	7
fat-free, 2 Tbsp	6
Millet	
○ cooked, 1 cup	6
○ uncooked, 2 oz	6
Miso	
1 Tbsp	1
Miso paste	
1 Tbsp	1
Mocha powder	
decaffeinated, with low-calorie sweetener, 1 Tbsp	4
with low-calorie sweetener, 1 Tbsp	5
Mochi	
1 (1 ¼ oz)	4

"We Like This!" item

○ No Count	SmartPoints® value
Molasses	
1 Tbsp	4
blackstrap, 1 Tbsp	3
light, 1 Tbsp	3
Mongolian beef	
4 ⅓ oz	9
Moo goo gai pan	
10 oz	7
Moo shoo	
chicken, 4 ¾ oz	9
pork, 4 ¾ oz	9
tofu, 5 ¼ oz	10
Moussaka	
8 ⅓ oz	16
Mozzarella, breaded	
mozzarella, breaded, frozen, prepared without fat, 1 oz	3
Mozzarella, fried	
1 piece (1 ¾ oz)	6
Muffin	
any type other than those listed here, 1 (3 ¾ oz)	10
any type, fast food, 4 ¼ oz	14
any type, mini, store-bought, 1 (1 oz)	5
any type, store-bought, 1 (4 oz)	17
banana-walnut, restaurant-type, 1 (5 oz)	23
blueberry, commercially prepared, 1 (2 oz)	5
blueberry, reduced-fat, restaurant-type, 1 (5 oz)	17
blueberry, toaster-type, 1 (1 oz)	3
chocolate chip, restaurant-type, 1 (5 oz)	22
corn, commercially prepared, 1 (2 ⅓ oz)	7
corn, restaurant-type, 1 (5 oz)	16
corn, toaster-type, 1 (1 oz)	4
cranberry-orange, restaurant-type, 1 (5 oz)	19

○ No Count	SmartPoints® value
fat-free, store-bought, 1 (2 oz)	5
oat bran, 1 (2 oz)	5
orange, 1 (2 oz)	9
pumpkin, restaurant-type, 1 (5 oz)	18
wheat bran, toaster-type, with raisins, 1 (1⅓ oz)	4
Muffin mix	
blueberry, 1 oz	5
corn, prepared, 1 (1¾ oz)	6
Mun doo	
fried, 1 (1⅔ oz)	1
steamed, 1 (1½ oz)	1
Mung dal	
9⅓ oz	8
Mushrooms	
breaded, prepared without fat, 7 (3 oz)	4
marinated, ½ cup	3
○ porcini, dried, ¼ oz	1
stuffed, 4 (2¾ oz)	4
Mussels Marinière	
4¼ oz	7
Mustard	
dijon, 1 Tbsp	0
honey, 1 Tbsp	2
honey-dijon, 1 Tbsp	1
regular, 1 Tbsp	0
Mutter paneer	
9⅓ oz	15

N

Nachos	
beef, 8⅔ oz	19
cheese, 3 oz	12
cheese and bean, 6½ oz	14
chicken, 8½ oz	16
with cheese sauce, 2¾ oz	8
with cheese, fast food, 2¾ oz	9

○ No Count	SmartPoints® value
Natto	
1 cup	10
Nectar	
any type, 8 fl oz	8
Noodles	
cellophane, cooked, 1 cup	6
cellophone, uncooked, 2 oz	6
egg, cooked, 1 cup	6
egg, no yolk, uncooked, 2 oz	6
egg, spinach, cooked, 1 cup	6
egg, spinach, dry, 2 oz	6
egg, uncooked, 2 oz	6
fried, 8 oz	8
○ Japanese, soba (100% buckwheat), dry, 2 oz	6
Japanese, soba, cooked, 1 cup	3
Japanese, soba, uncooked, 2 oz	5
Japanese, somen, cooked, 1 cup	6
Japanese, somen, dry, 2 oz	6
lasagna, dry, 2½ (2 oz)	6
lasagna, no cook, 2 oz	6
Oriental (bean thread), cooked, 1 cup	7
potato (dang myeon), 2 oz	6
ramen, fresh, uncooked, 1½ oz	6
rice, cooked, 1 cup	5
rice, dry, 2 oz	6
rice, packaged, 2 oz	6
udon, uncooked, 2 oz	6
○ whole-wheat, egg, uncooked, 2 oz	5
Noodles and sauce mix	
prepared, 4¼ oz	5
Noodles and sauce, soba	
8 oz	13
Nuts, mixed	
dry-roasted, ¼ cup	6
oil-roasted, ¼ cup	7
shelled, ¼ cup	6

No Count	SmartPoints® value

O

Oil	
canola, 1 Tbsp	4
corn, 1 Tbsp	4
flaxseed, 1 Tbsp	4
olive, 1 Tbsp	4
peanut, 1 Tbsp	4
safflower, 1 Tbsp	4
sesame, 1 Tbsp	4
sunflower, 1 Tbsp	4
vegetable, 1 Tbsp	4
Okra	
breaded, frozen, prepared without fat, 3 oz	3
fried, 7 oz	11
Olives	
black, ripe, canned, jumbo, 4 (1 oz)	1
black, ripe, canned, large, 4 (1¼ oz)	1
black, ripe, canned, small, 6 (⅔ oz)	1
black, ripe, canned, super-colossal, 4 (2 oz)	2
green, pickled, canned or bottled, 6 (½ oz)	1
oil-cured, 1 oz	4
pimiento-stuffed, 4 (¾ oz)	1
Omelet	
cheese, 4⅓ oz	11
ham and cheese, 5⅓ oz	12
herb or plain, 3⅔ oz	8
vegetable, 12¾ oz	8
Onion flakes	
dehydrated, 1 Tbsp	1
Onion rings	
breaded, frozen, prepared without fat, 2½ oz	10
breaded, frozen, unprepared, 3 oz	8
fast food, 1 (¼ oz)	1
fried, 3 oz	8
Onion, blooming	
5 oz	6
Orange-ginger beef	
1 cup	18
Osso bucco	
10⅓ oz	12
Oysters	
battered or breaded and fried, fast food, 5 oz	11
fried, 5¼ oz	9
Oysters Rockefeller	
2 oz	4

P

Pad si-iew (stir-fried beef with noodles)	
7⅓ oz	8
Pad Thai (rice noodles with chicken and shrimp)	
8 oz	12
Pad Thai, chicken	
restaurant-type, 1¼ cups	14
Paella	
8½ oz	9
Pajun (Korean green onion and shrimp pancake)	
7 oz	9
Pakora, vegetable	
1 (1¾ oz)	4
Palak paneer	
11 oz	15
Palak vada (vegetable dumpling)	
fried, 1 (2½ oz)	6
steamed, 1 (2¼ oz)	3
Panang curry with beef	
11 oz	19
Panang curry with chicken	
11 oz	18
Pancake	
any type, from mix (4"), 1 (1⅓ oz)	2
any type, frozen, 1 (1⅓ oz)	3

"We Like This!" item

No Count		SmartPoints® value
	buckwheat, dry mix, incomplete, ⅓ cup	4
	buttermilk, restaurant-type, with butter and syrup, 2 (6 oz)	17
	Chinese, 1 (1 oz)	2
	mini, frozen, without syrup, 6 (2⅓ oz)	5
	prepared from scratch, 1 (2 oz)	4
	with butter and syrup, fast food, 2 (8⅓ oz)	17
	Pancetta	
	1 oz	4
	Pancit canton (sautéed egg noodles)	
	5¼ oz	7
	Panettone	
	1 piece (1⅔ oz)	10
	Panini	
	chicken, 8 oz	13
	ham and cheese, 7⅔ oz	15
	vegetable, 13⅓ oz	12
	Paprikash	
	9⅓ oz	10
	Parfait, fruit and yogurt	
	restaurant-type, 8⅔ oz	10
	Parsnips	
O	cooked, canned, ½ cup	2
O	uncooked, ½ cup	2
	Pasta	
	brown rice, cooked, 1 cup	6
O	brown rice, dry, 2 oz	6
	cooked, 1 cup	5
	corn, cooked, 1 cup	5
	corn, dry, 2 oz	6
	fresh-refrigerated, plain, as purchased, 3 oz	6
	fresh-refrigerated, plain, cooked, 1 cup	8
	fresh-refrigerated, spinach, as purchased, 3 oz	7
	fresh-refrigerated, spinach, cooked, 1 cup	8

No Count		SmartPoints® value
	homemade, made with egg, cooked, 1 cup	8
	homemade, made without egg, cooked, 1 cup	8
	uncooked, 2 oz	6
O	whole-wheat, cooked, 1 cup	5
O	whole-wheat, uncooked, 2 oz	5
	Pasta e fagioli	
	1 cup	7
	Pasta primavera	
	with cream sauce, 11¾ oz	19
	with marinara sauce, 10 oz	7
	Pasta shells, stuffed with ricotta cheese	
	without sauce, frozen, 5⅓ oz	6
	Pasta with garlic and oil	
	5¾ oz	9
	Pastelitos de carne (Cuban meat pastry)	
	1 (2½ oz)	13
	Pastitsio	
	10⅓ oz	19
	Pastrami	
	beef, 3 oz	3
O	beef, 98% fat-free, 2 oz	1
	made from turkey, 2 oz	2
	Pâté	
	liver, 3 oz	5
	chicken liver, canned, 1 Tbsp	1
	fish, store-bought, 2 oz	4
	meat, store-bought, 1 Tbsp	2
	Pâté de foie gras	
	duck liver, canned, 1 Tbsp	2
	goose liver, smoked, 1 Tbsp	2
	Peach	
	canned, extra light syrup, ½ cup	3
	canned, heavy syrup pack, ½ cup	6
	canned, light syrup pack, ½ cup	4
	dried, halves, uncooked, ¼ cup	5
	dried, stewed, with added sugar, ½ cup	8

Peach (cont'd)

○ No Count	SmartPoints® value
dried, stewed, without added sugar, ¼ cup	3
spiced, canned, heavy syrup pack, ½ cup	5
with sugar, frozen, 1 cup	14
Peanut butter	
chunky, 2 Tbsp	6
creamy, 2 Tbsp	6
creamy, reduced-fat, 2 Tbsp	6
creamy, with omega-3, 2 Tbsp	6
reduced-sodium, 2 Tbsp	6
Peanut butter powder	
2 Tbsp	1
chocolate, 2 Tbsp	1
Peanuts	
¼ cup	6
chocolate-covered, 1	1
cooked, shelled, ¼ cup	4
dry-roasted, ¼ cup	7
heat peanuts, Cajun, ¼ cup	5
honey, reduced-fat, ¼ cup	3
oil-roasted, ¼ cup	6
raw, ¼ cup	6
Pears	
canned, extra light syrup pack, ½ cup	2
canned, heavy syrup pack, ½ cup	5
canned, light syrup pack, ½ cup	4
dried, uncooked, ¼ cup	7
Peas and rice	
Bahamian-style, 7 oz	10
Jamaican, 7¾ oz	12
Peas, black-eyed	
○ canned, ½ cup	3
○ fresh, cooked, ½ cup	3
○ fresh, raw, ¼ cup	1
Peas, green	
○ baby, frozen, ½ cup	2
○ canned, drained solids, ½ cup	2

○ No Count	SmartPoints® value
○ cooked, ½ cup	2
○ frozen, cooked, ½ cup	2
○ frozen, unprepared, ½ cup	2
○ raw, ½ cup	2
Peas, pigeon	
○ cooked, ½ cup	3
Peas, split	
○ cooked, ½ cup	3
○ dry, ¼ cup	5
Pecans	
chopped, ¼ cup	6
dry-roasted, ¼ cup	6
halves, ¼ cup	6
oil-roasted, ¼ cup	6
Peking duck	
5½ oz	13
Penne a la vodka	
10¾ oz	12
Pepper steak	
7 oz	16
Chinese, 3 oz	3
Pepper, chipotle	
in adobo sauce, canned, ½ cup	3
Pepperoni	
2 oz	10
turkey, 1 oz	2
Peppers, stuffed	
with beef and rice, 8 oz	11
with beef, in tomato sauce, frozen, 7 oz	7
Persimmon	
Japanese, dried, 1 (1¼ oz)	3
Pesarattu	
6¼ oz	8
Pesto	
sun-dried tomato, 2 Tbsp	5
Pheasant	
○ breast, raw, without skin and bone, 4 oz	2
cooked, 3 oz	4

"We Like This!" item

● No Count	SmartPoints® value
Picadillo	
2 Tbsp	2
Pickle	
dill, ¼ cup	0
dill, low-sodium, ¼ cup	0
sour, ¼ cup	0
sour, low-sodium, ¼ cup	0
sweet, ¼ cup	3
Pico de gallo	
● fat-free	0
Pie crust	
chocolate, ¾ oz	4
frozen, ready-to-bake, ¾ oz	3
graham cracker, 1⅓ oz	9
graham cracker, reduced-fat, ¾ oz	4
Pie filling	
fruit, canned, ¼ cup	3
fruit, light, canned, ¼ cup	2
Pie mix	
pumpkin, canned, ¼ cup	4
Pie, dessert	
apple, commercially prepared, 1 slice (4½ oz)	12
blueberry, commercially prepared, 1 slice (4 oz)	10
cherry, commercially prepared, 1 slice (4 oz)	12
chocolate crème, commercially prepared, 1 slice (3½ oz)	17
coconut cream, commercially prepared, ⅛ pie (1¾ oz)	6
coconut custard, 1 slice (6 oz)	17
coconut custard, commercially prepared, 1 slice (3¾ oz)	12
cream, with fruit, 1 slice (7 oz)	17
cream, with or without fruit, frozen, 1 slice (4¾ oz)	15
cream, without fruit, 1 slice (6 oz)	17
egg custard, commercially prepared, 1 slice (3¾ oz)	8

● No Count	SmartPoints® value
fried, fruit, 1 (4½ oz)	16
fruit, any type, frozen, 1 slice (4½ oz)	13
fruit, fast food, 1 slice (3¾ oz)	13
fruit, one-crust, 1 slice (5 oz)	13
fruit, two-crust, 1 slice (5¾ oz)	18
individual, 1 (4½ oz)	16
key lime, 1 slice (5⅓ oz)	25
key lime, commercially prepared, 1 slice (4½ oz)	22
lemon meringue, commercially prepared, 1 slice (4 oz)	13
meringue, 1 slice (6⅓ oz)	21
peach, 1 slice (4 oz)	10
pecan, 1 slice (4⅓ oz)	21
pecan, commercially prepared, 1 slice (4 oz)	21
pecan, frozen, 1 slice (4½ oz)	23
pumpkin, 1 slice (6⅔ oz)	17
pumpkin, commercially prepared, 1 slice (4¾ oz)	13
pumpkin, frozen, 1 slice (5 oz)	13
rhubarb, 1 slice (6 oz)	21
Pie, dessert, prepared from mix	
banana cream, no-bake type, 1 slice (3¼ oz)	10
chocolate mousse, no-bake type, 1 slice (3⅓ oz)	11
coconut cream, no-bake type, 1 slice (3⅓ oz)	11
Pierogies	
cabbage, 2½ oz	9
cheese, 2½ oz	10
meat, 2½ oz	10
potato, 2½ oz	10
potato and cheese or onion, low-fat, frozen, 4½ oz	5
potato and cheese, frozen, 4 oz	5
Pignolias (pine nuts)	
¼ cup	6

◎ No Count	SmartPoints® value
Pineapple	
canned, in heavy syrup, ½ cup	6
canned, in juice, ½ cup	4
canned, in light syrup, ½ cup	4
chunks, frozen, sweetened, 1 cup	13
dried, rings, 1 oz	4
Pistachio nuts	
dry-roasted, without shells, ¼ cup	5
without shells, ¼ cup	5
Pita	
pocketless, 1 (2 oz)	5
white, 1 (1 oz)	2
whole-wheat, 1 (1 oz)	2
Pizza	
14", cheese and pepperoni, regular crust, restaurant-type, 1 slice (4 oz)	10
14", cheese and pepperoni, thick crust, restaurant-type, 1 slice (4 ¼ oz)	11
14", cheese and pepperoni, thin crust, restaurant-type, 1 slice (2 ¾ oz)	9
14", cheese and sausage, regular crust, restaurant-type, 1 slice (4 oz)	11
14", cheese and sausage, thick crust, restaurant-type, 1 slice (4 ½ oz)	12
14", cheese and sausage, thin crust, restaurant-type, 1 slice (3 oz)	9
14", cheese, meat, and vegetable, regular crust, restaurant-type, 1 slice (4 ¾ oz)	11
14", cheese, regular crust, restaurant-type, 1 slice (3 ¾ oz)	9
14", cheese, stuffed crust, restaurant-type, 1 slice (4 oz)	11
14", cheese, thick crust, restaurant-type, 1 slice (4 oz)	10
14", cheese, thin crust, restaurant-type, 1 slice (2 ¾ oz)	8

"We Like This!" item

◎ No Count	SmartPoints® value
Canadian style bacon, frozen, 5 oz	10
one-meat topping, deep-dish, restaurant-type, 4 oz	10
one-meat topping, thin crust, restaurant-type, 2 ¾ oz	6
pepperoni, frozen, 5 ¼ oz	13
Sicilian, cheese, small, 3 oz	6
single serving, cheese, frozen, 6 ¾ oz	16
single serving, pepperoni, frozen, 7 oz	14
single serving, sausage, frozen, 7 oz	13
single serving, supreme, frozen, 7 ⅓ oz	15
supreme, frozen, 5 oz	12
vegetable, frozen, 5 oz	9
Pizza bagel	
mini, any type, 3 oz	6
Pizza crust dough	
refrigerated, frozen or ready-made, 1 oz	3
whole-wheat (refrigerated), ⅛ pie (2 oz)	3
Pizza crust dough mix	
¼ cup	5
Pizza pieces	
frozen, prepared without fat, 3 oz	7
Plantain	
baked or boiled, 1 cup	8
fried, ½ cup	4
raw, 1 medium (6 ⅓ oz)	10
Plátanos maduros (fried sweet plantains)	
1 ¾ oz	4
Plum	
canned, purple, heavy syrup pack, 1 (1 ⅔ oz)	2
canned, purple, juice pack, 1 (1 ⅔ oz)	2
canned, purple, light syrup pack, 1 (1 ⅔ oz)	2

◯ No Count	SmartPoints® value
Poi	
◯ ½ cup	4
Polenta	
◯ cooked, ½ cup	4
◯ ready-to-eat, in tube, 1 oz	1
Polenta mix	
◯ instant, dry, ¼ cup	4
Popcorn	
buttered, popped, 2 cups	5
butter-flavored, popped, 1 cup	1
caramel-coated, with peanuts, 2 cups	15
caramel-coated, without peanuts, 1 cup	12
cheese-flavored, popped, 1 cup	2
kettle, popped, 2 cups	5
◯ kettle, reduced-fat (94% fat-free), popped, 5 cups	3
light, butter-flavored, popped, 3 cups	3
light, caramel-coated, popped, 1 cup	6
light, cheese-flavored, popped, 2 cups	4
◯ light, microwave-popped, 3 cups	2
light, plain, popped, 2 cups	2
microwave, regular flavor, oil-popped, 1 cup	2
movie, without butter, 3 cups	5
◯ plain, air-popped, 2 cups	2
◯ plain, microwave-popped, 2 cups	3
plain, oil-popped, 2 cups	3
plain, packaged, popped, 2 cups	3
◯ reduced-fat (94% fat-free), microwave-popped, 2 cups	2
◯ white, air-popped, 2 cups	2
white, oil-popped, 1 cup	2
Popover	
1 (1⅔ oz)	3

◯ No Count	SmartPoints® value
Pork	
backribs, cooked, barbecued, 1 rib (3¼ oz)	10
backribs, lean and fat, cooked, 1 rib (2⅔ oz)	6
barbecue, 8½ oz	9
center loin, lean and fat, cooked, 3 oz	4
center loin, lean and fat, raw, 4 oz	6
◯ center loin, lean only, cooked, 3 oz	3
◯ center loin, lean only, raw, 4 oz	3
chop, center loin, raw, 4 oz	4
◯ chop, lean, without bone, cooked, 3 oz	3
◯ chop, lean, without bone, trimmed, raw, 4 oz	3
chop, loin, center rib, bone-in, lean, cooked, 3 oz	4
chop, loin, center rib, boneless, lean, cooked, 3 oz	4
◯ chop, sirloin, bone-in, lean, cooked, 3 oz	2
◯ chop, top loin, boneless, lean, cooked, 1 (5 oz)	5
country-style ribs, cooked, 3 oz	6
country-style ribs, loin, lean, bone-in, cooked, 5 oz	7
country-style ribs, loin, lean, boneless, cooked, 5 oz	7
leg, cooked, 3 oz	6
leg, trimmed, cooked, 3 oz	4
loin, center rib, lean and fat, cooked, 3 oz	6
loin, lean and fat, cooked, 3 oz	5
loin, lean and fat, raw, 4 oz	5
◯ loin, lean only, raw, 4 oz	4
loin, trimmed, cooked, 3 oz	4
roast, loin, center rib, bone-in, lean, cooked, 3 oz	4

Pork (cont'd)

○ No Count	Food	SmartPoints® value
	roast, loin, center rib, boneless, lean, cooked, 3 oz	4
	roast, sirloin, bone-in, lean, cooked, 3 oz	4
○	roast, sirloin, boneless, lean, cooked, 3 oz	3
	roast, top loin, boneless, untrimmed, raw, 3 oz	3
	shoulder, lean and fat, cooked, 3 oz	6
	shoulder, lean and fat, raw, 4 oz	7
	shoulder, lean only, cooked, 3 oz	5
	shoulder, lean only, raw, 4 oz	4
○	shoulder, petite tender, boneless untrimmed, raw, 1 piece (3 ¾ oz)	2
	sirloin, cooked, 3 oz	5
	sirloin, lean and fat, raw, 4 oz	4
○	sirloin, lean only, cooked, 3 oz	2
○	sirloin, lean only, raw, 4 oz	2
○	tenderloin, cooked, 3 oz	2
○	tenderloin, lean only, cooked, 3 oz	2
○	tenderloin, lean only, raw, 4 oz	2
○	tenderloin, raw, 4 oz	2
○	top loin, lean only, cooked, 3 oz	3
○	top loin, lean only, raw, 4 oz	2
	top loin, lean, untrimmed, cooked, 3 oz	3
	Pork and beans	
	canned, 4 ½ oz	4
	Pork and broccoli	
	6 ½ oz	3
	Pork in barbecue sauce	
	frozen, 2 oz	4
	Pork rinds/skins	
	barbecue-flavor, 1 oz	4
	plain, 1 oz	4
	Pork, ground	
	84% lean/16% fat, cooked, 3 oz	7
	84% lean/16% fat, raw, 4 oz	7

○ No Count	Food	SmartPoints® value
○	96% lean/4% fat, cooked, 3 oz	2
○	96% lean/4% fat, raw, 4 oz	2
	cooked, 3 oz	7
	raw, 4 oz	10
	Portuguese sweet bread	
	1 slice (3 oz)	10
	Pot pie	
	beef, chicken, or turkey, frozen, 7 oz	15
	chicken, homemade, 8 ½ oz	14
	Pot sticker (filled wontons)	
	pork or vegetable, frozen, 1 ½ oz	3
	vegetarian, fried, 3 oz	4
	vegetarian, steamed, 3 oz	4
	Potato	
○	baby, cooked, 1 (5 oz)	4
○	baby, uncooked, ½ cup	2
○	bliss, cooked, 6 oz	5
○	bliss, uncooked, ½ cup	2
○	boiled, ½ cup	2
○	canned, drained, ½ cup	2
○	new, cooked, 6 ½ oz	5
○	new, uncooked, ½ cup	2
○	red, cooked, ½ cup	2
○	red, uncooked, 1 medium (7 ⅔ oz)	4
	roasted, frozen, uncooked, 3 oz	3
○	roasted, with 1 tsp olive oil, ¾ cup	3
○	russet, baked, with or without skin, 1 large (10 ⅔ oz)	8
○	russet, uncooked, with or without skin, 1 oz	1
	shoestring, canned, ½ cup	5
○	uncooked, ½ cup	2
○	white, cooked, ½ cup	2
○	white, whole, uncooked, ½ cup	2
○	whole new, canned, drained, ½ cup	2
○	whole new, canned, with liquid, ½ cup	2

"We Like This!" item (shaded rows)

No Count	Food	SmartPoints® value
○	whole, frozen, uncooked, ½ cup	2
○	Yukon gold, uncooked, ½ cup	2
	Potato flakes	
	dehydrated, prepared, mashed, whole milk and butter added, ½ cup	4
	dry, ¼ cup	2
	Potato mix	
	flavored, prepared, ½ cup	4
	Potato pancake	
	3 ⅓ oz	3
	frozen, 2 oz	3
	Potato pancake mix	
	2 oz	6
	Potato puffs (appetizer pastry)	
	frozen, 1 (1 oz)	2
	frozen, prepared, 1 (⅓ oz)	1
	Potato skins	
	"loaded," frozen, 2 (4 oz)	8
○	frozen, uncooked, 1 ⅓ oz	1
	with cheese, bacon, and sour cream, 1 (3 ½ oz)	7
	Potato sticks	
	1 oz	5
	Potato, baked	
○	plain, 1 medium (6 oz)	5
	stuffed with bacon and cheese, 9 ¾ oz	17
	stuffed with vegetables and cheese, 13 ½ oz	14
	topped with cheese sauce and broccoli, fast food, 12 oz	15
	with cheese sauce and bacon, fast food, 10 ⅔ oz	16
	with cheese sauce and chili, fast food, 14 oz	17
	with cheese sauce, fast food, 10 ½ oz	17
	with sour cream and chives, fast food, 10 ¾ oz	15
	with vegetables and cheese, fast food, 13 ⅓ oz	14

No Count	Food	SmartPoints® value
	Potato, home-fried	
	5 ¾ oz	7
	Potato, mashed	
	fast food, 2 ¾ oz	2
	garlic, 5 oz	7
	home-prepared with whole milk added, 1 cup	5
	store-bought, refrigerated or frozen, 3 ¾ oz	4
	Potato, stuffed	
	stuffed with cheese, 5 ½ oz	7
	stuffed with sour cream and chives, 5 ½ oz	6
	Potato, sweet	
○	baked, mashed, ½ cup	4
	candied, ½ cup	8
	canned, in syrup, ½ cup	5
	canned, in syrup, drained, ½ cup	4
○	canned, mashed, 9 oz	9
○	canned, vacuum-pack, ½ cup	4
○	cooked, ½ cup	3
○	cooked, mashed, ½ cup	6
	French fries, frozen, unprepared, 3 oz	6
○	frozen, cooked, ½ cup	4
○	frozen, unprepared, ½ cup	2
○	uncooked, ½ cup	2
	Potatoes au gratin	
	dry mix, prepared with water, whole milk and butter, 5 oz	5
	dry mix, unprepared, 1 ¾ oz	5
	Potatoes O'Brien	
	frozen, prepared without fat, 4 ⅓ oz	3
	home-prepared, ½ cup	2
	Potatoes, scalloped	
	5 ¾ oz	6
	dry mix, prepared with water, whole milk and butter, ½ cup	4
	Poutine	
	12 oz	23

No Count	SmartPoints® value
Pozole (pork and hominy soup)	
1 cup	5
Preserves	
dietetic, any flavor, 1 Tbsp	1
fruit, 1 Tbsp	3
preserves, low-sugar, 1 Tbsp	1
Pretzel	
1 oz	3
Bavarian, 1 oz	3
chocolate-covered, 1 oz	6
hard, chocolate-coated, 1 oz	6
hard, plain, 1 oz	3
Philadelphia (soft), 1 oz	2
rods, 1 oz	3
soft, 1 oz	3
soft, 1 large (5 oz)	14
thins, plain, 1 oz	3
twists, 1 oz	3
whole-wheat, 1 oz	3
yogurt-covered, 1 oz	6
Profiterole	
1 (1½ oz)	5
Prosciutto	
2 oz	6
Protein powder	
1 Tbsp	1
Prunes	
¼ cup	5
canned, heavy syrup pack, ½ cup	7
dried, stewed, with added sugar, ½ cup	9
dried, stewed, without added sugar, ½ cup	8
Pubhouse battered halibut	
3½ oz	4
Pudding	
any flavor other than those listed here, ½ cup	7
banana, ½ cup	4

"We Like This!" item

No Count	SmartPoints® value
chocolate, prepared with fat-free milk, ½ cup	7
chocolate, ready-to-eat, 1 oz	2
lemon, ready-to-eat, ½ cup	4
plum, with 1 Tbsp sauce, ½ cup	20
ready-made, reduced-calorie, ½ cup	5
tapioca, fat-free, ready-to-eat, 1 container (4 oz)	5
vanilla, fat-free, ready-to-eat, 3½ oz	4
vanilla, prepared with fat-free milk, ½ cup	8
vanilla, ready-to-eat, ½ cup	3
Pudding mix	
banana, fat-free, sugar-free, instant, ¼ package (⅓ oz)	1
banana, instant, ¼ package (¾ oz)	5
banana, regular, ¼ package (¾ oz)	4
butterscotch, fat-free, ¼ package (¾ oz)	2
butterscotch, fat-free, sugar-free, instant, ¼ package (⅓ oz)	1
chocolate, fat-free, instant, ¼ package (½ oz)	1
chocolate, fat-free, sugar-free instant, ¼ package (⅓ oz)	1
chocolate, instant, ¼ package (1 oz)	5
chocolate, regular, ¼ package (¾ oz)	5
coconut cream, instant, ¼ package (¾ oz)	5
lemon, instant, ¼ package (¾ oz)	6
lemon, regular, ¼ package (¾ oz)	4
vanilla, fat-free, ¼ package (¾ oz)	2
vanilla, fat-free, sugar-free, instant, ¼ package (¼ oz)	1
vanilla, instant, ¼ package (¾ oz)	6
vanilla, regular, ¼ package (¾ oz)	5

No Count		SmartPoints® value
	Pudding, prepared from dry mix	
	any flavor, from fat-free, sugar-free mix, prepared with fat-free milk, ½ cup	3
	any flavor, from regular mix, prepared with fat-free milk, ½ cup	7
	banana, instant, prepared with whole milk, ½ cup	7
	banana, regular, prepared with whole milk, ½ cup	8
	chocolate, fat-free, sugar-free, instant, prepared with fat-free milk, ½ cup	3
	chocolate, regular, prepared with whole milk, ½ cup	7
	coconut cream, instant, prepared with whole milk, ½ cup	9
	coconut cream, regular, prepared with whole milk, ½ cup	8
	lemon, instant, prepared with whole milk, ½ cup	8
	lemon, regular, prepared with sugar, egg yolk and water, ½ cup	7
	puddings, vanilla, instant, prepared with whole milk, ½ cup	8
	vanilla, regular, prepared with whole milk, ½ cup	8
	Puff pastry	
	frozen, ready-to-bake, 1 shell (1⅔ oz)	9
	Puff pastry shell	
	frozen, baked, 1 (1½ oz)	7
	Pulled pork	
	in barbecue sauce, 9 oz	15
	Pumpkin bread	
	1 slice (3 oz)	13
	Pumpkin butter	
	1 Tbsp	2
	Pupusas	
	with beans, restaurant-type, 4½ oz	9
	with cheese, restaurant-type, 4 oz	10
	with pork, restaurant-type, 4⅓ oz	8

Q

No Count		SmartPoints® value
	Quesadilla	
	beef, 4 oz	9
	cheese, 2¼ oz	8
	chicken, 3¾ oz	8
	vegetable, 3⅔ oz	8
	with chicken, fast food, 6½ oz	17
	Quiche	
	appetizer, frozen, any type, ¾ oz	2
	Lorraine, 4½ oz	16
	vegetable, 6⅓ oz	14
	Quinoa	
○	cooked, 1 cup	6
○	uncooked, 2 oz	6

R

No Count		SmartPoints® value
	Rabbit	
○	domesticated, cooked, 3 oz	3
○	wild, cooked, 3 oz	2
	Raisins	
	¼ cup	6
	chocolate-covered, ¼ cup	10
	yogurt-covered, 2 oz	12
	Raita	
	1 cup	7
	Rajmah	
	1 cup	8
	Raspberries	
	canned, red, heavy syrup pack, ½ cup	7
	frozen, red, sweetened, 1 cup	14
	Ratatouille	
	8½ oz	3
	Ravioli	
	beef or chicken, without sauce, frozen, 4 oz	8
	beef, breaded, frozen, 4 oz	7
	beef, in meat sauce, canned, 9 oz	8
	cheese, breaded, frozen, 4 oz	10
	cheese, low-fat, 4 oz	6

No Count		SmartPoints® value
	cheese, with tomato sauce, entrée, frozen, uncooked, 1 cup	6
	cheese, without sauce, 9 oz	20
	cheese, without sauce, frozen, 4 oz	8
	cheese, without sauce, store-bought, 5 ¼ oz	10
	cheese-filled, canned, 8 ⅔ oz	7
	meat, with tomato sauce, 13 ⅓ oz	18
	meat, without sauce, 7 oz	16
	meat, without sauce, store-bought, 4 ¼ oz	9
	meat-filled, with tomato sauce or meat sauce, canned, 1 cup	9
	mushroom, without sauce, 4 ⅔ oz	9
	vegetable and cheese, without sauce, store-bought, 4 ¼ oz	8
	Red snapper Veracruz	
	11 ¾ oz	11
	Relish	
	¼ cup	4
	pickle, hot dog, ¼ cup	2
	pickle, sweet, ¼ cup	3
	Rhubarb	
	cooked, with sugar, ½ cup	8
	Rice	
	arborio rice, 2 oz	6
	basmati, uncooked, 2 oz	6
○	black, cooked, 1 cup	5
○	black, uncooked, 2 oz	6
○	brown, cooked, 1 cup	7
○	brown, instant, uncooked, 2 oz	6
○	brown, medium-grain, cooked, 1 cup	6
○	brown, medium-grain, uncooked, 2 oz	6
○	brown, quick-cooking, uncooked, 2 oz	6
○	brown, uncooked, 2 oz	6
	Chinese, white, steamed, restaurant-type, 1 cup	6
	jasmine, cooked, 1 cup	6
	jasmine, uncooked, 2 oz	6
	sushi, cooked, 3 oz	4
	white, cooked, 1 cup	6
	white, glutinous, cooked, 1 cup	5
	white, long-grain, instant, cooked, 1 cup	6
	white, long-grain, instant, uncooked, 2 oz	6
	white, medium-grain, cooked, 1 cup	7
	white, medium-grain, uncooked, 2 oz	6
	white, short-grain, cooked, 1 cup	7
	white, short-grain, uncooked, 2 oz	6
	white, uncooked, 2 oz	6
○	wild, cooked, 1 cup	5
○	wild, uncooked, 2 oz	5
	Rice and vermicelli mix	
	rice and vermicelli mix, beef flavor, prepared with margarine, 1 cup	9
	rice and vermicelli mix, beef flavor, unprepared, ⅓ cup	6
	rice and vermicelli mix, chicken flavor, prepared with margarine, 1 cup	10
	rice and vermicelli mix, chicken flavor, unprepared, ⅓ cup	6
	Rice bowl	
	with chicken, frozen, prepared, 12 oz	13
	Rice cakes	
	brown rice, buckwheat, 1 cake (⅓ oz)	1
	brown rice, multi-grain, 1 (⅓ oz)	1
	brown rice, plain, 1 cake (⅓ oz)	1
	brown rice, sesame seed, 1 (⅓ oz)	1
	cracker, 1 piece (¼ oz)	0
	mini, cheddar, 5 (½ oz)	2

"We Like This!" item

No Count		SmartPoints® value
	other than plain, 1 (½ oz)	1
	plain, 1 (⅓ oz)	1
	rye, 1 (⅓ oz)	1
	sesame seed, 1 (⅓ oz)	1
	Rice drink/rice beverage	
	chocolate, 8 fl oz	8
	fat-free, 8 fl oz	4
	plain, 8 fl oz	5
	unsweetened, 8 fl oz	5
	Rice mix	
	flavored, any type, prepared, 4 ¼ oz	5
	long-grain and wild rice, 2 oz	5
	Milan-style risotto, 2 oz	6
	Spanish, prepared with oil blend, 1 cup	8
	Spanish, unprepared, ½ cup	7
	white rice with pasta, prepared, 1 cup	7
	white rice with pasta, unprepared, 2 oz	6
	with black beans, prepared, 8 ⅔ oz	7
	with red beans, prepared, 8 ⅔ oz	7
	yellow, with seasoning, unprepared, 2 oz	6
	Rice pilaf	
	7 ⅓ oz	8
	Rice pilaf mix	
	2 oz	5
	Rice pudding	
	½ cup	7
	kheer, 8 oz	13
	ready-to-eat, ½ cup	8
	Rice pudding mix	
	¼ package (1 oz)	5
	prepared with whole milk, ½ cup	8
	Rice with pigeon peas (arroz con gandules)	
	8 oz	11
	Risotto	
	1 cup	15

No Count		SmartPoints® value
	Rocky mountain oysters	
	2 oz	13
	Rogan josh	
	8 ¾ oz	11
	Roll dough	
	crescent, reduced-fat, 1 piece (1 oz)	3
	Rolls	
	bollilo, 1 (3 ½ oz)	9
	crescent dinner, store-bought, 1 (1 oz)	4
	dinner, 1 (2 oz)	5
	dinner, egg, 1 (1 ¼ oz)	3
	dinner, oat bran, 1 (1 oz)	2
	dinner, rye, 1 (1 ½ oz)	3
	dinner, wheat, 1 (1 oz)	2
	dinner, whole-wheat, 1 (1 ½ oz)	4
	French, 1 (1 ⅓ oz)	3
	hard, 1 (2 oz)	5
	high fiber (3 grams or more dietary fiber per roll), 1 (2 oz)	5
	Kaiser, restaurant-type, 1 (2 oz)	5
○	light, 1 (1 ½ oz)	2
	potato, mini, 1 oz	2
	yeast, Parker House, 1 (1 oz)	3
	Ropa vieja	
	6 ½ oz	9
	Rotisserie chicken	
	barbecue, with skin, 3 oz	11
	Runza	
	1 (5 ½ oz)	11

S

No Count		SmartPoints® value
	Saag gosht	
	8 ½ oz	5
	Saag paneer	
	9 oz	9
	Saganaki	
	1 (2 ¾ oz)	10

No Count		SmartPoints® value
	Salad	
	beef, Thai, 11 oz	17
	Caesar, 6 oz	8
	Caesar chicken, grilled, restaurant-type, 6½ oz	9
	carrot and raisin, 4 oz	10
	chef's, fast food, 11½ oz	7
	chef's, with dressing, 8⅔ oz	11
	chef's, without dressing, 8⅔ oz	8
	chicken, grilled, southwestern, restaurant-type, 13⅓ oz	6
	chicken, grilled, without dressing, fast food, 12⅓ oz	5
	chicken, homemade, 3 oz	6
	chicken, Oriental, 10 oz	5
	chicken, restaurant-type, 3½ oz	7
	chicken, store-bought, 3½ oz	8
	chicken, Thai, 15½ oz	12
	chicken-macaroni, 6 oz	7
	cobb, without dressing, 12¾ oz	12
	conch, 5 oz	2
	egg, 4 oz	9
●	fruit (mixed fruits without added sugar)	0
	fruit, canned in juice, ½ cup	3
	fruit, canned, extra heavy syrup, ½ cup	7
	fruit, canned, heavy syrup, ½ cup	6
	fruit, canned, light syrup, ½ cup	4
	garden, restaurant-type, 6¼ oz	3
	grape and apple with yogurt and candied walnuts, 5¾ oz	8
	Greek, restaurant-type, 12¾ oz	13
	Greek, with dressing, 11½ oz	11
	Greek, without dressing, 10 oz	3
	green papaya, with pork and shrimp, 5 oz	2
●	green papaya, without meat, 8½ oz	0
	herring, store-bought, 2 oz	4
	lobster, 2⅔ oz	4

"We Like This!" item

No Count		SmartPoints® value
	macaroni, 3⅔ oz	8
	macaroni, store-bought, ½ cup	7
●	mixed greens	0
	Niçoise, without dressing, 16½ oz	8
	pasta, 3½ oz	5
	pasta, store-bought, 3¾ oz	3
	poke (Hawaiian fish salad), ahi, 3¼ oz	1
	poke (Hawaiian fish salad), tako, 3¼ oz	2
	potato, 3⅓ oz	4
	potato, German, 3¾ oz	4
	potato, homemade, ½ cup	6
	potato, hot, with ham, 8¾ oz	9
	potato, store-bought, 4 oz	4
	potato, with egg, ½ cup	7
	potato-macaroni, 4½ oz	12
	salmon, kippered, with mayonnaise, store-bought, 2 oz	7
	seafood, store-bought, 3½ oz	8
	seafood, Thai, 9⅓ oz	11
	seaweed, ½ cup	2
	shrimp, 2⅔ oz	4
●	side, without dressing, fast food	0
	spinach, with dressing, 8 oz	8
	taco, fast food, 7 oz	9
	taco, with chili con carne, fast food, 9⅓ oz	10
	taco, without shell and dressing, fast food, 14 oz	12
	three-bean, 5 oz	7
	three-bean, canned, without oil, 4½ oz	4
	tomato and mozzarella, without dressing, 6⅓ oz	6
●	tossed, without dressing	0
	tropical, canned, heavy syrup, ½ cup	6
	tuna, 3⅔ oz	5
	tuna, store-bought, 3½ oz	7
	tuna-macaroni, 6 oz	6

◯ No Count	SmartPoints® value
turkey cobb, restaurant-type, 11 ½ oz	11
turkey-macaroni, 6 oz	6
vegetable, tossed, with pasta and seafood, without dressing, fast food, 15 oz	11
vegetable, with cheese and egg, without dressing, fast food, 7 ¾ oz	3
vegetable, with chicken, without dressing, fast food, 7 ¾ oz	2
vegetable, with shrimp, without dressing, fast food, 8 ½ oz	2
vegetable, with turkey, ham and cheese, without dressing, fast food, 11 ⅔ oz	8
Waldorf, 4 ¾ oz	8
whitefish, store-bought, 2 oz	6
yogurt and cucumber, 3 ⅓ oz	2
Salad mix	
pasta, prepared according to package directions, 3 ¼ oz	5
Salami	
beef, 2 oz	5
beef and pork, 2 oz	6
beef and pork, dry or hard, 1 piece (⅓ oz)	1
beef and pork, Italian, dry, sliced, 50% less sodium, 2 oz	6
beef and pork, less sodium, 2 oz	8
pork, dry or hard, 2 oz	8
pork, Italian, 2 oz	8
turkey, 2 oz	2
Salisbury steak	
6 oz	14
with gravy, frozen, 4 ¾ oz	7
Salsa	
black bean and corn, 2 Tbsp	1
◯ fat-free	0
◯ fat-free, gluten-free	0
mango, 2 Tbsp	1

◯ No Count	SmartPoints® value
peach, 2 Tbsp	1
pineapple, 2 Tbsp	1
Salsa con queso	
store-bought, 2 Tbsp	2
Salsa verde	
◯ fat-free	0
Samosa	
1 (1 oz)	4
Sandwich	
bacon, lettuce, and tomato, 9 ¼ oz	16
bagel, with ham, egg and cheese, fast food, 6 ¾ oz	15
barbecue beef, frozen, 5 oz	14
chicken breast, grilled, on bun, 6 ½ oz	11
chicken fillet, crispy, with lettuce and mayonnaise, fast food, 5 ½ oz	13
chicken fillet, grilled, with lettuce, tomato, and spread, fast food, 8 ¼ oz	10
chicken fillet, plain, fast food, 6 ⅔ oz	13
chicken salad, reduced-calorie bread, 5 ⅓ oz	9
chicken salad, regular bread, 5 ½ oz	11
chicken, fried, fast food, 7 ⅓ oz	14
chicken, grilled, fast food, 6 ¾ oz	10
chicken, grilled, frozen, 4 ⅓ oz	9
croque-monsieur, 6 ½ oz	15
Cuban, 5 ¾ oz	14
egg and cheese, fast food, 5 ¼ oz	11
egg salad, 6 oz	15
fish fillet, frozen, 4 ½ oz	12
fish, with tartar sauce and cheese, fast food, 4 ¾ oz	12
fish, with tartar sauce, fast food, 7 ¾ oz	17
grinder, 2 ¾ oz	8

Sandwich (cont'd)

No Count	SmartPoints® value
ham and cheese, 4 oz	12
ham and cheese, fast food, 5 ¼ oz	11
ham and Swiss cheese, restaurant-type, 9 ¼ oz	10
ham, egg, and cheese, fast food, 5 oz	11
hero, 11 ⅓ oz	8
hoagie, 2 ¾ oz	8
lobster roll, 4 oz	6
lobster salad, 4 ½ oz	10
Monte Cristo, 3 ¾ oz	9
peanut butter and jelly, 3 ⅓ oz	11
peanut butter and jelly, restaurant-type, 4 ⅓ oz	15
Philly cheese steak, 9 oz	17
poor boy, 2 ¾ oz	8
roast beef, 7 ¾ oz	10
roast beef with cheese, fast food, 6 ¼ oz	15
roast beef, open-face, with gravy, 6 oz	12
roast beef, plain, fast food, 5 oz	10
shrimp salad, 4 ⅔ oz	9
sloppy Joe, 6 oz	10
steak, fast food, 7 ¼ oz	12
submarine, 2 ¾ oz	8
submarine, turkey and cheese, 6", no mayonnaise, restaurant-type, 8 ¾ oz	11
submarine, with cold cuts, fast food, 8 oz	15
submarine, with roast beef, fast food, 7 ¾ oz	12
submarine, with tuna salad, fast food, 9 oz	17
toasted cheese, 3 ¾ oz	12
tuna melt, 5 ¾ oz	11
tuna salad, 6 ⅓ oz	12
turkey, 4 oz	7

No Count	SmartPoints® value
Sashimi	
● all varieties except mackerel and salmon, 2 oz	1
mackerel, 2 oz	3
salmon, 2 oz	2
Satay	
beef, with peanut sauce, 2 (6 oz)	15
beef, without peanut sauce, 2 (3 oz)	5
chicken, with peanut sauce, 2 (5 ⅓ oz)	12
chicken, without peanut sauce, 2 (3 oz)	2
Sauce	
a la vodka, ½ cup	5
adobo, store-bought, 2 Tbsp	1
Alfredo, ½ cup	14
Alfredo, light, store-bought, ½ cup	7
Alfredo, regular, store-bought, ½ cup	14
arrabbiata, ½ cup	4
Asian stir-fry, 1 Tbsp	1
barbecue, 2 Tbsp	3
Béarnaise, 2 Tbsp	6
béchamel (white), 2 Tbsp	2
black bean, 2 Tbsp	2
Bolognese, ½ cup	7
brown, Chinese, 2 Tbsp	1
cheese, 2 Tbsp	2
cheese, store-bought, 2 Tbsp	2
chili, 2 Tbsp	1
chili, green, 2 Tbsp	0
chili, red, 2 Tbsp	1
chipotle, canned, 2 Tbsp	1
clam, red, ¼ cup	2
clam, red, store-bought, ¼ cup	1
clam, white, ¼ cup	3
clam, white, store-bought, ¼ cup	2
cocktail, store-bought, ¼ cup	3

"We Like This!" item

No Count		SmartPoints® value
	curry, Hawaiian-style, 1 Tbsp	2
	curry, jarred, 1 Tbsp	1
	donair, 2 Tbsp	4
	duck, 1 Tbsp	2
	enchilada, canned, 2 Tbsp	0
	fish, ready-to-serve, ¼ cup	1
	hoisin, 1 Tbsp	2
	hollandaise, 2 Tbsp	6
	hollandaise, store-bought, 1 Tbsp	1
	horseradish, store-bought, 1 Tbsp	2
	hot, 2 Tbsp	0
	hot dog, 2 Tbsp	1
	hot, Asian, 1 Tbsp	0
	kung pao, 1 Tbsp	2
	marinara with meat, homemade, ½ cup	6
	marinara, fat-free, jarred, ½ cup	2
	marinara, gluten-free, store-bought, ½ cup	2
	marinara, homemade, ½ cup	3
	marinara, store-bought, ½ cup	3
	mole poblano, 2 Tbsp	3
	mole, brown, store-bought, 2 Tbsp	2
	mornay, 2 Tbsp	3
	nuoc cham, 2 Tbsp	1
	oyster, ¼ cup	1
	pasta, bottled, any type, ½ cup	5
	pasta, bottled, any type, reduced-fat, ½ cup	2
	peanut, spicy, 1 Tbsp	2
	peanut, Thai, canned, 1 Tbsp	2
	pepper, 2 Tbsp	0
	pesto, ½ cup	19
	pesto, reduced-fat, ¼ cup	8
	pizza, store-bought, 2 Tbsp	0
	plum, 2 Tbsp	2
	puttanesca, ½ cup	13
	remoulade, 2 Tbsp	4

No Count		SmartPoints® value
	sambal oelek, 1 Tbsp	0
	satay, 1 Tbsp	1
	sloppy Joe, store-bought, 2 Tbsp	1
	sofrito, 2 Tbsp	2
	soy (shoyu), 1 Tbsp	0
	soy, gluten-free, 1 Tbsp	0
	spaghetti, bottled, any type, ½ cup	5
	spaghetti, bottled, any type, reduced-fat, ½ cup	3
	Spanish, 2 Tbsp	0
	sriracha, hot, 1 Tbsp	0
	steak, 1 Tbsp	1
	sweet and sour, 1 Tbsp	1
	taco, 2 Tbsp	1
	tamari, 2 Tbsp	0
	tartar, ¼ cup	5
	tartar, fat-free, ¼ cup	2
	teriyaki, 1 Tbsp	1
	teriyaki, gluten-free, 1 Tbsp	1
	teriyaki, reduced-sodium, 1 Tbsp	1
●	tomato, canned	0
●	tomato, canned, Spanish style	0
	tomato, Italian, ½ cup	3
	tomato, with herbs and cheese, canned, ½ cup	3
●	tomato, with mushrooms, canned	0
●	tomato, with onions, canned	0
	tomato, with onions, green peppers, and celery, canned, ½ cup	3
●	tomato, with roasted garlic	0
●	tomato, with tomato tidbits, canned	0
	tzatziki, 2 Tbsp	1
	Vietnamese spring roll dipping, ½ oz	0
	wine, 2 Tbsp	2
	Worcestershire, 1 Tbsp	1

○ No Count	SmartPoints® value
Sauerbraten	
4 ¾ oz	7
Sauerkraut	
fresh or canned	0
Sausage	
50% venison, 50% pork, uncooked, 3 oz	5
60% venison, 40% pork, uncooked, 3 oz	4
andouille, 3 oz	6
beef or pork, cooked, 3 oz	9
boudin, store-bought, 3 oz	4
bratwurst, 1 (3 oz)	9
chicken, beef and pork, skinless, smoked, 2 oz	4
chicken, cooked, 3 oz	3
chicken, uncooked, 4 oz	4
Italian, pork, cooked, 3 oz	10
Italian, sweet, cooked, 2 oz	2
Italian, sweet, turkey, uncooked, 1 link (3 ¾ oz)	3
Italian, turkey, smoked, 2 oz	3
lamb, 3 oz	7
low-fat (1 gram fat or less per oz), 3 oz	3
Polish, beef with chicken, hot, 2 oz	5
Polish, pork and beef, smoked, 2 oz	6
turkey, breakfast links, mild, 2 oz	4
turkey, cooked, 3 oz	4
turkey, hot, smoked, 2 oz	3
turkey, reduced-fat, brown and serve, cooked, 3 oz	4
turkey, uncooked, 4 oz	4
Sausage biscuit	
fast food, 4 ⅓ oz	15
frozen, 2 oz	8
Sausage on a roll	
plain, 5 ⅓ oz	16

○ No Count	SmartPoints® value
Scallion pancake	
1 (2 ¼ oz)	9
Scallops	
breaded and fried, 3 oz	5
breaded and fried, fast food, 3 oz	7
fried, 3 oz	5
fried, frozen, prepared without fat, 3 oz	6
Schaum torte	
with whipped cream, 1 oz	2
without whipped cream, 1 oz	2
Scone	
blueberry, restaurant-type, 1 (4 ¼ oz)	17
chocolate, restaurant-type, 1 (4 ¼ oz)	20
cinnamon, restaurant-type, 1 (4 ¼ oz)	20
cranberry, restaurant-type, 1 (4 ¼ oz)	16
orange, restaurant-type, 1 (4 ¼ oz)	18
plain, 1 (1 ½ oz)	5
raspberry, restaurant-type, 1 (4 ¼ oz)	18
Scrapple	
1" square, 3 oz	6
Seafood cakes (haw mok thalay)	
5 ¾ oz	14
Seafood mix	
○ frozen, 4 oz	1
Seasoning mix	
chili, dry, 1 Tbsp	1
taco, dry, 1 Tbsp	1
Seasonings and spices	
1 tsp	0
Seeds	
chia seeds, dried, ¼ cup	6
flax seeds, ¼ cup	7
lotus seeds, raw, 1 oz	1

"We Like This!" item

No Count		SmartPoints® value
	pumpkin seeds (pepitas), 1 Tbsp	1
	pumpkin seeds (pepitas), roasted, ¼ cup	5
	sesame seeds, 1 tsp	1
	sunflower seeds, ¼ cup	6
	sunflower seeds, dry-roasted, ¼ cup	6
	sunflower seeds, oil-roasted, ¼ cup	6
	sunflower seeds, toasted, ¼ cup	6
	Seitan	
	2 oz	1
	dry mix, prepared, 2 oz	1
	Sesame butter (tahini)	
	2 Tbsp	6
	Sesame chicken	
	7 oz	11
	Sesame noodles	
	1 cup	9
	Shabu shabu	
	9 oz	9
	Shake	
	chocolate, fast food, 1 cup	12
	strawberry, fast food, 1 cup	13
	vanilla, fast food, 1 cup	11
	Shawarma	
	chicken, 2 oz	5
	Shellfish	
○	clams, canned, 3 oz	2
○	clams, cooked, 3 oz	2
○	clams, littleneck, raw, 4 oz	1
○	clams, raw, 4 oz	1
○	crab, Alaska king, cooked, 3 oz	1
○	crab, Alaska king, raw, 4 oz	1
○	crab, blue, canned, 3 oz	1
○	crab, blue, cooked, 3 oz	1
○	crab, blue, raw, 4 oz	1
○	crab, dungeness, cooked, 3 oz	1
○	crab, dungeness, raw, 4 oz	1
○	crab, queen, cooked, 3 oz	1

No Count		SmartPoints® value
○	crabmeat, canned, 3 oz	1
○	crabmeat, cooked, 3 oz	1
○	crabmeat, lump, 3 oz	1
○	crayfish, cooked, 3 oz	1
○	crayfish, wild, cooked, 3 oz	1
○	lobster, cooked, 3 oz	1
○	lobster, spiny, cooked, 3 oz	2
○	lobster, steamed (1 ¼ pounds in the shell), 3 oz shelled	1
○	mussels, cooked, 3 oz	3
○	mussels, raw, in shell, 4 oz	2
○	octopus, common, cooked, 3 oz	2
○	oyster, canned, 3 oz	1
○	oyster, cooked, 3 oz	2
○	oyster, Pacific, cooked, 3 oz	3
○	oyster, raw, 4 oz	2
○	scallops, cooked, 3 oz	1
○	scallops, raw, 3 oz	1
○	shrimp, canned, 3 oz	1
○	shrimp, cooked, 3 oz	1
○	shrimp, frozen, 3 oz	1
○	shrimp, raw, 3 oz	1
○	squid, cooked, 3 oz	1
○	squid, raw, 4 oz	2
	Shephard's pie	
	9 ¾ oz	12
	Sherbet	
	½ cup	6
	Sherry	
	dry, 3 ½ fl oz	5
	sweet, 3 ½ fl oz	7
	Shish kabob	
	4 ¾ oz	9
	Shoyu chicken	
	3 ⅓ oz	7
	Shrimp	
	barbecued, 3 oz	15
	breaded and fried, 3 oz	5
	breaded and fried, fast food, 3 pieces (1 ⅓ oz)	4

Shrimp (cont'd)

No Count		SmartPoints® value
	broiled, stuffed, 3 oz	12
	butterfly, breaded, frozen, prepared without fat, 3 oz	7
	fried, 3 oz	5
	fried, stuffed, 9½ oz	9
	popcorn, breaded, frozen, prepared without fat, 3 oz	7
	Shrimp and broccoli	
	6½ oz	2
	Shrimp Cantonese	
	7¾ oz	9
	Shrimp puffs	
	1 (⅓ oz)	1
	Shrimp remoulade	
	3¾ oz	10
	Shrimp scampi	
	3⅔ oz	13
	Shrimp toast	
	1 oz	3
	Shumai	
	fried, 1 (¾ oz)	2
	steamed, 1 (¾ oz)	2
	Smoothie	
	8 fl oz	6
	Snack mix	
	Oriental, low-fat, store-bought, 1 oz	3
	Oriental, rice-based, 1 oz	4
	reduced-fat, store-bought, 1 oz	4
	store-bought, 1 oz	4
	Snack pack	
	cheese and breadstick, 1 oz	4
	cheese and pretzel, 1 oz	3
	Snack sticks	
	meat-based, smoked, 1 (¾ oz)	4
	Snow cone	
	1 (8 oz)	6

No Count		SmartPoints® value
	Soft drink, carbonated	
	any flavor other than those listed here, sweetened with sugar, 8 fl oz	7
	any flavor, diet, 8 fl oz	0
	cola, 12 fl oz	9
	cream, 8 fl oz	8
	ginger ale, 8 fl oz	5
	lemon-lime, 8 fl oz	6
	pepper-type, 8 fl oz	6
	root beer, 8 fl oz	6
	seltzer, plain or flavored, unsweetened, 8 fl oz	0
	Sopaipillas	
	2 (1 oz)	3
	Sorbet	
	any flavor, ½ cup	5
	Sorghum	
●	2 oz	5
	Soufflé	
	cheese, 3⅓ oz	7
	fruit, 2 oz	5
	Soup, beef	
	beef mushroom, canned, prepared with equal volume water, 1 cup	2
	beef stroganoff, chunky style, canned, 1 cup	8
	beef, chunky, canned, ready-to-serve, 1 cup	5
	beef-mushroom, canned, condensed, ½ cup	2
●	beef-mushroom, chunky style, low-sodium, 1 cup	6
	beef-noodle, canned, condensed, ½ cup	3
	beef-noodle, canned, prepared with equal volume water, 1 cup	3
	beef-noodle, dehydrated, prepared with water, 1 cup	1

"We Like This!" item

No Count		SmartPoints® value
	beef-vegetable, canned, prepared with equal volume water, 1 cup	2
	chili beef, canned, condensed, ½ cup	5
	chili beef, canned, prepared with equal volume water, 1 cup	5
	sirloin burger with vegetable, ready-to-serve, 1 cup	5
	tomato-beef with noodle, canned, condensed, ½ cup	4
	tomato-beef with noodle, canned, prepared with equal volume water, 1 cup	4
	vegetable-beef, microwavable, ready-to-serve, 10 ⅓ oz	2
	Soup, chicken	
	chicken and stars, canned, prepared with equal volume water, 1 cup	2
	chicken corn chowder, chunky style, ready-to-serve, 8 ½ oz	8
	chicken gumbo, canned, condensed, ½ cup	2
	chicken gumbo, canned, prepared with equal volume water, 1 cup	2
	chicken with dumplings, canned, condensed, ½ cup	3
	chicken with dumplings, canned, prepared with equal volume water, 1 cup	3
	chicken with matzo balls, 1 cup	4
	chicken with rice, canned, condensed, ½ cup	3
	chicken with rice, canned, prepared with equal volume water, 1 cup	2
	chicken with wild rice, canned, prepared with equal volume water, 1 cup	2
	chicken, chunky, canned, ready-to-serve, 1 cup	5
	chicken, without matzo balls (broth only), 1 cup	1

No Count		SmartPoints® value
	chicken-enchilada, 8 ¾ oz	6
	chicken-mushroom, canned, condensed, ½ cup	4
	chicken-mushroom, canned, prepared with equal volume water, 1 cup	4
○	chicken-noodle, 1 cup	3
	chicken-noodle in a cup, 1 (⅓ oz)	1
	chicken-noodle mix, prepared, 1 cup	2
	chicken-noodle, canned, condensed, ½ cup	2
	chicken-noodle, canned, prepared with equal volume water, 1 cup	2
	chicken-noodle, chunky, canned, ready-to-serve, 1 cup	3
	chicken-noodle, dehydrated, 1 packet (½ oz)	1
○	chicken-noodle, low-sodium, canned, prepared with equal volume water, 1 cup	2
○	chicken-noodle, reduced-sodium, ready-to-eat, 1 cup	3
	chicken-noodle, with meatballs, chunky, canned, ready-to-serve, 1 cup	3
	chicken-rice mix, dehydrated, 1 packet (½ oz)	2
	chicken-rice, chunky, canned, ready-to-serve, 1 cup	3
	chicken-rice, dehydrated, prepared with water, 1 cup	2
	chicken-vegetable in cup, 1 (1 oz)	3
	chicken-vegetable with potato and cheese, chunky, ready-to-eat, 1 cup	6
	chicken-vegetable, canned, condensed, ½ cup	2
	chicken-vegetable, chunky, canned, ready-to-serve, 1 cup	2
○	chicken-vegetable, chunky, reduced-fat and sodium, ready-to-serve, 8 ½ oz	2

Soup, chicken (cont'd)

No Count	SmartPoints® value
chicken-vegetable, dehydrated, 1 packet (⅓ oz)	1
cream of chicken, canned, condensed, ½ cup	4
cream of chicken, canned, made with fat-free milk, 1 cup	5
cream of chicken, canned, made with low-fat milk, 1 cup	6
cream of chicken, canned, made with whole milk, 1 cup	7
cream of chicken, canned, prepared with equal volume water, 1 cup	4
cream of chicken, dehydrated, 1 packet (⅔ oz)	3
cream of chicken, dehydrated, prepared with water, 1 cup	5
cream of chicken, low-fat, canned, made with fat-free milk, 1 cup	4
cream of chicken, low-fat, canned, made with low-fat milk, 1 cup	5
cream of chicken, reduced-sodium, canned, condensed, ½ cup	2
hot and spicy chicken, 1 cup	3
knefla, 1 cup	8
Thai chicken-coconut, 1 cup	12
with tortilla strips and shredded cheese, 1 cup	5
Soup, seafood	
asparagus-crab, 1 cup	2
bouillabaisse, 1 cup	4
cioppino, 1 cup	5
crab, canned, ready-to-serve, 1 cup	2
cream of shrimp, canned, condensed, ½ cup	3
cream of shrimp, canned, prepared with equal volume reduced-fat (2%) milk, 1 cup	6
cream of shrimp, canned, prepared with equal volume water, 1 cup	3
lobster bisque, 11 oz	7

No Count	SmartPoints® value
lobster bisque, canned, made with fat-free milk, 1 cup	4
lobster bisque, canned, made with low-fat milk, 1 cup	5
lobster bisque, canned, made with whole milk, 1 cup	6
lobster bisque, restaurant-type, 1 cup	16
Manhattan clam chowder, 6 ½ oz	4
Manhattan clam chowder, canned, condensed, ½ cup	3
Manhattan clam chowder, canned, prepared with equal volume water, 1 cup	3
Manhattan clam chowder, chunky, canned, ready-to-serve, 1 cup	4
Manhattan clam chowder, restaurant-type, 1 cup	5
New England clam chowder, 1 cup	6
New England clam chowder canned, ready-to-eat, 1 cup	6
New England clam chowder, canned, condensed, ½ cup	3
New England clam chowder, canned, made with fat-free milk, 1 cup	4
New England clam chowder, canned, made with low-fat milk, 1 cup	5
New England clam chowder, canned, made with whole milk, 1 cup	6
New England clam chowder, condensed, prepared with water, 8 ¾ oz	3
New England clam chowder, low-fat, canned, made with fat-free milk, 1 cup	4
New England clam chowder, low-fat, canned, made with low-fat milk, 1 cup	5
New England clam chowder, low-sodium, canned, ready-to-eat, 1 cup	5

"We Like This!" item

No Count		SmartPoints® value
	New England clam chowder, restaurant-type, 1 cup	11
	oyster stew, canned, condensed, ½ cup	2
	oyster stew, canned, made with fat-free milk, 1 cup	4
	oyster stew, canned, made with low-fat milk, 1 cup	4
	oyster stew, canned, made with whole milk, 1 cup	6
	Soup, turkey	
	turkey, chunky, ready-to-eat, 1 cup	3
	turkey-noodle, canned, prepared with equal volume water, 1 cup	4
	turkey-vegetable, canned, condensed, ½ cup	2
	turkey-vegetable, canned, prepared with equal volume water, 1 cup	2
	Soup, vegetable and other	
	avgolemono, 1 cup	4
	baked potato, restaurant-type, 1 cup	8
	bean with bacon, canned, prepared with equal volume water, 1 cup	5
	bean with bacon, dehydrated, 1 packet (1 oz)	3
	bean with bacon, dehydrated, prepared with water, 1 cup	3
	bean with ham, canned, prepared with equal volume water, 1 cup	8
	bean with ham, chunky, canned, ready-to-serve, 1 cup	7
	bean with ham, reduced-sodium, canned, 1 cup	6
	bean with pork, canned, condensed, ½ cup	5
	bean with pork, canned, prepared with equal volume water, 1 cup	5
	beef and vegetable, canned, 1 cup	4

No Count		SmartPoints® value
●	beef and vegetable, reduced-sodium, canned, ready-to-serve, 1 cup	3
	black bean in a cup, dry, 1 container (2 oz)	6
	black bean, canned, 1 cup	6
	black bean, canned, condensed, ½ cup	3
	black bean, canned, prepared with equal volume water, 1 cup	3
	black bean, homemade, 1 cup	3
	black bean, restaurant-type, 1 cup	7
	broccoli-cheese, 1 cup	10
	broccoli-cheese, canned, condensed, 4 ⅓ oz	4
	broccoli-cheese, canned, made with fat-free milk, 1 cup	6
	broccoli-cheese, canned, made with low-fat milk, 1 cup	6
	broccoli-cheese, canned, made with whole milk, 1 cup	7
	broccoli-cheese, low-fat, canned, made with fat-free or low-fat milk, 1 cup	4
	cabbage, 1 cup	1
	cauliflower, dehydrated, prepared with water, 1 cup	2
	cheddar cheese, canned, made with fat-free milk, 1 cup	5
	cheddar cheese, canned, made with low-fat milk, 1 cup	5
	cheddar cheese, canned, made with whole milk, 1 cup	7
	cheese, canned, condensed, ½ cup	4
	corn chowder in a cup, 1 container (1 oz)	4
	cream of asparagus, canned, condensed, ½ cup	3
	cream of asparagus, canned, prepared with equal volume milk, 1 cup	5

Soup, vegetable and other (cont'd)

No Count		SmartPoints® value
	cream of asparagus, canned, prepared with equal volume water, 1 cup	3
	cream of asparagus, dehydrated, 1 packet (2 ¼ oz)	7
	cream of asparagus, dehydrated, prepared with water, 1 cup	3
	cream of broccoli, 1 cup	9
	cream of broccoli, canned, made with fat-free milk, 1 cup	5
	cream of broccoli, canned, made with low-fat milk, 1 cup	6
	cream of broccoli, canned, made with whole milk, 1 cup	7
	cream of broccoli, low-fat, canned, made with fat-free milk, 1 cup	5
	cream of broccoli, low-fat, canned, made with low-fat milk, 1 cup	5
	cream of celery, canned, condensed, ½ cup	3
	cream of celery, canned, made with fat-free milk, 1 cup	5
	cream of celery, canned, made with low-fat milk, 1 cup	5
	cream of celery, canned, made with whole milk, 1 cup	6
	cream of celery, canned, prepared with equal volume water, 1 cup	3
	cream of celery, dehydrated, prepared with water, 1 cup	2
	cream of celery, low-fat, canned, made with fat-free milk, 1 cup	4
	cream of celery, low-fat, canned, made with low-fat milk, 1 cup	4
	cream of mushroom, 1 cup	13
	cream of mushroom, canned, condensed, ½ cup	3
	cream of mushroom, canned, made with fat-free milk, 1 cup	6
	cream of mushroom, canned, made with low-fat milk, 1 cup	7
	cream of mushroom, canned, made with whole milk, 1 cup	8

No Count		SmartPoints® value
	cream of mushroom, canned, prepared with equal volume water, 1 cup	3
	cream of mushroom, low-fat, canned, made with fat-free milk, 1 cup	4
	cream of mushroom, low-fat, canned, made with low-fat milk, 1 cup	5
	cream of mushroom, low-sodium, canned, ready-to-eat, 1 cup	5
	cream of mushroom, reduced-sodium, canned, condensed, 1 cup	5
	cream of onion, canned, condensed, ½ cup	4
	cream of onion, canned, prepared with equal volume milk, 1 cup	6
	cream of onion, canned, prepared with equal volume water, 1 cup	3
	cream of potato, canned, condensed, ½ cup	3
	cream of potato, canned, made with fat-free milk, 1 cup	4
	cream of potato, canned, made with low-fat milk, 1 cup	5
	cream of potato, canned, made with whole milk, 1 cup	6
	cream of potato, canned, prepared with equal volume water, 1 cup	2
	cream of potato, restaurant-type, 1 cup	6
	cream of tomato, 1 cup	6
	cream of vegetable, dehydrated, 1 packet (⅔ oz)	3
	cream of vegetable, dehydrated, prepared with water, 1 cup	4
○	egg drop, homemade, 1 cup	1
	egg drop, restaurant-type, 1 cup	2
	escarole, canned, 1 cup	1
	escarole, canned, ready-to-serve, 1 cup	1
	French onion au gratin, 1 cup	9

"We Like This!" item

◯ No Count	SmartPoints® value
◯ gazpacho, 1 cup	3
gazpacho, canned, prepared with equal volume water, 1 cup	1
gazpacho, canned, ready-to-serve, 1 cup	1
green pea, canned, prepared with equal volume water, 1 cup	5
herb with garlic, dehydrated, 1 packet (1¼ oz)	4
hot and sour, homemade, 1 cup	3
hot and sour, restaurant-type, 1 cup	2
Italian wedding, 1 cup	6
leek, dehydrated, 1 packet (2¾ oz)	9
lentil, 1 cup	5
lentil in a cup, 1 container (2 oz)	6
lentil with ham, canned, ready-to-serve, 1 cup	4
lentil-vegetable, 1 cup	5
matzo ball, canned, ready-to-serve, 1 cup	5
minestrone, 1 cup	7
minestrone in a cup, 1 container (1½ oz)	4
minestrone, canned, condensed, ½ cup	2
minestrone, canned, prepared with equal volume water, 1 cup	2
minestrone, chunky, canned, ready-to-serve, 1 cup	4
minestrone, dehydrated, 1 packet (⅔ oz)	2
minestrone, low-fat, canned, prepared with equal volume water, 1 cup	3
minestrone, reduced-sodium, canned, ready-to-eat, 1 cup	4
miso, 1 cup	2
mulligatawny, 1 cup	9
mushroom with beef stock, canned, condensed, ½ cup	3

◯ No Count	SmartPoints® value
mushroom with beef stock, canned, prepared with equal volume water, 1 cup	3
mushroom, dehydrated, prepared with water, 1 cup	3
mushroom-barley, 1 cup	4
mushroom-barley, canned, condensed, ½ cup	2
mushroom-barley, canned, prepared with equal volume water, 1 cup	2
onion, canned, condensed, ½ cup	2
onion, dehydrated, ¼ packet (⅓ oz)	1
onion, dehydrated, prepared with water, 1 cup	1
Oriental in a cup, 1 container (1 oz)	3
oxtail, 1 cup	2
oxtail, dehydrated, 1 packet (2⅔ oz)	9
oxtail, Hawaiian-style, 1 cup	6
pasta with vegetables, canned, prepared with equal volume water, 1 cup	3
pea, green, canned, condensed, ½ cup	5
pea, green, dehydrated, 1 packet (1 oz)	3
pea, green, dehydrated, prepared with water, 1 cup	4
◯ pea, low-sodium, canned, prepared with equal volume water, 1 cup	5
pepperpot, canned, prepared with equal volume water, 1 cup	3
Persian noodle, store-bought, 1 cup	5
Persian pomegranate, store-bought, 1 cup	8
petite marmite, 1 cup	3
pigeon pea and dumpling, 1 cup	8
Portuguese bean, 1 cup	7

Soup, vegetable and other (cont'd)

No Count		SmartPoints® value
	potato, dehydrated, ⅓ cup	4
●	potato, frozen, 1 (7½ oz)	3
	potato-leek in a cup, 1 container (1 oz)	4
	ramen noodle, dehydrated, 1 packet (3 oz)	13
	ramen noodle, low-fat, dehydrated, 1 packet (3 oz)	6
	ramen noodle, prepared with water, 1 cup	6
	ramen, low-fat, in a cup, 1 container (2 oz)	6
	red beans and rice in a cup, 1 container (2 oz)	5
	saimin, 1 cup	6
●	sambhar (Indian lentil), 1 cup	3
	schav, canned, 1 cup	0
	Scotch broth, 1 cup	6
	shark fin, restaurant-type, 1 cup	3
	split pea, 1 cup	4
	split pea in a cup, 1 container (2 oz)	5
	split pea with ham, canned, prepared with equal volume water, 1 cup	5
	split pea with ham, chunky, canned, ready-to-serve, 1 cup	6
	split pea with ham, chunky, reduced-fat and sodium, ready-to-serve, 1 cup	5
	split pea with ham, reduced-sodium, canned, prepared with equal volume water, 1 cup	5
	split pea, reduced-sodium, canned, prepared with equal volume water, 1 cup	6
	split pea, with ham condensed, ½ cup	5
	Thai coconut ginger, canned, 1 cup	8
	tomato bisque, canned, condensed, ½ cup	4

No Count		SmartPoints® value
	tomato bisque, canned, prepared with equal volume milk, 1 cup	6
	tomato bisque, canned, prepared with equal volume water, 1 cup	4
	tomato, canned, condensed, 1 cup	4
	tomato, canned, made with fat-free milk, 1 cup	5
	tomato, canned, made with low-fat milk, 1 cup	6
	tomato, canned, prepared with equal volume reduced-fat (2%) milk, 1 cup	6
	tomato, canned, prepared with equal volume water, 1 cup	3
	tomato, canned, prepared with equal volume whole milk, 1 cup	7
	tomato, dehydrated, prepared with water, 1 cup	3
	tomato, dehydrated, prepared with water, 1 cup	4
	tomato, homemade, 1 cup	3
●	tomato, low-sodium, canned, prepared with equal volume water, 1 cup	3
	tomato, reduced-sodium, canned, condensed, ½ cup	3
	tomato-rice, canned, condensed, ½ cup	4
	tomato-rice, canned, prepared with equal volume water, 1 cup	4
	tomato-vegetable, dehydrated dry, 1 packet (1⅓ oz)	4
●	tomato-vegetable, dehydrated, prepared with water, 1 cup	2
	tortilla, 1 cup	8
	turtle, 1 cup	3
	vegetable, 1 cup	3
	vegetable with beef broth, canned prepared with equal volume water, 1 cup	2
	vegetable with beef broth, canned, condensed, ½ cup	3

"We Like This!" item

○ No Count		SmartPoints® value
	vegetable, canned, prepared with equal volume water, 1 cup	2
	vegetable, chunky, canned, ready-to-serve, 1 cup	3
	vegetable, dehydrated, 1 packet (1 ¾ oz)	5
	vegetable, low-sodium, canned, condensed, ½ cup	3
○	vegetable, low-sodium, canned, prepared with equal volume water, 1 cup	3
	vegetable-beef, canned, prepared with equal volume water, 1 cup	2
	vegetable-beef, dehydrated, prepared with water, 1 cup	2
○	vegetable-chicken, low-sodium, canned, prepared with equal volume water, 1 cup	5
	vegetarian vegetable in a cup, 1 container (2 oz)	5
	vegetarian vegetable, canned, condensed, ½ cup	3
	vegetarian vegetable, canned, prepared with equal volume water, 1 cup	2
	vichyssoise, 1 cup	4
○	Vietnamese beef-noodle, 1 cup	3
	wonton, restaurant-type, 1 cup	2
○	yogurt and cucumber, 1 cup	4
	nebeyaki udon, 1 cup	3
	suimono, 1 cup	2
	Souse, chicken	
	4 ⅔ oz	9
	Souvlaki	
	chicken, 4 ½ oz	4
	chicken, in pita bread, 6 ½ oz	9
	lamb, 4 ¾ oz	9
	lamb, in pita bread, 6 ½ oz	11
	Soy beverage	
	light, original or vanilla, unsweetened, 8 fl oz	2
	reduced-fat, 8 fl oz	4
	regular, original or vanilla, 8 fl oz	4

○ No Count		SmartPoints® value
	Soy burger	
	2 ⅔ oz	3
	Soy cheese	
○	fat-free, ½ cup	1
○	regular, 1 oz	1
	Soy crumbles	
○	meatless, ½ cup	1
	Soy milk	
	chocolate, fat-free, 8 fl oz	4
	flavored, 8 fl oz	5
○	plain, fat-free, 8 fl oz	3
○	plain, low-fat, 8 fl oz	4
○	plain, unsweetened, 8 fl oz	2
	Soy protein isolate	
	3 oz	1
	Soy yogurt	
	flavored, ¾ cup	7
○	plain, ¾ cup	4
	Soybean nuts	
	¼ cup	3
	Spaetzle	
	1 cup	14
	Spaghetti Bolognese	
	11 oz	13
	Spaghetti with marinara sauce	
	10 ½ oz	8
	Spaghetti with meat sauce	
	10 oz	13
	frozen, 10 oz	7
	Spaghetti with tomato sauce	
	with meatballs, canned, 9 oz	8
	Spaghetti, spinach	
	cooked, 5 oz	5
	dry, 2 oz	6
	Spam musubi	
	1 (4 oz)	9
	Spanakopita	
	5 ¾ oz	12
	frozen, 1 piece (1 oz)	5

No Count	SmartPoints® value
Spanish rice	
canned, 9 oz	4
homemade, 14 oz	7
Spareribs	
barbecued, 4 ¼ oz	12
Chinese, barbecued, 1½ oz	5
pork, lean and fat, cooked, 3 oz	10
pork, lean and fat, raw, 4 oz	10
Spelt	
cooked, 1 cup	6
Spinach, creamed	
restaurant-type, 4 ⅓ oz	8
Spoon bread	
1 cup	15
Sports drink	
8 fl oz	3
Spread	
buttery soy, 1 Tbsp	4
caviar, store-bought, 1 Tbsp	1
cheese, pasteurized process, American, 1 oz	3
cheese, reduced-fat (American or cheddar), 1 oz	2
cheese, with garlic and herb, reduced-fat, 2 Tbsp	3
chicken, 2 oz	2
chocolate, 1 Tbsp	3
chopped pickle, 1 Tbsp	2
ham and cheese, 1 Tbsp	1
ham salad, 1 oz	2
hazelnut and chocolate, 2 Tbsp	11
liverwurst, 1 Tbsp	2
margarine-like, approximately 40% fat, 1 Tbsp	2
meat, canned, 2 ¼ oz	5
olive, store-bought, 1 Tbsp	2
pimiento-cheese, reduced-fat, store-bought, 1 oz	2
pimiento-cheese, regular, store-bought, 1 oz	3
pork or beef, 1 Tbsp	1

No Count	SmartPoints® value
roast beef, 1 Tbsp	1
vegetable oil and butter, reduced-calorie, 1 Tbsp	2
vegetable oil, 37% fat, 1 Tbsp	2
Spring roll	
beef or pork, 1 (2 ½ oz)	7
chicken, 1 (2 ½ oz)	5
fresh, Vietnamese, 1 (1 ¾ oz)	2
fried, Vietnamese, 1 (2 ½ oz)	5
lumpia, Filipino, 1 (2 ½ oz)	6
shrimp, 1 (2 ½ oz)	5
Thai, 1 (2 ½ oz)	5
Sprinkles	
any type, 1 Tbsp	1
Spumoni	
½ cup	13
Squid	
fried, 3 oz	3
Steak	
sandwich, sliced, frozen, prepared, 3 oz	10
Steak au poivre	
3 oz	7
Stew	
bean and lentil stew (dal maharani), 1 cup	9
beef, 7 ½ oz	5
beef, canned, 1 cup	7
beef, frozen, 1 cup	5
Brunswick, 1 ½ cups	6
burgoo, 1 cup	5
carne guisado (Cuban beef stew), 1 cup	6
chicken, canned, 8 ½ oz	7
Irish brown, 1 cup	6
lamb, 1 cup	5
vegetarian, 1 cup	6
Stir-fried vegetables	
1 cup	5
○ frozen, uncooked, 3 oz	1
with beef, 1 cup	5

"We Like This!" item

No Count		SmartPoints® value
	with chicken, 1 cup	3
	with pork, 1 cup	4
○	without sauce, 4 ⅓ oz	1
	Stir-fry, broccoli	
	5 ½ oz	4
	Stir-fry, mung bean sprouts	
	½ cup	1
	Stir-fry, with garlic or black bean sauce	
	beef, with garlic or black bean sauce, 11 ½ oz	8
	chicken, with garlic or black bean sauce, 11 ¾ oz	8
	pork, with garlic or black bean sauce, 11 ¾ oz	9
	shrimp, with garlic or black bean sauce, 11 ¾ oz	7
	Stock	
○	beef (bone broth), homemade, 1 cup	1
○	chicken (bone broth), homemade, 1 cup	3
	chicken, store-bought, 1 cup	0
○	fish, homemade, 1 cup	1
	Strawberries	
	canned, heavy syrup pack, ½ cup	7
	frozen, sliced, sweetened, ½ cup	7
	organic, dried, ¼ cup	4
	with sugar, 1 cup	12
	Stromboli	
	2 ¾ oz	6
	Strudel	
	any type, 1 (6 oz)	18
	Stuffing	
	½ cup	6
	Stuffing mix	
	bread, 1 oz	3
	bread, prepared, ½ cup	6
	Succotash	
○	cooked, 1 cup	7
○	frozen, unprepared, ½ cup	2

No Count		SmartPoints® value
○	with corn and limas, frozen, cooked, ½ cup	2
	with cream-style corn, canned, ½ cup	3
○	with whole-kernel corn, canned, ½ cup	2
	Sugar	
	white or brown, any type, 1 tsp	1
	Sugar substitute	
	1 tsp	0
	aspartame, 1 packet	0
	saccharin, 1 packet	0
	stevia, 1 packet	0
	sucralose, 1 tsp	0
	Sugar substitute, baking	
	brown sugar and sucralose, 1 Tbsp	2
	white sugar and sucralose, 1 Tbsp	2
	Sukiyaki	
	with sauce, 15 ¼ oz	15
	Summer squash casserole	
	7 ½ oz	11
	Sunflower seed butter	
	1 Tbsp	3
	Sunomono	
	2 ½ oz	1
	Sushi	
	Alaskan roll, 3 oz	4
	California roll, 5 ⅓ oz	5
	cone, 2 ¾ oz	4
	inari, 2 ¾ oz	4
	kappa maki (cucumber roll), 4 medium pieces (5 oz)	3
	maki (vegetables and rice rolled with seaweed), 1 piece (¾ oz)	1
	nigiri (sliced raw fish over rice), 6 small pieces (4 oz)	2
	nori maki (raw fish and rice rolled with seaweed), 4 ½ oz	3
	Philadelphia roll, 2 ¾ oz	4
	rainbow roll, 3 pieces (4 oz)	3

Sushi (cont'd)

No Count	SmartPoints® value
shrimp tempura roll, 8 ½ oz	10
spider roll, 9 ⅔ oz	10
tuna roll, 4 oz	3
tuna roll, spicy, 7 oz	7
uni maki, 4 oz	3
vegetable tempura roll, 7 ⅔ oz	6
yellowtail roll, 4 oz	3
Sweet and sour	
chicken, homemade, 8 ¾ oz	14
chicken, restaurant-type, 2 oz	5
pork, restaurant-type, 1 ½ oz	4
shrimp, 8 ½ oz	14
Sweet potato pie	
6 ¾ oz	16
Sweet potato puffs	
frozen, unprepared, 3 oz	5
Sweet roll	
1 (4 oz)	9
cheese, 1 (2 ⅓ oz)	9
cinnamon, refrigerated dough with frosting, baked, 1 (1 oz)	4
pecan-swirl, store-bought, 1 (1 oz)	5
store-bought, 1 (2 oz)	9
Sweetbreads	
○ cooked, 3 oz	2
Syrup	
agave, ¼ cup	15
chocolate, ¼ cup	11
chocolate fudge-type, ¼ cup	12
corn, dark, ¼ cup	15
corn, high fructose, ¼ cup	14
corn, light, ¼ cup	15
dietetic, 1 Tbsp	0
flavored, ¼ cup	10
grenadine, ¼ cup	11
maple, ¼ cup	12
pancake, low-calorie, ¼ cup	5
pancake, regular, ¼ cup	8
pancake, with butter, ¼ cup	13

"We Like This!" item

No Count	SmartPoints® value
simple syrup from table sugar, ¾ oz	4
sorghum, ¼ cup	15
table blend, ¼ cup	10
Szechuan chicken	
frozen, 7 oz	9
Szechuan pork hotpot	
8 oz	7

T

Tabouli	
3 ¼ oz	7
Taco	
beef, 1 (3 ⅔ oz)	7
breakfast, 3 ¾ oz	7
chicken, 1 (3 ⅔ oz)	6
fish, 1 (4 ⅓ oz)	5
hard, dinner kit in a box, prepared, 2 (5 ½ oz)	9
hard, fast food, 1 (3 oz)	5
pork, 1 (3 ½ oz)	5
soft, fast food, 1 (3 ½ oz)	4
Taco salad shells	
large, store-bought, 2 (2 oz)	8
small, store-bought, 2 (1 ½ oz)	6
Tamago-yaki (omelet roll)	
1 (1 ½ oz)	2
Tamales	
beef, canned, 2 (4 oz)	5
beef, frozen, 1 (1 ⅔ oz)	3
chicken, canned, 1 (2 oz)	3
chicken, frozen, 1 (2 oz)	3
corn, restaurant-type, 6 oz	11
pork, frozen, 1 (1 ½ oz)	3
pork, restaurant-type, 5 oz	8
Tandoori chicken	
breast, without skin, 4 ½ oz	4
thigh, without skin, 1 (3 oz)	4

No Count	SmartPoints® value
Tandoori fish	
5 ½ oz	5
Tandoori shrimp	
5 ½ oz	3
Tangerine (mandarin orange)	
canned, light syrup pack, ½ cup	5
Tapenade	
olive, prepared, 1 Tbsp	1
Tapioca	
ready-to-eat, ½ cup	6
Thai, ½ cup	7
Tapioca mix	
¼ package (¾ oz)	4
prepared with whole milk, ½ cup	7
Taquitos	
beef, 3 oz	5
chicken, 3 oz	3
frozen, 1 (1 oz)	2
Taro	
◎ cooked, ½ cup	3
Tart shell	
1 (2 oz)	10
store-bought, 1 (1 ½ oz)	10
Tarte aux fruits	
1 slice (5 ⅔ oz)	17
Tater tots	
cooked, 3 oz	5
Tea	
decaffeinated or regular, sweetened, 8 fl oz	5
decaffeinated or regular, unsweetened, 8 fl oz	0
instant, artificially sweetened, lemon-flavored, prepared, 8 fl oz	0
instant, sweetened with sugar, lemon-flavored, prepared, 8 fl oz	5
instant, sweetened with sugar, powder, 1 Tbsp	5
Tempeh	
cooked, 3 oz	4

No Count	SmartPoints® value
Tempura	
shrimp, 3 ¾ oz	13
vegetable, 4 ½ oz	9
Tempura batter mix	
⅓ cup	4
Teppan yaki (mixed grill of beef, chicken, shrimp and vegetables)	
9 ½ oz	12
Teriyaki	
beef, 5 ½ oz	8
chicken, 5 ½ oz	6
fish (except salmon), 5 ½ oz	5
salmon, 5 ⅓ oz	9
tofu, 5 ⅓ oz	5
Texas trash (cereal and nut mix)	
1 oz	4
Textured vegetable protein	
3 oz	5
Thai chicken with basil	
3 ¾ oz	4
Thai chili beef (neua pad prik)	
8 oz	6
Thai coffee or tea	
8 fl oz	16
Thai crisp noodles	
1 cup	10
Thai curry paste	
1 Tbsp	2
Thai grilled beef (nuea nam tok)	
5 ¾ oz	6
Tiramisu	
1 piece (6 ⅓ oz)	15
restaurant-type, 1 piece (4 ¾ oz)	20
Toaster pastry	
brown sugar-cinnamon flavor, 1 oz	4
fruit, 1 (2 oz)	8
fruit, frosted, 1 (2 oz)	8
low-fat, 1 (1 ¾ oz)	8

No Count		SmartPoints® value
	Tofu	
	aburage, bean curd, fried, 3 oz	8
	agedashi, fried, 5 oz	7
●	extra firm, 3 oz	2
●	firm, light, 3 oz	1
●	firm, regular, 3 oz	1
	fried, 3 oz	6
●	silken, 3 oz	1
●	silken, light, 3 oz	1
●	soft, regular, 3 oz	1
	Tofu, frozen	
	dessert, 3 oz	11
	Tom yum kung	
	9 ⅓ oz	2
	Tomato paste	
	canned, ¼ cup	2
	Tomatoes	
●	dried, not packed in oil, drained, ½ cup	0
	dried, packed in oil, drained, ½ cup	4
	fried green, 2 slices (5 oz)	5
	Tonkatsu	
	beef, 3 ⅔ oz	8
	chicken, 3 ⅔ oz	7
	pork, 3 ½ oz	10
	Topping, dessert	
	butterscotch or caramel, 2 Tbsp	5
	caramel, fat-free, 2 Tbsp	6
	fruit, 2 Tbsp	5
	fudge, fat-free, 2 Tbsp	5
	fudge, regular, 2 Tbsp	7
	nuts, in syrup, 2 Tbsp	7
	Topping, whipped	
	dairy or nondairy, light or fat-free, aerosol or frozen, 2 Tbsp	1
	fat-free, 2 Tbsp	1
	frozen, low-fat, 1 cup	9
	light, 1 Tbsp	1

"We Like This!" item

No Count		SmartPoints® value
	Tortellini	
	beef, chicken, or pork, without sauce, frozen, 3 ¼ oz	8
	cheese, fresh, refrigerated, store-bought, ¾ cup	7
	cheese, without sauce, 3 oz	7
	cheese, without sauce, frozen, 3 ¾ oz	9
	cheese, without sauce, store-bought, 4 ¼ oz	9
	meat, without sauce, 3 oz	5
	meat, without sauce, store-bought, 4 ½ oz	10
	mushroom, without sauce, frozen, 3 ¼ oz	10
	sausage, without sauce, frozen, 3 ¼ oz	11
	vegetable and cheese, without sauce, 3 ¾ oz	9
	Tortellini, spinach	
	cheese, without sauce, store-bought, 4 oz	10
	Tortilla	
	corn, 1 (¾ oz)	2
●	corn, reduced-fat, 2 (1 ⅔ oz)	3
	flour, 1 medium (1 oz)	3
	flour, 8", 1 (1 ¾ oz)	5
	flour, burrito-size, 1 large (2 ¼ oz)	3
	flour, fat-free, 1 (½ oz)	1
	multi-grain, 8", 1 (1 ¾ oz)	5
	whole-wheat, 1 (1 ⅓ oz)	2
	whole-wheat, 96% fat-free (7"-8"), 1 (1 ⅔ oz)	4
	Tortoni	
	2 ½ oz	12
	Tostada	
	beef, 1 (8 ½ oz)	13
	chicken, 1 (8 ⅓ oz)	11
	with beans and cheese, fast food, 1 (5 oz)	7
	with beef and cheese, fast food, 5 ¾ oz	11

○ No Count		SmartPoints® value
	Tostada shells	
	corn, 1 (½ oz)	2
	store-bought, 1 (½ oz)	2
	Tourtière (Canadian meat pie)	
	5 oz	11
	Trail mix	
	1 oz	5
	tropical, 1 oz	5
	with chocolate chips, 1 oz	5
	Trifle	
	½ cup	5
	Tripe	
○	cooked, 3 oz	2
	Tropical fruit	
	canned, in passionfruit juice, ½ cup	4
	Tuna noodle casserole	
	8 oz	10
	Tuna steak	
○	grilled, frozen, 3 oz	1
	Turkey	
	canned, 3 oz	3
	dark meat, cooked, with skin, 3 oz	4
	dark meat, cooked, without skin, 3 oz	2
	light and dark meat, seasoned, 3 oz	2
○	light meat, cooked, without skin, 3 oz	1
	light meat, rotisserie, deli-type, 2 oz	1
	meat only, roasted, 3 oz	2
	with gravy, frozen, 3 oz	1
	Turkey breast	
	sliced, prepackaged, 1 slice (½ oz)	0
○	smoked, 3 oz	2
	smoked, lemon-pepper flavor, 97% fat-free, 1 slice (1 oz)	0
	with skin, cooked, 3 oz	3
○	without skin, cooked, 3 oz	1
○	without skin, raw, 4 oz	1

○ No Count		SmartPoints® value
	Turkey breast, ground	
○	99% fat-free, cooked, 3 oz	1
○	99% fat-free, raw, 4 oz	1
○	raw, 4 oz	2
	Turkey burger	
	frozen, prepared, 3 oz	4
	Turkey croquette	
	breaded, frozen, 3½ oz	7
	Turkey drumstick	
	without skin, cooked, 3 oz	2
	Turkey leg	
	with skin, cooked, 3 oz	4
	Turkey neck	
	cooked, 3 oz	2
	Turkey patty	
	93% lean/7% fat, cooked, 3 oz	4
	breaded, battered, fried, 3 oz	7
○	fat-free, cooked, 3 oz	1
	Turkey roast	
	boneless, frozen, seasoned, raw, 3 oz	2
	light and dark meat, seasoned, roasted, 3 oz	3
	Turkey roll	
	2 oz	2
	Turkey thigh	
	with skin, cooked, 3 oz	4
	with skin, pre-basted, roasted, 3 oz	3
	without skin, raw, 4 oz	2
	Turkey wing	
	meat and skin, cooked, 3 oz	4
○	meat only, cooked, 3 oz	1
	without skin and bone, smoked, cooked, ⅔ oz	1
	Turkey, deli-sliced	
	2 oz	1
	turkey-ham, extra-lean, sliced, deli-type, pieces, 2 oz	1

No Count		SmartPoints® value
	Turkey, ground	
	85% lean/15% fat, pan-broiled crumbles, 3 oz	6
	85% lean/15% fat, raw, 3 oz	4
	93% lean/7% fat, pan-broiled crumbles, 3 oz	4
	93% lean/7% fat, raw, 4 oz	3
	regular, cooked, 3 oz	5
	regular, raw, 4 oz	4
	Turnover	
	fruit, any type, 1 (3 ½ oz)	8
	fruit, any type, fast food, 1 (4 oz)	13
	Twice-cooked pork	
	3 oz	6
	Tyropitas	
	frozen, 1 (1 oz)	3
	Tzimmes, vegetable	
	6 ⅔ oz	5

V

No Count		SmartPoints® value
	Veal	
	leg, cooked, 3 oz	3
	leg, top round, lean and fat, cooked, 3 oz	3
	leg, top round, lean and fat, pan fried, breaded, 3 oz	5
	leg, top round, lean only, pan-fried, breaded, 3 oz	4
○	leg, top round, lean only, raw, 4 oz	1
○	leg, top round, lean, cooked, 3 oz	2
○	leg, trimmed, cooked, 3 oz	3
○	leg, trimmed, raw, 4 oz	1
	loin, cooked, 3 oz	6
	loin, lean and fat, raw, 4 oz	5
○	loin, trimmed, cooked, 3 oz	3
○	loin, trimmed, raw, 4 oz	2
	rib, cooked, 3 oz	5
	rib, lean only, cooked, 3 oz	3
	rib, lean only, raw, 4 oz	2
	rib, raw, 4 oz	5
○	shank, cooked, 3 oz	3
○	shank, lean and fat, raw, 4 oz	2
○	shank, lean only, cooked, 3 oz	2
○	shank, lean only, raw, 4 oz	2
	shoulder, cooked, 3 oz	4
○	shoulder, lean only, raw, 4 oz	2
○	shoulder, trimmed, cooked, 3 oz	3
○	shoulder, trimmed, raw, 4 oz	2
	sirloin, cooked, 3 oz	5
○	sirloin, lean only, raw, 4 oz	2
○	sirloin, lean, cooked, 3 oz	3
	Veal breast	
	cooked, 3 oz	6
	lean and fat, cooked, 3 oz	6
	lean and fat, raw, 4 oz	7
	trimmed, cooked, 3 oz	4
	Veal chop	
	cooked, 3 oz	6
○	lean, cooked, 3 oz	4
○	lean, raw, 4 oz	2
	loin, grilled, 3 oz	4
○	loin, lean, grilled, 3 oz	2
	raw, 4 oz	5
	Veal cutlet	
	breaded, fried, 4 oz	8
	cooked, 3 oz	3
○	lean, cooked, 3 oz	3
○	lean, raw, 4 oz	2
○	raw, 4 oz	2
	Veal parmigiana	
	with sauce, 13 ¾ oz	14
	without sauce, 5 ½ oz	12
	Veal piccata	
	6 oz	12
	Veal scaloppine	
	4 ⅔ oz	8

"We Like This!" item

○ No Count		SmartPoints® value
	Veal with peppers	
	9 ¾ oz	11
	Veal, ground	
	cooked, 3 oz	3
	raw, 4 oz	6
	Vegetable burger on bun	
	restaurant-type, 7 ¼ oz	14
	Vegetable pulao	
	5 oz	5
	Vegetables	
○	most individual or mixed vegetables: fresh, frozen, canned, or jarred, without added sugar or oil	0
	Vegetables in sauce	
	frozen, ½ cup	2
	Vegetables, Chinese	
	prepared with oil, 7 oz	6
	prepared without oil, 7 oz	3
	Vegetables, creamed	
	except creamed corn, ½ cup	1
	Vegetables, fried	
	3 oz	5
	Vegetables, mixed	
○	canned, drained (corn, peas, carrots), ½ cup	1
	carrots and parsnips, 1 cup	1
○	drained, ½ cup	2
○	frozen, unprepared, ½ cup	1
○	gumbo-style vegetables, frozen, 1 cup	5
○	peas and carrots, canned, solids and liquids, ½ cup	1
○	peas and carrots, cooked or uncooked, ½ cup	1
○	peas and onions, canned, solids and liquids, ½ cup	1
○	peas and onions, cooked, ½ cup	1
○	peas and onions, unprepared, ½ cup	2

○ No Count		SmartPoints® value
	Vegetables, oven-roasted	
○	with 1 tsp olive oil, 1 cup	2
	with pan drippings, ½ cup	2
	Vegetables, sautéed	
○	with 1 tsp olive oil, 1 cup	2
	Vegetarian breakfast link	
	sausage-type, 1 ½ oz	3
	Vegetarian breakfast patty	
	sausage-type, 1 ⅓ oz	1
	Vegetarian breakfast strips	
	1 (⅓ oz)	1
	Vegetarian burger	
	black bean, frozen, 1 ½ oz	3
○	fat-free, frozen, 2 ¾ oz	1
	vegetarian burger, frozen, 2 ¾ oz	3
○	with 2 g fat or less, 1 (3 oz)	2
	Vegetarian chicken	
○	patty, frozen, 1 (3 oz)	3
	pieces, nugget-style, frozen, 2 ¾ oz	4
	Vegetarian chili	
	1 cup	7
	Vegetarian deli slices	
	frozen, 2 ¾ oz	1
	Vegetarian ground meat	
○	frozen, ½ cup	1
	Vegetarian luncheon meat	
	1 ½ oz	1
	Vegetarian sausage	
	frozen, 1 ⅓ oz	2
	Vegetarian topping	
○	made with soy, 1 ½ oz	1
	Venison	
○	cooked, 3 oz	2
○	raw, 4 oz	2
	Venison, ground	
	cooked, 3 oz	4
	raw, 4 oz	4

◯ No Count	SmartPoints® value
Vindaloo	
chicken, 8 oz	7
lamb, 8 ⅓ oz	20
pork, 8 ⅓ oz	9
Vinegar	
any type except balsamic, 1 Tbsp	0
balsamic, 1 Tbsp	1
seasoned rice wine, 1 Tbsp	2

W

◯ No Count	SmartPoints® value
Waffle	
any type, frozen, 2 (2 ½ oz)	6
any type, low-fat, frozen, 2 (2 ¾ oz)	5
Belgian, frozen (2"-3"), 1 (1 oz)	3
made from mix (7" round), 1 (2 ⅔ oz)	7
mini, frozen, 4 (1 ¾ oz)	4
whole-grain, frozen, 2 (2 ⅔ oz)	5
Walnuts	
¼ cup	6
black, dried, ¼ cup	5
chopped, ¼ cup	6
glazed, 1 oz	5
Wasabi paste	
prepared, 1 Tbsp	1
Wasabi powder	
1 Tbsp	1
Water	
8 fl oz	0
Wheat berries	
◯ cooked, 1 cup	5
◯ raw, 2 oz	5
Wheat germ	
2 Tbsp	1
Whitefish and pike	
store-bought, 3 oz	3
Wiener schnitzel	
3 oz	10
Wine	
dessert, dry, 3 ½ fl oz	5
dessert, sweet, 3 ½ fl oz	7
light, 5 fl oz	2
prosecco, 5 fl oz	4
red, 5 fl oz	4
white, 5 fl oz	4
Wine cooler	
5 fl oz	4
Wine spritzer	
8 fl oz	3
Wine, cooking	
1 Tbsp	1
Wine, non-alcoholic	
5 fl oz	0
Wontons	
boiled, 6 (6 oz)	7
fried, 6 (4 oz)	13
Wrap	
chicken Caesar, restaurant-type, 10 ½ oz	18
lettuce, beef, 1 (3 oz)	2
lettuce, chicken, 1 (3 oz)	2
Wrapper	
egg roll, 1 (½ oz)	1
lumpia, 1 oz	2
spinach, 1 wrap (2 ½ oz)	6
wonton, 5 (1 ½ oz)	3
wonton/egg roll, 1 oz	2

Y

Yaki-soba	
beef, 5 ⅔ oz	5
chicken, 5 ⅔ oz	5
pork, 5 ⅔ oz	6
Yakitori	
7 ½ oz	5

"We Like This!" item

No Count	Food	SmartPoints® value
	Yam	
	canned, in syrup, ½ cup	5
●	cooked, ½ cup	2
●	uncooked, ½ cup	3
	Yam patty	
	frozen, 1 (4 oz)	3
	Yogurt	
	fat-free, flavored (vanilla, lemon, coffee), sweetened with sugar, 1 cup	7
	fat-free, fruit-flavored, sweetened with sugar, 1 cup	11
●	fat-free, plain, 1 cup	5
●	light (artificially sweetened), 1 cup	5
	low-fat, plain, 1 cup	6
	low-fat, sweetened with sugar, flavored (vanilla, lemon, coffee), 1 cup	10
	low-fat, sweetened with sugar, fruit-flavored, 1 cup	12
	low-fat, vanilla, 1 cup	10
	whole milk, plain, 1 cup	6
	Yogurt drink	
	1 cup	9
	mango lassi, 1 cup	8
	Yogurt parfait	
	low-fat, with fruit and granola, 1 (5 ⅓ oz)	6
	Yogurt, Greek	
●	fat-free, plain, 1 cup	3
	fat-free, vanilla, 1 cup	5
	low-fat, plain, 1 cup	4
	low-fat, vanilla, 1 cup	9
	Yorkshire pudding	
	1 (5 oz)	9
	Yosenabe	
	13 ¼ oz	3
	Yucca (cassava)	
	raw, ½ cup	5

Z

No Count	Food	SmartPoints® value
	Zabaglione	
	½ cup	7
	Zeppole	
	1 (3 oz)	9
	Ziti, baked	
	with meat, 8 ⅔ oz	13
	without meat, 8 oz	9
	Zucchini	
	breaded, prepared without fat, 6 pieces (3 oz)	6
●	Italian-style, canned, ½ cup	1
	Zucchini bread	
	1 slice (2 oz)	9
	Zuppa di pesce	
	14 oz	10
	Zwieback	
	4 (1 oz)	4

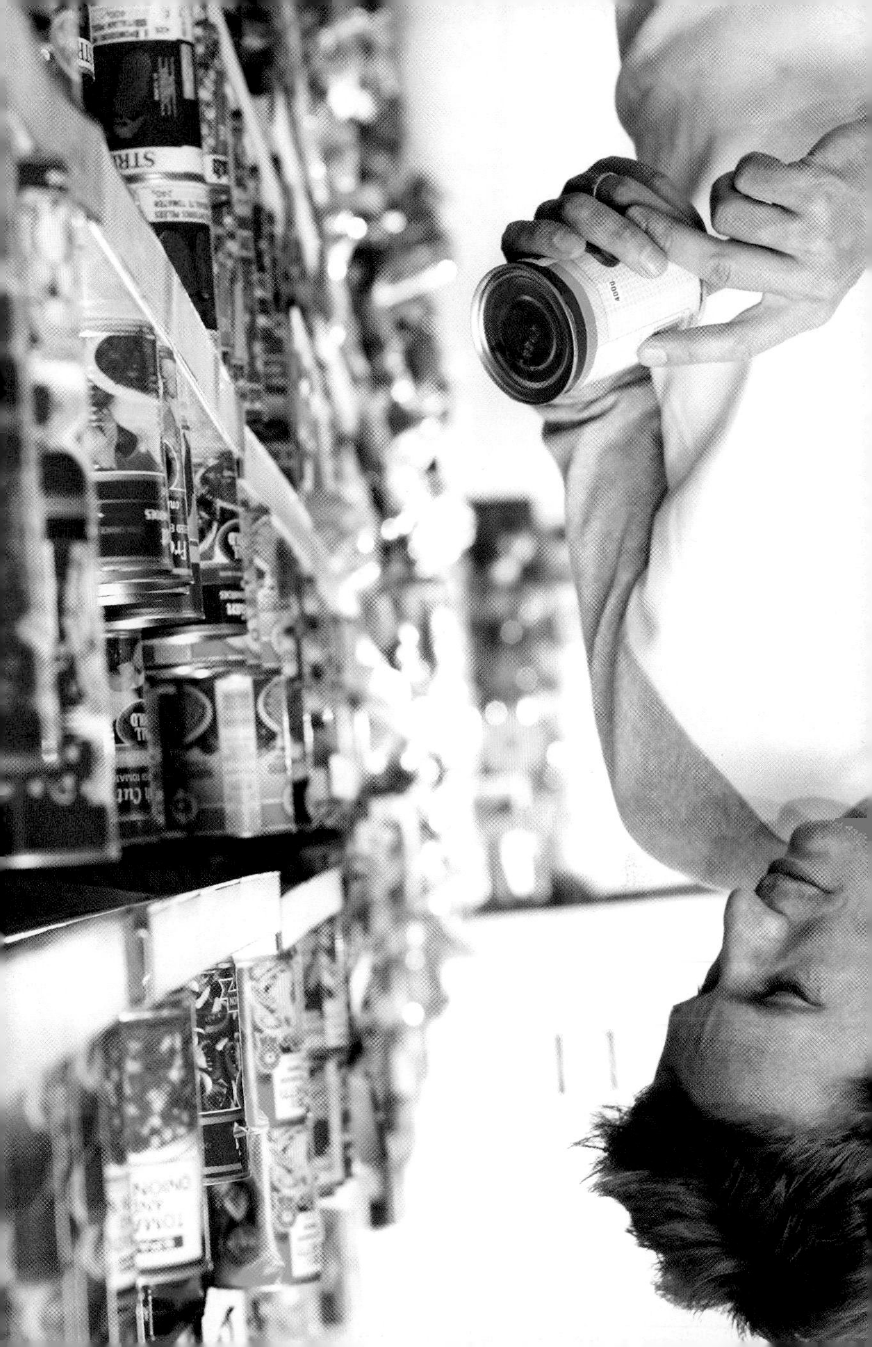

brand name food list

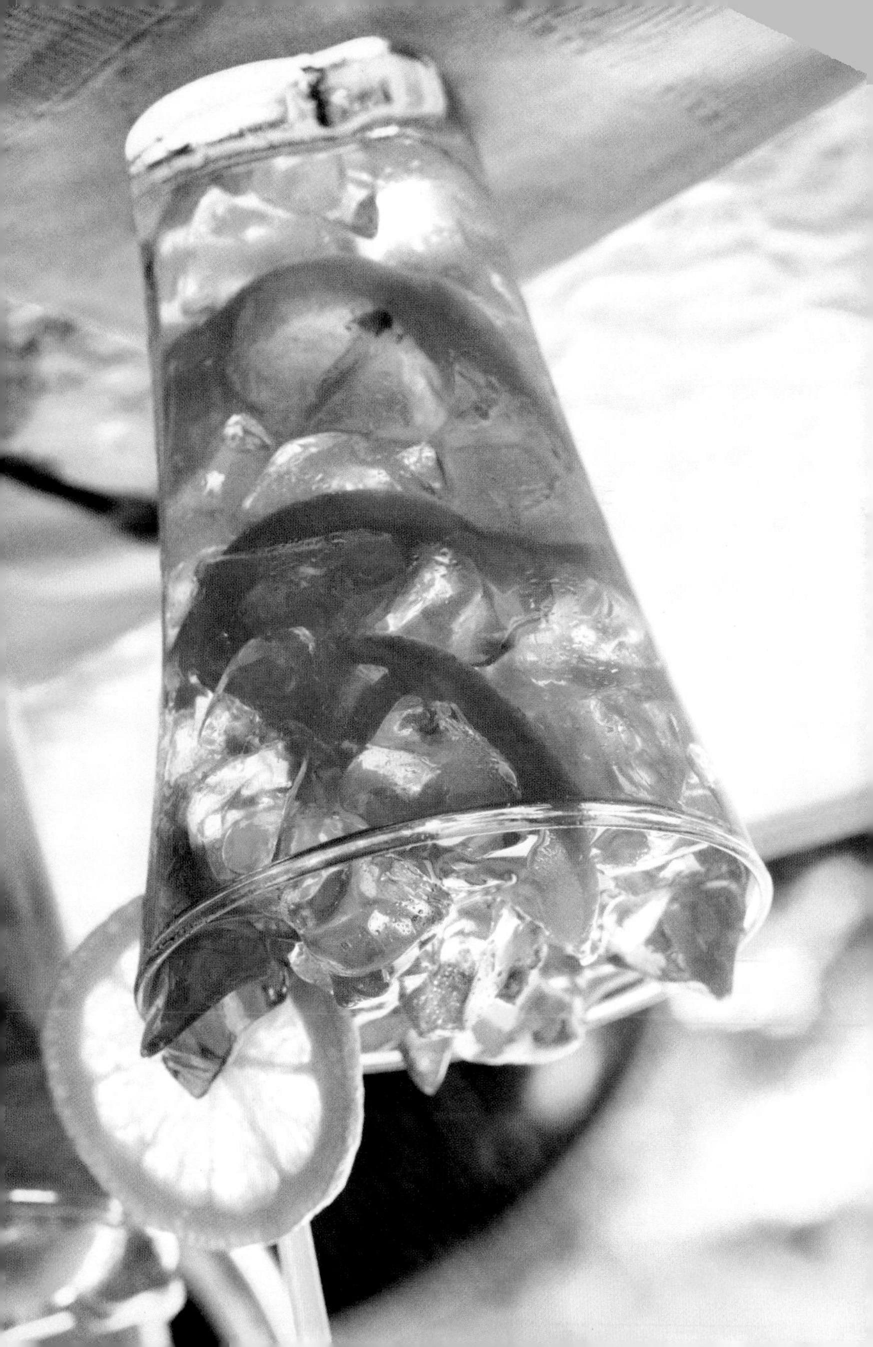

beverages

	SmartPoints® value
Alcoholic Beverages	
Absolut	
Vodka, 1½ fl oz	3
Bacardi	
Puerto Rican rum, 1½ fl oz	3
Bacardi Superior	
Puerto Rican rum, 1½ fl oz	3
Bailey's	
The original Irish cream liqueur, 3½ fl oz	15
Captain Morgan	
Spiced rum, original, 1½ fl oz	3
Crown Royal	
Regal apple flavored whisky, 1½ fl oz	3
Whisky, 1½ fl oz	3
Fireball	
Red hot cinnamon whiskey, 1½ fl oz	4
Grey Goose	
Vodka, 1½ fl oz	3
Henry's Hard Soda	
Hard ginger ale, 12 fl oz	7
Hard orange soda, 12 fl oz	6
Jack Daniel's Old No. 7 Brand	
Tennessee whiskey, 1 fl oz	3
Jose Cuervo	
Margarita, golden, 1½ fl oz	2
Malibu	
Caribbean rum with natural coconut flavor, 1½ fl oz	3
Redd's	
Wicked apple ale, 12 fl oz	9
Seagram's	
7 crown blended whiskey, 1½ fl oz	4
Skinnygirl	
Margarita, 1½ fl oz	1
Smirnoff	
Ice peach bellini, 1 bottle (336 ml)	10

	SmartPoints® value
Beer/Ale	
Amstel	
Lager, light, 12 fl oz	3
Angry Orchard Hard Cider	
Crisp apple, 12 fl oz	9
Beck's	
Beer, premier light, 12 fl oz	2
Blue Moon	
Ale, Belgian-style wheat, Belgian white, 1 bottle (355 ml)	5
Belgian pale ale, 12 fl oz	5
Belgian white, 1 can or bottle (340.19 g)	5
Bud Light	
Beer, 12 fl oz	4
Beer, lime, 12 fl oz	3
Beer, platinum, 12 fl oz	5
Platinum beer, 12 fl oz	5
Budweiser	
Beer, 12 fl oz	5
Bud light, 12 fl oz	4
Select, 12 fl oz	3
Busch	
Light beer, 12 fl oz	3
Coors	
Light, 1 can or bottle (340.19 g)	3
Coors Light	
Beer, 12 fl oz	3
Corona Extra	
Beer, 1 can (355 ml)	5
Corona Light	
Beer, 12 fl oz	3
Dos Equis XX	
Beer, lager especial, 1 bottle (355 ml)	5
Fat Tire	
Ale, amber, 1 bottle (355 ml)	5
Fat tire draft beer, 14 fl oz	6
Guinness	
American blonde lager, 12 fl oz	5
Beer, draught, 12 fl oz	4

	SmartPoints® value
Guinness Draught	
Stout, pasteurized, 1 can (441 ml)	6
Heineken	
Beer, lager, 1 bottle (355 ml)	5
Heineken Light	
Imported premium lager beer, 1 bottle (354 ml)	3
Labatt Blue Light	
Beer, Canadian pilsner, 12 oz	4
Lagunitas Brewing	
India pale ale, 12 fl oz	6
Leinenkugel's	
Summer shandy, 12 fl oz	4
Sunset wheat beer, 12 fl oz	5
Michelob	
Michelob ultra brand beer, 12 fl oz	3
Michelob Light	
Beer, 12 oz	4
Michelob Ultra	
Superior light beer, 1 bottle (355 ml)	3
Superior light beer, 1 can (354 ml)	3
Miller	
Beer, lite, 12 fl oz	6
Henry Weinhard's woodland pass ipa, 1 can or bottle (340.19 g)	6
Mgd 64, 12 fl oz	2
Miller 64, 1 can or bottle (340.19 g)	2
Miller Lite	
Pilsner beer, 1 can (354 ml)	3
Modelo Especial	
Beer, imported, especial, 1 bottle (355 ml)	5
Natural Light	
Beer, 1 can (354 ml)	3
O Doul's	
Malt beverage, premium, non-alcoholic brew, 12 oz	2
Redd's	
Apple ale, 1 bottle (355 ml)	5

	SmartPoints® value
Sam Adams	
Beer, light, 12 oz	4
Samuel Adams	
Lager, Boston, 1 bottle (355 ml)	5
Select 55	
Beer, premium light, 12 fl oz	2
Shiner Bock	
Beer, 1 bottle (355 ml)	5
Shock Top	
Ale, Belgian white, 1 bottle (355 ml)	5
Sierra Nevada	
Pale ale, 1 bottle (355 ml)	5
Stella Artois	
Beer, premium lager, imported, 1 bottle (331 ml)	5
Yuengling	
Draft beer, 14 fl oz	6
Lager, light, 1 bottle (355 ml)	3
Lager, traditional, original amber, 1 bottle (355 ml)	5

Cider, Hard

Angry Orchard	
Hard cider, crisp apple, 1 bottle (355 ml)	9
Crispin	
Hard apple cider, 12 fl oz	6
Hard apple cider, natural, brut, 12 fl oz	6
Johnny Appleseed	
Hard apple cider, 12 fl oz	9

Cocktail Mixes

Margaritaville	
Margarita, skinny, 4 fl oz	3
Mr & Mrs T	
Bloody Mary mix, bold & spicy, 4 fl oz	2
On the Border	
Mexican grill & cantina frozen margarita drink mix, 5 fl oz	7

Cocktail Mixes (cont'd)

	SmartPoints® value
Wegman's	
Cocktail mixer, lemon drop martini, 3 fl oz	4
Weight Watchers In-Meeting/ Online Products: Cocktail Mixers	
Cosmopolitan city, 3 fl oz	0
Margarita mambo, 3 fl oz	0
Zing Zang	
Bloody Mary mix, 3 fl oz	1

Cocoa and Chocolate Drinks

	SmartPoints® value
Beaumont Cocoa Grocery	
Instant dark chocolate hot chocolate, 1 packet (28 g)	6
Café Escapes	
K-cups, hot cocoa, dark chocolate, 1 pack (15 g)	3
K-cups, hot cocoa, milk chocolate flavored, 1 portion pack (15 g)	3
Caffe D'Vita	
Hot cocoa mix, 3 Tbsp	6
Dunkin' Donuts	
Milk chocolate hot cocoa k-cups, 1 k-cup	3
FLAVIA®	
Dove® hot chocolate, 1 serving (20 g)	4
Gevalia	
Peppermint mocha latte, 1 serving (8 g)	4
Grove Square	
Hot cocoa (single serve cup), 1 serving (15 g)	3
Ideal Protein	
Chocolate drink mix, 1 packet (33 g)	2
Kroger	
Hot cocoa mix, Dutch, fat free, milk chocolate, 1 packet (8 g)	1
Nestlé	
Chocolate flavor drink mix, 2 Tbsp	3
Dark chocolate hot cocoa mix, 1 packet (20 g)	4
Fat free hot cocoa mix, 2 Tbsp	1
Hot cocoa mix, rich milk chocolate flavor, 1 envelope (20 g)	4
Hot cocoa mix, rich milk chocolate flavor, fat free, 2 Tbsp	1
Rich milk chocolate fat free hot chocolate mix, 1 envelope (28 g)	1
Nestlé Nesquik	
Chocolate flavor no sugar added powder drink mix, 2 Tbsp	1
Chocolate flavor powder mix, 2 Tbsp	3
Nutrisystem Nutricrush	
Chocolate shake mix, 1 packet (41 g)	5
Nutrisystem Turbo Shake	
Chocolate shake mix, 1 packet (36 g)	4
Ovaltine	
Drink mix, chocolate malt, 4 Tbsp (21 g)	4
Rich chocolate drink mix, 2 Tbsp	2
Publix	
No sugar added hot cocoa mix, 1 pouch (15 g)	2
Slimfast 3-2-1 Plan	
Shake mix, chocolate royale, 1 scoop (26 g)	4
Starbucks	
Classic hot cocoa k-cup, 1 k-cup	5
Starbucks Grocery	
Classic hot cocoa, 1 serving (21 g)	5
Gourmet hot cocoa, 1 pouch (35 g)	7
White chocolate mocha instant latte, 1 packet (35 g)	7
Stephen's	
Milk chocolate gourmet hot cocoa, 3 Tbsp	8
Sugar Babies	
Premium hot cocoa, 1 serving (15 g)	3

	SmartPoints® value
Swiss Miss	
Hot cocoa mix, milk chocolate, ¼ cup	3
Marshmallow hot cocoa mix, 1 packet (21 g)	4
Milk chocolate hot cocoa, 1 serving (15 g)	3
Milk chocolate hot cocoa mix, 1 pouch (21 g)	4
Milk chocolate hot cocoa mix, 3 Tbsp	5
Milk chocolate hot cocoa mix k-cup, 1 serving (15 g)	3
Sensible sweets diet hot chocolate mix, 1 envelope (8 g)	1
Sensible sweets no sugar added hot chocolate mix, 1 envelope (16 g)	3
Simply cocoa dark chocolate flavor hot cocoa mix, 1 envelope (27 g)	5
Swiss Miss Classics	
Hot cocoa mix, milk chocolate flavor, 1 envelope (21 g)	4
Milk chocolate hot chocolate k-cup, 1 k-cup	3
Tootsie Roll	
Hot cocoa mix, 1 serving (15 g)	3

Coffee, Cappuccino, and Latte

	SmartPoints® value
Atkins	
Mocha latte shake, 11 fl oz	4
Atkins Advantage	
Mocha latte shake, 11 fl oz	4
Big Train	
Chamba chai latte drink mix, 3 Tbsp	8
Bolthouse Farms	
Salted caramel latte, 11 fl oz	8
Café Bustelo	
Cafe espresso, 1 oz	0
Espresso coffee, 1 fl oz	0
Café Escapes	
Cafe caramel, 1 serving (15 g)	3
Cafe caramel k-cups, 1 k-cup	3
Chai latte k-cup packs, 1 k-cup	3
K-cups, coffee, cafe mocha, 1 k-cup	3
Califia Farms	
Pure cafe latte iced coffee with almond milk, 8 fl oz	4
Coffee People	
K-cup, extra bold, medium roast, donut shop coffee, 1 cup	0
Coffee People Donut Shop	
K-cups, coffee, flavored medium roast, coconut mocha, 1 cup	0
Daily Chef	
French vanilla cappuccino beverage mix, 1 scoop (19 g)	4
French vanilla cappuccino mix, 1 serving (15 g)	4
Donut House Collection Keurig Brewed	
Donut house coffee light roast k-cups, 1 k-cup	0
Dunkin' Donuts	
Coffee, ground, French vanilla, 1 cup	0
Coffee, ground, original blend, 1 cup	0
Hazelnut flavored coffee, 1 cup	0
Original blend coffee k-cups, 1 k-cup	0
Eight O'Clock	
Hazelnut coffee k-cups, 1 single serve cup (9.5 g)	0
Folgers	
100% Colombian med-dark roast ground coffee, brewed, 6 fl oz	0
100% Colombian medium dark ground coffee, 1 cup	0
Black silk dark roast ground coffee, brewed, 6 fl oz	0
Cappuccino, French vanilla, 8 oz	4

Beverages

Coffee, Cappuccino, and Latte, Folgers (cont'd)

	SmartPoints® value
Classic medium roast coffee k-cups, 1 k-cup	0
Classic roast coffee crystals, 1 serving (2 g)	0
Classic roast instant coffee crystals, 6 fl oz	0
Coffee, medium, classic roast, 1 cup	0
Folgers Gourmet Selections	
Vanilla biscotti flavored coffee k-cup, 1 k-cup	0
General Foods International	
Coffeehouse beverage mix, cafe francais, 1⅓ Tbsp	3
Gevalia	
Cappuccino, 2-step, 1 coffee cup (27 g)	5
Mocha latte, 2-step, 1 serving (169 g)	4
Gloria Jeans	
Butter toffee medium roast coffee k-cups, 6 fl oz	0
Green Mountain Coffee	
Breakfast blend k-cups, 1 k-cup	0
Caramel vanilla cream flavored k-cup, 1 k-cup	0
Hazelnut k-cup coffee, 1 k-cup	0
Green Mountain Coffee Keurig Brewed	
Nantucket blend medium roast coffee k-cups, 1 k-cup	0
Grove Square	
French vanilla cappuccino k-cup, 1 k-cup	4
French vanilla cappuccino mix, 1 single serve cup (15 g)	4
Hazelnut cappuccino (k-cup), 1 k-cup	4
Hills Bros.	
Cappuccino drink mix, English toffee, 3 Tbsp	6
Cappuccino drink mix, sugar free, French vanilla, 2 Tbsp	2

	SmartPoints® value
French vanilla cappuccino cafe style drink mix, 1 serving (20 g)	5
International Delight	
Iced coffee, sweet & creamy light, mocha, 1 cup	5
Keurig Café Escapes	
Chai latte, 1 latte (14 g)	3
Keurig Cinnabon	
Classic cinnamon roll k-cups, 1 k-cup	0
Kirkland Signature	
Fine grind dark roast supremo bean 100% Colombian coffee (prepared), 8 fl oz	0
Kroger	
French vanilla k-cup cappuccino, 1 serving (15 g)	4
Hazelnut cappuccino, 1 serving (15 g)	4
Maxwell House	
Breakfast blend ground coffee, 6 fl oz	0
Original roast ground coffee, 6 fl oz	0
Maxwell House International Café	
Beverage mix, cafe-style, cafe Vienna, 1⅓ Tbsp	4
Beverage mix, cafe-style, French vanilla, 1⅓ Tbsp	1
Beverage mix, cafe-style, hazelnut, 1⅓ Tbsp	4
Beverage mix, cafe-style, sugar free, decaffeinated, suisse mocha cafe, 1⅓ Tbsp	1
Beverage mix, sugar free, decaffeinated, French vanilla, 1⅓ Tbsp	1
Beverage mix, cafe-style, vanilla caramel, 1⅓ Tbsp	3
McCafé	
Medium roast coffee k-cup packs, 1 k-cup	0
Milton's	
Pacific bold dark roast coffee, 1 serving (30 g)	4

	SmartPoints® value
Nescafé	
Clasico pure instant coffee, 1 tsp	0
Nescafé Taster's Choice	
Coffee, gourmet instant, original, 1 cup	0
House blend instant coffee (prepared), 6 fl oz	0
Starbucks	
Bottled mocha lite frappuccino coffee drink (9.5 fl oz), 1 bottle (281 ml)	4
Caramel flavor coffee k-cup, 1 k-cup	0
Cinnamon dolce coffee k-cups, 1 k-cup	0
Espresso beverage, chilled, skinny caramel macchiato, 8 fl oz	3
Espresso beverage, chilled, skinny vanilla latte, 8 fl oz	3
K-cups, coffee, blonde roast, veranda blend, 1 k-cup	0
K-cups, coffee, dark, French roast, 1 cup	0
K-cups, coffee, medium, breakfast blend, 1 cup	0
K-cups, coffee, medium, house blend, 1 cup	0
K-cups, coffee, medium, pike place roast, 1 cup	0
Lightly sweetened premium iced coffee beverage, 1 cup	3
Low calorie iced coffee and milk, 1 bottle (330 g)	2
Skinny vanilla latte chilled espresso beverage, 8 fl oz	3
Unsweetened premium iced coffee beverage, 1 cup	0
Starbucks Coffee Doubleshot	
Coffee drink, premium, espresso & cream, 1 can (190 ml)	7
Starbucks Coffee Doubleshot Light	
Coffee drink, premium, espresso & cream, 6½ fl oz	3

	SmartPoints® value
Starbucks Frappuccino	
Coffee drink, light, vanilla, 1 bottle (281 ml)	4
Mocha coffee drink, 1 bottle (281 ml)	9
Starbucks Grocery	
Skinny caramel macchiato, 8 fl oz	3
Tazo	
Chai latte black tea concentrate, ½ cup	4

Flavorings/Nutrient Enhancers for Water

Fit & Active	
Strawberry watermelon water enhancer, ½ tsp	0
Weight Watchers In-Meeting/ Online Products: Water Enhancers	
Berry pomegranate, 2 ml	0
Pink punch, 2 ml	0
Southern sweet tea, 2 ml	0

Fruit Juices and Drinks

Alpine Sugar Free	
Spiced apple cider instant drink mix, 1 pouch (4 g)	0
Bai Antioxidant Infusions	
Antioxidant beverage, Brasilia blueberry, 8 fl oz	0
Antioxidant beverage, Costa Rica clementine, 8 fl oz	0
Antioxidant beverage, Ipanema pomegranate, 8 fl oz	0
Beverage, Molokai coconut, 8 fl oz	0
BluePrint Cold Pressed Juice	
Beet, apple, carrot, lemon, ginger juice, 1 bottle (295 ml)	6
Crystal Light Energy	
Drink mix, grape, ½ packet (2 g)	0
Emergen-C	
Raspberry flavored fizzy drink mix with vitamins, 1 packet (9.1 g)	1

Fruit Juices and Drinks, Emergen-C (cont'd)

	SmartPoints® value
Super orange flavored fizzy drink mix, 1 packet (8.8 g)	1
Florida's Natural	
Juice, orange, no pulp, 8 fl oz	6
Premium orange juice, 8 fl oz	6
Florida's Natural Fit & Delicious	
Valencia orange juice beverage with calcium and vitamin D, 8 fl oz	3
Goya	
Diet pear nectar, 1 can (284 ml)	4
Great Value	
Orange juice with calcium, 8 fl oz	6
Juicy Juice	
100% apple juice, 8 fl oz	6
Kirkland Signature	
Organic coconut water, 11 fl oz	3
Kroger	
Lite orange juice, 8 fl oz	2
Member's Mark	
100% apple juice, 8 fl oz	7
Minute Maid	
100% orange juice, 8 fl oz	6
Juice beverage, light, pure squeezed, orange, 8 fl oz	3
Minute Maid Light	
Orange juice beverage, light, pure squeezed, no pulp, 8 fl oz	3
Mountain Dew Kickstart	
Sparkling juice beverage, energizing, black cherry, 1 can (473 ml)	5
Ocean Spray	
100% cranberry juice, 8 fl oz	7
100% cranberry juice, 8 fl oz	7
Apple white cranberry juice drink, 8 fl oz	5
Cran pomegranate juice drink, 1 bottle (295 ml)	9
Cran-grape juice drink, 8 fl oz	7
Juice beverage, diet, cranberry, 8 fl oz	0

	SmartPoints® value
Juice beverage, diet, cranberry grape, 8 fl oz	0
Juice drink, diet, cranberry pomegranate, 8 fl oz	0
Juice drink, diet, cran-mango, 8 fl oz	0
Light cranberry juice cocktail, 8 fl oz	2
Ocean Spray Diet	
Cranberry and concord grape juice drink, 8 fl oz	3
Juice drink, cranberry, 8 fl oz	3
Juice drink, cran-raspberry (64 oz container, "light"), 8 fl oz	2
Juice drink, ruby red, 8 fl oz	2
Pom Wonderful	
Pomegranate juice, 8 fl oz	8
ReaLemon	
Lemon juice, natural strength, 1 tsp	0
Silk Pure Coconut	
Coconutmilk, unsweetened, 1 cup	2
Original coconut milk, 1 cup	4
Simple Truth	
Unsweetened coconut milk, 1 cup	3
Simply Grapefruit	
Grapefruit juice, pulp free, original, 8 fl oz	5
Simply Orange	
100% orange juice, pulp free, 1 bottle (340 ml)	9
Juice blend, 100%, with mango, 8 oz	6
Orange juice, country stand, calcium, medium pulp, 8 fl oz	6
Orange juice, high pulp, 8 fl oz	6
Orange juice, pulp free, 1 bottle (400 ml)	10
So Delicious	
Coconut milk beverage, unsweetened vanilla, 1 cup	2
Coconut milk, beverage, unsweetened, 1 cup	3

	SmartPoints® value
Unsweetened coconut milk beverage, 1 cup	2
Unsweetened vanilla flavor coconut milk, 4 fl oz	3
Suja Essentials	
Organic daybreak probiotic fruit juice drink, 1 bottle (354 ml)	6
Sunsweet	
Juice, prune, 8 fl oz	8
Prune juice cocktail, light, 8 fl oz	4
Trader Joe's	
Unpasteurized fresh squeezed orange juice, 8 fl oz	6
Unsweetened coconut milk beverage, 8 fl oz	3
Tropicana	
Juice, orange, no pulp, original, 8 fl oz	6
Orange juice, low acid, 8 fl oz	6
Tropicana Pure Premium	
100% juice, orange, no pulp original, 8 fl oz	6
100% juice, orange, no pulp, calcium + vitamin D, 8 fl oz	6
100% juice, orange, some pulp homestyle, 8 fl oz	6
Tropicana Trop50	
Juice beverage, orange, no pulp, 8 fl oz	3
Juice beverage, orange, some pulp, 8 fl oz	3
Orange juice, calcium + vitamin D, no pulp, 8 fl oz	3
V8 V-Fusion	
+energy beverage blend, orange pineapple, 8 fl oz	3
Zico	
Coconut water, pure premium, 8 oz	3

Lemonade

	SmartPoints® value
Crystal Light	
Lemonade, 8 fl oz	0
Minute Maid Just 15 Calories	
Lemonade, 8 fl oz	1
Minute Maid Light	
Lemonade, 8 fl oz	0
Wawa Grocery	
Strawberry lemonade, 1 bottle (480 ml)	14

Smoothies

	SmartPoints® value
Bolthouse Farms	
Green goodness fruit smoothie, 8 fl oz	8
Multi v goodness fruit juice smoothie, 8 fl oz	7
Strawberry banana fruit juice smoothie, 8 fl oz	7
Concord Foods	
Kale and apple smoothie mix, 5 tsp	2
Dannon Light & Fit	
Mixed berry protein smoothie, 1 bottle (281 ml)	4
Raspberries and cream protein smoothie, 9½ fl oz	4
Salted caramel protein smoothie, 1 bottle (281 ml)	4
Dole Shakers	
Smoothie, fruit, strawberry, 4 oz	4
Fresh & Easy	
Smoothie, primary greens, 8 fl oz	1
Fresh Start Organic	
Berries kale spinach smoothie blend, 1 pouch (227 g)	4
Kroger CARBmaster	
Blueberry cream protein smoothie, 1 bottle (296 ml)	2
Raspberry cream protein smoothie, 1 bottle (296 ml)	2
Strawberry protein smoothie, 1 bottle (296 ml)	2
Tropical mango protein smoothie, 1 bottle (296 ml)	2

Smoothies, Kroger CARBmaster (cont'd)

	SmartPoints® value
Vanilla cream protein smoothie, 1 bottle (296 ml)	2
Lifeway	
Kefir cultured milk smoothie, lowfat, blueberry, 1 cup	6
Kefir cultured milk smoothie, lowfat, plain, unsweetened, 1 cup	4
Kefir cultured milk smoothie, lowfat, strawberry, 1 cup	6
Market Pantry	
Berry fruit smoothie, ½ fl oz	6
Naked	
100% juice smoothie, boosted, green machine, 8 fl oz	7
Berry almond almond milk juice smoothie, 1 bottle (450 ml)	14
Green machine juice smoothie, 10 fl oz	9
Peachy almond almond milk juice smoothie, 1 bottle (450 ml)	12
Premier Protein	
High protein shake, chocolate, 11 fl oz	2
Strawberry creme high protein shake, 1 shake (325 ml)	2
Private Selection	
Triple berry medley smoothie blend, 1 cup	3
Slimfast Smoothie	
Creamy chocolate high protein meal replacement beverage mix, 1 scoop (26 g)	2
Vega	
Choc-a-lot protein smoothie, 1 scoop (26 g)	2
Vega One	
Viva vanilla protein smoothie drink mix, 1 scoop (22 g)	1
Weight Watchers In-Meeting/ Online Products: Smoothies	
Creamy chocolate, 1 slim pack	2
French vanilla, 1 slim pack	2

	SmartPoints® value
Salted caramel super smoothie, 1 slim pack	3
Triple berry super smoothie, 1 slim pack	3
Weight Watchers Smart Ones Smart Delights	
Mixed berry smoothie, 1 cup	5
Strawberry banana smoothie, 1 cup	5
Tropical fruit smoothie, 1 cup	5

Soft Drinks, Carbonated

7 Up	
Soda, 8 fl oz	6
Soda, diet, 1 can (57 ml)	0
A&W	
Root beer, 8 fl oz	7
Root beer, diet, 1 bottle (236 ml)	0
A&W Ten	
Root beer, 1 can (355 ml)	1
Canada Dry	
Cranberry ginger ale, 1 can (355 ml)	9
Ginger ale, 1 can (221 ml)	5
Ginger ale, diet, 1 can (355 ml)	0
Clear American	
Wild cherry sparkling water beverage, 8 fl oz	0
Clear American Zero	
Black cherry sparkling water, 1 can (355 ml)	0
Coca-Cola	
Cherry, 12 fl oz	10
Diet coke, 1 can (355 ml)	0
Vanilla zero calorie cola, 1 can (355 ml)	0
Coca-Cola / Coke	
Cola, 12 fl oz	9
Coca-Cola Zero	
Caffeine free zero calorie cola, 1 can (355 ml)	0
Cherry calorie free, 8 fl oz	0
Cola zero calorie, 1 bottle (237 ml)	0

	SmartPoints® value
Coke	
Cola, diet, 12 fl oz	0
Coke Zero	
Cola, 12 fl oz	0
Dr Pepper	
Soda, 1 bottle (500 ml)	13
Soda, 8 fl oz	6
Soda, diet, 1 can (355 ml)	0
Soda, diet, 12 fl oz	0
Soda, diet, cherry, 1 can (355 ml)	0
Dr Pepper Ten	
10 bold tasting calories soda, 8 fl oz	0
Soda, 1 can (355 ml)	1
Fanta	
Soda, orange, 12 fl oz	10
Fresca	
Sparkling citrus flavored beverage, 8 fl oz	0
Izze	
Blackberry pear sparkling water beverage, 12 fl oz	1
Raspberry watermelon sparkling water beverage, 12 fl oz	1
La Croix	
Cherry lime sparkling water, 1 can (355 ml)	0
Coconut sparkling water, 1 can (355 ml)	0
Mountain Dew	
Soda, 12 fl oz	10
Soda, diet, 12 fl oz	0
Mountain Dew Kickstart	
Blueberry pomegranate sparkling juice, 1 can (355 ml)	4
Energizing watermelon soda, 1 can (355 ml)	4
Midnight grape sparkling juice, 1 can (473 ml)	5
Ocean Spray	
Diet sparkling cranberry fruit juice drink, 1 can (248 ml)	1

	SmartPoints® value
Sparkling cranberry fruit juice drink, 1 can (248 ml)	5
Pepsi	
Cola, 12 fl oz	10
Cola, diet, 1 bottle (355 ml)	0
Cola, diet, 1 can (237 ml)	0
Cola, diet, 12 fl oz	0
Cola, diet, 8 oz	0
Cola, diet, caffeine free, 1 can (355 ml)	0
Cola, wild cherry, diet, 8 fl oz	0
Soda, diet, wild cherry, 8 fl oz	0
Wild cherry soda, 1 can (355 ml)	10
Pepsi Max	
Cola, 0 calorie, 8 oz	0
Polar	
Cranberry and clementine seltzer, 8 fl oz	0
Schweppes	
Tonic water, diet, 1 bottle (296 ml)	0
Seagram's	
Ginger ale, 12 fl oz	6
Sierra Mist	
Diet lemon lime soda, 1 can (355 ml)	0
Lemon lime soda caffeine free, 1 can (355 ml)	7
Soy 7	
Lemon lime soda, 1 can (355 ml)	1
Sparkling ICE	
Orange mango sparkling water, 1 bottle (240 ml)	0
Sparkling water, peach nectarine, 8 fl oz	0
Spindrift	
Grapefruit seltzer, 12 fl oz	1
Sprite	
Cranberry lemon lime soda, 1 can (355 ml)	9
Cranberry soda, 1 can (355 ml)	9
Soda, 12 fl oz	9

Soft Drinks, Carbonated (cont'd)

	SmartPoints® value
Sprite Zero	
Soda, diet, 8 fl oz	0
Soda, lemon-lime, zero calorie, 1 can (355 ml)	0
Sunkist	
Soda, diet, orange, 1 can (355 ml)	0
Talking Rain Sparkling Ice	
Cherry limeade sparkling beverage, 8 fl oz	0
Villa Italia	
Italian blood orange soda, 8 fl oz	7

Soy, Rice, and Nut Drinks

	SmartPoints® value
365 Everyday Value	
Organic unsweetened almond milk, 8 fl oz	1
Unsweetened organic almond milk, 1 cup	1
365 Everyday Value Organic	
Unsweetened vanilla almond milk, 1 cup	1
Ahold	
Unsweetened vanilla almond milk, 1 cup	1
Almond Breeze Reduced Sugar	
Original almond milk, 1 cup	1
Vanilla almond milk, 1 cup	3
Almond Breeze Unsweetened	
Almond coconut almond milk coconutmilk blend, 1 cup	2
Chocolate almond milk, 1 cup	1
Vanilla almond coconut almond milk coconutmilk blend, 1 cup	2
Vanilla almond milk, 1 cup	1
Blue Diamond Almond Breeze	
Original almond milk, 1 container (325 ml)	3
Original reduced sugar almond milk, 1 cup	1
Unsweetened almond cashew milk blend, 1 cup	1
Unsweetened original almond milk, 1 cup	1
Unsweetened vanilla almond cashew milk blend, 1 cup	1
Califia Farms	
Chocolate coconut almond milk blend, 8 fl oz	5
Pure toasted coconut almond milk blend, 8 fl oz	2
Califia Farms Pure	
Almond milk, creamy original, 8 fl oz	2
Almond milk, unsweetened, 8 fl oz	1
Almond milk, vanilla, 8 fl oz	2
Calnaturale Svelte	
Protein shake, organic, cappuccino, 11 fl oz	5
Friendly Farms Original	
All natural almond milk, 8 fl oz	3
Giant	
Unsweetened almond milk, 1 cup	1
Giant Eagle	
Unsweetened almond milk, 1 cup	1
Original unsweetened almond milk, 1 cup	1
Vanilla flavored almond milk, 1 cup	4
H-E-B	
Original almond milk, 1 cup	3
Unsweetened almond milk, 1 cup	1
Unsweetened vanilla almond milk, 1 cup	1
Hiland	
Unsweetened almond milk, 1 cup	1
Unsweetened vanilla almond milk, 1 cup	1
Hills Bros.	
Cappuccino drink mix, sugar free, double mocha, 2 Tbsp	2
Hy-Vee	
Unsweetened almond milk, 1 cup	1
Vanilla unsweetened almond milk, 1 cup	1
Kirkland Signature	
Organic vanilla soy milk, 1 cup	3

	SmartPoints® value
Organic vanilla soymilk, 1 fl oz	0
Original organic ricemilk, 1 cup	4
Plain organic soymilk, 1 cup	3
Lucerne Farms	
Unsweetened vanilla almond milk, 1 cup	1
Market Basket	
Unsweetened vanilla almond milk, 1 cup	1
Meijer	
Original unsweetened almond milk, 1 cup	1
Nature's Place	
Unsweetened original almond milk, 1 cup	1
Unsweetened vanilla almond milk, 1 cup	1
ShopRite	
Unsweetened vanilla almond milk, 1 cup	1
Silk	
Almond coconut blend beverage, 8 fl oz	2
Almond coconut blend, unsweetened, 1 cup	1
Cashewmilk, original, 1 cup	3
Cashewmilk, unsweetened, no sugar added, 1 cup	1
Chocolate light soymilk, 1 cup	4
Dark chocolate almond milk, 1 cup	5
Light vanilla soymilk, 1 cup	2
Organic almond milk, 1 cup	3
Original soymilk, 1 cup	3
Soymilk, light, original, 1 cup	2
Unsweetened cashewmilk, 1 cup	1
Unsweetened organic almond milk, 1 cup	1
Unsweetened organic soymilk, 1 cup	2
Unsweetened original almond milk, 1 cup	1

	SmartPoints® value
Unsweetened vanilla flavored almond milk, 1 cup	1
Vanilla almond milk, 1 cup	5
Vanilla soymilk, 1 cup	4
Silk Nutchello	
Caramel almonds + cashews nut based beverage, 1 cup	3
Silk Nutchello	
Rich dark chocolate and walnuts nut based beverage, 1 cup	4
Silk Pure Almond	
Almond milk, dark chocolate, 1 container (236 ml)	6
Almond milk, original, unsweetened, 1 cup	1
Almond milk, vanilla, 1 container (236 ml)	4
Almond milk, vanilla, unsweetened, 1 cup	1
Light original almond milk, 1 cup	2
Light, vanilla almond milk, 1 cup	3
Original almond milk, 1 cup	3
Simple Truth	
Almond milk, 1 cup	3
Chocolate almond milk, 1 cup	3
Unsweetened almond milk, 1 cup	1
Unsweetened vanilla almond milk, 1 cup	1
Vanilla almond milk, 1 cup	3
Simple Truth Organic	
Unsweetened almond milk, 1 cup	1
Unsweetened vanilla almond milk, 1 cup	1
Simply Balanced	
Original unsweetened almond milk, 1 cup	1
Simply Nature	
Organic original soymilk, 1 cup	3
Simply Nature Organic	
Original unsweetened almond milk, 1 cup	1
So Delicious	
Cashew milk, unsweetened, 1 cup	1

Soy, Rice, and Nut Drinks, So Delicious (cont'd)

	SmartPoints® value
Coconut-almond milk blend, 1 cup	2
Unsweetened almond milk, 1 cup	1
Vanilla almond milk, 1 cup	2
Trader Joe's	
Original almond milk, 1 cup	3
Original non-dairy coconut creamer, 1 Tbsp	0
Unsweetened original almond beverage, 1 cup	1
Unsweetened vanilla almond beverage, 1 cup	1
Trader Joe's Refrigerated	
Almond milk - vanilla unsweetened (half gallon), 1 cup	1
Wegman's Organic	
Unsweetened vanilla almond milk, 1 cup	1

Sports and Energy Drinks

	SmartPoints® value
Gatorade G Series	
Fruit punch flavor thirst quencher, 1 bottle (355 ml)	5
Glacier cherry gatorade frost thirst quencher, 1 bottle (355 ml)	5
Orange thirst quencher, 1 bottle (355 ml)	5
Gatorade G2	
Low calorie fruit punch flavored thirst quencher, 12 fl oz	2
Glaceau Vitaminwater Zero	
Vitamin water, power-c, dragonfruit, 1 bottle (591 g)	0
Xxx acai blueberry pomegranate enhanced beverage, 1 bottle (591 g)	0
GTs Enlightened	
Kombucha, organic raw, gingerade, 8 fl oz	1
Kellogg's Special K	
Raspberry cheesecake protein shake, 1 bottle (296 ml)	7
Monster	
Lo-carb energy supplement, 8 fl oz	1
Rehab tea and pink lemonade energy drink, 8 fl oz	1
Monster Energy	
Zero ultra beverage, 8 fl oz	0
Powerade Ion4	
Mountain berry blast sports drink, 1 bottle (355 ml)	5
Red Bull	
Energy drink, the blue edition, 1 can (250 ml)	7
Energy shot, sugar free, 1 bottle (59 ml)	0
Starbucks Refreshers	
Energy drink, sparkling green coffee, raspberry pomegranate, 1 can (355 ml)	3
Energy drink, sparkling green coffee, strawberry lemonade, 1 can (355 ml)	3
Synergy Enlightened	
Kombucha, organic & raw, cosmic cranberry, 8 fl oz	1
Kombucha, organic & raw, trilogy, 8 fl oz	1
V8 V-Fusion	
Cranberry raspberry diet energy drink, 8 fl oz	1

Tea and Iced Tea

	SmartPoints® value
Argo Tea	
Hibiscus tea sangria, 8 fl oz	3
Arizona	
Green tea, diet, with ginseng, 8 fl oz	0
Green tea, with ginseng and honey, 8 fl oz	4
Arizona Arnold Palmer	
Half & half iced tea/lemonade, lite, 8 fl oz	3
Half & half, iced tea/lemonade, zero, 8 fl oz	0

	SmartPoints® value
Bigelow	
Green tea, bags, 8 fl oz	0
Tea, English breakfast, 8 oz	0
Tea, plantation mint, 8 fl oz	0
Brisk	
Iced tea, raspberry flavor, 12 fl oz	4
Celestial Seasonings	
Herbal tea, cinnamon apple spice, 1 tea bag	0
Herbal tea, peppermint, 1 tea bag	0
Celestial Seasonings Sleepytime	
Herbal tea, caffeine free, 1 tea bag	0
Crystal Light	
Beverage, iced tea, 8 oz	0
Gold Peak	
Iced tea, diet, 8 fl oz	0
Iced tea, sweet tea, 12 fl oz	8
Good Earth Sweet & Spicy	
Tea & herb blend, original, bags, 1 tea bag	0
Green Foods	
Green tea, organic, matcha, 2 tsp	1
Honest Tea	
Green tea, organic, honey, 8 fl oz	2
Orange mango flavored herbal tea, 1 bottle (500 ml)	6
Lipton	
Black tea, premium blend, 1 tea bag	0
Diet mixed berry green tea, 1 bottle (500 ml)	0
Green tea with citrus, diet, 8 fl oz	0
Green tea, diet, citrus, 8 fl oz	0
Green tea, naturally decaffeinated, 1 tea bag	0
Iced tea, sweet tea, 8 oz	5
Tea bags, green tea, 1 tea bag	0
Tea, bags, 1 tea bag	0
Lipton Brisk	
Half and half iced tea and lemonade, 1 can (355 ml)	4

	SmartPoints® value
Lipton Pure Leaf	
Peach iced tea, 1 bottle (547 ml)	11
Ice tea, diet, peach, 8 fl oz	0
Oregon Chai	
Original chai tea latte, sugar-free, ½ cup	0
Pure Leaf	
Tea, sweet tea, 8 fl oz	4
Tea, unsweetened, 8 fl oz	0
Red Diamond	
Tea, unsweet, 8 fl oz	0
Snapple	
Diet iced tea, lemon, 1 can (340 ml)	0
Diet peach tea, 1 bottle (473 ml)	0
Lemonade iced tea, half & half, diet, 1 bottle (473 ml)	0
Tea, raspberry, diet, 1 cup	0
Snapple Diet	
Half 'n half, 12 fl oz	0
Tazo	
Black tea, awake English breakfast, filterbags, 1 cup	0
Black tea, organic, chai, filterbags, 1 cup	0
Green tea, zen, filterbags, 1 tea bag	0
Herbal tea, passion, 1 tea bag	0
Tradewinds	
Unsweet tea, 8 fl oz	0
Twinings	
Chai tea, 8 fl oz	0
English breakfast tea, prepared, 6 fl oz	0
Green tea, 1 tea bag	0
Yogi	
Caffeine free detox tea bags, 1 tea bag	0
Ginger tea bag, 1 tea bag	0

Vegetable Juices and Drinks

	SmartPoints® value
Bolthouse Farms	
Carrot juice, 8 fl oz	4
Campbell's	
Juice, tomato, 1 can (163 ml)	1
Tomato juice, 8 fl oz	2
Clamato	
Tomato cocktail, 8 fl oz	3
Nature's Nectar	
100% tomato juice, 8 fl oz	2
Suja Essentials Carrot Crush	
Carrot juice, 1 bottle (354 ml)	7
V8	
100% vegetable juice, low sodium, original, 5½ fl oz	1
100% vegetable juice, low sodium, spicy hot, 8 fl oz	2
Healthy greens juice, 1 bottle (360 ml)	4
Healthy greens veggie blend, 8 fl oz	3
Original 100% vegetable juice, 8 fl oz	2
Original vegetable juice, 1 can (340 ml)	3
Spicy hot 100% vegetable juice, 8 fl oz	2
Spicy hot 100% vegetable juice, 1 can (340 ml)	3
Spicy hot vegetable juice, 8 fl oz	2
Vegetable juice, 8 fl oz	2
V8 Energy	
Original 100% vegetable juice, 1 can (237 g)	2
V8 Splash	
Juice beverage, tropical blend, diet, 8 fl oz	1
V8 V-Fusion Light	
Peach mango beverage blend, 8 fl oz	3
Strawberry banana beverage blend, 8 fl oz	3

Water

	SmartPoints® value
Arrowhead	
Water, 100% mountain spring, 16.9 fl oz	0
Dasani	
Purified water, 1 bottle (355 ml)	0
Water, purified, 8 fl oz	0
Deer Park	
Spring water, 100% natural, 16.9 fl oz	0
Glaceau Vitaminwater Zero	
Water beverage, nutrient enhanced, rise, naturally sweetened, orange, 8 fl oz	0
Water beverage, nutrient enhanced, xxx, naturally sweetened, acai-blueberry-pomegranate, 8 fl oz	0
Ice Mountain	
Water, 100% natural spring, 9 fl oz (266 ml)	0
Kirkland	
Purified drinking water, 1 bottle (500 ml)	0
La Croix	
Natural mango essenced sparkling water, 1 can (355 ml)	0
Sparkling water, 12 fl oz	0
Sparkling water, grapefruit, 1 can (355 ml)	0
Sparkling water, lime, 8 fl oz	0
Nestlé Pure Life	
Water, purified, 16.9 fl oz	0
Ozarka	
Spring water, 100% natural, 16.9 fl oz	0
Perrier	
Mineral water, sparkling, natural, 8 fl oz	0
Poland Spring	
Water, natural spring, 16.9 fl oz	0
Protein 2 O	
Grape splash protein enhanced water, 1 bottle (500 ml)	1

	SmartPoints® value
PurAqua	
Purified water, 8 fl oz	0
S. Pellegrino	
Mineral water, sparkling natural, 1 bottle (250 ml)	0
Sam's Choice	
Purified drinking water, 8 fl oz	0
Sam's Choice Clear American	
Naturally flavored sparkling water beverage, 8 fl oz	0
Schweppes	
Black cherry sparkling seltzer water, 1 can (360 ml)	0
Sparkling ICE	
Black raspberry sparkling water, 1 cup	0
Vita Coco	
Coconut water, 100% pure, 1 bottle (330 ml)	4

Wine and Wine Coolers

	SmartPoints® value
Barefoot® Cellars	
Moscato wine, 5 fl oz	5
Pink moscato, 5 fl oz	5
Riesling wine, 5 fl oz	4
Sauvignon blanc, 5 fl oz	4
Sweet red wine, 5 fl oz	4
Bella Sera	
Pinot grigio, 5 fl oz	4
Beringer	
2003 white zinfandel, 4 fl oz	4
Black Box	
Cabernet sauvignon wine, 5 fl oz	5
Cupcake Vineyards	
Marlborough sauvignon blanc, 5 fl oz	4
Folie A Deux	
Sauvignon blanc, 5 fl oz	4
Franzia	
Sunset blush, 5 fl oz	4
Franzia House Wine Favorites	
Sangria, fruity red, 5 fl oz	4
Il Conte	
Stella rosa red wine, 5 fl oz	4
Kendall-Jackson Vintner's Reserve	
2002 California chardonnay, 5 fl oz	4
Menage a Trois	
2013 midnight dark red wine blend, 5 fl oz	4
Redwood Creek Wine	
White zinfandel, 5 fl oz	4
Risata	
Moscato d'asti, 8 fl oz	10
Skinnygirl The Wine Collection	
California red, 2011, 5 fl oz	3
California white, 2011, 5 fl oz	3
Sutter Home	
Moscato, 5 fl oz	4
White zinfandel, 5 fl oz	4
Woodbridge	
Cabernet sauvignon, California, 2001, 5 fl oz	4
Woodbridge Robert Mondavi	
2010 California chardonnay, 5 fl oz	4
Yellow Tail	
Shiraz wine, 6 fl oz	4

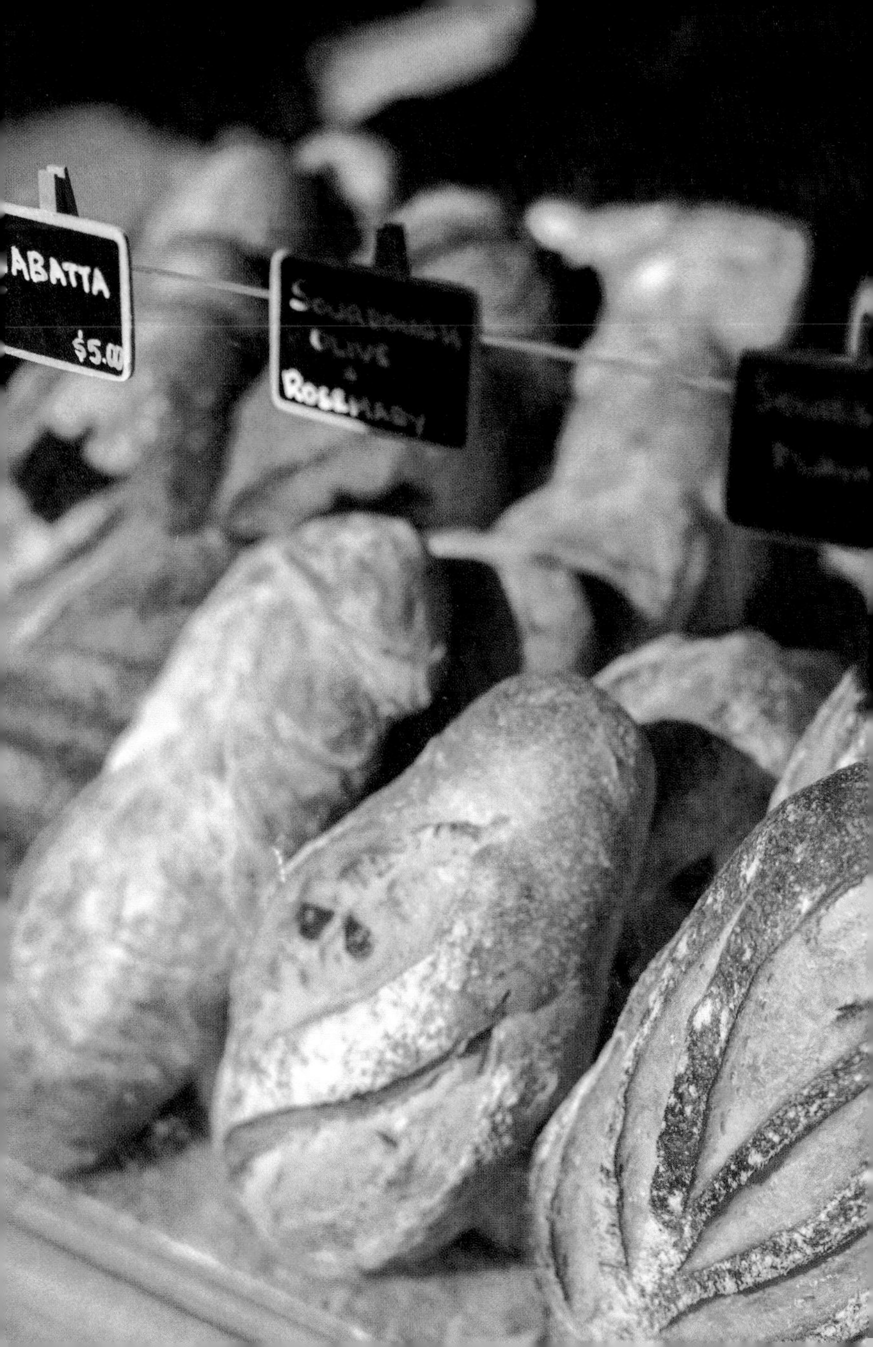
ABATTA
$5.00

bread & baked goods

Bagels

	SmartPoints® value
Bagel House	
Bagels, whole wheat, 1 bagel (83 g)	5
Bubba's	
100% whole wheat honey bagel, 1 bagel (85 g)	6
Everything skinny bagels, 1 bagel (46 g)	3
Plain bagels, 1 bagel (85 g)	6
Plain skinny bagels, 1 bagel (46 g)	3
Skinny bagels, 1 bagel (46 g)	3
Cobblestone Bread Co.	
100% whole wheat bagels, 1 bagel (95 g)	6
100% whole wheat bagel, 1 bagel (46 g)	3
Original bagel, 1 bagel (46 g)	3
David's Deli	
Egg bagels, 1 bagel (81 g)	7
Onion bagels, 1 bagel (81 g)	6
H-E-B	
Everything thin bagels, 1 bagel (46 g)	3
Plain thin bagels, 1 bagel (46 g)	3
Itty Bitty Bagels	
Cinnaraisin bagels, 1 bagel (38 g)	3
Kroger	
Mini plain bagels, 1 bagel (43 g)	3
Lender's	
Original plain bagel, 1 bagel (57 g)	4
Lender's Bagel Shop Bagels	
Bagels, 100% whole wheat, 1 bagel (81 g)	5
Bagels, cinnamon raisin swirl, pre-sliced, 1 bagel (81 g)	7
Bagels, pre-sliced, onion, 1 bagel (81 g)	6
Blueberry bagel, 1 bagel (81 g)	7
Plain bagel, 1 bagel (81 g)	6

	SmartPoints® value
Market Basket	
Everything bagel slims, 1 bagel slim (46 g)	3
Whole wheat bagel slims, 1 bagel slim (46 g)	3
Market Pantry	
Plain bagels, 1 bagel (81 g)	6
Nature's Own	
100% whole wheat thin sliced bagel, 1 bagel (46 g)	3
Nutrisystem	
Honey wheat bagel, 1 package (57 g)	5
Nutrisystem Breakfast	
Honey wheat bagel, 1 package (57 g)	5
O' Doughs Bagel Thins	
Sprouted whole grain flax gluten free, 1 bagel (50 g)	3
Pepperidge Farm	
Mini bagels, whole grain, 100% whole wheat, 1 bagel (40 g)	3
Plain bagel flats, 1 bagel flat (43 g)	3
Plain mini bagel, 1 bagel (40 g)	3
Publix	
Premium bagels, 1 bagel (95 g)	9
Premium cinnamon raisin swirl bagels, 1 bagel (95 g)	8
Sara Lee Deluxe	
Plain bagel, 1 bagel (95 g)	7
Shaw's	
Plain bagels, 1 bagel (104 g)	7
Thomas'	
Blueberry pre-sliced bagel, 1 bagel (95 g)	9
Cinnamon raisin pre-sliced bagel, 1 bagel (95 g)	8
Cinnamon swirl pre-sliced bagel, 1 bagel (95 g)	9
Everything pre-sliced bagel, 1 bagel (95 g)	8

	SmartPoints® value
Onion pre-sliced bagel, 1 bagel (95 g)	8
Plain bagel pre sliced, 1 bagel (95 g)	8
Plain pre-sliced bagel, 1 bagel (95 g)	8
Thomas' Bagel Thins	
100% whole wheat pre-sliced bagel, 1 bagel (46 g)	3
Cinnamon raisin, 1 bagel (46 g)	4
Cinnamon raisin pre-sliced bagel, 1 bagel (46 g)	4
Everything pre-sliced bagel, 1 bagel (46 g)	3
Plain pre-sliced bagel, 1 bagel (46 g)	3
Thomas' Hearty Grains	
100% whole wheat bagel, 1 bagel (95 g)	7
Thomas' Mini Bagels	
100% whole wheat pre-sliced, 1 bagel (43 g)	3
Blueberry pre-sliced, 1 bagel (43 g)	4
Brown sugar cinnamon pre-sliced, 1 bagel (43 g)	4
Cinnamon raisin pre-sliced, 1 bagel (43 g)	4
Plain pre-sliced, 1 bagel (43 g)	4
Toufayan Bakeries	
Classic plain bagels, 1 bagel (43 g)	3
Toufayan Bakeries Smart Bagel	
Plain bagel, 1 bagel (45 g)	3
Trader Joe's	
100% whole wheat everything bagel slims, 1 bagel (46 g)	3
Bagel Josef's wheat bagels, 1 bagel (85 g)	6
Cinnamon raisin bagels, 1 bagel (85 g)	8

	SmartPoints® value
Biscuits	
Bake House	
Buttermilk biscuits, 2 biscuits (43 g)	3
BelVita	
Breakfast biscuits, blueberry, 1 pack (50 g)	8
Breakfast biscuits, cinnamon brown sugar, 4 biscuits (50 g)	8
Breakfast biscuits, golden oat, 1 pack (50 g)	8
Cinnamon brown sugar breakfast biscuits, 4 biscuits (50 g)	8
BelVita Bites	
Chocolate mini breakfast biscuits, 1 pack (50 g)	8
Mixed berry breakfast biscuits, 1 biscuit (50 g)	7
BelVita Soft Baked	
Banana bread breakfast biscuits, 1 pack (50 g)	7
Breakfast biscuit, oats & chocolate, 1 pack (50 g)	7
Great Value	
Buttermilk jumbo biscuits, 1 biscuit (57 g)	7
Mary B's	
Buttermilk biscuits (unprepared), 1 biscuit (62 g)	6
Nature Valley	
Breakfast biscuits, blueberry, 4 biscuits (50 g)	8
Pillsbury	
Biscuits, buttermilk, 3 biscuits (64 g)	5
Flaky layers biscuits, 3 biscuits (64 g)	6
Pillsbury Grands!	
Biscuits, big, buttermilk, 1 biscuit (58 g)	6
Biscuits, buttermilk, 1 biscuit (59 g)	5

Biscuits, Pillsbury Grands! (cont'd)

	SmartPoints® value
Biscuits, southern style, 1 biscuit (59 g)	5
Southern homestyle buttermilk biscuits, 1 biscuit (59 g)	6
Pillsbury Grands! Flaky Layers	
Biscuits, honey butter, 1 biscuit (58 g)	6
Biscuits, original, 1 biscuit (58 g)	6
Pillsbury Grands! Jr. Golden Layers	
Biscuits, flaky, buttermilk, 1 biscuit (34 g)	3
Shredded Wheat	
Big biscuit, original, 2 biscuits (47 g)	4
THINaddictives	
Blueberry oat almond thins, 1 package (21 g)	3

Bread

	SmartPoints® value
365 Everyday Value	
Early bird seed bread, 1 slice (33 g)	2
Whole wheat sandwich bread, 1 slice (43 g)	3
Ahold	
Light multigrain bread, 2 slices (41 g)	2
Light wheat bread, 2 slices (41 g)	2
Alexia Artisan Breads	
Garlic baguette, twin pack, 2 pieces (43 g)	4
Alpine Valley Breads	
Honey oat bran bread, 1 slice (28 g)	2
Alpine Valley Breads Organic	
Omega 3 multigrain sandwich bread, 1 slice (28 g)	2
Sprouted honey wheat with flaxseed bread, 1 slice (28 g)	2
Alpine Valley Breads Super Grains	
Organic power seeds: quinoa, teff and kamut bread, 1 slice (28 g)	3
Alpine Valley Organic	
12 grain with omega-3 bread, 1 slice (23 g)	2
Honey chia bread, 1 slice (28 g)	2
Multi grain bread with omega-3, 1 slice (28 g)	2
Raisin cinnamon whole wheat bread, 1 slice (28 g)	2
Alvarado St	
Bread, California style complete protein, 1 slice (34 g)	2
Bread, sprouted multi - grain, 1 slice (34.1 g)	2
Bread, sprouted whole wheat, 1 slice (38 g)	3
Essential flax seed bread, 2 slices (45 g)	3
Angelic Bakehouse	
Sprouted seven grain bread, 1 slice (28 g)	2
Sprouted wheat bread, 1 slice (28 g)	2
Arnold	
Bread, premium Italian, 1 slice (32 g)	2
Bread, real Jewish rye with seeds, 1 slice (30 g)	2
Marble rye bread, rye & pump, 1 slice (30 g)	3
Arnold Bakery Light	
Bread, 100% whole wheat, 2 slices (43 g)	2
Arnold Classic	
100% whole wheat bread, 1 slice (35 g)	3
Arnold Country	
100% whole wheat bread, 1 slice (43 gs)	3

	SmartPoints® value
Arnold Grains & More	
Bread, 100% whole wheat, double fiber, 1 slice (43 g)	3
Arnold Healthfull	
9 grain flax and fiber thins, 1 roll (43 g)	3
Flax & sunflower 100% whole grain bread, 1 slice (32 g)	2
Multigrain bread, 2 slices (46 g)	2
Arnold Hearty & Delicious	
Extra grainy flax & sesame seed bread, 1 slice (43 g)	4
Arnold Nature's Harvest	
Bread, 100% stone ground whole wheat, 2 slices (52 g)	4
Bread, butter top, whole grain wheat, 2 slices (52 g)	4
Bread, light, multigrain, 2 slices (43 g)	2
Honey wheat bread, 2 slices (52 g)	4
Light multigrain bread, 2 slices (43 g)	2
Arnold Whole Grains	
Bread, health nut, 1 slice (43 g)	4
Bread, healthy multi-grain, 1 slice (43 g)	3
Bread, honey whole wheat, 1 slice (43 g)	3
Aunt Millie's	
Bread, cracked wheat with whole grain, homestyle, 1 slice (34 g)	2
Bread, homestyle, 100% whole wheat, 1 slice (34 g)	2
Butter top wheat bread, 2 slices (57 g)	4
German rye bread, 2 slices (43 g)	3
Multi whole grain wheat bread 97% fat free, 2 slices (52 g)	4
Aunt Millie's 35 Calorie	
Light 100% whole wheat bread, 2 slices (47 g)	2

	SmartPoints® value
Aunt Millie's Healthy Goodness	
Bread, whole grain, white, 2 slices (45 g)	3
Fiber and flavor potato bread, 2 slices (52 g)	4
Fiber for life light potato bread, 2 slices (47 g)	2
Bake Shoppe	
100% whole wheat thin rounds, 1 roll (43 g)	3
Classic white bread, 1 slice (28 g)	2
Bavarian Bakery	
Sunflower whole wheat bread, 1 slice (28 g)	1
Beefsteak	
Pumpernickel bread, 2 slices (57 g)	4
Seeded hearty rye bread, 2 slices (57 g)	4
Soft rye bread no seeds, 2 slices (57 g)	4
Bimbo	
Bread, soft wheat, family, 2 slices (47 g)	3
Soft white bread, 2 slices (47 g)	4
Braum's Grocery	
Light wheat bread, 2 slices (43 g)	3
Sugar free light wheat bread, 2 slices (43 g)	2
Bread Alone Bakery	
Organic whole wheat sourdough bread, 1 slice (33 g)	2
Brownberry	
Bread, natural wheat, 1 slice (36 g)	3
Brownberry Country	
Bread, white, 1 slice (43 g)	4
Brownberry Whole Grains	
Bread, 100% whole wheat, 1 slice (43 g)	3
Bread, 12 grain, 1 slice (43 g)	3

Bread, Brownberry Whole Grains (cont'd)

	SmartPoints® value
Bread, oatnut, 1 slice (43 g)	4
Hearty wheatberry bread, 1 slice (43 g)	3
Bunny	
Bread, 100% whole wheat, original, 2 slices (50 g)	3
Bread, thin sandwich, giant, white enriched, 1 slice (26.2 g)	2
Bunny Soft-Twist	
Bread, white enriched, 2 slices (45.4 g)	3
Bunny Ultra-Soft	
Bread, whole grain white, 2 slices (56.7 g)	4
Butternut	
Bread, all whole grain 100% whole wheat, 2 slices (57 g)	4
California Goldminer	
Sourdough square bread, 2 oz	3
Canyon Bakehouse	
Gluten free 100% whole grain bread, 1 slice (34 g)	3
Gluten free deli rye style bread, 1 slice (34 g)	2
Canyon Bakehouse Gluten Free	
7 grain bread, 1 slice (34 g)	3
Mountain white bread, 1 slice (34 g)	3
Cobblestone Bread Co.	
Complete wheat bread, 1 slice (46 g)	3
Cobblestone Bread Co. Right Sized	
24 whole grains and seeds bread made with honey, 1 slice (46 g)	3
Cole's	
Garlic toast, pre-sliced, 1 piece (33.1 g)	4
Country Hearth	
Dakota style 12 grain bread, 1 slice (34 g)	3

	SmartPoints® value
Country Hearth Lite	
100% whole wheat bread, 2 slices (41 g)	2
Country Kitchen	
Enriched bread, light Italian, pre-priced, 1 slice (27 g)	1
Light wheat bread, 2 slices (42 g)	2
Country Kitchen Light	
Oatmeal bread, 2 slices (42 g)	2
Country Oven	
Sourdough French bread, 1 slice (38 g)	3
Cub Foods	
Light wheat bread, 2 slices (46 g)	2
Daily Chef	
French baguette (serves 5), 1 piece (48 g)	3
Dave's Killer Bread	
Bread, 21 whole grains, 1 slice (45 g)	4
Bread, 21 whole grains, thin-sliced, 1 slice (28 g)	2
Bread, good seed, 1 slice (45 g)	4
Bread, good seed, thin-sliced, 1 slice (28 g)	2
Bread, powerseed, 1 slice (50 g)	3
Good seed organic bread, 1 slice (45 g)	4
Powerseed thin sliced organic bread, 1 slice (32 g)	2
Sprouted whole grains organic bread, 1 slice (37 g)	3
Dave's Killer Bread Thin-Sliced	
Powerseed organic bread, 1 slice (28 g)	2
100% whole wheat organic bread, 1 slice (28 g)	2
D'Italiano	
Light Italian bread, sliced, 2 slices (45 g)	2

	SmartPoints® value
Eureka!	
Grainiac organic sandwich bread, 1 slice (28 g)	2
Saaa-wheat! Organic sandwich bread, 1 slice (28 g)	2
Seeds the day organic sandwich bread, 1 slice (28 g)	3
Sweet baby grains organic bread, 1 slice (28 g)	2
Top seed organic bread, 1 slice (28 g)	2
Fabulous Flats	
Tandoori naan, 1 serving (63 g)	5
Tandoori naan, garlic, ¼ package (62 g)	5
Fantini	
Bread, enriched Italian, scali, with sesame, 2 slices (41.5 g)	3
Fiber One	
Honey whole wheat bread, 2 slices (50 g)	3
Fiber One 100 Calorie	
Multigrain bread, 2 slices (50 g)	3
White bread, 2 slices (50 g)	3
First Street	
Wheat sandwich bread, 1 slice (28 g)	2
Fit & Active	
Wheat bread, 1 slice (28 g)	1
Fit & Active 40 Calorie	
Wheat bread, 2 slices (41 g)	2
Flatout Hungry Girl Foldit	
Flatbread, traditional white, 1 flatbread (43 g)	3
Food For Life	
Bread, sprouted 100% whole grain, cinnamon raisin, 1 slice (34 g)	3
Ezekiel 4:9 flax bread, 1 slice (34 g)	2
Sprouted grain bread, 1 slice (34 g)	2

	SmartPoints® value
Food For Life Ezekiel 4:9	
100% whole grain sprouted bread, 1 slice (34 g)	2
Bread, sprouted grain, low sodium, 1 slice (34 g)	2
Bread, sprouted, sesame, organic, 1 slice (34 g)	2
Bread, sprouted100% whole grain, 1 slice (34 g)	2
Cinnamon raisin 100% sprouted whole grain bread, 1 slice (34 g)	3
Food Lion	
White sandwich bread, 2 slices (44 g)	3
Francisco International	
Long sourdough bread, sliced, 1 slice (41.2 g)	3
Franz	
Bread, 100% whole wheat, 2 slices (45 g)	3
Bread, gluten free, 7 grains, 1 slice (34 g)	3
Bread, organic twenty-four, thin sliced, 1 slice (28 g)	2
Brioche bread, 1 slice (37 g)	3
Cinnamon vanilla raisin bread, 1 slice (32 g)	4
Nine grain bread, 1 slice (38 g)	3
Organic thin sliced great seed bread, 1 slice (28 g)	2
Thin sliced honey oat bread, 1 slice (26 g)	2
Thin sliced nine grain San Juan island bread, 1 slice (26 g)	2
Fred Meyer	
100% whole wheat sandwich slims, 1 piece (43 g)	3
Hawaiian sandwich slims, 1 piece (43 g)	3
Honey wheat sandwich slims, 1 piece (42 g)	3
White bread, 1 slice (29 g)	2

Bread (cont'd)

	SmartPoints® value
Freihofer's	
100% whole wheat bread, stone ground, pre-priced, 1 slice (36 g)	3
Premium Italian seeded bread, 1 slice (32 g)	3
Freihofer's D'Italiano	
Italian bread, no seeds, 1 slice (32 g)	2
Giant	
Lavash bread whole wheat and oat bran, 1 piece (56 g)	2
Light wheat bread, 2 slices (41 g)	2
Wheat sandwich bread, 2 slices (43 g)	3
Giant Eagle	
King size enriched bread, 2 slices (47 g)	4
Light wheat bread, 2 slices (42 g)	2
Glutino	
White gluten free sandwich bread, 1 slice (29 g)	2
Glutino Genius	
Gluten free multigrain sandwich bread, 1 slice (29 g)	2
Grandma Sycamore	
Bread, white, 1 slice (40 g)	3
Great Grains Bakery	
Double fiber and honey bread, 1 slice (45 g)	3
Great Value	
100% whole wheat bread, 1 slice (27 g)	2
Enriched sandwich bread, 1 slice (26 g)	2
Garlic Texas toast, 1 slice (40 g)	5
Round top white bread, 2 slices (45 g)	4
Thick slice bread, 1 slice (40 g)	3
Wheat bread, 2 slices (45 g)	2
Whole wheat and honey bread, 1 slice (45 g)	3

	SmartPoints® value
Greenlee's	
Cinnamon bread, 1 slice (59 g)	8
Harper's Homemade	
Bran bread, 1 slice (36 g)	2
Healthy Life	
Bread, 100% whole wheat whole grain, flaxseed, 2 slices (41 g)	2
Bread, 100% whole wheat, southern country style, 2 slices (56.7 g)	3
Bread, 100% whole wheat, whole grain, 2 slices (41 g)	2
Bread, Italian, 2 slices (41 g)	2
Bread, white, 2 slices (41 g)	2
Sourdough bread, 2 slices (41 g)	2
H-E-B	
Thin rounds flatbread, 1 roll (43 g)	3
Heidelberg Baking Co.	
Sliced cracked wheat bread, 1 slice (57 g)	3
Heiner's	
Bread, reduced calorie, 35, hearty wheat, 2 slices (41.2 g)	2
Heiner's 35	
Bread, reduced calorie, vegetable fiber, wheat, 2 slices (38 g)	2
Hill Country Fare	
Thin sliced enriched bread, 1 slice (28 g)	2
Wheat bread, 1 slice (28 g)	2
Hillbilly	
Old fashion bread, 1 slice (25.5 g)	2
Home Bake Value	
Wheat bread, 2 slices (46 g)	3
Home Pride	
Bread, wheat, butter top, 1 slice (26 g)	2
Hy-Vee	
Sandwich wheat bread, 1 slice (28 g)	2

	SmartPoints® value
Hy-Vee 40 Calorie	
Soft and delicious light wheat bread, 2 slices (43 g)	2
Ingles	
Wheat bread, 2 slices (45 g)	2
Jessica's Brick Oven	
Artisan tuscan pane wheat bread, 1 slice (38 g)	2
Joseph's	
Garlic and herb flatbread, 1 flatbread (56 g)	2
Lavash bread, flax, oat bran & whole wheat flour, ½ lavash (32 g)	1
King's Hawaiian	
Bread, Hawaiian sweet, original, 1 slice (38 g)	5
Kirkland Signature	
Demi baguettes, ⅓ roll (50 g)	4
Multigrain bread, 1 slice (53 g)	4
Split top wheat bread, 1 slice (34 g)	2
Koepplinger's Recipe	
All natural cracked whole grain wheat bread, 2 slices (62 g)	5
Kroger	
Enriched white sandwich bread, 2 slices (47 g)	4
Hawaiian sandwich slims, 1 sandwich slim (43 g)	3
Multigrain sandwich slims, 1 sandwich slim (43 g)	2
Texas toast enriched bread, 1 slice (52 g)	4
Wheat sandwich bread, 2 slices (47 g)	4
La Brea Bakery	
Baguette, French demi, ½ baguette (57 g)	4
Sourdough loaf, 2 oz	4

	SmartPoints® value
Levy's	
Bread, real Jewish rye, 1 slice (32 g)	2
Soft rye seedless bread, 1 slice (27 g)	2
Lewis Shop	
Nutty oat special recipe bread, 1 slice (28 g)	2
LiveGfree	
Gluten free white bread, 2 slices (52 g)	4
L'oven Fresh	
100% whole wheat bread, 1 slice (45 g)	3
Bread, 100% whole wheat, 1 slice (28 g)	2
Wheat sandwich bread, 2 slices (47 g)	3
White sandwich bread, 2 slices (47 g)	3
Maiers	
Bread, Italian, premium, 1 slice (32 g)	2
Market Basket	
Corn bread mini loaves, 2 oz	8
Honey wheat deli slims, 1 deli slim (43 g)	3
Light Italian enriched bread, 1 slice (26.7 g)	1
Light oatmeal bread, 2 slices (42 g)	2
Light wheat bread, 2 slices (42 g)	2
Light white bread, 2 slices (42 g)	2
Multigrain deli slims buns, 1 deli slim (43 g)	3
Split top wheat bread, 1 slice (28 g)	2
Whole wheat deli slims, 1 deli slim (43 g)	3

	SmartPoints® value
Market Pantry	
100% whole wheat round top bread, 1 slice (26 g)	1
Demi French bread, 3" slice (57 g)	4
Wheat round top bread, 1 slice (28 g)	2
White enriched round top bread, 1 slice (28 g)	2
Marketside	
Italian loaf bread, 2 oz	3
Martin's	
100% whole wheat potato bread, 1 slice (35 g)	2
Enriched potato sandwich bread, 1 slice (32 g)	2
Master	
English muffin toasting bread, 1 slice (30.3 g)	2
Meijer	
Bread, light wheat, 2 slices (47 g)	2
Merita	
Old fashioned enriched bread, 1 slice (26 g)	2
Mestemacher	
Bread, fitness, 1 piece (72 g)	3
Milton's	
Bread, healthy whole grain, 1 slice (38 g)	3
Bread, multi-grain, 1 slice (43 g)	3
Mrs Baird's	
Honey wheat bread, 1 slice (30.9 g)	3
Mrs Baird's	
Whole grain white bread, 2 slices (57 g)	4
Natural Ovens Bakery Organic	
100% whole grain wheat bread, 1 slice (43 g)	3
Natural Ovens Weight Sense	
Bread, right wheat, 2 slices (45 g)	3

	SmartPoints® value
Nature's Harvest	
100% whole wheat bread, 1 slice (28 g)	1
Honey 7 grain bread, 2 slices (57 g)	5
Light 100% whole wheat bread, 2 slices (44 g)	2
Nature's Own	
Bread, 100% whole wheat, 2 slices (45 g)	3
Bread, double fiber wheat, 1 slice (28 g)	1
Bread, wheat, enriched, 2 slices (45 g)	2
Bread, white, enriched, 2 slices (45 g)	2
Bread, whole grain, 1 slice (43 g)	3
Butterbread bread, 1 slice (26 g)	2
Enriched bread, whitewheat, 1 slice (28 g)	2
Honey oat bread, 1 slice (26 g)	2
Honey wheat enriched bread, 1 slice (26 g)	2
Sugar free 100% whole wheat whole grain bread, 1 slice (25 g)	1
Nature's Own 40 Calories	
Honey wheat enriched bread (per slice), 2 slices (45 g)	2
Nature's Own Whitewheat	
Whole grain enriched bread, 2 slices (52 g)	3
New York	
Texas toast, the original, five cheese, 1 slice (48 g)	6
Texas toast, the original, lite, 1 slice (40 g)	4
The original Texas toast with garlic, 1 slice (40 g)	5
Nickles	
Honey wheat split top bread, 2 slices (49 g)	4
Split top wheat bread, 1 slice (25 g)	2

	SmartPoints® value
Oasis	
Low carb flaxseed sprouted bread, 1 serving (22 g)	1
Orlando	
Deli Italian bread, 1 slice (27 g)	2
Oroweat	
Bread, 100% whole wheat, 2 slices (50 g)	4
Bread, 12 grain, 1 slice (38 g)	3
Bread, country buttermilk, 1 slice (38 g)	3
Bread, double fiber, 1 slice (38 g)	2
Bread, health nut, 1 slice (38 g)	3
Bread, healthy multi-grain, 1 slice (38 g)	3
Bread, Jewish rye, 1 slice (32 g)	3
Bread, original oatnut, 1 slice (38 g)	3
Bread, russian rye, 1 slice (28 g)	2
Dill rye bread, 1 piece (28 g)	2
Double fiber bread, 1 slice (38 g)	2
Extra grainy 17 grains and seeds bread, 1 slice (43 g)	3
Oatnut bread, 1 slice (38 g)	3
Schwarzwalder dark rye bread, 1 oz	2
Oroweat Dutch Country	
Bread, 100% whole wheat, 1 slice (38 g)	3
Oroweat Healthfull	
100% whole wheat thins, 1 roll (43 g)	3
Steel cut oats & honey 100% whole grain bread, 1 slice (32 g)	2
Papa Pita	
Thinwich, pre-sliced, 100% whole wheat & honey, 1 thinwich (43 g)	3
Thinwich, pre-sliced, multi-grain with flax seeds, 1 thinwich (43 g)	2
Papa's Organic Thinwich	
Multigrain bread, 1 piece (43 g)	3

	SmartPoints® value
Pepperidge Farm	
3 cheese Italian bread, 1 slice (44 g)	4
Carb style bread, 7 grain, 1 slice (25.8 g)	1
Chocolate banana swirl bread, 1 slice (34 g)	3
Chocolatey chip swirl bread, 1 slice (26 g)	3
French toast swirl bread, 1 slice (33 g)	4
Garlic bread, 2 ½" slice (50 g)	6
Garlic bread, five cheese, 2 ¼" slice (55 g)	6
Italian white bread, 1 slice (32 g)	2
Jewish rye seeded bread, 1 slice (32 g)	2
Jewish rye seedless bread, 1 slice (32 g)	2
Sliced enriched white sandwich bread, 2 slices (45 g)	4
Pepperidge Farm Carb Style	
Soft 100% whole wheat bread, 1 slice (25.8 g)	1
Pepperidge Farm Deli Swirl	
Rye and pump bread, 1 slice (32 g)	2
Pepperidge Farm Farmhouse	
12 grain bread, 1 slice (43 g)	4
Hearty white bread, 1 slice (43 g)	3
Oatmeal bread, 1 slice (43 g)	4
Sourdough bread, 1 slice (43 g)	3
Pepperidge Farm Light Style	
100% whole wheat bread, 3 slices (57 g)	4
7 grain bread, 3 slices (57 g)	4
Oatmeal bread, 3 slices (57 g)	4
Pepperidge Farm Pumpernickel	
Dark pump bread, 1 slice (32 g)	2
Pepperidge Farm Rye	
Jewish rye whole grain seeded bread, 1 slice (32 g)	2

	SmartPoints® value
Pepperidge Farm Soft	
Seedless rye bread, 1 SLICE (32 g)	2
Pepperidge Farm Swirl	
100% whole wheat cinnamon with raisins bread, 1 slice (28 g)	3
Cinnamon bread, 1 slice (28 g)	3
Raisin cinnamon bread, 1 slice (28 g)	3
Pepperidge Farm Texas Toast	
Garlic bread, 1 slice (40 g)	5
Pepperidge Farm Very Thin	
100% whole wheat bread, 3 slices (45 g)	3
White bread, 3 slices (45 g)	3
Pepperidge Farm Whole Grain	
100% whole wheat bread, 1 slice (43 g)	3
15 grain bread, 1 slice (43 g)	3
Ancient grains hearty multi grain bread, 1 slice (43 g)	3
Oatmeal bread, 1 slice (43 g)	3
Private Selection	
100% whole wheat bread, 1 slice (38 g)	3
Dark rye wide pan bread, 1 slice (45 g)	3
Deli style dark Jewish rye bread, 2 slices (37 g)	3
Light Jewish rye bread, 2 slices (37 g)	3
Olde Chicago rye deli style bread with caraway seeds, 1 slice (28 g)	2
Rustic pugliese loaf, ⅛ loaf (57 g)	3
Private Selection Sugar Free	
100% whole wheat bread, 1 slice (45 g)	3
Publix	
Bread, reduced calorie, wheat enriched, 2 slices (45 g)	2

	SmartPoints® value
Publix Premium	
Bread, 100% stoneground, whole wheat, 1 slice (28 g)	2
Bread, honey wheat, 1 slice (26 g)	2
Bread, multi-grain, 1 slice (43 g)	3
Rudi's	
Multigrain sandwich bread, 1 slice (37 g)	3
Rudi's	
Sprouted multigrain bread, 2 slices (51 g)	3
Rudi's Organic	
Artisan breads, rosemary olive oil, sliced, 1 slice (41.5 g)	3
S Rosens	
Bohemian style rye bread, thin sliced, unseeded, 2 slices (37.8 g)	3
Rye bread with caraway seeds, thin sliced, 2 slices (37.8 g)	3
Sacramento Bake	
Bread, sliced, sourdough, 1 slice (42 g)	2
Safeway Kitchens	
Bread, sourdough, sliced long loaf, 1 slice (26 g)	2
San Luis Sourdough	
Bread, 1 piece (48.6 g)	4
Bread, deli, sourdough, 1 slice (45 g)	3
Bread, sourdough, cracked wheat, 1 slice (28 g)	2
Sara Lee	
100% whole wheat bread, 2 slices (57 g)	5
Artesano style bread, 1 slice (38 g)	3
Honey wheat bread, 2 slices (57 g)	5
Sara Lee 45 Calories & Delightful	
100% multi-grain bread, 2 slices (44 g)	2
100% whole wheat bread, 2 slices (45 g)	2

	SmartPoints® value
100% whole wheat with honey bread, 2 slices (44 g)	2
Healthy multi-grain bread, 2 slices (45 g)	2
Sara Lee Classic	
100% whole wheat bread, 1 slice (26 g)	2
100% whole wheat bread, 1 slice (28 g)	2
Butter bread, 1 slice (26 g)	2
Honey wheat bread, 1 slice (26 g)	2
Sara Lee Delightful	
45 calories wheat bread, 2 slices (45 g)	2
Healthy multigrain bread, 2 slices (45 g)	2
Sara Lee Soft & Smooth	
White bread made with whole grain, 2 slices (52 g)	4
Schar	
Bread, multigrain, 1 slice (30 g)	2
Schmidt Old Tyme	
647 wheat bread, 1 slice (28 g)	1
647 white bread, 1 slice (28 g)	1
Bread, split-top wheat, 1 slice (31 g)	2
Wheat bread made with honey, 1 slice (28 g)	1
Schwebel's	
Bread, enriched lite wheat, 2 slices (41 g)	2
Bread, Italiano, sliced Italian, 1 slice (26.7 g)	2
Bread, sweet harvest wheat, 1 slice (27 g)	2
Shaw's	
Light multi-grain bread, 2 slices (41 g)	2
Light seedless rye bread, 1 slice (28 g)	1

	SmartPoints® value
ShopRite	
Bread, light, hearth baked Jewish rye, no seeds, 1 slice (32 g)	2
Bread, light, hearth baked Jewish rye, seeded, 1 slice (32 g)	2
Silver Hills	
Little big bread, 2 slices (43 g)	3
Simply Nature	
Reduced sodium sprouted 7 grain bread, 1 slice (28 g)	2
Sprouted 7 grain bread, 1 slice (28 g)	2
Simply Nature Organic	
Seedtastic bread, 1 slice (45 g)	3
Sprouts Farmers Market	
Raisin cinnamon whole wheat, 1 slice (28 g)	2
Wheat bread, 1 slice (23 g)	2
Stop & Shop	
Bread, light wheat, 2 slices (41 g)	2
Light rye bread, seeded, 1 slice (32 g)	1
Light rye bread, seedless, 1 slice (32 g)	1
Stroehmann	
Small white bread, 2 slices (50 g)	4
Stroehmann Dutch Country	
Bread, 100% whole wheat, 1 slice (38 g)	3
Sunbeam	
Bread, enriched white, 2 slices (45 g)	3
Bread, enriched, giant, 2 slices (57 g)	5
Sun-Maid	
Bread, raisin, cinnamon swirl, 1 slice (32 g)	4
Texas Toast	
Bread, enriched, 1 slice (43 g)	3

	SmartPoints® value
The Essential Baking Company Gluten Free	
Super seeded multi grain bread, 1 slice (41 g)	3
Thomas'	
English muffin toasting bread, 1 slice (30 g)	2
Thomas' Limited Edition Swirl	
Maple French toast breakfast bread, 1 slice (32 g)	3
Today's Temptations	
Whole grain bread, 1 oz	1
Trader Joe's	
99% fat free cracked wheat sourdough bread, 1 slice (50 g)	4
Clay oven baked lavash bread, ½ piece (38 g)	3
Gluten free white sandwich bread, 2 slices (49 g)	4
Gluten free whole grain bread, 2 slices (49 g)	4
Harvest whole wheat bread, 1 slice (42 g)	3
Lavash flatbread, 1 lavash (36 g)	2
Multigrain brown rice bread, 1 slice (37 g)	3
Organic multigrain sandwich bread, 1 slice (34 g)	2
Sodium free sprouted whole grain daily bread, 1 slice (34 g)	2
Soft 10 grain bread, 1 slice (34 g)	3
Sourdough sandwich bread, 1 slice (49 g)	3
Sprouted rye bread, 1 slice (28 g)	1
Sprouted wheat bread, 1 slice (28 g)	1
Whole grain bread, 1 slice (43 g)	3
Whole wheat lavash flatbread, 1 lavash (36 g)	2
Trader Joe's Frozen	
Garlic naan, 1 piece (85 g)	6

	SmartPoints® value
Trader Joe's Grocery	
Low calorie light wheat bread, 1 slice (28 g)	1
Soft multigrain rustico bread, 1 slice (28 g)	2
Sprouted flourless whole wheat berry bread, 1 slice (34 g)	2
Sprouted multigrain bread, 1 slice (34 g)	2
Turano	
Italian bread, pane turano, 1 piece (56.7 g)	4
Twenty Third Psalm	
Soft whole wheat bread, 1 slice (34 g)	3
Udi's	
Bread, cinnamon raisin, 2 slices (60 g)	6
Bread, sandwich, white, 2 slices (57 g)	5
Bread, whole grain, 2 slices (57 g)	5
Gluten free millet chia bread, 2 slices (58 g)	4
Gluten free omega flax and fiber bread, 2 slices (58 g)	4
Udi's Gluten Free	
Rich and hearty whole grain bread, 2 slices (49 g)	4
Soft and hearty whole grain bread, 2 slices (49 g)	4
Soft and hearty whole grain bread, 2 slices (67 g)	6
White sandwich bread, 2 slices (61 g)	5
Van de Kamp's	
Sliced sourdough bread, 1 slice (26 g)	2
Vermont	
Bread, soft whole wheat, 1 slice (38 g)	2

	SmartPoints® value
Village Hearth Light	
12 grain bread, 2 slices (46 g)	2
Italian bread, 2 slices (43 g)	3
Wheat bread, 2 slices (46 g)	2
Wegman's	
Bread, lite, white, 2 slices (43 g)	2
Wegman's Food You Feel Good About	
Bread, lite, wheat, 2 slices (42 g)	2
Wellsley Farms	
Soft wheat bread, 2 slices (47 g)	3
Wheat Montana	
Big sky wheat bread, 1 slice (31 g)	2
When Pigs Fly	
Low carb whole wheatbread, 1 slice (32 g)	2
Whole Foods Market	
Organic seeded 6 sprout bread, 2 slices (57 g)	3
WinCo Foods	
White enriched bread, 1 slice (31 g)	2
Winn-Dixie	
100% whole wheat bread, 1 slice (26 g)	1
Old fashioned white bread, 1 slice (26 g)	2
Wonder	
Bread, 100% whole wheat, 1 slice (25 g)	1
Bread, classic white, 2 slices (57 g)	4
Bread, whole grain white, 2 slices (57 g)	3
Calcium fortified enriched white bread, 2 slices (57 g)	4
Zomick's	
Egg challah, 1 roll (61 g)	6

Breadsticks

	SmartPoints® value
New York	
Bread sticks, the original, garlic, 1 breadstick (50 g)	5
Safeway Select	
Sea salt grissini breadsticks, 2 sticks (13 g)	1
Wawa Grocery	
Pretzel braid, 1 pretzel (113 g)	9

Croissants

L'oven Fresh	
Mini butter croissants, 1 croissant (24 g)	4
The Bakery	
Cocktail croissants, 1 croissant (28 g)	4

Croutons

Chatham Village	
Croutons, traditional cut, fat free, garlic & onion, 2 Tbsp	1
Garlic and butter croutons, 2 Tbsp	1
Fresh Gourmet	
Croutons, premium, cheese & garlic, 6 croutons (7 g)	1
Organic seasoned croutons, 2 Tbsp	1
Premium croutons, butter & garlic, ¼ oz	1
Premium croutons, classic Caesar, 6 croutons (7 g)	1
Premium croutons, Italian seasoned, 6 croutons (7 g)	1
Premium Italian seasoned croutons, 1 packet (14 g)	2
Roasted garlic focaccia croutons, 2 Tbsp	1
Kroger	
Croutons, homestyle, cheese & garlic, 2 Tbsp	1

	SmartPoints® value
Kroger Homestyle	
Croutons, seasoned herb, 2 Tbsp	1
Marzetti	
Seasoned baked croutons, 2 Tbsp	1
Mrs. Cubbison's	
Croutons, restaurant style, classic seasoned, 5 croutons (7 g)	1
Croutons, restaurant style, fat free, seasoned, 2 Tbsp	1
New York	
Gluten free seasoned herb croutons, 2 Tbsp	1
New York The Original Texas Toast	
Croutons, Caesar, 2 Tbsp	1
Croutons, cheese & garlic, 2 Tbsp	1
Croutons, garlic & butter flavored, 2 Tbsp	1
Croutons, seasoned, 2 Tbsp	1
Olive Garden	
Garlic and Romano seasoned croutons, 2 Tbsp	1
Olive Garden Signature Recipe	
Garlic and Romano seasoned croutons, 2 Tbsp	1
Rothbury Farms	
Croutons, cheese garlic, 2 Tbsp	1
Croutons, fat free, seasoned, 2 Tbsp	1
Croutons, seasoned, Italian style, 2 Tbsp	1
Seasoned croutons, 2 Tbsp	1
Simply Nature Organic	
Seasoned croutons, 2 Tbsp	1
Tuscan Garden	
Caesar gourmet restaurant style croutons, 2 Tbsp	1
Cheese garlic croutons, 2 Tbsp	1
Italian seasoned croutons, 1 Tbsp	1
Wellsley Farms	
Caesar style croutons, 2 Tbsp	1

Danish, Sweet Rolls, and Pastries

	SmartPoints® value
Bahama	
Sweet rolls, 1 roll (35 g)	3
Bake House	
Cinnamon rolls with icing, 1 roll (44 g)	6
Butter Braid	
Cherry braided pastry, 1" slice (57 g)	6
Cinnamon braided pastry with white icing, 2 oz	7
Churros	
Churros pastry stix, 1 churro (28.3 g)	4
Creme Curls Bakery	
Cream puffs, mini, filled, 1 cream puff (18 g)	2
Delizza Patisserie	
Belgian mini cream puffs, 6 cream puffs (75 g)	13
Fresh Bakery	
Hot cross buns, 2 oz	6
Ozery Bakery Morning Rounds	
Cranberry orange toastable fruit and grain buns, 1 bun (60 g)	5
Pillsbury	
Cinnamon rolls, cream cheese icing, 1 roll (44 g)	6
Cinnamon rolls, reduced fat, with icing, 1 roll (44 g)	6
Sweet rolls, orange, with icing, 1 roll (49 g)	6
Pillsbury Cinnabon	
Cinnamon rolls with icing, 1 roll with icing (44 g)	6
Rhodes	
Cinnamon rolls, 1 roll (74 g)	8
Safeway	
Cinnamon roll, 1 roll (71 g)	9

	SmartPoints® value
Svenhard's Swedish Bakery	
Berry horn, 1 horn (57 g)	10
Breakfast claw, 1 claw (57 g)	11
The Bakery	
Pecan tarts, 1 tart (76 g)	13
Trader Joe's	
Mini cinnamon sugar churros, 10 mini churros (56 g)	9
Salted caramel bread pudding, 1 slice (128 g)	16
Trader Joe's Grocery	
Mini café twists, 4 twists (26 g)	5
Two-Bite	
Spiced pumpkin cupcakes, 4 cupcakes (83 g)	14
Wal-Mart Bakery	
White sub rolls, 1 roll (75 g)	6

Doughnuts

Concord Bakery	
Assorted donut holes, 2 donut holes (57 g)	10
Entenmann's	
Classic rich frosted donuts, 1 donut (55 g)	13
Golden Donut	
Glazed donuts, 1 donut (40 g)	7
Great Value	
Donut sticks, 1 stick (47 g)	10
Hostess Donettes	
Frosted mini donuts, 6 donuts (85 g)	19
Powdered mini donuts, 4 donuts (60 g)	10
Krispy Kreme	
Doughnuts, 1 doughnut (49 g)	9
Original glazed doughnut, 1 doughnut (49 g)	8
Kroger	
Powdered donuts, 1 donut (28 g)	5

	SmartPoints® value
Little Debbie	
Donuts, mini powdered, 4 donuts (53 g)	10
Safeway	
Donut bar, maple, 1 bar (78 g)	10
Safeway Kitchens	
Donut holes, glazed, old fashioned, 4 holes (48 g)	9
The Bakery	
Chocolate donut holes with sprinkles, 4 doughnuts (57 g)	10
Wegman's	
Donut holes, glazed, 4 donut holes (57 g)	10

English Muffins

365 Everyday Value	
Whole wheat English muffins, 1 muffin (71 g)	3
Ahold	
Light English muffin, 1 muffin (56 g)	2
Light multigrain English muffin, 1 muffin (57 g)	3
Aunt Millie's	
Multi whole grain English muffins, 1 muffin (57 g)	3
Bays	
English muffins, multi-grain, 1 muffin (57 g)	4
English muffins, original, 1 muffin (57 g)	4
English muffins, sourdough, 1 muffin (57 g)	4
Big Y	
Lite plain English muffin, 1 muffin (57 g)	2
Bubba's	
Lite English muffins, 1 muffin (57 g)	2

English Muffins (cont'd)

	SmartPoints® value
Cascade Pride	
English muffins, 1 muffin (56 g)	3
Extra crispy English muffins, 1 muffin (56 g)	3
Sour dough muffins, 1 muffin (56 g)	3
Cobblestone Bread Co.	
Original English muffins, 1 muffin (57 g)	3
Wheat English muffins, 1 muffin (57 g)	4
Crystal Farms	
Wheat English muffins, 1 muffin (57 g)	3
Essential Everyday	
English muffins, 1 muffin (56 g)	3
Fareway	
Lite English muffins, 1 muffin (57 g)	2
Farm Country	
Crumpets, 1 serving (44 g)	2
Fiber One	
100% whole wheat English muffin, 1 muffin (57 g)	3
Hearty wheat multigrain English muffin, 1 muffin (66 g)	3
Multigrain English muffin, 1 muffin (57 g)	3
Original English muffin, 1 muffin (57 g)	3
Food For Life	
English muffins, 7-sprouted grains, ½ muffin (37.8 g)	2
English muffins, sprouted grain, ½ muffin (38 g)	2
Multi seed gluten free English muffins, 1 muffin (85 g)	4
Food For Life Ezekiel 4:9	
English muffins, cinnamon raisin, ½ muffin (37.8 g)	3

	SmartPoints® value
Franz	
English muffins, 100% whole wheat, 1 muffin (61.3 g)	3
English muffins, extra crisp, 1 muffin (61 g)	4
English muffins, extra sourdough, 1 muffin (61 g)	3
English muffins, premium, healthy multigrain, 1 muffin (61 g)	3
Fred Meyer	
Extra crispy English muffins, 1 muffin (56 g)	3
Original English muffins, 1 muffin (56 g)	3
Sourdough English muffins, 1 muffin (56 g)	3
Whole wheat English muffins, 1 muffin (64 g)	4
Glutino	
English muffins, gluten free, 1 muffin (80 g)	6
Grain Power	
Original English muffins, 1 muffin (56 g)	3
Great Value	
Original English muffins, 1 muffin (57 g)	3
Hannaford	
100 calorie English muffins, 1 muffin (57 g)	3
Plain English muffins, 1 muffin (57 g)	3
Healthy Life	
English muffins, light, 1 muffin (57 g)	2
English muffins, light, multi-grain, 1 muffin (57 g)	2
Hy-Vee	
Light English muffins, 1 muffin (57 g)	2

	SmartPoints® value
L'oven Fresh	
Light multi grain English muffins, 1 muffin (57 g)	3
Pre sliced English muffins, 1 muffin (57 g)	3
Whole wheat English muffins, 1 muffin (57 g)	3
Market Basket	
Fork split light English muffins, 1 muffin (57 g)	2
Whole wheat English muffins, 1 muffin (57 g)	3
Nature's Own 100 Calorie	
English muffins, multi grain, 1 muffin (57 g)	3
Old Fashion Hearth	
English muffins, 1 muffin (57 g)	3
Oroweat	
English muffins, 100% whole wheat, 1 muffin (65 g)	5
English muffins, double fiber, 1 muffin (59 g)	4
English muffins, extra crisp, 1 muffin (59 g)	4
Rudi's Organic	
English muffins, organic whole grain wheat, 1 muffin (56.7 g)	3
Safeway Kitchens	
English muffins, extra crisp, 1 muffin (57 g)	3
English muffins, sourdough, 1 muffin (57 g)	3
Shaw's	
Light English muffins, 1 muffin (56 g)	2
Light multi-grain English muffin, 1 muffin (56 g)	3
ShopRite	
English muffins, fork split, light, 1 muffin (56 g)	2

	SmartPoints® value
Thomas'	
100% whole wheat English muffins, 1 muffin (57 g)	3
Cinnamon raisin English muffin, 1 muffin (61 g)	5
Corn English muffin, 1 muffin (61 g)	4
Cranberry English muffin, 1 muffin (61 g)	5
High fiber plain English muffin, 1 muffin (57 g)	3
Honey wheat English muffin, 1 muffin (57 g)	4
Original English muffins, 1 muffin (57 g)	3
Pumpkin spice English muffins, 1 muffin (61 g)	5
Sourdough English muffin, 1 muffin (57 g)	4
Thomas' Double Protein	
Oatmeal English muffin, 1 muffin (61 g)	4
Thomas' Light	
Multigrain English muffin, 1 muffin (57 g)	3
Multigrain English muffin, 1 muffin (57 g)	3
Thomas' Original	
English muffin, 1 muffin (57 g)	3
Sandwich size English muffin, 1 muffin (92 g)	5
Whole grain English muffin, 1 muffin (57 g)	4
Thomas' Whole Grain	
100% whole wheat English muffin, 1 muffin (57 g)	3
Trader Joe's	
British style crumpets, 1 crumpet (42 g)	3
Fat free English muffins, 1 muffin (57 g)	3
San francisco style extra sour sourdough English muffins, 1 muffin (57 g)	3

	SmartPoints® value
Trader Joe's Grocery	
British style crumpets, 1 crumpet (52 g)	3
Whole wheat British muffins, 1 muffin (57 g)	3
Whole wheat multigrain British muffins, 1 muffin (57 g)	3
Vermont Bread Company	
100% whole wheat English muffins, 1 muffin (61 g)	3
Village Hearth	
White English muffins, 1 muffin (57 g)	4
Village Hearth Light	
English muffins, 1 muffin (47 g)	2

Flatbread and Pita

	SmartPoints® value
Aladdin's	
Small plain pocket pita, 1 pita (47 g)	3
Arnold Pocket Thins	
100% whole wheat flatbread, ½ flatbread (42 g)	3
Best Pita	
Pocket pita bread, 1 pita (37 g)	2
White pocket pita bread, 1 pita (37 g)	2
Cobblestone Bread Co. Flatbread Rounds	
100% whole grain roll, 1 roll (43 g)	3
100% whole wheat roll, 1 roll (43 g)	3
Multigrain roll, 1 roll (43 g)	3
Daily Chef	
Original naan flatbread, ½ flatbread (50 g)	5
Ephraim's	
Whole wheat pita bread, 1 pita (57 g)	3
Flatout	
Flatbread, thin crust, artisan pizza, rosemary & olive oil, 1 flatbread (48 g)	3
Flatout Flatbread	
Light original flatbread, 1 flatbread (53 g)	2
Flatout Flatbread Pizza Crust	
Rustic white artisan thin, 1 crust (48 g)	3
Flatout Foldit	
5 grain flax artisan flatbread, 1 flatbread (43 g)	2
Artisan rosemary and olive oil flatbread, 1 flatbread (43 g)	3
Everything artisan flatbreads, 1 flatbread (43 g)	3
Flatbread, artisan, traditional country, 1 flatbread (51 g)	4
Flatout Foldit Protein	
Ancient grains flatbread, 1 flatbread (51 g)	3
Flatout Healthy Grain	
Flatbread wraps, honey wheat, 1 flatbread (53 g)	3
Flatbread wraps, multi-grain with flax, 1 flatbread (53 g)	2
Flatout Hungry Girl Foldit	
Whole wheat with flax flatbread, 1 flatbread (43 g)	2
Flatout Light	
Flatbread wraps, garden spinach, 1 flatbread (53 g)	2
Flatbread wraps, Italian herb, 1 flatbread (53 g)	2
Flatbread wraps, low-fat, original, 1 flatbread (53 g)	2
Flatbread wraps, sundried tomato, 1 flatbread (53 g)	2
Flatout Protein Up Carb Down	
Core 12 flatbread, 1 flatbread (57 g)	3
Flatout Soft Wraps	
100% whole wheat flatbreads, 1 flatbread (53 g)	2

	SmartPoints® value
Flatout Thin Crust Flatbreads	
Artisan pizza rustic white, 1 flatbread (48 g)	3
Artisan pizza spicy Italian, 1 flatbread (48 g)	4
Giant	
White pita bread, 1 pita (56 g)	4
Global Bakeries	
Whole wheat pita bread, ½ pita (43 g)	2
Joseph's	
Enriched syrian bread, middle east style, 1 pita (30.3 g)	2
Flax, oat bran & whole wheat pita bread, 1 pita (28 g)	1
Flax, oat bran and whole wheat flour pita bread, 1 pita (38 g)	1
Honey wheat flatbread, 1 flatbread (56 g)	3
Multi-grain flatbread, 1 flatbread (56 g)	2
Pita bread, ½ pita (39 g)	2
Tomato and basil flatbread, 1 flatbread (56 g)	2
Joseph's Heart Friendly	
Pita bread, 1 pita (40 g)	1
Kangaroo	
Pita pockets, sliced halves, original white, ½ pita (34 g)	3
Pita pockets, sliced halves, whole wheat, ½ pita (34 g)	2
Kronos	
Original white pita flat bread, 1 flat bread (71 g)	4
Lawash	
Lower carb white flatbread, 1 slice (57 g)	2
Lawash Original Recipe	
Low carb wheat flatbread, 1 flatbread (57 g)	1
Masada Bakery	
Kosher pocket bread, 1 bread (85 g)	3

	SmartPoints® value
Mediterranean	
Pita bread, white, 1 pita (57 g)	4
Middle East Bakery	
Mediterranean flat bread, 1 flat bread (91 g)	6
Oroweat Pocket Thins 100 Calories	
Healthy multi-grain flatbread, ½ pocket (42 g)	3
Papa Filin's	
Pita, 1 pita (100 g)	2
Paramount	
White pita bread, 1 oz	2
Pita Gourmet	
Flat bread, white, ½ pita (42.5 g)	3
Sajouna	
White baby pita, 1 pita (18 g)	1
Specially Selected	
Garlic cheese flatbread, ¼ piece (73 g)	10
Garlic naan, ½ slice (63 g)	6
Stonefire	
Tandoor baked naan, 1 naan (69 g)	6
Thomas' Sahara	
100% whole wheat regular size pita pocket, 1 loaf (57 g)	4
Toufayan	
Pita bread, white, 1 loaf (56 g)	4
Whole wheat pita bread, 1 loaf (57 g)	4
Toufayan Bakeries Lavash Plus	
Whole wheat and flax hearth baked, 1 piece (40 g)	2
Toufayan Bakeries Pitettes	
Whole wheat pita bread, 1 pita (28 g)	2
Toufayan Bakeries Small Pockets	
100% whole wheat with multigrain pocket pita bread, 1 pita (43 g)	2
Tourza Baking Company	
Lebanese style pita bread, ½ pita (34 g)	2

Flatbread and Pita (cont'd)

	SmartPoints® value
Trader Joe's	
Clay oven baked whole wheat lavash bread, ½ lavash (38 g)	3
Mini pita pockets, 1 piece (28 g)	2
Pita bread whole wheat pockets, 1 pita (43 g)	3
Tandoori garlic naan, 1 piece (85 g)	7
Whole wheat pita bread, 1 pita (60 g)	4
Whole wheat tandoori naan, 1 piece (85 g)	7

Muffins

	SmartPoints® value
Amaral's	
Portuguese raisin muffins, 1 muffin (65 g)	7
Betty Crocker	
Muffin mix, banana nut, 1 serving (30 g)	5
Muffin mix, blueberry, 1 serving (30 g)	5
Butterfly Bakery	
Muffins, pumpkin, ½ muffin (51 g)	3
Café Valley Bakery	
Chocolate chip mini muffins, 1 muffin (25 g)	4
Entermann's Little Bites	
Banana muffins, 1 pouch (47 g)	8
Flap Jacked	
Double chocolate mighty muffin with probiotics, 1 container (55 g)	7
Garden Lites	
Veggie muffins, zucchini chocolate, 1 muffin (56 g)	5
Garden Lites Veggie Muffins	
Zucchini chocolate muffins, 1 muffin (56 g)	5
Nutrisystem	
Blueberry muffin, 1 package (57 g)	5
Nutrisystem Breakfast	
Blueberry muffin, 1 muffin (57 g)	5
Cinnamon streusel muffin, 1 muffin (51 g)	7
Otis Spunkmeyer	
Banana nut muffin, ½ muffin (57 g)	9
Quaker	
Wild blueberry homestyle oatmeal muffins, 1 muffin (71 g)	9
Safeway Kitchens	
Muffins, mini, blueberry, 1 muffin (25 g)	4
Signature Bakery	
Chocolate chip muffin, 1 muffin (99 g)	15
The Bakery	
Blueberry streusel mini muffins, 2 muffins (56 g)	9
Trader Joe's	
Apple cranberry fiber mini cakes, 1 cake (57 g)	2
Classic British muffins, 1 muffin (57 g)	5
Trader Joe's Grocery	
Apple cranberry bran muffins, 1 muffin (57 g)	2
Blueberry wheat bran muffins (99% fat free), 1 oz	2
Vitalicious VitaTops	
Banana choco chip muffin top, 1 muffin top (55 g)	4
Chocolate chip, 1 vitatop (55 g)	4
Chocolate chip muffin top, 1 vitatop (55 g)	4
Cran bran, 1 vitatop (55 g)	4
Wild blueberry, 1 vitatop (55 g)	4
Vitalicious VitaTops 100 Calories	
Cran bran muffin top, 1 vitatop (55 g)	4
Deep chocolate muffin top, 1 vitatop (55 g)	4

	SmartPoints® value
Fudgy peanut butter chip muffin top, 1 vitatop (55 g)	4
Sugar free velvety chocolate muffin top, 1 vitatop (55 g)	3
VitaMuffin VitaTops	
Deep chocolate muffin top, 1 muffin top (55 g)	4

Rolls and Buns

	SmartPoints® value
Ahold	
Light hamburger roll, 1 roll (43 g)	2
Albertsons	
Enriched hamburger buns, 1 bun (43 g)	3
Amorosos	
Rolls, club, 1 roll (57 g)	4
Arnold	
100 calorie everything sandwich thins, 1 roll (43 g)	3
100% whole wheat with flax and fiber sandwich thins, 1 roll (43 g)	3
Multi-grain pre-sliced sandwich thins, 1 roll (43 g)	3
Potato rolls sandwich thins, 1 roll (43 g)	3
Sandwich thins, 100% whole grain, 1 roll (43 g)	3
Arnold Sandwich Thins	
Honey wheat rolls, 1 roll (43 g)	3
Rolls, 100% whole wheat flax & fiber, 1 roll (43 g)	3
Arnold Select	
Whole wheat sandwich thins, 1 roll (43 g)	3
Arnold Select Fill 'ems	
Sandwich thins, multi-grain, 1 roll (43 g)	3
Aunt Millie's Hearth	
Hamburger buns, whole grain, 1 bun (60 g)	4
Aunt Millie's Slimwiches	
Buns, slim, pre-sliced, 100% whole wheat, 1 bun (42 g)	3
Bake House	
Crescent rolls, 1 roll (28 g)	4
Ball Park	
Hamburger buns, 1 bun (50 g)	4
Pre-sliced hot dog bun, 1 bun (46 g)	4
Brooklyn Bred	
Country potato bistro buns, 1 bun (42 g)	3
Brownberry	
100% whole wheat sandwich thins, 1 oz	2
Honey wheat sandwich thin, 1 roll (43 g)	3
Multi-grain sandwich thin, 1 roll (43 g)	3
Bunny	
Enriched hamburger buns, 1 bun (47 g)	3
Calise & Sons	
Rolls, bulkie, enriched, deli, 1 roll (61.3 g)	5
Calise Bakery	
Split sub rolls, 1 roll (71 g)	5
Chabaso Bakery	
Ciabatta rolls, classic, 1 roll (57 g)	4
Cobblestone Bread Co.	
Sweet party rolls, 1 roll (28 g)	3
White grinder sub roll, 1 roll (90 g)	7
Coborn's Signature	
White dollar buns, 1 bun (39 g)	3
Daily Chef	
Yeast dinner roll, 1 roll (30 g)	4
Damascus Bakeries Roll-Up	
Flax flatbread, 1 roll up (57 g)	2
Earth Grains	
100% whole wheat thin bun, 1 bun (43 g)	3
Equate Bread	
Hot dog buns, 1 bun (39 g)	3

Rolls and Buns (cont'd)

	SmartPoints® value
Euro Classic Imports	
Pre sliced authentic French brioche hamburger buns, 1 bun (50 g)	5
Fiber One 90 Calorie	
12 grain thin sandwich roll, 1 roll (43 g)	3
Whole wheat thin sandwich roll, 1 roll (43 g)	3
Food Club	
Pretzel rolls, soft, 1 roll (49 g)	4
Fred Meyer	
Hot dog enriched buns, 1 bun (43 g)	3
Multigrain sandwich slims, 1 piece (43 g)	2
Fresh Bakery	
Hoagie rolls, 1 roll (57 g)	5
Giant	
White rolls, 1 roll (38 g)	3
Giant Eagle	
Brown and serve rolls, 1 roll (26 g)	2
Whole grain wheat buns, 1 bun (46 g)	4
Great Value	
100% whole wheat hot dog bun, 1 roll (46 g)	3
Hamburger buns, 1 bun (43 g)	4
Whole wheat hamburger bun, 1 roll (53 g)	4
Healthy Life	
Hot dog buns, wheat, light, 1 bun (43 g)	2
Hot dog buns, white, light, 1 bun (43 g)	2
Sandwich buns, light, wheat, 1 bun (43 g)	2
Sandwich buns, light, white, 1 bun (43 g)	2
H-E-B	
Wheat hamburger buns, 1 bun (63 g)	6

	SmartPoints® value
Hill Country Fare	
Hamburger buns, 1 bun (46 g)	4
Hostess	
Soft white hamburger buns, 1 bun (43 g)	4
Joseph's	
Thin sandwich rolls, 1 roll (43 g)	2
Kasanof's	
Onion rolls, 1 roll (66.2 g)	5
King's Hawaiian	
Hawaiian sweet roll(12 pack), 1 roll (31 g)	4
Original Hawaiian sweet roll, 1 roll (28 g)	3
Rolls, honey wheat, 1 roll (28 g)	3
Rolls, savory butter, 1 roll (28 g)	3
Kroger	
Hamburger enriched buns, 1 bun (57 g)	5
Hot dog buns, 1 bun (39 g)	3
Original yeast dinner roll dough, 1 roll (38 g)	3
White hoagie enriched rolls, 1 roll (68 g)	5
La Brea Bakery Take and Bake	
Telera sandwich roll, 1 roll (85 g)	6
Lakeland	
Hamburger buns, 1 bun (38 g)	3
L'oven Fresh	
Brown and serve rolls, 1 roll (29 g)	2
Hamburger buns, 1 bun (43 g)	3
L'oven Fresh Sandwich Skinnys	
Pre sliced multigrain buns, 1 roll (43 g)	3
Maiers	
Rolls, hoagie, Italian style, 1 roll (85 g)	7
Maplehurst	
Split top sweet multigrain dinner rolls, 1 roll (35 g)	2

	SmartPoints® value
Market Basket	
Light wheat hamburger rolls, 1 roll (41 g)	2
Marketside	
Multigrain ciabatta rolls, 1 roll (85 g)	6
Savory garlic knots, 1 knot (37 g)	3
Martin's	
100% whole wheat potato roll, 1 roll (42 g)	3
Enriched dinner rolls, potato, 1 roll (35.4 g)	3
Long potato rolls, 1 roll (53 g)	4
Potato roll, 1 roll (53 g)	4
Meijer	
Pretzel hamburger bun, 1 roll (85 g)	7
Mrs Baird's	
Large hamburger buns, 1 bun (65 g)	5
Nature's Harvest	
100% whole wheat hamburger bun, 1 roll (57 g)	4
Nature's Own	
100% whole wheat sandwich rounds, 1 roll (43 g)	3
Hot dog rolls, 100% whole wheat, 1 roll (46 g)	3
Sandwich rolls, 100% whole wheat, 1 roll (53 g)	4
Sandwich rounds, 100% whole grain, 1 roll (43 g)	3
Sandwich rounds, healthy multi-grain, 1 roll (43 g)	3
Whitewheat enriched sliced hamburger bun, 1 bun (50 g)	3
Nature's Own Butter Buns	
Hamburger rolls, 1 bun (57 g)	4
Nature's Own Whitewheat	
Hot dog buns, 1 bun (46 g)	3

	SmartPoints® value
New French Bakery	
Ciabatta roll, 1 roll (57 g)	4
New York	
Garlic knots, hand-tied, 1 knot (35 g)	4
Nickles	
Dinner rolls, 1 roll (26 g)	2
Enriched sandwich buns, 1 bun (42 g)	4
Oroweat	
100% whole wheat sandwich thins, 1 roll (43 g)	3
Hamburger buns, 100% whole wheat, 1 bun (74 g)	6
Sandwich thins, pre-sliced, whole grain white, 1 roll (43 g)	3
Oroweat Naturals Sandwich Thins	
Rolls, pre-sliced 100% whole wheat, flax & fiber, 1 roll (43 g)	3
Oroweat Sandwich Thins	
Rolls, pre-sliced, 1 roll (43 g)	3
Oroweat Select	
Sandwich rolls, wheat, 1 roll (57 g)	5
Ozery Bakery One Bun	
100 calorie whole wheat thin sandwich buns, 1 bun (40 g)	3
Papa Ciro's	
Garlic knots, 1 knot (36 g)	3
Pepperidge Farm	
Bakery classics golden potato slider bun, 1 roll (36 g)	3
Dinner rolls, stone baked artisan, French, 1 roll (50 g)	3
Hot dog buns, top sliced, classic, 1 Bun (50 g)	4
Pepperidge Farm Bakery Classics	
100% whole wheat hamburger bun, 1 bun (51 g)	4
Golden potato hamburger bun, 1 bun (53 g)	5

Rolls and Buns, Pepperidge Farm Bakery Classics (cont'd)

	SmartPoints® value
Hamburger buns, sesame topped, 1 bun (46 g)	5
Soft white hamburger bun, 1 bun (51 g)	4
Sweet and soft sliders, 1 bun (36 g)	3
Pepperidge Farm Classic	
Sandwich buns, mini, sliders, 1 bun (36 g)	3
Sandwich buns, mini, wheat sliders, 1 bun (36 g)	3
Sandwich buns, onion with poppy seeds, 1 roll (53 g)	4
Pepperidge Farm Deli Flats	
Thin rolls, 7 grain, 1 roll (43 g)	3
Thin rolls, soft 100% whole wheat, 1 roll (43 g)	3
Pillsbury	
Dinner rolls, crescent, butter flake, 1 roll (28 g)	4
Original crescent rolls, 1 roll (28 g)	4
Reduced fat crescent dinner rolls, 1 roll (28 g)	3
Publix	
Hamburger buns, 1 bun (46 g)	4
Rainbo	
Brown 'n serve enriched rolls, 1 roll (28 g)	2
White dinner rolls, 1 roll (40 g)	4
Rhodes	
French crusty rolls, 1 roll (54 g)	3
Rhodes Bake-N-Serv	
Dinner rolls, white, 1 roll (37.8 g)	3
White dinner rolls, 1 roll (37.8 g)	3
Artisan mini baguettes, 1 roll (99 g)	6
Roll-Up	
Whole wheat rolls, 2 oz	3

	SmartPoints® value
Sandwich Thins	
100% whole wheat no artificial sandwich thins, 24 count, 1 serving	3
100% whole wheat sandwich thins, 8 count, 1 serving	3
100% whole wheat sandwich thins, 16 count, 1 serving	3
100% whole wheat sandwich thins, 24 count, 1 serving	3
Flax & fiber sandwich thins, 8 count, 1 serving	3
Honey wheat sandwich thins, 8 count, 1 serving	3
Multi grain sandwich thins, 8 count, 1 serving	3
Multi grain sandwich thins, 16 count, 1 serving	3
Multi grain sandwich thins, 24 count, 1 serving	3
No artificial 9 grain flax & fiber sandwich thins, 24 count, 1 serving	3
Potato sandwich thins, 8 count, 1 serving	3
Sara Lee	
Sesame seed hamburger buns, 1 bar (40 g)	5
Sweet Hawaiian roll, 1 roll (35 g)	3
Wheat with honey dinner rolls, 1 roll (40 g)	3
Sara Lee 80 Calories & Delightful	
Wheat hamburger bun, 1 bun (43 g)	2
Wheat hot dog bun, 1 bun (43 g)	2
Sara Lee Classic	
Dinner roll, 1 roll (40 g)	4
Schwebel's	
Buns, sandwich, lite, 1 bun (42 g)	3

	SmartPoints® value
Shaw's	
Light sliced hamburger rolls, 1 roll (43 g)	2
Light wheat hot dog rolls, 1 roll (43 g)	3
Shop 'n Save	
Sliced hot dog buns, 1 bun (43 g)	3
ShopRite	
Rolls, hamburger, light, enriched, 1 roll (42.5 g)	2
Sister Schubert's	
Dinner yeast rolls, 1 roll (42.5 g)	5
Sister Schubert's Warm & Serve	
Yeast rolls, parker house style, 2 rolls (41 g)	5
Stater Bros.	
Hot dog buns, 1 bun (43 g)	3
Stop & Shop	
Hamburger rolls, enriched, light, 1 roll (43 g)	2
The Bakery	
Hard rolls, 1 roll (54 g)	4
Yeast rolls, 1 roll (40 g)	3
The Bakery Baked With Pride	
Mini ciabatta rolls, 2 rolls (56 g)	5
The HoneyBaked Ham Company	
Wheat dinner rolls, 1 roll (31 g)	3
Trader Joe's Artisan Breads	
Ciabatta rolls, 1 roll (57 g)	3
Trader Joe's Grocery	
Multigrain slims sandwich bread, 1 roll (43 g)	3
Whole wheat hamburger buns, 1 bun (43 g)	3
Whole wheat slims sandwich bread, 1 roll (43 g)	3
Udi's	
Classic French dinner rolls, 1 roll (35 g)	2

	SmartPoints® value
Udi's Gluten Free	
Hamburger buns, classic, 1 bun (77 g)	6
Seeded whole grain dinner rolls, 1 roll (40 g)	3
Vermont Bread Company	
Potato hot dog buns, 1 roll (57 g)	4
Village Hearth	
Light Italian hamburger buns, 1 roll (46 g)	2
Village Hearth Slender Rounds	
Multi-grain pre-sliced roll, 1 roll (43 g)	2
Wegman's	
Rolls, kaiser, 1 roll (66 g)	3
WinCo Foods	
Enriched hamburger buns, 1 bun (43 g)	3

Stuffing

Chef Karlin	
Chicken stuffing mix (unprepared), 1 oz	3
Great Value	
Chicken flavored stuffing mix, 1 oz	3
Pepperidge Farm	
Stuffing, herb seasoned, ¾ cup	5
Reser's Fine Foods	
Homestyle stuffing, ½ cup	4
Stove Top	
Cornbread stuffing mix (serves 6), 1 serving (28 g)	3
Stuffing mix for chicken (serves 6), 1 serving (28 g)	3
Stuffing mix for pork (serves 6), 1 serving (28 g)	3
Stuffing mix for turkey (serves 6), 1 serving (28 g)	3

	SmartPoints® value
Taco/Tostada Shells	
Guerrero	
Tostadas, caseras amarillas, 2 tostadas (32 g)	5
H-E-B	
Baked tostadas horneadas, 3 tostadas (34 g)	3
Corn tostadas de maiz, 2 tostadas (23 g)	4
Old El Paso	
Taco shells, crunchy, 3 shells (32 g)	5
Old El Paso Stand 'n Stuff	
Taco shells, 2 shells (27 g)	4
Ortega	
Taco shells, whole grain corn, 2 shells (28 g)	3
Taco shells, yellow corn, 2 shells (28 g)	4
Yellow corn taco shells, 2 shells (28 g)	3
Ortega Fiesta Flats	
Flat bottom taco shells, 2 taco shells (27 g)	4
Tortillas	
365 Everyday Value	
Corn tortillas, 3 tortillas (57 g)	4
Soft corn tortillas, 1 tortilla (25 g)	2
Ahold	
Medium soft taco size multigrain tortilla, 1 serving (50 g)	4
Azteca	
Soft taco size flour tortillas, 2 tortillas (48 g)	4
Benita	
Medium flour tortillas, 1 tortilla (49 g)	4
Small fajita flour tortillas, 1 tortilla (37 g)	2
Carlita	
Burrito style 10 flour tortillas, 1 tortilla (68 g)	6

	SmartPoints® value
Chi-Chi's	
Flour tortilla, burrito size, 1 tortilla (60 g)	5
Tortillas, flour, soft taco size, 1 tortilla (28 g)	3
Whole wheat fajita style tortillas, 1 tortilla (57 g)	5
Chi-Chi's 100 Calorie	
Fajita style tortilla, 1 tortilla (43 g)	3
El Milagro	
Corn tortillas, 1 tortilla (24 g)	1
Tortillas, corn, 1 tortilla (24 g)	1
Fit & Active	
100% whole wheat flour tortillas (soft taco), 1 tortilla (45 g)	4
Multi grain wraps, 1 wrap (53 g)	2
Food For Life	
Tortillas, brown rice, 1 tortilla (57 g)	4
Food For Life Ezekiel 4:9	
Sprouted grain tortillas, new Mexico style, 1 tortilla (57 g)	4
Guerrero	
4.5″ tortillas de maíz blanco (white corn tortillas), 3 tortillas (45 g)	3
6″ tortillas de maíz blanco (white corn tortillas), 2 tortillas (50 g)	3
8″ tortillas de harina integral tortillas (whole wheat flour tortilla), 1 tortilla (41 g)	4
Tortilla de harina, 1 tortilla (32 g)	3
Tortillas de harina caseras, 1 tortilla (59 g)	6
Tortillas de harina riquisimas, 1 tortilla (41 g)	4
H-E-B	
100% whole wheat flour tortillas, 1 tortilla (38 g)	3
Flour tortillas, 1 tortilla (34 g)	3
Hy-Vee	
Multigrain tortillas, 1 tortilla (50 g)	5

	SmartPoints® value
Joseph's	
Oat bran and whole wheat flour tortilla, 1 tortilla (43 g)	2
Kroger	
100% whole wheat soft taco size tortillas, 1 tortilla (45 g)	4
La Banderita	
Extra large burrito grande flour tortilla, 1 tortilla (71 g)	7
Fajitas flour tortilla, 1 tortilla (31 g)	2
Fat free soft taco flour tortilla, 1 tortilla (39 g)	3
Flour tortilla (family pack), 1 tortilla (33 g)	2
Large soft taco flour tortilla, 1 tortilla (45 g)	4
Mini taco corn tortilla, 2 tortillas (36 g)	3
Whole wheat fajita flour tortilla, 1 tortilla (28 g)	3
Whole wheat soft taco tortilla, 1 tortilla (45 g)	4
La Banderita Carb Counter	
Low carb tortilla, 1 tortilla (42 g)	3
La Banderita Low Carb	
Soft taco tortilla, 1 tortilla (45 g)	2
La Banderita Xtreme Fiber	
Soft taco flour tortilla, 1 tortilla (45 g)	1
La Burrita	
Corn tortillas, 2 tortillas (78 g)	5
La Tortilla	
100 calorie 100% whole wheat tortilla, 1 tortilla (58 g)	3
Tortillas, corn, hand made style, green chile, 1 tortilla (41 g)	2
Tortillas, white corn, 1 tortilla (41 g)	2
Tortillas, yellow corn, 1 tortilla (41 g)	2
La Tortilla Factory	
Organic tortillas, 1 tortilla (43 g)	4
White corn organic tortillas, 1 tortilla (41 g)	2

	SmartPoints® value
La Tortilla Low Carb High Fiber	
Traditional flour tortilla, 1 tortilla (42 g)	2
La Tortilla Smart & Delicious	
Large whole wheat gourmet tortilla, 1 tortilla (62 g)	2
Tortillas low carb high fiber original made with whole wheat, 1 tortilla (37 g)	1
Tortillas, flour, light, 1 tortilla (39 g)	2
La Tortilla Soft Wraps	
Tortillas, mini, white whole wheat, 1 wrap (29 g)	1
Late July Organic	
Snack chips, multigrain, mild green mojo, 13 chips (28 g)	3
Snack chips, multigrain, sea salt by the seashore, 13 chips (28 g)	3
Mama Lupe's	
98% fat free flour tortillas, 1 tortilla (50 g)	3
Flour tortillas, 1 tortilla (51 g)	4
Low carb tortillas, 1 serving (36 g)	1
Maria and Ricardo's Tortilla Factory	
Wheat tortillas, 1 tortilla (28 g)	1
Market Basket	
Mexicali flour tortillas, 1 tortilla (45 g)	4
Whole wheat tortillas, 1 tortilla (45 g)	4
Mi Rancho Taco Sliders	
Tortillas, organic corn, 4 tortillas (59 g)	3
Mission 96% Fat Free	
Medium soft taco whole wheat tortillas, 1 tortilla (50 g)	4
Mission Carb Balance	
Large whole wheat tortilla burrito, 1 tortilla (70 g)	6
Medium soft taco flour tortillas, 1 tortilla (42.5 g)	4
Soft taco whole wheat tortillas, 1 tortilla (42 g)	4

Tortillas, Mission Carb Balance (cont'd)

	SmartPoints® value
Tortillas, flour, medium, soft taco, 1 tortilla (42 g)	4
Tortillas, flour, small fajita, 1 tortilla (28 g)	2
Whole wheat tortillas (small fajita size), 1 tortilla (28 g)	2
Mission®	
100% whole wheat flour tortilla burrito, 1 tortilla (70 g)	7
100% whole wheat soft taco flour tortilla, 1 tortilla (45 g)	4
Corn tortillas street tacos, 3 tacos (44 g)	3
Flour tortilla fajita, 1 tortilla (36 g)	3
Gluten free tortillas, 1 tortilla (49 g)	4
Large burrito flour tortilla, 1 tortilla (70 g)	6
Soft taco size flour tortilla, 1 tortilla (49 g)	5
Tortillas, artisan style, corn & whole wheat blend, 1 tortilla (36 g)	3
Tortillas, flour, burrito, large, 1 tortilla (70 g)	7
Tortillas, flour, fajita, extra fluffy, 1 tortilla (32 g)	3
Tortillas, flour, medium, soft taco, 1 tortilla (49 g)	4
Tortillas, flour, multi-grain, medium, 1 tortilla (49 g)	5
Tortillas, flour, small, 1 tortilla (36 g)	3
Tortillas, flour, small, fajita, 1 tortilla (32 g)	3
Tortillas, white corn, super size, 1 tortilla (33 g)	2
White corn tortillas, 2 tortillas (42 g)	3
Yellow corn tortillas, 2 tortillas (51 g)	3
Old El Paso	
Flour tortilla, 2 tortillas (46 g)	5
Mini soft tortilla taco boats, 4 boats (48 g)	5

	SmartPoints® value
Tortillas, flour, for burritos, 1 tortilla (39 g)	4
Old El Paso Stand 'n Stuff	
Soft flour tortilla shell taco boats, 2 tortilla shells (47 g)	5
Olé	
Whole wheat tortilla wrap, 1 tortilla (45 g)	4
Olé Mexican Foods Xtreme Wellness!	
High fiber low carb tortilla wrap, 1 wrap (45 g)	1
Spinach and herbs tortilla wrap, 1 tortilla (45 g)	1
Tomato basil tortilla wrap, 1 tortilla (45 g)	2
Ortega	
Whole wheat tortilla, 1 tortilla (45 g)	4
Psst	
Flour tortillas, 1 tortilla (45 g)	4
Rudi's	
Tortillas, gluten-free, plain, 1 tortilla (32 g)	3
Sahara	
Wheat tortilla wraps, 1 tortilla (43 g)	4
Santa Fe Tortilla Company	
Homestyle whole grain tortillas, 1 tortilla (57 g)	2
Santa Fe Tortilla Company Carb Chopper	
Flour tortillas, 1 tortilla (36 g)	2
Sprouts Farmers Market	
Artisan corn tortillas, 1 tortilla (49 g)	2
Whole wheat tortillas, 1 tortilla (32 g)	2
Tortilla Land	
Tortillas, uncooked, corn, 1 tortilla (40 g)	2
Uncooked flour tortilla, 1 piece (47 g)	4

	SmartPoints® value
Tortillas Del Comai	
Flame cooked flour tortillas, 1 tortilla (57 g)	5
Trader Joe's	
Whole wheat tortillas, 1 tortilla (33 g)	4
Trader Joe's Grocery	
Brown rice tortillas, 1 tortilla (57 g)	4
Corn tortillas, 2 tortillas (52 g)	4
Reduced carb whole wheat flour tortilla, 1 tortilla (28 g)	1
Trader Jose's	
100% whole wheat flour tortillas, 1 tortilla (33 g)	3
Stone ground white corn tortillas, 1 tortilla (28 g)	2
Trader Jose's Organic	
Whole wheat and corn flour tortillas, 1 tortilla (42 g)	3
Wrap-itz	
Savory spinach tortilla wraps, 1 tortilla (43 g)	3

Wraps

Banh Trang	
Spring rolls skin (serves 5), 1 serving (68 g)	7
Cedar's	
Whole wheat wrap, 1 wrap (43 g)	2
Wraps, whole wheat, 1 wrap (71 g)	7
Fiber One	
Vegetable garden wrap, 1 wrap (43 g)	2
Fiber One 80 Calorie	
Honey wheat wrap, 1 wrap (43 g)	2
Traditional white wrap, 1 wrap (43 g)	2
La Tortilla Smart & Delicious	
Soft wraps, multi grain, 1 wrap (62 g)	2

	SmartPoints® value
LiveGfree	
Plain gluten free wrap, 1 wrap (52 g)	4
Mission®	
Garden spinach herb wrap, 1 tortilla (70 g)	7
Wraps, sun-dried tomato basil, 1 tortilla (70 g)	6
Yellow corn extra thin tortillas, 3 tortillas (38 g)	4
Nasoya	
Won ton wraps, 8 wrappers (60 g)	4
Olé Mexican Foods Xtreme Wellness!	
High fiber low carb tortilla wraps (8"), 1 wrap (45 g)	2
Toufayan	
Gluten free wraps, 1 wrap (52 g)	4
Low carb low sodium wrap, 1 wrap (57 g)	2
Toufayan Bakeries	
Savory tomato wraps, 1 wrap (52 g)	4
Tumaros Low-in-Carb	
New York deli style everything wrap, 1 wrap (60 g)	2
Wraps, 9 grain with chia, 1 wrap (40 g)	1
Wraps, ancient grain, 1 wrap (40 g)	1
Wraps, garden veggie, 1 wrap (40 g)	1
Wraps, honey wheat, 1 wrap (40 g)	2
Wraps, multi-grain, 1 wrap (40 g)	1
Wraps, premium white, 1 wrap (40 g)	1
Wraps, sundried tomato basil, 1 wrap (40 g)	1
Wraps, whole wheat, 1 wrap (40 g)	1
Wing Hing	
Egg roll wraps, 1 piece (28 g)	2

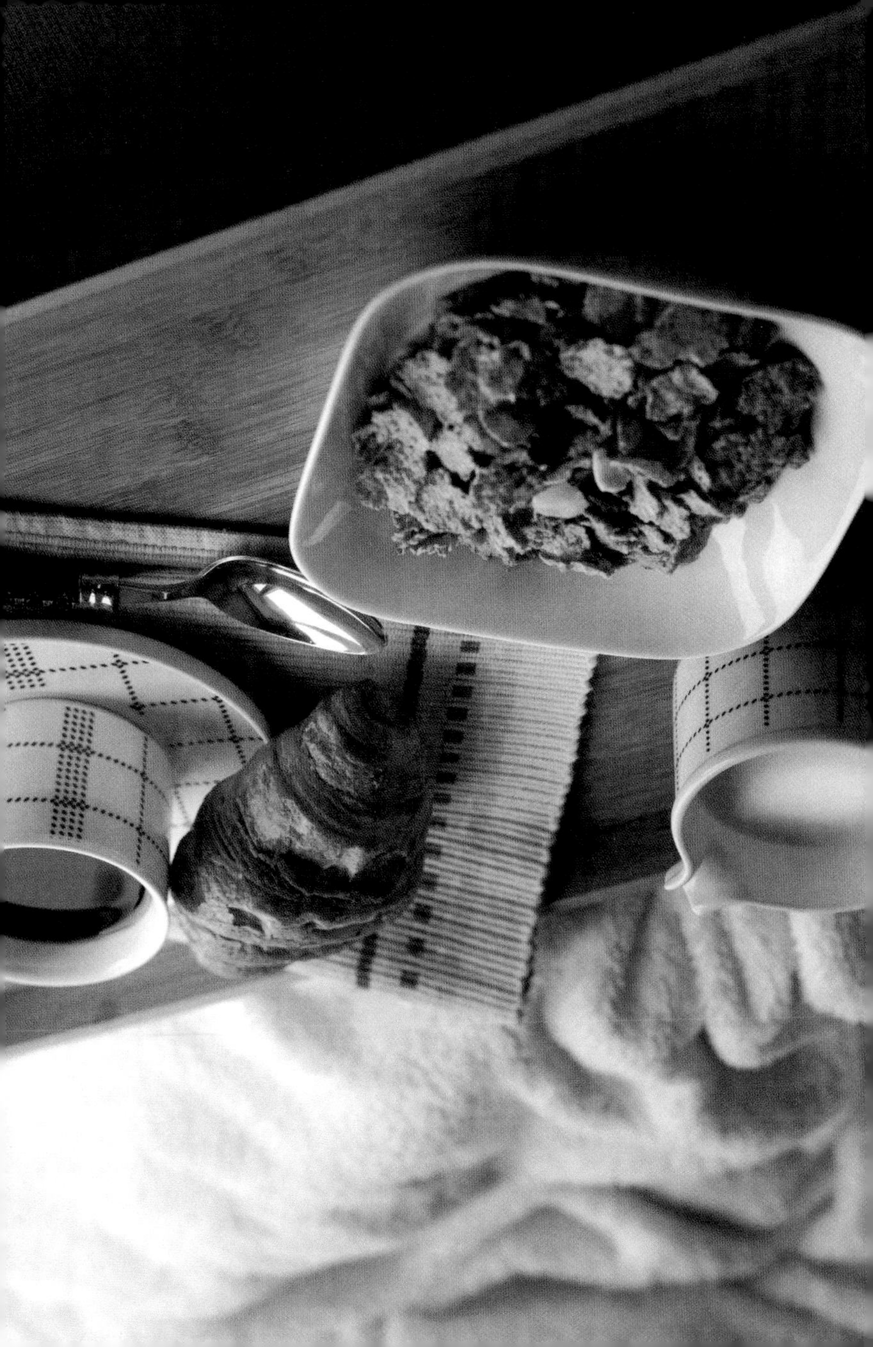

breakfast

Cereal, Hot

	SmartPoints® value
365 Everyday Value	
Multigrain with flax instant hot cereal, 1 packet (40 g)	4
Original organic instant oatmeal, 1 packet (40 g)	4
365 Everyday Value Organic	
Old fashioned rolled oats, ½ cup	4
Ahold Sugar Free	
Apples and cinnamon instant oatmeal, 1 packet (28 g)	3
Maple and brown sugar instant oatmeal, 1 packet (28 g)	3
Archer Farms	
Chai spice multigrain oatmeal, 1 container (48 g)	7
Better Oats OatFit	
100 calories cinnamon roll instant oatmeal with flax, 1 oz	3
Instant oatmeal with flax apples and cinnamon, 1 pouch (28 g)	3
Instant oatmeal with flax maple and brown sugar, 1 pouch (28 g)	3
Oatmeal, instant, maple & brown sugar, 1 pouch (28 g)	3
Better Oats Oat Revolution!	
Maple and brown sugar steel cut instant oatmeal with flax, 1 pouch (43 g)	6
Steel cut oats, with flax, classic, 1 pouch (33 g)	4
Steel cut oats, with flax, maple & brown sugar, 1 pouch (43 g)	6
Better Oats Raw Pure & Simple	
Maple and brown sugar multigrain hot cereal with flax (variety pack), 1 pouch (41 g)	6
Organic bare instant multigrain hot cereal with flax, 1 pouch (42 g)	4
Bob's Red Mill	
Hot cereal, oat bran, ⅓ cup	3
Hot cereal, rolled whole grain, 5 grain, ⅓ cup	3
Rolled oats, extra thick whole grain, ½ cup dry	5
Steel cut oats, ¼ cup dry	5
Steel cut oats, quick cooking, ¼ cup dry	4
Bob's Red Mill Gluten Free	
Quick cooking oats, ½ cup dry	5
Rolled oats, whole grain, ½ cup dry	5
Clover Valley	
Old fashioned oats, ½ cup	4
Cream of Wheat	
Instant hot cereal cinnabon flavor, 1 packet (35 g)	5
Instant hot cereal maple brown sugar, 1 packet (35 g)	5
Instant hot cereal original flavor, 1 packet (28 g)	3
Maple brown sugar instant hot cereal, 1 packet (35 g)	5
Cream of Wheat Original	
2 ½ minute cook time hot cereal, 3 Tbsp dry	3
Cream of Wheat Whole Grain	
2 ½ minute cook time hot cereal, 3 Tbsp	3
Essential Everyday	
Instant oatmeal, lower sugar, maple & brown sugar, 1 packet (34 g)	4
Giant	
Instant oatmeal, original flavor, 1 packet (28 g)	3
Great Value	
Apple cinnamon sugar free instant oatmeal, 1 packet (28 g)	3
Enriched instant grits butter flavor, 1 packet (28 g)	3
Fruit and cream variety pack instant oatmeal, 1 packet (35 g)	5
Instant oatmeal, 1 packet (28 g)	3

	SmartPoints® value
Maple and brown sugar instant oatmeal, 1 packet (43 g)	6
Oven toasted quick oats, ½ cup dry	4
Peaches & cream instant oatmeal, 1 packet (35 g)	5
Sugar free instant oatmeal, 1 packet (28 g)	3
Toasted whole grain oat cereal, 1 oz	3
Hannaford	
Apples and cinnamon instant oatmeal, 1 packet (31 g)	4
Harris Teeter Organics Grocery	
Steel cut oats, ¼ cup	4
H-E-B	
Blueberry instant oatmeal, 1 packet (36 g)	3
Maple and brown sugar instant oatmeal, 1 packet (28 g)	3
Old fashioned oats, ½ cup	4
Original instant oatmeal, 1 packet (28 g)	3
Quick oats, ½ cup	4
Sugar free apple cinnamon instant oatmeal, 1 packet (28 g)	3
Hodgson Mill	
Hot cereal, oat bran, ¼ cup	3
Hy-Vee	
Sugar free maple and brown sugar instant oatmeal, 1 packet (28 g)	3
I Love Oats	
Quick oats, ½ cup	4
John McCann's	
Irish oatmeal, steel cut, ¼ cup	4
Kashi Go Lean	
Instant hot cereal, truly vanilla, 1 packet (40 g)	4
Kathleen's	
Cranberry granola quick oats, 1 serving (57 g)	8

	SmartPoints® value
Kroger	
Instant oatmeal, apple cinnamon, 1 pouch (31 g)	4
Lower sugar instant maple & brown sugar oatmeal, 1 pouch (33 g)	4
Maple & brown sugar instant oatmeal, 1 pouch (43 g)	6
Oatmeal, instant, apple cinnamon, 1 pouch (35 g)	5
Oats, 100% whole grain, ½ cup	4
Old fashioned oats, 100% whole grain, ½ cup	4
Original instant oatmeal, 1 pouch (28 g)	3
Whole grain steel cut oats, 1 cup	4
Malt O Meal	
Hot wheat cereal, quick cooking, chocolate, 3 Tbsp dry	4
Hot wheat cereal, quick cooking, original, 3 Tbsp	3
Market Pantry	
Old fashioned oats, ½ cup	4
Quick oats, ½ cup	4
Toasted oats cereal, 1 cup	3
McCann's	
Irish oatmeal, instant, regular flavor, 1 packet (28 g)	3
Irish oatmeal, quick cooking, ½ cup	4
Irish oatmeal, steel cut, ¼ cup	4
Quick & easy steel cut Irish oatmeal (unprepared), ¼ cup	4
Medifast	
Maple and brown sugar oatmeal, 1 packet (32.2 g)	2
Meijer	
Instant oatmeal, sugar free, maple & brown sugar, 1 packet (28 g)	3
Minsley	
Cooked steelcut oatmeal with dried berries and seeds, 5 oz	5
Steelcut oatmeal, 5 oz	5

Cereal, Hot (cont'd)

	SmartPoints® value
Mom's Best Cereals	
Choco chimp cookie dough instant oatmeal, 1 container (42 g)	6
Oatmeal, old fashioned oats, ½ cup dry	4
Mom's Best Naturals	
Quick oats, ½ cup dry	4
My Essentials	
Old fashioned oats, ½ cup	4
Nature's Path Organic	
Apple cinnamon pumpkin seeds premium oatmeal (variety pack), 1 packet (40 g)	5
Cinnamon pumpkin seed oatmeal, 1 packet (38 g)	4
Instant hot oatmeal flax 'n oats, 1 packet (50 g)	7
Instant hot oatmeal, original, 1 packet (50 g)	5
Oatmeal, brown sugar maple, with ancient grains, 1 packet (40 g)	5
Nature's Path Organic Qi'a	
Gluten free creamy coconut oatmeal, 1 packet (38 g)	5
Nature's Place	
Steel cut quick cook oats, ¼ cup	4
Nutrisystem	
Apple cinnamon oatmeal, 1 package (37 g)	5
Maple brown sugar oatmeal, 1 package (38 g)	5
Private Selection	
Cranberry apple walnut rolled oatmeal, 1 package (73 g)	10
Private Selection Organic All Natural No Preservatives	
Instant oatmeal, 1 pouch (28 g)	3
Publix	
Lower sugar maple and brown sugar instant oatmeal, 1 packet (34 g)	4

	SmartPoints® value
Organic maple brown sugar instant oatmeal, 1 packet (41 g)	6
Original flavor instant oatmeal, 1 packet (28 g)	3
Quaker	
100% natural whole grain old fashioned oats, ½ cup	4
American cheese flavored instant grits, 1 packet (28 g)	3
Apples and cranberries instant oatmeal, 1 packet (43 g)	6
Butter flavor instant grits, 1 packet (28 g)	3
Cheddar cheese flavored instant grits, 1 packet (28 g)	3
Cinnamon and spice instant oatmeal, 1 packet (43 g)	6
Cinnamon pecan instant oatmeal (50% less sugar), 1 container (40 g)	5
Country bacon flavored instant grits, 1 packet (28 g)	3
Fruit & cream instant oatmeal variety pack (strawberries & cream flavor), 1 packet (35 g)	5
Maple and brown sugar classic recipe instant oatmeal, 1 packet (43 g)	6
Maple and brown sugar instant oatmeal, 1 packet (43 g)	6
Maple and brown sugar instant oatmeal (variety pack), 1 packet (43 g)	6
Oat bran instant hot cereal, ½ cup dry	4
Oatmeal, steel cut, blueberries & cranberries, 1 packet (46 g)	6
Oats, steel cut, ¼ cup	4
Oats, steel cut, quick 3-minute, ⅓ cup	5
Old fashioned oats, ½ cup dry	4
Original instant grits, 1 packet (28 g)	3

	SmartPoints® value
Original instant oatmeal, 1 packet (28 g)	3
Original instant oatmeal, 1 packet (35 g)	3
Quick 3 minute steel cut oats, ⅓ cup	5
Quick 3-minute oatmeal, steel cut, brown sugar & cinnamon, 1 packet (48 g)	7
Raisin date and walnut instant oatmeal, 1 packet (37 g)	5
Raisins and spice instant oatmeal, 1 packet (43 g)	6
Quaker Express	
Butter instant grits, 1 package (42 g)	4
Quaker Fruit & Cream	
Peaches and cream instant oatmeal, 1 packet (35 g)	5
Strawberries and cream instant oatmeal, 1 packet (35 g)	5
Quaker High Fiber	
Cinnamon swirl instant oatmeal, 1 packet (45 g)	5
Maple and brown sugar instant oatmeal, 1 packet (45 g)	5
Quaker Lower Sugar	
Apples and cinnamon instant oatmeal, 1 packet (31 g)	4
Cinnamon and spice instant oatmeal, 1 packet (34 g)	4
Fruit and cream variety pack instant oatmeal, 1 packet (35 g)	4
Maple and brown sugar instant oatmeal, 1 packet (34 g)	4
Quaker Oatmeal Cups	
Apples and cinnamon flavored instant oatmeal to go, 1 container (43 g)	6
Apples and cranberries flavored instant oatmeal to go, 1 container (51 g)	7

	SmartPoints® value
Honey and almonds flavored instant oatmeal, 1 cup	6
Maple and brown sugar instant oatmeal, 1 cup	7
Quaker Oats	
Oatmeal, ½ cup	4
Original instant oatmeal, 1 packet (28 g)	3
Quaker Oats Select Starts	
Gluten free maple brown sugar instant oatmeal, 1 packet (43 g)	6
Quaker Oats Select Starts Gluten Free	
Quick 1 minute oats, ½ cup	4
Quaker Organic	
Maple and brown sugar instant oatmeal, 1 packet (41 g)	6
Regular instant oatmeal, 1 packet (28 g)	3
Quaker Original	
Quick instant grits, ¼ cup dry	4
Quaker Protein	
Banana nut instant oatmeal, 1 packet (61 g)	8
Cranberry almond instant oatmeal, 1 packet (62 g)	8
Quaker Quick Oats	
1 minute hot cereal, ½ cup	4
Quaker Safari Animals	
Strawberry instant oatmeal, 1 packet (50 g)	7
Quaker Select Starts	
Apples and cinnamon super grains instant hot cereal, 1 pouch (57 g)	7
Honey almond super grains instant hot cereal, 1 pouch (56 g)	7
Quaker Weight Control	
Banana bread instant oatmeal, 1 packet (45 g)	4
Cinnamon instant oatmeal, 1 packet (45 g)	4

Cereal, Hot, Quaker Weight Control (cont'd)

	SmartPoints® value
Maple and brown sugar instant oatmeal (variety pack), 1 packet (45 g)	4
ShopRite	
Instant oatmeal, original, 1 packet (28 g)	3
Maple & brown sugar instant oatmeal, 1 packet (43 g)	6
Oatmeal, instant, sugar free, maple & brown sugar, 1 packet (28 g)	3
Simply Nature	
Apple cinnamon organic instant oatmeal, 1 packet (40 g)	6
Oats and flax instant oatmeal, 1 packet (40 g)	5
Special K Nourish	
Hot cereal, maple brown sugar crunch, 1 container (52 g)	6
Maple brown sugar crunch hot cereal, 1 container (52 g)	6
Sprouts Farmers Market	
Spiced cran orange instant oatmeal, 1 packet (43 g)	6
Think Thin	
Farmer's market berry crumble protein & fiber hot oatmeal, 1 packet (50 g)	6
Madagascar vanilla, almonds, pecans protein & fiber hot oatmeal, 1 packet (50 g)	6
Trader Joe's	
Maple and brown sugar instant oatmeal, 1 pouch (43 g)	6
Oatmeal complete, 1 packet (40 g)	5
Organic cinnamon spice instant oatmeal, 1 packet (40 g)	4
Organic oats and flax instant oatmeal, 1 packet (40 g)	5
Quick cook steel cut oats, ¼ cup dry	4
Quinoa and steel cut oatmeal, 1 packet (227 g)	6

	SmartPoints® value
Rolled oats, ½ cup dry	4
Toasted oat bran, ⅓ cup	4
Triple ginger instant oatmeal, 1 packet (38 g)	5
Trader Joe's Frozen	
Steelcut oatmeal, 1 packet (227 g)	5
Trader Joe's Grocery	
Organic multigrain hot cereal, ½ cup	4
Wegman's	
Oatmeal, instant, weight control, maple & brown sugar, 1 packet (45 g)	4
Weight Watchers In-Meeting/ Online Products: Oatmeal	
Apple cinnamon, 1 container	3
Blueberry vanilla, 1 container	3
Maple brown sugar, 1 container	3
Strawberry 'n' cream, 1 container	3
Weight Watchers Smart Ones Smart Beginnings	
Apple and cinnamon oatmeal, 1 cup	7
Maple and brown sugar oatmeal, 1 cup	7
Peaches and cream oatmeal, 1 cup	6

Cereal, Ready-to-Eat

All-Bran	
Buds cereal, ⅓ cup	3
Original wheat bran cereal, ½ cup	3
All-Bran Complete	
Cereal, wheat flakes, ¾ cup	3
Alpen	
Muesli, no sugar added, ⅔ cup	7
Apple Jacks	
Cereal, 1 cup	5
Arrowhead Mills	
Cereal, puffed kamut, organic, 1 cup	1

	SmartPoints® value
Back To Nature	
Granola, classic, ½ cup	7
Barbara's	
Cereal, puffins, original, ¾ cup	3
Barbara's Original	
Multigrain spoonfuls cereal, ¾ cup dry	4
Barbara's Puffins	
Cereal, cinnamon, ⅔ cup	3
Cereal, peanut butter & chocolate, ¾ cup	4
Basic 4	
Cereal, 1 cup dry	8
Bear Naked	
Fruit and nut granola, ¼ cup dry	5
Granola, all natural, maple pecan, ¼ cup	5
Honey and almond granola, ¼ cup	4
Original cinnamon granola, ¼ cup	4
Bear Naked Fit	
100% pure & natural granola, vanilla almond crunch, ¼ cup	4
Triple berry crunch granola, ¼ cup dry	4
Better Oats Mmm...Muffins	
Thick & hearty blueberry muffin instant thick cut oats with flax, 1 pouch (43 g)	6
Bob's Red Mill	
Muesli, old country style, ¼ cup	4
Cap'n Crunch	
Cereal, berries, ¾ cup	5
Cereal, sweetened corn & oat, ¾ cup	5
Cap'n Crunch Peanut Butter Crunch	
Sweetened corn and oat cereal, ¾ cup	5
Cascadian Farm Organic	
Cinnamon crunch cereal, ¾ cup	4
Granola, oats and honey, ⅔ cup	9

	SmartPoints® value
Cheerios	
Ancient grains cereal, ¾ cup	4
Chocolate flavored whole grain corn and oat cereal, ¾ cup dry	4
Honey nut medley crunch, ¾ cup	4
Multi grain cereal, 1 cup dry	4
Original toasted whole grain oat cereal, 1 cup	3
Original toasted whole grain oat cereal single serve cup, 1 container (39 g)	4
Cheerios Apple Cinnamon	
Naturally sweetened whole grain oat and corn cereal, ¾ cup dry	5
Cheerios Frosted	
Whole grain oat and corn cereal, ¾ cup dry	4
Cheerios Honey Nut	
Sweetened whole grain oat cereal with real honey and natural almond flavor, ¾ cup dry	4
Sweetened whole grain oat cereal with real honey and natural almond flavor single serve container, 1 container (52 g)	8
Sweetened wholegrain oat cereal with honey and almond flavor, ¾ cup	4
Whole grain oats cereal, 1 pouch (32 g)	5
Cheerios Multi Grain	
Peanut butter flavored whole grain toasted oats cereal, ¾ cup dry	4
Cheerios Multi Grain Dark Chocolate Crunch	
Chocolate flavored whole grain corn and oat cereal, ¾ cup	4
Cheerios Protein	
Cereal, oats & honey, 1¼ cups	8
Cinnamon almond flavored cereal, 1¼ cups	8
Oats and honey cereal, 1¼ cups	8

	SmartPoints® value
Chex	
Cereal, honey nut, ¾ cup	5
Cereal, vanilla, gluten free, ¾ cup	5
Cereal, wheat, ¾ cup	5
Gluten free corn cereal, 1 cup	4
Gluten free honey nut corn cereal, ¾ cup	5
Gluten free oven toasted rice cereal, 1 cup	3
Gluten free rice cereal with natural chocolate flavor, ¾ cup	5
Cinnamon Toast Crunch	
Cereal, ¾ cup	5
Cocoa Pebbles	
Sweetened rice cereal with real cocoa, ¾ cup	5
Cocoa Puffs	
Frosted puffs, reduced sugar, 1 cup	4
Corn Pops	
Cereal, 1 cup	5
Crispix	
Cereal, 1 cup	4
Engine 2 Plant Strong	
Organic morning blend grain medley, 1 cup	8
Fiber One	
Cereal, honey clusters, 1 cup	6
Nutty clusters and almonds cereal, 1 cup	7
Original bran cereal, ½ cup dry	2
Raisin bran clusters cereal, 1 cup dry	7
Fit & Active	
Low-fat multigrain granola with raisins, ⅔ cup	7
Froot Loops	
Sweetened multi-grain cereal, 1 cup	5

	SmartPoints® value
Frosted Mini Wheats	
Original lightly sweetened whole grain cereal, 21 pieces (54 g)	7
Strawberry flavored cereal, 25 biscuits (55 g)	7
Frosted Mini Wheats Little Bites	
Original lightly sweetened whole grain cereal, 1 cup	7
Fruity Cheerios	
Sweetened whole grain corn and oat cereal, ¾ cup dry	4
Fruity Pebbles	
Cereal, ¾ cup	5
General Mills Cinnamon Toast Crunch	
Crispy sweetened whole wheat and rice cereal, 1 pouch (39 g)	6
General Mills French Toast Crunch	
Crispy sweetened corn cereal, ¾ cup	4
General Mills Multi-Grain Cheerios	
5 whole grains lightly sweetened cereal, 1 cup	4
Giant Oats & O's	
Toasted whole grain oat cereal, 1 cup	3
Golden Grahams	
Cereal, ¾ cup	5
Granola Unleashed	
French vanilla almond granola, 1 container (55 g)	9
Grape-Nuts	
Cereal, ½ cup	6
Cereal, flakes, ¾ cup	4
The original cereal, ½ cup	6
Great Grains	
Raisins dates and pecans cereal, ¾ cup	8
Great Grains Selects	
Banana nut crunch cereal, 1 cup dry	8
Crunchy pecans cereal, ¾ cup	7

	SmartPoints® value
Great Value	
Bran flakes cereal, ¾ cup	4
Crisp rice cereal, 1¼ cups	4
Shredded wheat cereal, 1 cup	5
Strawberry awake cereal, 1 cup	4
Toasted multi grain spins cereal, 1 cup	4
Toasted rice cereal, 1 cup	3
Toasted whole grain oat spins cereal, 1 cup	3
Great Value Awake	
Crunchy rice and wheat flakes with strawberries cereal, 1 cup	4
Great Value Crunchy Nuggets	
Whole grain wheat with barley cereal, ½ cup	6
Great Value Frosted Shredded Wheat	
Cereal, 1 cup	6
Honey Bunches of Oats	
Cereal with real apples and cinnamon bunches, ¾ cup	4
Cereal, honey roasted, ¾ cup	4
Cereal, with almonds, ¾ cup	4
Cereal, with cinnamon bunches, ¾ cup	4
Crunchy honey roasted cereal, ¾ cup	4
Whole grain honey crunch cereal, 1 cup	8
Honey Comb	
Cereal, 1½ cups	5
Hospitality	
Toasted oats cereal, 1 cup	3
Kashi	
Berry fruitful cereal, 28 biscuits (55 g)	6
Cereal, autumn wheat, 29 biscuits (54 g)	6
Cinnamon harvest organic whole wheat biscuits, 28 biscuits (55 g)	6
Sunflower and pepita overnight muesli, 1 container (60 g)	8

	SmartPoints® value
Kashi Go Lean	
Cereal, 1 cup	4
Cereal, crunch, protein & high fiber, 1 cup	7
Crunch, 1 cup	6
Crunch honey almond flax, 1 cup	7
Vanilla graham clusters cereal, 1 cup	5
Vanilla pepita cereal, 1 cup	7
Kashi Go Lean Crisp!	
Cereal, toasted berry crumble, ¾ cup	6
Cinnamon crumble cereal, ¾ cup	6
Kashi Go Lean Crunch!	
Honey almond flax cereal, ⅔ cup	7
Kashi Heart to Heart	
Cinnamon, ¾ cup	4
Honey toasted oat cereal, ¾ cup	4
Oat flakes & blueberry clusters cereal, 1 cup	7
Warm cinnamon oat cereal, ¾ cup	4
Kashi Organic Promise	
Cinnamon harvest whole wheat biscuits, 28 biscuits (55 g)	6
Sprouted grains cereal, 1¼ cups	6
Kellogg's	
Cereal, 1 cup	3
Low-fat granola original multi-grain cereral, ½ cup	7
Raisin bran cereal, 1 cup	7
Kellogg's Cocoa Krispies	
Rice cereal, ¾ cup	5
Kellogg's Frosted Flakes	
Corn cereal, ¾ cup	5
Kellogg's Mini Wheats	
Blueberry with vanilla drizzle whole grain cereal, 27 pieces (55 g)	6
Kellogg's Mini Wheats Harvest Delights	
Cranberry with yogurt drizzle cereal, 27 pieces (55 g)	6

Cereal, Ready-to-Eat (cont'd)

	SmartPoints® value
Kellogg's Raisin Bran	
Cereal, 1 cup	7
Kellogg's Raisin Bran Crunch	
Toasted flakes, raisins and crunchy oat clusters cereal, 1 cup	8
Kellogg's Smart Start	
Original antioxidants cereal, 1 cup	7
Kellogg's Special K	
Apple cinnamon crunch cereal, ¾ cup	5
Chocolatey delight cereal, ¾ cup	5
Chocolatey strawberry cereal, ¾ cup	4
Cranberry granola, ⅔ cup	8
Limited edition apple cinnamon crunch cereal, ¾ cup	5
Oats and honey cereal, ⅔ cup	4
Oats and honey cereal, ⅔ cup	4
Protein cereal, ¾ cup	4
Vanilla almond cereal, ¾ cup	4
Kellogg's Special K Nourish	
Apple raspberry almond cereal, 1 cup	6
Coconut cranberry almond cereal, 1 cup	7
Kellogg's Special K Protein	
Cinnamon brown sugar crunch cereal, ¾ cup	4
Kind Healthy Grains	
Fruit and nut clusters, ⅓ cup	3
Maple quinoa clusters with chia seeds, ⅓ cup	4
Raspberry clusters with chia seeds, ⅓ cup	4
Kirkland Nature's Path Organic	
Ancient grains granola with almonds, ¾ cup	9
Kix	
Crispy corn puffs cereal, 1¼ cups	4
Krave	
Cereal, with chocolate flavored center, ¾ cup	5

	SmartPoints® value
Kroger	
Cereal, honey crisp medley, ¾ cup	4
Toasted flakes with strawberries, 1 cup	4
Vanilla flavored flakes with almonds, ¾ cup	4
Kroger Nutty Nuggets	
Crunchy wheat and barley cereal, ½ cup	6
Kroger Toasted Oats	
Whole grain oat cereal, 1 cup	3
Life	
Cereal, cinnamon, ¾ cup	4
Cereal, multigrain, original, ¾ cup	4
Lucky Charms	
Cereal, ¾ cup	4
Malt-O-Meal	
Honey nut scooters cereal, 1 cup	4
Malt-O-Meal Golden Puffs	
Sweetened puff wheat cereal, ¾ cup	5
Malt-O-Meal Oat Blenders	
Corn and whole wheat flakes cereal with honey and almonds, ¾ cup	4
Market Pantry Honey & Oat Mixers	
Crispy flakes crunchy oat clusters and honey cereal, ¾ cup	4
Medifast	
Cinnamon and brown sugar cereal crunch, 1 package (30 g)	2
Mixed berry cereal crunch, 1 packet (30 g)	2
Millville	
Bran flakes, ¾ cup	3
Crispy oats toasted whole grain oat cereal, 1 cup	3
Fruit rounds cereal, 1 cup	4
Honey nut crispy oats, 1 cup	4
Honey wheat puffs cereal, ¾ cup	5
Multigrain crispy oats, 1 cup	4
Pumpkin spice cranberry granola, ⅔ cup	9

	SmartPoints® value
Mini-Wheats	
Cereal, little bites, frosted, chocolate, 42 biscuits (55 g)	7
Mini-Wheats Frosted	
Cereal, bite-size, ¾ cup	3
Nature Valley	
Baked oat bites cereal, ¾ cup	8
Breakfast biscuits, honey, 4 biscuits (50 g)	8
Honey oat cluster cereal, 1 cup	8
Nature Valley Protein	
Oats 'n dark chocolate crunchy granola, ½ cup	8
Oats 'n honey crunchy granola, ½ cup	7
Peanut butter granola, ½ cup	8
Nature's Path Organic	
Cereal, smart bran with psyllium & oatbran, ⅔ cup	3
Heritage ancient grains multigrain cereal, ¾ cup	3
Heritage flakes cereal, ¾ cup	4
Organic granola, premium organic, love crunch, dark chocolate & red berries, ¼ cup	5
Sunrise, crunchy vanilla, ⅔ cup	4
Nature's Path Organic Flax Plus	
Cereal, multibran flakes, ¾ cup	3
Pumpkin flax granola (dry), 1 oz	5
Pumpkin flax granola cereal, ¾ cup	9
Nature's Promise	
Vanilla almond granola, ½ cup	7
Nutrisystem	
Granola cereal, 1 package (40 g)	5
Ohs	
Honey graham cereal, ¾ cup	5
Publix	
Fiber active bran cereal, ½ cup	2
Toasted oats whole grain oat cereal, 1 cup	3

	SmartPoints® value
Publix Fiber Active	
Bran cereal, ½ cup	2
Puffed Wheat Essentials	
Cereal, 1¼ cups	1
Quaker	
Cereal, oatmeal squares, with a hint of cinnamon, 1 cup	7
Corn bran crunch toasted corn cereal, ¾ cup dry	3
Oats honey and almonds simply granola cereal, ½ cup	7
Oats honey raisins and almonds simply granola cereal, ½ cup	8
Quaker Instant Oatmeal	
Bananas and cream, 1 packet (35 g)	5
Blueberries and cream, 1 packet (35 g)	5
Pumpkin spice, 1 packet (43 g)	6
Quaker Life	
Cinnamon multigrain cereal, ¾ cup	4
Original multigrain cereal, ¾ cup	4
Quaker Oatmeal Squares	
Hint of brown sugar cereal, 1 cup	7
Quaker Real Medleys	
Cinnamon apple walnut supergrains, ½ cup	8
Dark chocolate cranberry almond granola, ⅓ cup	5
Summer berry granola, ⅓ cup	4
Super grains blueberry pecan, ½ cup	8
Raisin Bran	
Cereal with cranberries, 1¼ cups	8
Cereal, whole grain wheat & bran, 1 cup	8
Raisin Nut Bran	
Cereal, ¾ cup	7
Reese's Puffs	
Cereal, ¾ cup	5

Cereal, Ready-to-Eat (cont'd)

	SmartPoints® value
Rice Krispies	
Cereal, 1¼ cups	4
ShopRite	
Raisin bran cereal, 1 cup	7
Shredded Wheat	
Cereal, lightly frosted, spoon size, 1 cup dry	7
Shredded Wheat Natural Advantage	
Cereal, original, spoon size, 1 cup dry	5
Cereal, wheat 'n bran, spoon size, 1¼ cups dry	5
Simple Truth Organic	
Toasted oats cereal, 1 cup	3
Simply Balanced	
Honey almond flax granola, ½ cup	8
Simply Nature Organic	
Dark chocolate macaroon premium granola, 1 cup	5
Special K	
Cereal, chocolate almond, ⅔ cup	4
Cereal, chocolatey delight, ¾ cup	5
Cereal, fruit & yogurt, ¾ cup	5
Cereal, low-fat, granola, touch of honey, ½ cup dry	6
Cereal, oats & honey, ⅔ cup	4
Chocolatey strawberry cereal, ¾ cup	4
Cinnamon pecan cereal, ¾ cup	4
Fruit and yogurt cereal, ¾ cup	5
Low-fat granola cereal, ½ cup	6
Original toasted rice cereal, 1 cup	4
Red berries cereal, 1 cup	4
Vanilla almond cereal, ¾ cup	4
Special K Protein	
Cereal, ¾ cup	4
The Silver Palate	
Grain berry cinnamon frosted cereal, 1 cup	7

	SmartPoints® value
Total	
Cereal, whole grain, ¾ cup	3
Trader Joe's	
Organic high fiber o's cereal, 1¼ cups	6
Trader Joe's Grocery	
Bran flakes, ¾ cup	3
High fiber cereal, ⅔ cup	3
Honey nut o's, ¾ cup	5
Joe's o's, 1 cup	3
Low-fat granola mixed berry, ¾ cup	8
Multigrain o's cereal, 1 cup	4
Shredded bite size wheats, 1 cup	5
Toasted oatmeal flakes, ¾ cup	4
Trix	
Corn puffs cereal, 1 pouch (31 g)	5
Udi's	
Granola, ¼ cup	4
Granola, vanilla, ¼ cup	4
Uncle Sam	
Cereal, original, value size, ¾ cup	5
Weetabix Organic	
Cereal, whole grain biscuit, 2 biscuits (35 g)	3
Weight Watchers Cereal	
Oat clusters with almonds cereal, ¾ cup	4
Wheaties	
Cereal, ¾ cup	3
Wild Oats Marketplace Organic	
Cinnamon squares cereal, 1 cup	4

French Toast

Aunt Jemima	
French toast, cinnamon, 2 slices (118 g)	7
Trader Giotto's	
Panettone French toast, 1 slice (113 g)	10

	SmartPoints® value
Pancakes	
Aunt Jemima	
Complete buttermilk pancake & waffle mix, ⅓ cup mix	5
Pancake & waffle mix, original, 4 pancakes (48 g)	5
Pancake & waffle mix, original, complete, 2 pancakes (45 g)	5
Birch Benders	
Protein pancake and waffle mix, ½ cup	5
Bisquick Shake 'N Pour	
Pancake mix, buttermilk, 3 pancakes (58 g)	7
Crepini by the Crepe Team	
Naked crepini, 1⅔ oz	3
De Wafelbakkers	
Blueberry pancakes, 3 pancakes (117 g)	9
Hungry Jack	
Complete buttermilk pancake & waffle mix, 3 4″ pancakes (44 g)	5
Complete extra light & fluffy pancake & waffle mix, 3 4″ pancakes (44 g)	5
Gluten free buttermilk pancake and waffle mix with candy bits, ⅓ cup	7
Kodiak Cakes	
Flapjack and waffle mix, frontier, original, ⅓ cup	4
Frontier flapjack and waffle mix, buttermilk & honey, ⅓ cup	4
Kodiak Cakes Power Cakes	
Whole grain buttermilk flapjack and waffle mix, ½ cup	5
Kroger	
Complete pancake and waffle mix (unprepared), ½ cup	8
Krusteaz	
Complete pancake mix, blueberry, 3 pancakes (66 g)	8
Pancake mix, complete, buttermilk, ½ cup mix	7

	SmartPoints® value
Maple Grove Farms of Vermont	
Whole wheat blend pancake and waffle mix (unprepared), ⅓ cup	4
Meijer	
Whole wheat pancake mix (unprepared), ⅓ cup	5
Toaster Pastries	
Kellogg's Special K Pastry Crisps	
Strawberry flavored pastry (variety pack), 2 crisps (25 g)	4
Pillsbury	
Pumpkin pie toaster strudel, 1 strudel (55 g)	8
Pillsbury Toaster Scrambles	
Ham toaster pastries, 1 pastry (51 g)	6
Pillsbury Toaster Strudel	
Pastries, strawberry, 1 pastry (54 g)	7
Pop-Tarts	
Toaster pastries, chocolate fudge, frosted, 2 pastries (104 g)	17
Toaster pastries, frosted blueberry, 1 pastry (52 g)	8
Toaster pastries, frosted strawberry, 1 pastry (52 g)	8
Toaster pastries, frosted, brown sugar cinnamon, value pack, 1 pastry (50 g)	9
Toaster pastries, frosted, cherry, 1 pastry (52 g)	8
Toaster pastries, s'mores, 2 pastries (104 g)	17
Toaster pastries, strawberry, 1 pastry (50 g)	8
Special K	
Blueberry fruit crisps, 2 crisps (25 g)	4
Blueberry pastry crisps, 2 crisps (25 g)	4
Pastry crisps, brown sugar cinnamon, 2 crisps (25 g)	4

Toaster Pastries, Special K (cont'd)

	SmartPoints® value
Pastry crisps, chocolatey delight, 2 crisps (25 g)	4
Pastry crisps, strawberry, 2 crisps (25 g)	4

Waffles

	SmartPoints® value
De Wafelbakkers	
European style waffles, 2 pieces (43 g)	8
Eggo	
Chocolate chip waffles, 2 waffles (70 g)	7
Cinnamon toast waffles (3 sets of 4), 3 waffles (92 g)	11
Strawberry waffles, 2 waffles (70 g)	7
Waffles, blueberry, 2 waffles (70 ml)	7
Waffles, buttermilk, family pack, 2 waffles (70 g)	6
Waffles, homestyle, 2 waffles (70 g)	6
Waffles, thick & fluffy, original recipe, 1 waffle (55 g)	5
Eggo Nutri-Grain	
Low-fat whole grain waffles, 2 waffles (70 g)	4
Whole wheat waffles, 2 waffles (70 g)	6
Fit & Active	
Multigrain waffles, 2 waffles (70 g)	6
Giant	
Raspberry waffles, 2 waffles (70 g)	7
Great Value	
Homestyle waffles, 2 pieces (70 g)	4
Kashi	
Waffles, 7 grain, 2 waffles (72 g)	5
Waffles, blueberry, 2 waffles (72 g)	5
Trader Joe's Frozen	
Multi grain toaster waffles, 2 waffles (78 g)	8
Van's	
Waffles, blueberry, 2 waffles (85 g)	8
Waffles, lite, totally natural, 2 waffles (76 g)	4
Waffles, totally natural, 2 waffles (85 g)	8
Whole grain organic waffles, 2 waffles (76 g)	6
Van's Natural Foods	
Gluten free ancient grains waffles, 2 waffles (76 g)	7
Van's Power Grains	
Waffles, totally natural, 2 waffles (85 g)	5
Van's Whole Grains	
Multigrain waffles, 2 waffles (76 g)	4

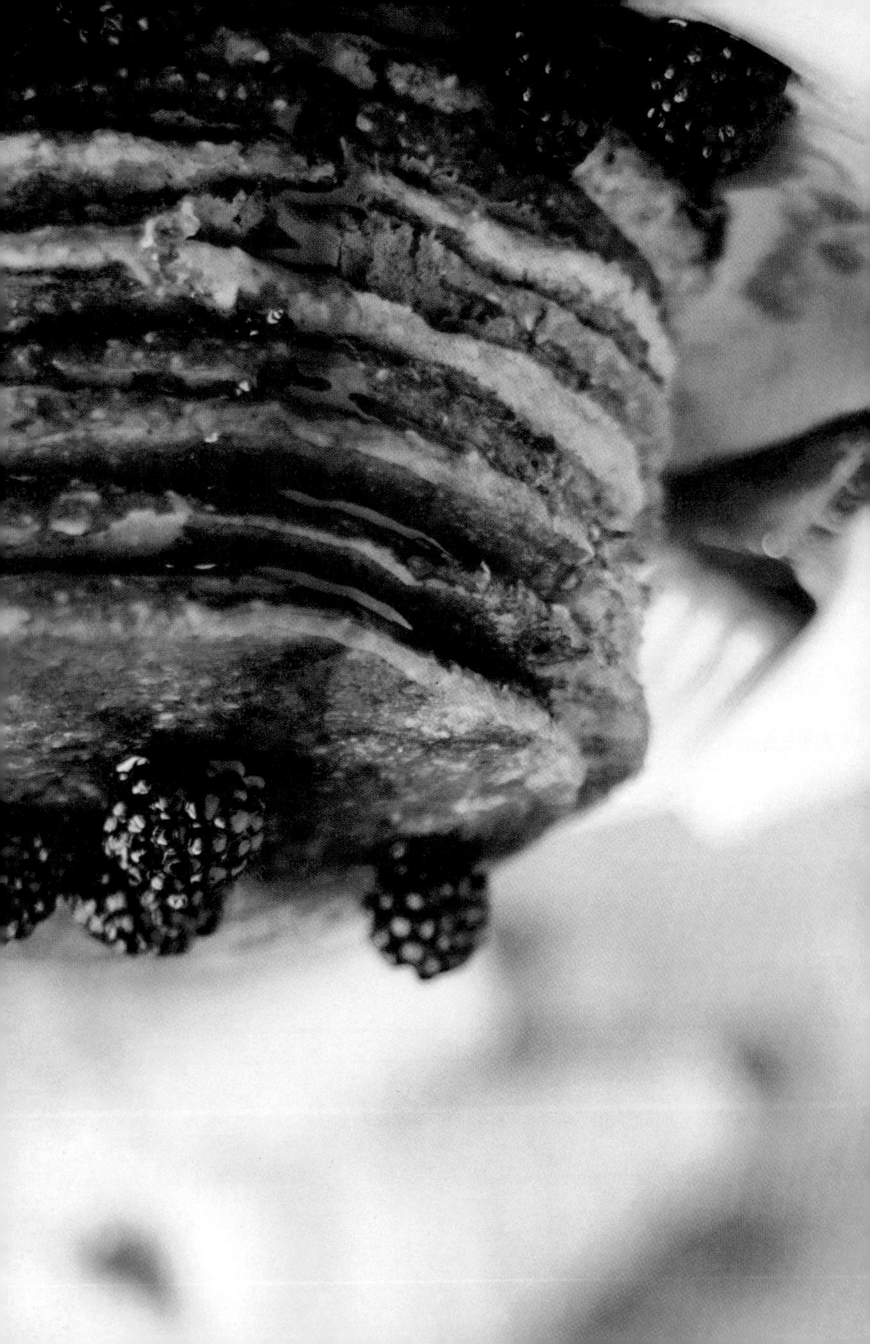

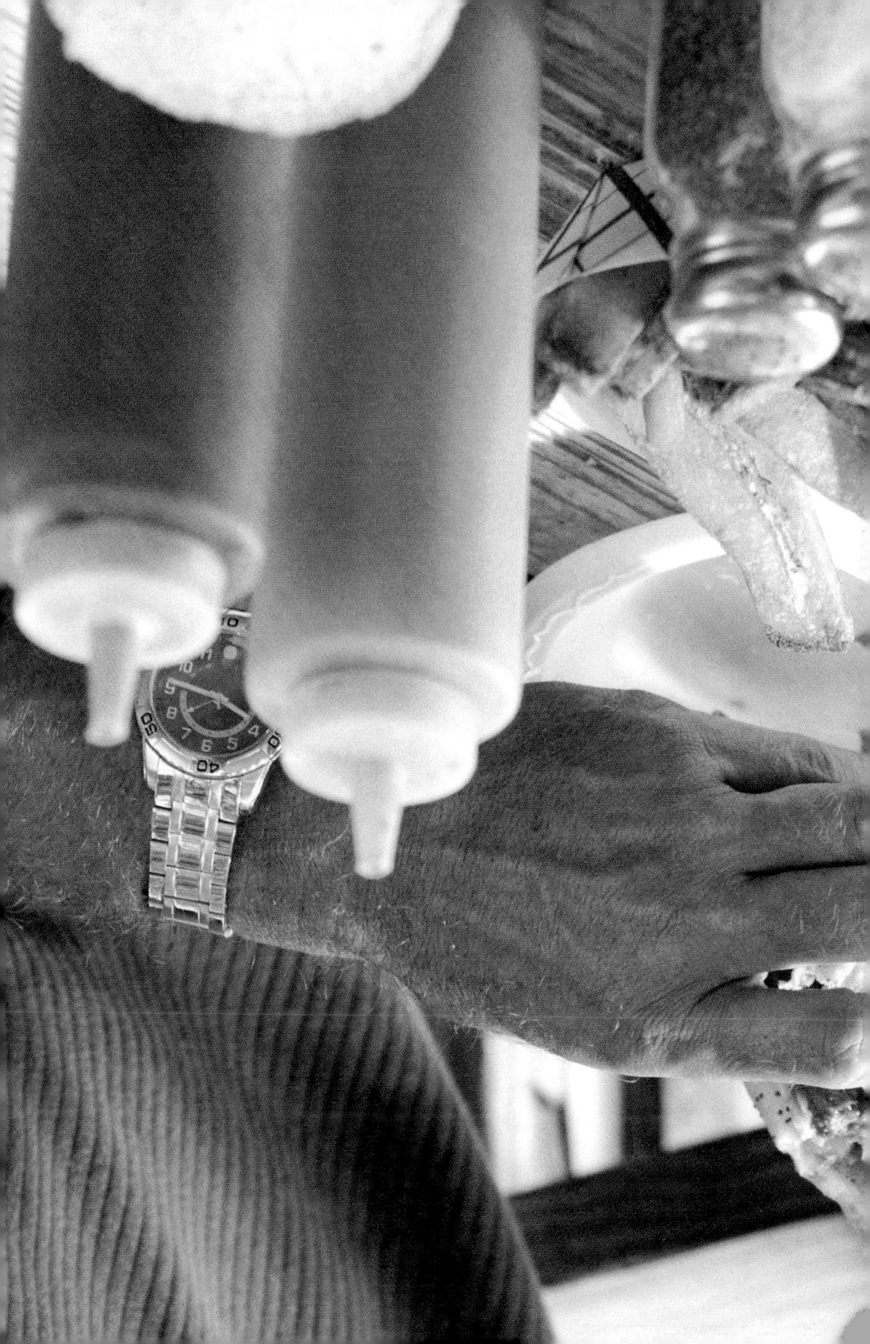

condiments, sauces & gravies

	SmartPoints® value
Asian Sauces and Condiments	
Archer Farms	
Tikka masala simmer sauce, ½ cup	5
House Of Tsang	
Stir-fry sauce, classic, 1 Tbsp	1
Stir-fry sauce, Szechuan spicy, 1 Tbsp	1
Kichigai	
Spicy mayo, all purpose, 1 tsp	1
Kikkoman	
Soy sauce, 1 Tbsp	0
La Choy	
Soy sauce, lite, 1 tsp	1
Lee Kum Kee	
Sriracha mayo, 1 Tbsp	3
Thai sweet chili sauce, 1 Tbsp	1
Saffron Road	
Thai red curry simmer sauce, 1 serving (30 g)	1
Terry Ho's	
Yum yum sauce, 2 Tbsp	6
Trader Joe's	
Island soyaki sauce, 1 Tbsp	1
Thai red curry sauce, ¼ cup	4
Thai yellow curry sauce, ¼ cup	4
Trader Joe's Grocery	
Sweet chili sauce, 1 Tbsp	1
Trader Ming's	
Gyoza dipping sauce, 2 Tbsp	1
Yoshida's	
Original marinade sauce, 1 Tbsp	2
Barbecue and Grilling Sauces	
Campbell's	
Cheddar applewood bacon chicken grill sauce, ¼ cup	3
Jim Beam	
Honey barbeque sauce, 2 Tbsp	2

	SmartPoints® value
KC Masterpiece	
Barbecue sauce, original, 2 Tbsp	3
KC Masterpiece Private Stock Reserve	
Original bbq sauce, 2 Tbsp	3
Kraft	
Original barbecue sauce, 2 Tbsp	3
Stubbs	
Bar-b-q sauce, original, 2 Tbsp	1
Sweet Baby Ray's	
Barbecue sauce, 2 Tbsp	4
Barbecue sauce, award winning, 2 Tbsp	4
Barbecue sauce, hickory & brown sugar, 2 Tbsp	4
Barbecue sauce, honey, 2 Tbsp	4
Honey barbecue sauce, 2 Tbsp	4
Fruit Sauces	
Great Value	
Whole berry cranberry sauce, ¼ cup	6
Ocean Spray	
Cran raspberry cranberry sauce, ¼ cup	6
Cranberry sauce, jellied, ¼ cup	6
Gravies	
Heinz Home Style	
Gravy, classic chicken, ¼ cup	1
Gravy, pork, ¼ cup	1
Gravy, roasted turkey, ¼ cup	1
Gravy, savory beef, ¼ cup	1
McCormick	
Country gravy mix, peppered, ¼ cup	2
Homestyle country gravy mix (unprepared), 2 tsp	0
Mix, brown gravy, 1 Tbsp dry mix	1

	SmartPoints® value
Horseradish Sauces	
Boar's Head	
Horseradish sauce, pub style (gluten free), 1 tsp	1
Kraft	
Horseradish sauce, creamy, 1 tsp	1
Woeber's Sandwich Pal	
Horseradish sauce, 1 tsp	1
Hot and Latin Sauces	
Cholula	
Hot sauce, original, 1 tsp	0
Frank's RedHot	
Cayenne pepper sauce, original, 1 tsp	0
Huy Fong	
Chili sauce, sriracha, hot, 1 tsp	0
Old El Paso	
Enchilada sauce, mild, ¼ cup	1
Ortega	
Taco sauce, original, medium, 1 Tbsp	0
Taco sauce, original, medium, thick & smooth, 1 Tbsp	0
Taco sauce, thick & smooth, original, mild, 1 Tbsp	0
Pace	
Mild original picante sauce, 2 Tbsp	1
Picante sauce, medium, 2 Tbsp	1
Silver Spring	
Spicy sriracha sauce, 1 Tbsp	3
Taco Bell	
Mild sauce, 1 tsp	0
Tapatio	
Hot sauce, 1 tsp	0
Trader Joe's	
Green dragon hot sauce, 1 tsp	0

	SmartPoints® value
Ketchup	
French's	
Tomato ketchup, 1 Tbsp	1
Great Value	
Tomato ketchup, 1 Tbsp	1
Heinz	
Ketchup, tomato, 1 Tbsp	1
Ketchup, tomato, reduced sugar, 1 Tbsp	0
Ketchup, tomato, value size, 1 Tbsp	1
Organic tomato ketchup, 1 Tbsp	1
Reduced sugar tomato ketchup, 1 Tbsp	0
Heinz Organic	
Tomato ketchup, 1 Tbsp	1
Heinz Simply Heinz	
Ketchup, tomato, 1 Tbsp	1
Ketchup, tomato simply Heinz (no high fructose corn syrup), 1 Tbsp	1
Tomato ketchup, 1 Tbsp	1
Hunt's	
Ketchup, tomatoes, perfect squeeze, 1 Tbsp	1
Tomato ketchup, 1 Tbsp	1
Kroger	
Tomato ketchup, 1 Tbsp	1
Simply Nature	
Organic ketchup, 1 Tbsp	1
Springfield	
Tomato catsup, 1 Tbsp	1
Marinades	
Bernstein's Light Fantastic	
Dressing & marinade, cheese fantastico, 2 Tbsp	1
Garlic Expressions	
Salad dressing & marinade, classic vinaigrette, 1 Tbsp	2

Marinades (cont'd)

	SmartPoints® value
Gazebo Room	
Salad dressing & marinade, Greek, lite, 1 Tbsp	1
Kikkoman	
Teriyaki marinade & sauce, 1 Tbsp	1
Teriyaki marinade & sauce, less sodium, 1 Tbsp	1
Lawry's 30 Minute	
Marinade, teriyaki with pineapple juice, 1 Tbsp	1
Olde Cape Cod	
Vinaigrette & marinade dressing, toasted sesame soy & ginger, fat free, 2 Tbsp	2
Soy Vay	
Marinade & sauce, veri veri teriyaki, 1 Tbsp	2
Sweet Baby Ray's	
Marinade & sauce, buffalo wing sauce, 1 Tbsp	0

Mayonnaise

	SmartPoints® value
Bama	
Light mayonnaise, 1 Tbsp	2
Best Foods	
Light mayonnaise, 1 Tbsp	1
Mayonnaise dressing with olive oil, 1 Tbsp	2
Mayonnaise dressing, low-fat, 1 Tbsp	1
Mayonnaise, light, 1 Tbsp	1
Real mayonnaise, 1 Tbsp	3
Blue Plate	
Light mayonnaise, 1 Tbsp	2
Light mayonnaise with olive oil, 1 Tbsp	1
Real mayonnaise, 1 Tbsp	3
Burman's	
Real mayonnaise, 1 Tbsp	3
Cains	
Mayonnaise, 1 Tbsp	3
Reduced calorie mayonnaise, light, 1 Tbsp	2
Duke's	
Mayonnaise, light, 1 Tbsp	2
Mayonnaise, real, 1 Tbsp	3
Duke's Light	
Mayonnaise, 1 Tbsp	2
Mayonnaise with olive oil, 1 Tbsp	2
Fit & Active	
Light mayonnaise, 1 Tbsp	1
Hellmann's	
Aioli, real, classic, 1 Tbsp	2
Canola mayonnaise, 1 Tbsp	1
Light mayonnaise, 1 Tbsp	1
Low-fat mayonnaise dressing, 1 Tbsp	1
Mayonnaise dressing with olive oil, 1 Tbsp	2
Mayonnaise, light, 1 Tbsp	1
Olive oil mayonnaise dressing, 1 Tbsp	2
Real mayonnaise, 1 Tbsp	3
Kraft	
Light mayo, 1 Tbsp	1
Mayo, fat free, 1 Tbsp	0
Mayo, homestyle, 1 Tbsp	3
Mayo, light, 1 Tbsp	1
Mayo, reduced fat, chipotle, 1 Tbsp	1
Mayo, reduced fat, with olive oil, 1 Tbsp	1
Mayonnaise, reduced fat, with olive oil, cracked pepper, 1 Tbsp	1
Reduced fat mayo with olive oil, 1 Tbsp	1
Kraft	
Reduced fat, light, 1 Tbsp	2

	SmartPoints® value
Kroger	
Olive oil mayo, 1 Tbsp	2
Portmann's	
Light mayonnaise, 1 Tbsp	2
Primal Kitchen	
Mayo made with avocado oil (sugar free), 1 Tbsp	3
ShopRite	
Real mayonnaise, 1 Tbsp	3
Smart Balance	
Light mayonnaise, 1 Tbsp	2
Spectrum Natural Naturals	
Light canola mayo, eggless, vegan, 1 Tbsp	1
Subway	
Mayonnaise, light, 1 pouch (12.4 g)	1
The HoneyBaked Ham Company	
Honey mustard mayonnaise, 1 tsp	1
Trader Joe's	
Organic mayonnaise, 1 Tbsp	3
Real mayonnaise, 1 Tbsp	4
Trader Joe's Grocery	
Reduced fat mayonnaise, 1 Tbsp	1
WinCo Foods	
Light mayonnaise, 1 Tbsp	2

Mustard

Boar's Head	
Honey mustard with pure golden honey (gluten free), 1 tsp	0
Burman's	
Dijon mustard, 1 tsp	0
Honey mustard, 1 tsp	0
Spicy brown mustard, 1 tsp	0
French's	
Mustard, classic yellow, 1 tsp	0
Mustard, honey, 1 tsp	0
Mustard, honey dijon, 1 tsp	0
Mustard, horseradish, 1 tsp	0
Mustard, spicy brown, 1 tsp	0

	SmartPoints® value
French's Classic	
Spicy yellow mustard with cayenne pepper, 1 tsp	0
Great Value	
Spicy brown mustard, 1 tsp	0
Grey Poupon	
Mustard, classic dijon, 1 tsp	0
Mustard, dijon, 1 tsp	0
Gulden's	
Mustard, spicy brown, 1 tsp	0
Heinz	
Yellow mustard, 1 tsp	0
Hellmann's	
Dijonnaise, 1 tsp	0
Dijonnaise creamy dijon mustard, 1 tsp	0
Kroger	
Yellow mustard, 1 tsp	0
Market Pantry	
Honey mustard, 1 tsp	0
Trader Joe's Grocery	
Aioli garlic mustard sauce, 1 tsp	0

Olives

Great Value	
Large pitted California ripe olives, 4 olives (15 g)	1
Manzanilla olives stuffed with minced pimento, 5 olives (15 g)	1
Sliced salad olives, 2 Tbsp	1
Kroger	
Manzanilla olives stuffed with pimiento, 5 olives (15 g)	1
Mario	
Reduced sodium pimiento stuffed Spanish olives, 5 olives (15 g)	1
Sliced black olives, 2 Tbsp	1
Spanish green olives stuffed with minced pimiento, 2 pieces (16 g)	1

Olives (cont'd)

	SmartPoints® value
Mezzetta	
Italian castelvetrano pitted green olives, 3 olives (15 g)	1
Olives, calamata, 4 olives (15 g)	1
Olives, kalamata, sliced Greek, 9 pieces (15 g)	1
Olives, pitted Greek kalamata, 4 olives (15 g)	1
Stuffed olives, garlic, 1½ olives (15 g)	1
Parthenon	
Pitted kalamata olives, 4 olives (14 g)	1
Pearls	
Olives, to go, ripe, black pitted California, large, 4 olives (15 g)	0
Pimiento stuffed Spanish green olives, 3 olives (14 g)	1
Pearls Olives to Go!	
Black pitted olives, 4 olives (15 g)	0
Kalamata pitted Greek olives, 3 olives (14 g)	1
Kalamata pitted Greek olives, 5 olives (15 g)	2
Pimiento stuffed Spanish green olives, 3 olives (14 g)	1
Pilaros	
Pitted kalamata gourmet Greek olives, 5 olives (14 g)	1
Private Selection	
Greek olive mix, 3 olives (15 g)	1
Seville	
Green olives, manzanilla Spanish, stuffed, 5 olives (15 g)	1
Tassos	
Olives, super mammoth, double stuffed jalapeño garlic, 2 olives (15 g)	1
Trader Joe's	
Pitted kalamata olives, 5 olives (15 g)	1

	SmartPoints® value
Trader Joe's Grocery	
Jumbo pitted Greek kalamata olives, 5 olives (15 g)	1
Tuscan Garden	
Hot and spicy pizza topping, 1 oz	2
Wegman's	
Kalamata olives, pitted, 5 olives (15 g)	1

Pasta Sauces

Barilla	
Sauce, traditional, ½ cup	3
Tomato and basil pasta sauce, ½ cup	3
Bertolli	
Sauce, garlic Alfredo, ¼ cup	4
Sauce, reduced fat, Alfredo, ¼ cup	2
Classico	
Pasta sauce, creamy Alfredo, ¼ cup	2
Pasta sauce, light, creamy Alfredo, ¼ cup	1
Classico Organic	
Tomato herbs and spices pasta sauce, ½ cup	3
Classico Signature Recipes	
Pasta sauce, asiago Romano Alfredo, light, ¼ cup	2
Classico Traditional Favorites	
Pasta sauce, tomato & basil, ½ cup	2
Tomato and basil pasta sauce, ½ cup	2
Colonna	
Traditional pasta sauce, ½ cup	2
Francesco Rinaldi	
Tomato & basil pasta sauce, ½ cup	3

	SmartPoints® value
Great Value	
Chunky mushrooms and green peppers pasta sauce, ½ cup	3
Hunt's	
Pasta sauce (no added sugar), ½ cup	1
Kirkland Signature	
Basil pesto, ¼ cup	11
Newman's Own	
Alfredo pasta sauce, ¼ cup	4
Marinara pasta sauce, ½ cup	3
Prego	
Italian sauce flavored with meat, ½ cup	4
Italian sauce traditional, ½ cup	3
Italian sauce, roasted garlic & herb, ½ cup	4
Meat sauce, Italian sausage & garlic, ½ cup	4
Traditional Italian sauce, ½ cup	3
Prego Chunky Garden	
Italian sauce, tomato, onion & garlic, ½ cup	4
Prego Heart Smart	
Traditional Italian sauce, ½ cup	3
Prego Light	
Homestyle Alfredo sauce, ¼ cup	2
Prego Traditional	
Italian sauce fresh mushroom, ½ cup	3
Italian sauce three cheese, ½ cup	4
Italian sauce tomato basil garlic, ½ cup	3
Priano	
Spinach and cheese pasta sauce, ½ cup	2
Tomato basil pasta sauce, 1 cup	4

	SmartPoints® value
Private Selection	
Arrabiatta spicy marinara sauce, ½ cup	2
Basil pesto Alfredo cream sauce, ¼ cup	3
Ragu	
Old world style traditional sauce, ½ cup	3
Sauce, classic Alfredo, ¼ cup	3
Ragu Cheese Creations	
Double cheddar sauce, ¼ cup	4
Ragu Chunky	
Garlic and onion tomato sauce, ½ cup	4
Sauce, tomato, garlic & onion, ½ cup	4
Ragu Old World Style	
Pasta sauce, smooth, traditional, ½ cup	3
Rao's Homemade	
Marinara sauce, sensitive formula, ½ cup	3
Simply Nature	
Organic marinara premium pasta sauce, ½ cup	2
Trader Giotto's	
Organic tomato basil marinara sauce, ½ cup	2
Tomato basil marinara sauce, ½ cup	4
Trader Joe's Grocery	
Marinara sauce, ½ cup	2
Victoria	
Marinara sauce, family size, ½ cup	2
Wellsley Farms	
All natural Italian style marinara sauce, ½ cup	2

	SmartPoints® value
Pickles	
Claussen	
Kosher dill pickle spears, 1 spear (34 g)	0
Kosher dill, halves, 1 pickle half (28 g)	0
Kosher dill, mini, 1 pickle (23 g)	0
Kosher dill, sandwich slices, 2 slices (34 g)	0
Kosher dill, wholes, ⅓ pickle (28 g)	0
Pickles, kosher dill, deli style, halves, ½ pickle (45 g)	0
Famous Dave's Signature Spicy	
Spicy pickle chips, 4 slices (28 g)	2
Great Gherkins	
Hamburger dill pickle chips, 4 slices (28 g)	0
Kosher dill sandwich slices, 1 slice (28 g)	0
Great Value	
Sweet gherkin pickles, 1 oz	2
Grillo's Pickles	
Bread and butter chips, 3 pieces (24 g)	1
Kroger	
Pickles, spears, kosher dill, 1 spear (28 g)	0
Mt. Olive	
Bread & butter chips, old fashioned sweet, fresh pack, 6 chips (28 g)	1
Dill petites, kosher, pickle pak, 1 pak (51 g)	0
That Pickle Guy	
Classic olive muffalata, 2 Tbsp	2

	SmartPoints® value
Vlasic	
Baby kosher dills pickles, 1 oz	0
Dill relish, 1 Tbsp	0
Pickles, kosher dill, 1 oz	0
Stackers, bread & butter, 1½ slices (28 g)	1
Stackers, kosher dill, 1½ slices (28 g)	0
Sweet gherkins, 3 pickles (28 g)	2
Sweet relish, 1 Tbsp	1
Vlasic Snak'mms	
Kosher dill, 3 pickles (28 g)	0
Pizza Sauces	
Classico Signature Recipes	
Pizza sauce, fire roasted, ¼ cup	1
Francesco Rinaldi	
Traditional pizza sauce, ¼ cup	1
H-E-B	
Traditional pizza sauce, ¼ cup	1
Prego	
Pizza sauce, ¼ cup	2
Prego	
Pizzeria style pizza sauce, ¼ cup	2
Reggano	
Traditional style pizza sauce, ¼ cup	1
Trader Giotto's	
Fat free pizza sauce, ¼ cup	1

	SmartPoints® value
Relish	
Great Value	
Sweet pickle relish, 1 oz	0
Sweet relish, 1 Tbsp	1
Heinz	
Relish, sweet, 1 Tbsp	1
Kroger	
No sugar added sweet relish, 1 Tbsp	0
Sweet relish, 1 Tbsp	1
Safeway	
Pickle relish, dill, 1 Tbsp	0
Tuscan Garden	
Hot diced giardiniera, 1 oz	2
Seafood Sauces	
Burman's	
Cocktail sauce, ¼ cup	2
Heinz	
Cocktail sauce, original, ¼ cup	3
Hellmann's	
Tartar sauce, 2 Tbsp	3
Kraft	
Tartar sauce, 2 Tbsp	2
Kroger	
Tartar sauce, squeezable, 2 Tbsp	4
McCormick	
Original cocktail sauce for seafood, ¼ cup	5
Shur Fine	
Tartar sauce, 2 Tbsp	2

	SmartPoints® value
Steak and Meat Sauces	
A1	
Steak sauce, 1 Tbsp	1
Campbell's Skillet Sauces	
Chicken marsala, ¼ cup	3
Frank's RedHot	
Wings sauce, buffalo, 1 Tbsp	0
Heinz 57	
Sauce, 1 Tbsp	1
Manwich	
Sloppy joe sauce, original, ¼ cup	2
Tahini	
Trader Joe's	
Tahini sauce, 2 Tbsp	3
Worcestershire Sauce	
Lea & Perrins	
Worcestershire sauce, the original, 1 tsp	0

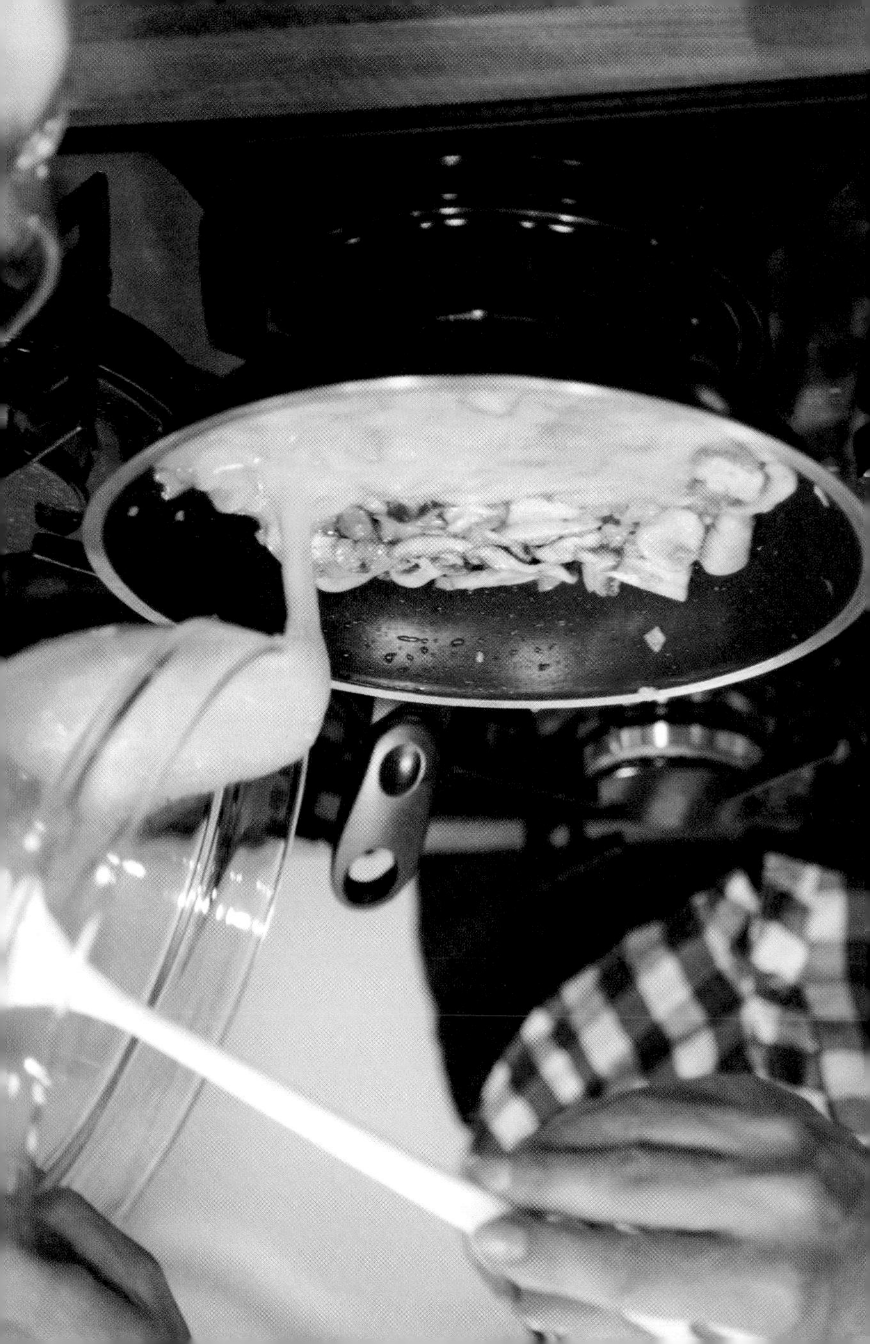

dairy & eggs

Butter and Butter Substitutes

	SmartPoints® value
Balade	
Light butter, 1 Tbsp	2
Breakstone's	
Whipped butter, salted, 1 Tbsp	3
Brummel & Brown	
Vegetable oil spread made with nonfat yogurt, 1 Tbsp	2
Challenge	
Butter, spreadable, with canola oil, 1 Tbsp	4
Butter, whipped, salted, 1 Tbsp	3
Country Crock	
Original spreadable butter with canola oil, 1 Tbsp	4
Earth Balance	
Buttery spread, natural, original, 1 Tbsp	4
Natural buttery spread, 1 Tbsp	3
Natural soy free buttery spread, 1 Tbsp	4
Hy-Vee	
Sweet cream spreadable butter with canola oil, 1 Tbsp	4
I Can't Believe It's Not Butter!	
Original spread, 1 Tbsp	2
Kerrygold	
Butter, pure Irish, 1 Tbsp	5
Butter, pure Irish, naturally softer, 1 Tbsp	5
Land O Lakes	
Butter spread, cinnamon sugar, 1 Tbsp	3
Butter spread, light, with canola oil, 1 Tbsp	2
Butter spread, with canola oil, 1 Tbsp	4
Butter spread, with olive oil, 1 Tbsp	4
Butter with canola oil, 1 Tbsp	4
Butter with olive oil & sea salt, 1 Tbsp	4
Butter, light, 1 Tbsp	2
Butter, salted, 1 Tbsp	5
Butter, whipped, 1 Tbsp	2
Olivio	
Spreadable butter with olive and canola oil, 1 Tbsp	4
Smart Balance	
Butter & canola oil blend, light, spreadable, 1 Tbsp	2
Buttery spread, 1 Tbsp	3
Buttery spread, light, original, 1 Tbsp	2
Buttery spread, made with extra virgin olive oil, 1 Tbsp	2
Buttery spread, non-hydrogenated, 1 Tbsp	3
Buttery spread, original, 1 Tbsp	3
Smart Balance Omega	
Buttery spread, light, 1 Tbsp	2

Cheese

365 Everyday Value	
Feta cheese crumbles, 1 oz	2
Grated parmesan, 1 Tbsp	1
Mozzarella cheese slices, 1 slice (28 g)	2
Shredded mild cheddar and Monterey Jack cheese, ¼ cup	4
Shredded mozzarella cheese, ¼ cup	2
365 Everyday Value Organic	
Fat free cottage cheese, ½ cup	2
Light string cheese, 1 stick (28 g)	2
4C	
Grated cheese, homestyle, parmesan - Romano, 1 Tbsp	1
Homestyle parmesan grated cheese, 1 Tbsp	1

	SmartPoints® value
Ahold	
Reduced fat mozzarella string cheese, 1 stick (28 g)	1
Reduced fat string cheese, 1 stick (28 g)	1
Sharp cheddar cheese cracker cuts, 4 slices (32 g)	5
Alouette	
Crumbled cheese, goat, ¼ cup	3
Garlic & herbs cheese spread (le petite fromage), 1 portion (17 g)	2
Parmesan and basil spreadable cheese, 1 portion (17 g)	2
Alouette Light	
Garlic and herb soft spreadable cheese, 2 Tbsp	2
Alpenrose	
2% lowfat cottage cheese, ½ cup	2
Fat free cottage cheese, ½ cup	1
Alpine Lace	
Cheese, deli thin, reduced fat provolone, 1 slice (23 g)	2
Cheese, deli thin, reduced fat Swiss, 1 slice (23 g)	2
Cheese, reduced fat Swiss, 1 oz	3
Swiss cheese, 1 slice (23 g)	2
Ambriola's Gourmet	
Grated pecorino Romano cheese, 1 Tbsp	1
American Heritage	
American cheese singles, 1 slice (21 g)	3
Amish Valley	
Shredded mozzarella cheese, ¼ cup	3
Anderson Erickson	
Low-fat 2% cottage cheese with sea salt, ½ cup	2
Argitoni	
Parmesan cheese, 1 Tbsp	1

	SmartPoints® value
Athenos	
Crumbled cheese, feta, traditional, ¼ cup	3
Crumbled cheese, reduced fat feta, ¼ cup	3
Crumbled cheese, traditional, reduced fat, feta, ¼ cup	2
Traditional crumbled fat free feta cheese, ¼ cup	0
Traditional crumbled feta cheese, ¼ cup	3
Babybel	
Semi soft cheese, mini, mozzarella style, reduced fat, 1 piece (21 g)	2
Baker	
Light string cheese, 1 stick (24 g)	1
String cheese, 1 piece (28 g)	2
BelGioioso	
Burrata, 1 oz	3
Cheese, all-natural fresh mozzarella, 1 oz	3
Cheese, fresh mozzarella, pearls, 1 oz	2
Fresh mozzarella, 1 oz	2
Fresh mozzarella snacking cheese (gluten free), 1 oz	2
Freshly shaved cheese, parmesan, 1 Tbsp	1
Salad blend cheese, 1 Tbsp	1
Shredded parmesan Romano cheese, 1 Tbsp	1
Snacking cheese, fresh mozzarella, 1 oz	2
Boar's Head	
25% lower fat, 25% lower sodium American cheese (gluten free), 1 oz	3
44% lower sodium provolone cheese (gluten free), 2 slices (28 g)	4
Bold horseradish cheddar cheese (gluten free), 1 oz	4

Cheese, Boar's Head (cont'd)

	SmartPoints® value
Cheese, muenster (gluten free), 1 oz	4
Cheese, Vermont cheddar (gluten free), 1 oz	4
Lacey Swiss cheese, 1 oz	3
Monterey Jack cheese, 2 slices (28 g)	4
Picante provolone cheese (gluten free), 1 oz	4
Sliced American cheese, 2 slices (28 g)	4
Sliced baby Swiss cheese, 2 slices (28 g)	4
Smoked gouda, pasteurized process gouda and cheddar cheese (gluten free), 1 oz	4
Swiss cheese, 1 slice (28 g)	3
Vermont cheddar cheese, 1 oz	4
Borden	
2% milk reduced fat singles, American, 1 slice (21 g)	2
Cheese product slices, American, 2% milk, reduced fat, 1 slice (19 g)	2
Cheese product, pasteurized prepared, 2% milk reduced fat, singles, sharp, 1 slice (21 g)	2
Cheese product, pasteurized prepared, fat free, singles, American, 1 slice (21 g)	1
Cheese product, pasteurized prepared, fat free, singles, sharp, 1 slice (21 g)	1
Fat free Swiss cheese singles, 1 slice (21 g)	1
Pepper Jack cheese, 1 slice (17 g)	2
String cheese, mozzarella cheese, 1 stick (24 g)	2
Borden Dairy Fat Free	
pepper Jack singles, 1 slice (21 g)	1
Borden Singles	
Cheese product, pastuerized prepared, American, 1 slice (21 g)	3

	SmartPoints® value
Boursin	
Spreadable cheese, gourmet, garlic & herbs, 2 Tbsp	3
Breakstone's	
2% lowfat small curd cottage cheese snack size, 1 container (113 g)	3
2% milkfat lowfat 30% less sodium cottage cheese, ½ cup	3
2% milkfat lowfat large curd cottage cheese, ½ cup	3
2% milkfat lowfat small curd cottage cheese, ½ cup	3
Fat free small curd cottage cheese, ½ cup	2
Fat free small curd cottage cheese snack size, 1 container (113 g)	2
Breakstone's 100 Calorie	
Cottage doubles, blueberry, 1 container (110 g)	4
Cottage doubles, peach, 1 container (110 g)	4
Cottage doubles, raspberry, 1 container (110 g)	4
Breakstone's Cottage Doubles	
2% milkfat lowfat cottage cheese & pineapple topping, 1 container (110 g)	4
2% milkfat lowfat cottage cheese & strawberry topping, 1 container (110 g)	4
Breakstone's LiveActive	
2% milkfat lowfat cottage cheese, 1 container (113 g)	2
Cabot	
75% reduce fat cheddar cheese, 1" cube (28 g)	1
Cheese slices, cheddar, 1 slice (28 g)	2
Cheese, cheddar, 50% reduced fat, 1 oz	2

	SmartPoints® value
Cheese, cheddar, extra sharp, 1 oz	4
Cheese, extra sharp aged cheddar, 1 oz	4
Cheese, sharp cheddar, 50% reduced fat, 1 oz	2
Cheese, sharp cheddar, 75% reduced fat, 1 oz	1
White oak cheddar cheese, 1 oz	4
Cabot Serious Snacking	
Sharp cheddar cheese, 1 bar (21 g)	3
Sharp cheddar cheese, 50% reduced fat, 1 bar (21 g)	2
Cabot Vermont	
50% reduced fat sharp cheddar cheese, 1 oz	2
Cheese, cheddar, 50% light, 1 oz	2
Cheese, seriously sharp cheddar, 1 oz	4
Cabot Vermont Snack Packs	
50% light cheddar cheese, 1 snack bar (21 g)	2
Cache Valley	
Lite string cheese, 1 stick (24 g)	1
Cacique	
Queso fresco, 1 oz	3
Cello	
Grated pecorino Romano cheese, 1 Tbsp	1
Shaved grana padano, 1 Tbsp	1
Chevre	
Cranberry cinnamon fresh goat cheese, 1 oz	4
Coburn Farms	
Low-fat cottage cheese, ½ cup	2
Cow Pals	
Snack cheese, 1 piece (21 g)	3

	SmartPoints® value
Cracker Barrel	
Cheddar Jack cheese sticks, 1 stick (21 g)	3
Cheese bars, extra sharp cheddar, 1 bar (21 g)	2
Cheese slices, extra sharp white cheddar, 1 slice (18 g)	3
Cheese, cheddar, extra sharp, 1 oz	4
Cheese, natural, sharp cheddar, slices, 1 slice (20 g)	3
Cracker cuts, sharp white cheddar, 4 slices (33 g)	5
Extra sharp cheddar cheese sticks, 1 stick (21 g)	3
Extra sharp cheddar cracker cuts, 4 slices (33 g)	5
Extra sharp reduced fat cheddar cheese sticks, 1 stick (21 g)	2
Extra sharp white cheddar cheese sticks, 1 stick (21 g)	3
Havarti cheese slices, 1 slice (20 g)	3
Jalapeño cheddar cheese sticks, 1 stick (21 g)	3
Provolone cheese with smoke flavor added, 1 slice (20 g)	2
Crystal Farms	
Fat free American cheese, 1 slice (21 g)	1
Neufchatel cheese, 1 oz	3
Pepper Jack thins, 3 slices (32 g)	5
Provolone cheese with natural smoke flavor, 3 slices (32 g)	4
Reduced fat marble Jack cheese, 1 oz	3
Reduced fat pepper Jack cheese, 1 oz	3
Reduced fat provolone cheese, 1 slice (23 g)	2
Reduced fat shredded sharp cheddar cheese, ¼ cup	3

	SmartPoints® value
Thins Swiss cheese, 3 slices (32 g)	4
Wisconsin string cheese, 1 piece (24 g)	2
Wisconsin string cheese, 1 stick (24 g)	2
Crystal Farms Cheezoids	
Reduced fat mozzarella string cheese, 1 stick (24 g)	2
Crystal Farms Light	
Wisconsin string cheese, 1 piece (24 g)	1
Crystal Farms Marble Jack	
Finely shredded colby and Monterey Jack cheese, ¼ cup	4
Crystal Farms Thins	
Marble Jack cheese, 3 slices (32 g)	5
Daily Chef	
2% low-fat small curd cottage cheese, ½ cup	2
American cheese slices, 2 slices (28 g)	4
Fancy shredded 4 cheese Mexican style blend, ⅓ cup	4
Mild cheddar & Monterey Jack cheese, ⅓ cup	4
Shredded colby and Monterey Jack cheese, ⅓ cup	4
Daisy	
2% milkfat small curd low-fat cottage cheese, ½ cup	2
Cottage cheese, small curd, ½ cup	3
Low-fat cottage cheese, ½ cup	2
Daiya	
Cheddar style slices, deliciously dairy free, 1 slice (20 g)	2
Darigold	
Cottage cheese, trim, ½ cup	3
Trim lowfat cottage cheese, ½ cup	2

	SmartPoints® value
Dean's	
Lowfat small curd cottage cheese, ½ cup	2
DiGiorno	
Shaved cheese, parmesan, ¼ cup	4
Dodoni	
Feta in brine, 1 oz	3
Dofino	
Creamy havarti deli slices, 1 oz	4
Einstein Bros	
Double whipped pumpkin shmear cream cheese spread, 2 Tbsp	4
Elli	
Bananas foster quark cheese, 1 container (170 g)	2
Cherry creamy German style quark cheese, 1 container (170 g)	2
Creamy German style blueberry quark, 1 container (170 g)	2
Creamy German style lemon quark, 1 container (170 g)	2
Creamy German style sea salt caramel quark, 1 container (170 g)	2
Creamy German style strawberry quark, 1 container (170 g)	2
Mint chocolate creamy German style quark cheese, 1 container (170 g)	2
Peach creamy German style quark cheese, 1 container (170 g)	2
Pineapple creamy German style quark cheese, 1 container (170 g)	2
Plain quark cheese, 1 container (170 g)	2
Vanilla bean creamy German style quark cheese, 1 container (170 g)	2
Elsie Borden Plus	
Natural sliced Swiss cheese, 1 slice (14 g)	2
Essential Everyday	
Shredded fat free mild cheddar cheese, ¼ cup	0

	SmartPoints® value
Fareway	
Small curd low-fat cottage cheese, ½ cup	2
Fiber One	
Lowfat cottage cheese with fiber, ½ cup	2
Finlandia	
Light Swiss cheese, 1 slice (22 g)	2
Muenster cheese, 1 slice (28 g)	4
Reduced fat havarti cheese slice, 1 slice (22 g)	1
Finlandia Deli Slices	
Muenster cheese, 1 slice (21 g)	3
Finlandia Heavenly Light	
Imported light Swiss cheese, 1 oz	2
Fit & Active	
2% milk Mexican shredded cheese blend, ¼ cup	3
Neufchatel cheese, 1 oz	3
Reduce fat provolone cheese deli slices, 1 slice (19 g)	2
Reduced fat colby Jack cheese deli slices, 1 slice (19 g)	2
Food Club	
Finely shredded mild cheddar cheese, ¼ cup	3
Food Lion	
Extra thin Swiss cheese slices, 3 slices (32 g)	4
Fancy shredded sharp cheddar cheese, ¼ cup	3
Fat free American singles, 1 slice (21 g)	1
Fat free cottage cheese, ½ cup	2
Lowfat cottage cheese, ½ cup	2
Mild cheddar cheese, 1 slice (21 g)	2
Mozzarella string cheese, 1 piece (28 g)	2
Shredded Mexican blend cheese, ¼ cup	3
Shredded mozzarella cheese, ¼ cup	2

	SmartPoints® value
Foodhold USA	
Thin sliced provolone cheese, 3 slices (32 g)	4
Fred Meyer	
Lowfat cottage cheese, ½ cup	3
Friendly Farms	
Low-fat small curd cottage cheese, ½ cup	2
Small curd fat free cottage cheese, ½ cup	2
Friendship	
1% milkfat whipped cottage cheese, ½ cup	2
Cottage cheese, 1% milkfat, no salt added, small curd, ½ cup	2
Cottage cheese, 1% milkfat, small curd, ½ cup	2
Cottage cheese, large curd, 2% milkfat, low-fat, pot style, ½ cup	2
Frigo Cheese Heads	
100% natural string cheese, 1 piece (28 g)	3
Cheese sticks, reduced fat, colby Jack, 1 piece (24 g)	2
Light string mozzarella cheese, 1 piece (24 g)	1
String cheese, 100% natural, light, mozzarella, 1 oz	1
String cheese, 100% natural, mozzarella, 1 package (28 g)	3
String cheese, natural, light swirls, 1 oz	1
Frigo Cheese Heads Light	
Low moisture part skim mozzarella string cheese, 1 stick (24 g)	1
Frigo Cheese Heads Premium Snacking	
Wisconsin colby Jack cheese sticks, 1 piece (24 g)	3
Frigo Cheese Heads String	
100% natural string cheese, 1 stick (28 g)	3

Cheese (cont'd)

	SmartPoints® value
Frigo Cheese Heads Swirls	
String cheese, natural, light, 1 oz	1
Galbani	
Mozzarella low moisture part skim organic string cheese, 1 string cheese (28 g)	3
Part skim mozzarella cheese, 1 oz	3
String cheese, 1 piece (28 g)	2
Variety pack snack cheese, 1 stick (24 g)	4
Genuine Locatelli	
Grated cheese, pecorino Romano, 1 Tbsp	1
Giant	
American cheese singles, 1 slice (19 g)	1
Colby Jack cracker cuts, 4 slices (32 g)	5
Pepper Jack cheese cracker cuts, 4 slices (32 g)	5
Sharp cheddar cheese cracker cuts, 4 slices (32 g)	2
Shredded cheese, reduced fat, mozzarella, ¼ cup	2
Thin sliced Swiss cheese, 3 slices (32 g)	4
Giant Eagle	
Fat free American singles, 1 slice (21 g)	1
Light mozzarella string cheese, 1 stick (24 g)	1
Low-fat cottage cheese, ½ cup	2
Mexican style fancy shredded cheese, ¼ cup	3
Mozzarella shredded cheese, ¼ cup	2
Provolone cheese slices, 3 slices (32 g)	4
Reduced fat milk cheddar shredded cheese, ¼ cup	3
Reduced fat provolone cheese slices, 1 slice (21 g)	2

	SmartPoints® value
Sharp cheddar cheese cracker cuts, 3 slices (28 g)	4
Shredded mozzarella cheese, ¼ cup	3
Thin provolone cheese slices, 3 slices (32 g)	4
Great Lakes Cheese	
Provalone shingle slice, 1 slice (19 g)	3
Great Value	
100% parmesan grated cheese, 1 Tbsp	1
Cheese product, pasteurized prepared, singles, white American, 1 slice (19 g)	2
Cheese, finely shredded, colby & Monterey Jack, ⅓ cup	4
Cheese, finely shredded, fiesta blend, ⅓ cup	4
Cheese, finely shredded, mozzarella, ⅓ cup	3
Cheese, finely shredded, sharp, cheddar, ⅓ cup	4
Cheese, pasteurized process, fat free, singles, 1 slice (21 g)	1
Cheese, shredded, mozzarella, ¼ cup	3
Cottage cheese, low-fat, ½ cup	2
Cottage cheese, low-fat, small curd, ½ cup	2
Cottage cheese, small curd, fat free, ½ cup	2
Deli style sliced colby and Monterey Jack cheese, 1 slice (19 g)	3
Deli style sliced provolone cheese, 1 slice (19 g)	2
Deluxe reduced fat American cheese, 1 slice (19 g)	2
Fat free cream cheese, 1 oz	1
Finely shredded cheese, fiesta blend, reduced fat, ⅓ cup	3
Finely shredded Italian style cheese, 1 oz	3

	SmartPoints® value
Light cream cheese spread, 1 oz	3
Low moisture part skim mozzarella string cheese, 1 stick (28 g)	3
Mild cheddar cheese, 1 oz	4
Pasteurized prepared cheese product, singles, American, 1 slice (19 g)	2
Sharp cheddar sliced cheese, 1 serving (20 g)	3
Sharp reduced fat cheddar cheese, 1 oz	3
Shredded cheese, mild cheddar, ¼ cup	4
Shredded colby and Monterey Jack cheese, ¼ cup	4
White American cheese, 1 slice (21 g)	3
Great Value Deli Style	
Sliced jalapeño and habanero pepper Jack cheese, 1 slice (21 g)	3
Swiss cheese slices, 1 slice (19 g)	3
Green Mountain Farms	
Greek cream cheese, 2 Tbsp	2
Hannaford	
Classic fat free American cheese singles, 1 slice (21 g)	1
Mozzarella string cheese, 1 piece (28 g)	2
Shredded mozzarella cheese, 1 cup	2
Happy Farms	
American cheese deluxe slices, 1 slice (19 g)	3
Colby Jack cheese cubes, 7 cubes (28 g)	4
Cream cheese spread, 2 Tbsp	5
Light spreadable cheese wedges, 1 wedge (19 g)	1
Low moisture part skim shredded mozzarella cheese, ¼ cup	3
Low-moisture part-skim mozzarella string cheese, 1 piece (24 g)	2

	SmartPoints® value
Part skim mozzarella cheese, 1 oz	3
Sliced provolone cheese, 1 slice (21 g)	3
Happy Farms Light	
Jalapeño pepper spreadable cheese wedge, 1 wedge (19 g)	1
Happy Farms Natural Cheese	
Deli sliced mild cheddar cheese, 1 slice (21 g)	3
Harris Teeter	
Fancy shredded colby Jack cheese, ¼ cup	3
Four cheese Mexican blend, ¼ cup	3
Light mozzarella string cheese, 1 string cheese (24 g)	1
Part skim mozzarella cheese, ¼ cup	2
Reduced fat sharp cheddar cheese snack sticks, 1 stick (21 g)	2
Sharp cheddar cheese, ¼ cup	3
Harris Teeter Deli Style	
Reduced fat sliced sharp cheddar cheese, 1 slice (19 g)	2
Reduced fat sliced Swiss cheese, 1 slice (19 g)	2
H-E-B	
2% milk cheddar cheese, 1 slice (21 g)	2
Bajo en grasa queso cottage, ½ cup	2
colby Jack cheese, 1 slice (21 g)	2
Fancy shredded cheddar cheese, ¼ cup	3
Fancy shredded colby Jack cheese, ¼ cup	3
Fancy shredded mozzarella cheese, ¼ cup	3
Fancy shredded sharp cheddar cheese made with 2% milk, ¼ cup	3
Fat free cottage cheese, ½ cup	2
Fat free process cheese product singles, 1 slice (21 g)	1

Cheese, H-E-B (cont'd)

	SmartPoints® value
Fat free shredded cheddar cheese, ¼ cup	0
Herb and garlic cheese wedges, 1 wedge (19 g)	1
Light pepper Jack cheese wedges, 1 wedge (19 g)	1
Light smoked gouda cheese wedges, 1 wedge (19 g)	1
Provolone cheese, 1 slice (21 g)	3
Queso cottage sin grasa, ½ cup	2
Reduced fat colby Jack cheese sticks, 1 stick (21 g)	2
Reduced fat mozzarella string cheese, 1 piece (24 g)	1
Reduced fat shredded mozzarella cheese, ¼ cup	2
Reduced fat whipped cream cheese spread, 2 Tbsp	3
Sharp cheddar cheese, 1 slice (21 g)	2
Shredded mozzarella cheese, ¼ cup	0
String cheese, 1 string cheese (24 g)	1
Thin sliced baby Swiss cheese, 1 slice (21 g)	3
Thin sliced Monterey Jack cheese, 1 slice (21 g)	2
Thin sliced sharp cheddar cheese, 1 slice (21 g)	3
White cheddar light cheese wedges, 1 wedge (19 g)	1
H-E-B Natural Cheese	
2% milk Mexican blend fancy shredded cheese, ¼ cup	3
Home Made Brand	
Cheese spread, pimento, 2 Tbsp	4
Hood	
Cottage cheese with chive, ½ cup	4
Cottage cheese, low-fat, ½ cup	2
Cottage cheese, with pineapple, fat free, ½ cup	4

	SmartPoints® value
Horizon Organic	
American cheese singles, 1 slice (19 g)	3
String cheese, mozzarella, 1 stick (28 g)	3
Hy-Vee	
1% lowfat small curd cottage cheese, ½ cup	2
2% milk provolone cheese, 1 slice (20 g)	2
2% milk reduced fat colby Jack cheese, ¼ cup	3
2% milk Swiss natural cheese, 1 slice (20 g)	2
Colby Jack cheese, 1 slice (20 g)	2
Colby Jack cheese, ¼ cup	4
Fat free cottage cheese, ½ cup	2
Finely shredded mozzarella cheese, ¼ cup	2
Finely shredded reduced fat cheddar Jack cheese, ¼ cup	3
Finely shredded sharp cheddar cheese, ¼ cup	4
Mozzarella string cheese, 1 piece (24 g)	1
Reduced fat sharp cheddar cheese, ¼ cup	3
Shredded Mexican blend cheese, ¼ cup	3
Small curd cottage cheese, ½ cup	4
Ultra thin colby Jack cheese, 3 slices (32 g)	5
Hy-Vee Light	
Strings mozzarella cheese, 1 piece (24 g)	1
Imos	
Shredded cheese, provel, ¼ cup	4
Jarlsberg	
Cheese, reduced fat, lite, Swiss, 1 oz	2
Cheese, Swiss, 1 oz	4
Reduced fat Swiss cheese, 1 slice (21 g)	1

	SmartPoints® value
Jarlsberg Lite	
Reduced fat Swiss cheese slices, 1 slice (21 g)	1
Sliced cheese, deli thin, reduced fat Swiss, 1 slice (23 g)	1
Kalona Supernatural	
Organic reduced fat 2% cottage cheese, ½ cup	2
Kaukauna	
Spreadable cheese, port wine, 2 Tbsp	4
Kemps	
1% lowfat cottage cheese, ½ cup	2
2% lowfat cottage cheese, ½ cup	2
Fat free cottage cheese, ½ Cup	2
Kerrygold	
Dubliner cheese, 1 oz	4
Kirkland Signature	
Colby Jack cheese, 1 oz	4
Deluxe American cheese slices, 1 slice (19 g)	3
Fresh and creamy goat cheese, 1 oz	3
Low moisture part skim shredded mozzarella cheese, ¼ cup	3
Mexican style shredded cheese, ⅓ cup	4
Mild cheddar cheese, 1 oz	4
Sharp cheddar cheese, 1 oz	4
Shredded parmigiano reggiano, 1 Tbsp	1
Knudsen	
2% milkfat small curd cottage cheese, ½ cup	2
Lowfat 2% milk fat small curd cottage cheese, ½ cup	3
Knudsen Cottage Doubles 100 Calorie	
Cottage cheese, 2% milkfat lowfat, and pineapple topping, 1 container (110 g)	4

	SmartPoints® value
Knudsen Free	
Nonfat cottage cheese, ½ cup	2
Knudsen on the Go!	
Cottage cheese, lowfat, 1 container (113 g)	3
Kraft	
100% grated parmesan cheese, 2 tsp	1
Cheese crumbles, blue cheese, 3 Tbsp	4
Cheese slices, big slice, American, 1 slice (23 g)	3
Cheese twists, made with 2% milk, mozzarella & cheddar, 1 stick (21 g)	1
Cheese twists, mozzarella & cheddar, 1 stick (21 g)	2
Cheese, shredded parmesan, ¼ cup	2
Finely shredded cheese, sharp cheddar, reduced fat, ¼ cup	3
Finely shredded sharp cheddar cheese, ¼ cup	4
Grated parmesan cheese, 2 tsp	1
Parmesan style grated topping, reduced fat, 2 tsp	1
Sharp cheddar cheese cuts, 4 slices (33 g)	5
Sharp cheddar shredded cheese, ¼ cup	4
Shredded cheese, Italian five cheese, ¼ cup	3
Shredded cheese, mozzarella, ¼ cup	3
Shredded cheese, mozzarella, fat free, ¼ cup	0
Shredded cheese, parmesan, Romano and asiago, ¼ cup	4
Shredded low moisture part skim mozzarella with cream cheese, ¼ cup	3
Shredded Mexican style four cheese, ¼ cup	4

Cheese, Kraft (cont'd)

	SmartPoints® value
Shredded Swiss cheese, ¼ cup	4
Shredded three cheese, ¼ cup	4
String cheese, jalapeño, 1 stick (24 g)	2
String cheese, low-moisture part-skim, mozzarella, 1 stick (28 g)	3
String cheese, made with 2% milk, mozzarella, 1 stick (24 g)	2
Swiss cheese slices, 1 slice (16 g)	2
Velveeta, made with 2% milk, ¼" slice (28 g)	2
Kraft Crumbles	
Three cheese, ¼ cup	4
Kraft Deli Deluxe	
American pasteurized process cheese, 1 slice (19 g)	3
Cheese slices, reduced fat pasteurized process, American, 1 slice (19 g)	2
Pasteurized process cheese, sharp cheddar, slices, 1 slice (19 g)	3
Kraft Natural Cheese	
2% milk shredded low moisture part skim mozzarella cheese, ¼ cup	2
Big cheese slices, colby Jack, 1 slice (23 g)	3
Big cheese slices, pepper Jack, medium heat, 1 slice (23 g)	3
Big cheese slices, sharp cheddar, 1 slice (23 g)	4
Cheese cubes, cheddar & Monterey Jack, 7 pieces (30 g)	5
Cheese cubes, mild cheddar, 7 pieces (30 g)	5
Cheese slices, extra thin, extra sharp white cheddar, slim cut, 3 slices (35 g)	4
Cheese slices, extra thin, Swiss, 1 slice (16 g)	2
Cheese slices, made with 2% milk, sharp cheddar, 1 slice (20 g)	2

	SmartPoints® value
Cheese slices, mozzarella, slim cut, 3 slices (33 g)	3
Cheese slices, Swiss, made with 2% milk, 1 slice (18 g)	2
Cheese, made with 2% milk, colby & Monterey Jack, 1 oz	3
Cheese, made with 2% milk, sharp cheddar, 1 oz	3
Cheese, mild cheddar, made with 2% milk, 1 oz	3
Cheese, provolone, 1 slice (19 g)	2
Cheese, Swiss, slices, 1 slice (23 g)	3
Fat free shredded cheddar, ¼ cup	0
Fat free shredded mozzarella, ¼ cup	0
Finely shredded cheese, made with 2% milk, Mexican style cheddar Jack, ¼ cup	3
Finely shredded cheese, made with 2% milk, Mexican style four cheese, ¼ cup	3
Finely shredded colby and Monterey Jack, ¼ cup	4
Finely shredded low moisture part skim mozzarella cheese, ¼ cup	3
Finely shredded Mexican style cheddar Jack, ¼ cup	4
Finely shredded Mexican style four cheese, ¼ cup	4
Finely shredded Mexican style taco cheese, ¼ cup	4
Finely shredded mild cheddar, ¼ cup	4
Finely shredded parmesan, ¼ cup	4
Finely shredded reduced fat Mexican style four cheese, ¼ cup	3
Finely shredded reduced fat sharp cheddar, ¼ cup	3
Finely shredded sharp cheddar, ¼ cup	4
Finely shredded triple cheddar, ¼ cup	4

	SmartPoints® value
Mexican style taco shredded cheese made with 2% milk, ¼ cup	3
Mozzarella string cheese, 1 stick (28 g)	3
Reduced fat shredded colby and Monterey Jack cheese, ¼ cup	3
Shredded cheese, made with 2% milk, mozzarella, ¼ cup	2
Shredded colby and Monterey Jack cheeses, ¼ cup	4
Shredded colby and Monterey Jack cheeses, ¼ cup	4
Shredded Italian five cheese, ¼ cup	3
Shredded low moisture part skim mozzarella cheese, ¼ cup	3
Shredded low moisture part skim mozzarella made with 2% milk, ¼ cup	2
Shredded mild cheddar cheese, ¼ cup	4
Shredded sharp cheddar, ¼ cup	4
Slim cut cheese slices, reduced fat, Swiss, 3 Slices (33 g)	4
Slim cut cheese, reduced fat, sharp cheddar, 3 Slices (35 g)	4
Kraft Simply	
Cottage cheese, small curd, 2% milkfat, low-fat, ½ cup	3
Cottage cheese, small curd, fat free, ½ cup	2
Kraft Singles	
American cheese pasteurized cheese product, 1 slice (19 g)	2
American cheese pasteurized prepared cheese product, 1 slice (19 g)	2
American cheese pasteurized prepared cheese product, 1 slice (21 g)	3
Cheese product slices, made with skim milk, sharp cheddar, 1 slice (19 g)	0

	SmartPoints® value
Cheese product slices, sharp cheddar, 1 slice (21 g)	2
Cheese product, made with 2% milk, Swiss, 1 slice (19 g)	2
Cheese product, pasteurized prepared, made with 2% milk, sharp cheddar, 1 slice (19 g)	2
Cheese product, pasteurized prepared, made with 2% milk, white American, 1 slice (19 g)	2
Cheese product, pasteurized prepared, made with skim milk, American, 1 slice (19 g)	0
Cheese product, pasteurized prepared, reduced fat 2%, American, 1 slice (19 g)	2
Cheese product, pasteurized prepared, reduced fat, 2% milk, American, 1 slice (21 g)	2
Cheese product, pasteurized prepared, white American, 1 slice (21 g)	3
Cheese product, pepperjack, made with 2% milk, 1 slice (19 g)	1
Kroger	
2% milk reduced fat American cheese product singles, 1 slice (21 g)	2
Cheese product, fat free singles, Swiss, 1 slice (21 g)	1
Cheese product, singles, American, 1 slice (19 g)	2
Cheese slices, aged sharp white cheddar, 1 slice (21 g)	3
Cheese slices, mild cheddar, 1 slice (21 g)	3
Cheese slices, mozzarella, 1 slice (21 g)	2
Cheese slices, pepper Jack, 1 slice (21 g)	3
Cheese spread, pimento, 1 Tbsp	3
Cheese, deli thin slices, aged Swiss, 1 slice (21 g)	3

Cheese, Kroger (cont'd)

	SmartPoints® value
Cheese, deli thin slices, medium cheddar, 1 slice (21 g)	3
Cheese, deli thin slices, smoke flavored provolone, 1 slice (21 g)	3
Cheese, Mexican style, finely shredded, ¼ cup	4
Cheese, slices, colby Jack, 1 slice (21 g)	3
Cheese, string, low moisture part skim mozzarella, twists, 1 piece (24 g)	2
Cheese, Swiss, reduced fat, slices, 1 slice (28 g)	2
Colby Jack cheese slices, 3 slices (32 g)	4
Colby Jack finely shredded cheese, ¼ cup	4
Fat free American cheese singles, 1 slice (21 g)	1
Fat-free cottage cheese, ½ cup	1
Finely shredded cheese, sharp cheddar, reduced fat, ¼ cup	3
Finely shredded Swiss cheese, ¼ cup	4
Greek cream cheese and Greek yogurt, 2 Tbsp	2
Italian blend cheese, ¼ cup	3
Light mozzarella string cheese, 1 stick (28 g)	2
Lowfat cottage cheese, ½ cup	3
Mexican style finely shredded cheese, ¼ cup	4
Mild cheddar Jack finely shredded cheese, ¼ cup	4
Mild cheddar shredded cheese, ¼ cup	4
Mozzarella part skim finely shredded cheese, ¼ cup	2
Parmesan finely shredded cheese, ¼ cup	3
Reduced fat 4 cheese Mexican blend finely shredded cheese, ¼ cup	3

	SmartPoints® value
Reduced fat mild cheddar finely shredded cheese, ¼ cup	3
Sharp cheddar shredded cheese, ¼ cup	4
Shredded cheese, Mexican style, ¼ cup	4
Smoke flavored provolone cheese slices, 3 slices (32 g)	4
Swiss cheese slices, 3 slices (32 g)	4
Whipped onion and chive cream cheese spread, 2 Tbsp	3
Kroger CowPals	
Snack cheese, mild cheddar, 1 piece (21 g)	3
String cheese, mozzarella, 1 piece (28 g)	3
Lactaid	
Cottage cheese, lowfat, ½ cup	2
Land O Lakes	
Cheese, American, 1 oz	4
Cheese, reduced fat, 2% milk, American, 1 oz	3
Deli cheese, American, 1 slice (18 g)	3
Deli cheese, American, slices, 1 slice (19 g)	3
Deli cheese, white American, 1 slice (19 g)	3
Deli cheese, yellow American, 1 slice (19 g)	3
Light string cheese, 1 stick (28 g)	2
Low-fat 1% milkfat small curd cottage cheese, ½ cup	2
String cheese, 1 oz	3
Variety pack snack cheese, 1 piece (21 g)	3
Land O Lakes Snack 'N Cheese To-Go!	
Cheese, natural, co-jack, 1 bar (21 g)	3
Cheese, natural, mild cheddar, 1 bar (21 g)	3

	SmartPoints® value
Laughing Cow	
Creamy asiago spreadable cheese wedge, 1 wedge (21 g)	1
Creamy spicy pepper Jack spreadable cheese wedges, 1 wedge (21 g)	1
Light creamy Swiss spreadable cheese wedges, 1 wedge (21 g)	1
Spreadable cheese wedges, creamy mozzarella sun-dried tomato & basil, 1 wedge (21 g)	1
Spreadable cheese wedges, creamy queso fresco chipotle, 1 wedge (21 g)	1
Spreadable cheese wedges, creamy Swiss French onion, 1 wedge (21 g)	1
Spreadable cheese wedges, creamy Swiss, light, 1 wedge (21 g)	1
Spreadable cheese wedges, creamy Swiss, original, 1 wedge (21 g)	2
Spreadable cheese wedges, white cheddar flavor, creamy, 1 wedge (21 g)	1
Laughing Cow Light	
Garlic and herb spreadable cheese wedge, 1 wedge (21 g)	1
Laughing Cow Mini Babybel	
Semi-soft cheese, gouda, 1 piece (21 g)	3
Semisoft cheeses, cheddar variety, 1 piece (21 g)	2
Semisoft cheeses, original, 1 piece (21 g)	3
Semisoft cheeses, sharp original, 1 piece (20 g)	2
Semisoft cheeses, white cheddar variety, 1 piece (20 g)	3
Lucerne	
Cheese product, 2% milk American slices, 1 slice (21 g)	2
Cheese sticks, sharp cheddar, reduced fat 2% milk, 1 stick (23 g)	2

	SmartPoints® value
Cheese, American, fat free slices, 1 slice (21 g)	1
Cheese, natural, 2% milk, reduced fat, sliced, provolone, 1 slice (21 g)	2
Cheese, natural, medium cheddar, 2% reduced fat, 1 oz	3
Cheese, natural, reduced fat, sliced, medium, ¾ oz	2
Cheese, natural, reduced fat, sliced, Swiss, 1 slice (21 g)	2
Cheese, smoked gouda, sliced, 1 slice (21 g)	3
Chive and onion whipped cream cheese, 2 Tbsp	2
Cottage cheese, 2% milkfat, lowfat, ½ cup	2
Fat free cottage cheese, ½ cup	2
Finely shredded cheese, Mexican, ¼ cup	4
Greek cream cheese and Greek yogurt blend, 2 Tbsp	2
Light string cheese, 1 stick (24 g)	1
Mozzarella fat free shredded cheese, ¼ cup	0
Shredded mozzarella cheese, ¼ cup	3
String cheese, 1 piece (28 g)	3
String cheese, light, 1 piece (24 g)	1
Lucerne Dairy Farms	
Colby Jack cheese, ¼ cup	3
Low moisture part skim mozzarella string cheese, 1 stick (24 g)	2
Lucerne Thin Slices	
Natural Swiss cheese slices, 3 slices (32 g)	4
Market Basket	
Fat free American singles, 1 slice (21 g)	1
Fat free sharp cheddar cheese, 1 slice (21 g)	1
Low-fat cottage cheese, ½ cup	2
Low-fat cottage cheese with chive and toasted onion, ½ cup	2

Cheese, Market Basket (cont'd)

	SmartPoints® value
Mozzarella and mild cheddar cheese blend, ¼ cup	3
Natural shredded mozzarella cheese, ¼ cup	3
Part skim mozzarella cheese, ¼ cup	3
Part skim mozzarella string cheese, 1 piece (24 g)	2
Shredded Mexican four cheese, ¼ cup	4
Market Pantry	
Cheese slices, deli-style, colby Jack, reduced fat, 2% milk, 1 slice (19 g)	2
Cheese slices, deli-style, mild cheddar, reduced fat, 2% milk, 1 slice (19 g)	2
Finely shredded cheddar Jack cheese, ¼ cup	4
Light part skim mozzarella string cheese, 1 string cheese (24 g)	1
Mozzarella string cheese, 1 piece (28 g)	3
Pepper Jack ultra thin cheese slices, 2 slices (25 g)	3
Reduced fat deli style provolone cheese slice, 1 slice (19 g)	2
Reduced fat Mexican-style shredded cheese, ¼ cup	3
Reduced fat sharp cheddar shredded cheese, ¼ cup	3
Reduced fat shredded mozzarella cheese, ¼ cup	2
String cheese, light, mozzarella, 1 piece (28 g)	2
Swiss cheese slices, 1 slice (20 g)	2
Marvel Avengers Hero Twists	
Mozzarella string cheese, 1 piece (24 g)	2
Meadow Gold	
Fat free small curd cottage cheese, ½ cup	2
Lowfat small curd cottage cheese, ½ cup	2

	SmartPoints® value
Meijer	
⅓ less fat cream cheese, 2 Tbsp	3
2% milk reduced fat provolone cheese, 1 slice (19 g)	2
Cottage cheese, small curd, 1% milkfat, ½ cup	2
Cottage cheese, small curd, fat free, ½ cup	2
Finely shredded mild cheddar cheese, ¼ cup	4
Mozzarella string cheese, 1 piece (24 g)	1
Shredded mozzarella cheese, ¼ cup	3
String cheese, light, 1 piece (28 g)	1
Mini Babybel	
Light semisoft cheese, 1 piece (21 g)	1
Mozzarella style semisoft cheese, 1 piece (21 g)	2
Original semisoft cheese, 1 piece (21 g)	3
My Essentials 2% milk	
Fancy shredded sharp cheddar cheese, ¼ cup	3
Organic Creamery	
colby Jack cheese, 1 slice (23 g)	3
Organic Valley	
Cottage cheese, lowfat, organic small curd, ½ cup	2
Our Family	
Cheese product, American, 2% milk, singles, 1 slice (21 g)	2
Palmetto	
Cheese spread, 2 Tbsp	5
Pimento cheese with jalapeños, 2 Tbsp	5
Philadelphia	
Blueberry cream cheese spread, 2 Tbsp	3
Brown sugar and cinnamon cream cheese spread, 2 Tbsp	4
Cheese, neufchatel, 1 oz	3

	SmartPoints® value
Chive and onion cream cheese spread, 2 Tbsp	4
Cream cheese, 1 oz	5
Cream cheese spread, whipped, mixed berry, 2 Tbsp	3
Cream cheese, ⅓ less fat, 2 Tbsp	3
Fat free cream cheese, 2 Tbsp	1
Garden vegetable cream cheese spread, 2 Tbsp	3
Garden vegetable cream cheese spread, 2 Tbsp	3
Honey pecan flavored cream cheese spread, 2 Tbsp	4
Original cream cheese, 2 Tbsp	4
Reduced fat chive and onion cream cheese, 2 Tbsp	3
Reduced fat cream cheese, 2 Tbsp	3
Reduced fat garden vegetable cream cheese, 2 Tbsp	3
Reduced fat strawberry cream cheese, 2 Tbsp	3
Smoked salmon cream cheese spread, 2 Tbsp	3
Spicy jalapeño cream cheese spread, 2 Tbsp	3
Strawberry cream cheese spread, 2 Tbsp	4
Philadelphia 2x Protein	
Regular cream cheese spread, 2 Tbsp	2
Philadelphia Fat Free	
Strawberry cream cheese, 2 Tbsp	2
Philadelphia Whipped	
Chive cream cheese spread, 2 Tbsp	2
Original cream cheese spread, 2 Tbsp	2
Polly-O	
Cheese, mozzarella, part skim, 1 oz	2
Low-moisture part-skim mozzarella cheese, 1 stick (28 g)	3

	SmartPoints® value
String cheese, mozzarella, reduced fat, 1 stick (24 g)	2
String cheese, mozzarella, reduced fat, family size, 1 stick (24 g)	2
Twists, mozzarella & cheddar cheeses, 1 stick (21 g)	2
Polly-O Snackables Twists	
Cheese, cheddar & mozzarella, 1 stick (21 g)	2
Polly-O String	
Mozzarella cheese, 1 stick (28 g)	3
Prairie Farms	
Cottage cheese, low-fat, ½ cup	2
Precious	
String cheese, mozzarella, 1 stick (28 g)	3
President	
Cheese, feta, 1 oz	3
Crumbled cheese, fat free, 1 oz	0
Crumbled feta, fat free, 1 oz	0
President Rondele	
Garden vegetable gourmet spreadable cheese, 2 Tbsp	3
Garlic and herbs light spreadable cheese, 2 Tbsp	2
President Wee Bries	
Spreadable cheese wedges, 1 wedge (17.5 g)	2
Price Chopper	
Fat free shredded mozzarella cheese, ⅓ cup	0
Private Selection	
Cheese, feta, reduced fat, crumbled, traditional, ¼ cup	3
Shaved parmesan cheese, 1 Tbsp	1
Shredded parmesan cheese, 1 Tbsp	1
Sliced Swiss cheese, 1 slice (22 g)	3
Pub Cheese	
Cheddar with horseradish, 2 Tbsp	3
Cheddar with jalapeño spreadable cheese, 2 Tbsp	3

Cheese (cont'd)

	SmartPoints® value
Publix	
2% milk reduced fat American cheese slices, 1 slice (21 g)	2
Colby Jack shredded cheese, ¼ cup	4
Cottage cheese, fat free, small curd, ½ cup	1
Cottage cheese, small curd, fat free, ½ cup	1
Goat crumbled cheese, ¼ cup	2
Low moisture part skim mozzarella shredded cheese, ¼ cup	3
Mozzarella string cheese, 1 stick (28 g)	2
Neufchatel cheese, 1 oz	3
Parmesan shaved cheese, ¼ cup	3
Reduced fat 2% milk Swiss cheese, 1 slice (21 g)	2
Shredded mozzarella cheese, ¼ cup	3
Raley's	
Low moisture part skim mozzarella cheese string, 1 piece (28 g)	2
Reggano	
2% reduced fat grated parmesan cheese, 2 tsp	1
Parmesan and Romano grated cheese, 1 Tbsp	1
Roundy's	
2% reduced fat sliced provolone cheese, 1 slice (19 g)	2
2% reduced fat sliced sharp cheddar cheese, 1 slice (19 g)	2
Light string cheese low moisture part skim 2% milk, 1 piece (28 g)	2
String cheese, reduced fat, 1 piece (24 g)	2
Safeway	
Grated cheese, 3 cheese blend, 1 Tbsp	1
Salemville	
Amish blue cheese crumbles, 1 oz	4

	SmartPoints® value
Sam's Choice	
Mozzarella and asiago cheese sticks, 1 piece (35 g)	4
Sargento	
Cheese sticks, natural, mild cheddar, reduced fat, 1 piece (21 g)	2
Cheese, 4 cheese Mexican, reduced fat, shredded, ¼ cup	3
Cheese, extra sharp cheddar, natural, 1 slice (20 g)	3
Cheese, reduced fat, pepper Jack, 1 slice (19 g)	2
Chipotle bbq cheddar snack bites, 7 pieces (30 g)	5
Colby pepper Jack snack cheese bites, 7 pieces (30 g)	4
Colby-jack cheese stick, 1 piece (21 g)	3
Garlic and herb Jack sliced cheese, 1 slice (17 g)	2
Light mozzarella string cheese, 1 piece (21 g)	1
Natural deli style sliced aged Swiss cheese, 1 slice (18 g)	2
Natural deli style sliced baby Swiss cheese, 1 slice (18 g)	3
Natural deli style sliced colby-jack cheese, 1 slice (19 g)	3
Natural deli style sliced gouda cheese, 1 slice (20 g)	3
Natural deli style sliced medium cheddar cheese, 1 slice (21 g)	3
Natural deli style sliced muenster cheese, 1 slice (21 g)	3
Natural deli style sliced provolone cheese, 1 slice (19 g)	2
Natural deli style sliced Swiss cheese, 1 slice (18 g)	2
Natural deli style sliced Vermont sharp white cheddar cheese, 1 slice (20 g)	3
Natural reduced fat colby-jack snacks, 1 piece (21 g)	2

	SmartPoints® value
Natural sharp cheddar cheese sticks, 1 piece (21 g)	3
Pepper Jack cheese sticks, 1 piece (21 g)	3
Reduced fat 4 cheese Italian shredded cheese, ¼ cup	2
Reduced fat 4 cheese Mexican, ¼ cup	3
Reduced fat 4 cheese Mexican shredded cheese, ¼ cup	3
Reduced fat colby Jack cheese snacks, 1 piece (21 g)	2
Reduced fat colby-jack cheese slices, 1 slice (19 g)	2
Reduced fat medium cheddar cheese slices, 1 slice (19 g)	2
Reduced fat mild cheddar cheese snacks, 1 piece (21 g)	2
Reduced fat sharp cheddar cheese snacks, 1 piece (21 g)	2
Reduced fat shredded cheddar Jack cheese, ¼ cup	3
Reduced fat shredded colby Jack cheese, ¼ cup	3
Reduced fat shredded low moisture mozzarella cheese, ¼ cup	2
Reduced fat shredded mild cheddar cheese, ¼ cup	3
Reduced fat shredded mozzarella cheese, ¼ cup	2
Reduced fat shredded sharp cheddar cheese, ¼ cup	3
Reduced fat sliced provolone cheese, 1 slice (19 g)	2
Reduced fat Swiss cheese slices, 1 slice (21 g)	2
Reduced sodium pepper Jack cheese slices, 1 slice (19 g)	3
Savory garlic and herb Jack snack cheese bites, 7 pieces (30 g)	4
Sharp cheddar cheese, ¼ cup	3
Tomato and basil Jack sliced cheese, 1 slice (17 g)	2

	SmartPoints® value
Ultra thin provolone cheese slices, 3 slices (32 g)	5
Ultra thin sliced natural Swiss baby cheese, 3 slices (30 g)	4
Sargento Artisan Blends	
Shredded parmesan cheese (stand up pouch), 2 tsp	1
Sargento Chef Blends	
Shredded taco cheese blend, ¼ cup	4
Sargento Classic	
4 cheese Mexican, ¼ cup	4
Sargento Deli Style	
Natural deli style sliced sharp cheddar cheese, 1 slice (21 g)	3
Sargento Natural Blends	
Cheddar mozzarella cheese sticks, 1 piece (21 g)	3
Colby-pepper Jack cheese slices, 1 slice (19 g)	3
Provolone-mozzarella cheese slices, 1 slice (19 g)	2
Sharp cheddar-jack cheese slices, 1 slice (19 g)	3
Sargento Off the Block	
Fine cut shredded 4 cheese Mexican blend, ¼ cup	4
Fine cut shredded mild cheddar cheese, ¼ cup	4
Fine cut shredded sharp cheddar cheese (8 oz bag), ¼ cup	4
Sharp cheddar traditional cut shredded cheese, ¼ cup	4
Shredded cheese, sharp cheddar, traditional cut, ¼ cup	4
Traditional cut extra sharp cheddar shredded cheese, ¼ cup	4
Sargento Snacks	
Cheese sticks, natural, extra sharp cheddar, 1 piece (21 g)	3
Colby Jack cheese cubes, 7 cubes (30 g)	4

Cheese, Sargento Snacks (cont'd)

	SmartPoints® value
Mozzarella string cheese, 1 piece (21 g)	2
Sharp cheddar cheese stick, 1 piece (21 g)	3
Wisconsin sharp cheddar cheese, 7 pieces (30 g)	5
Sargento Tastings	
Smoky chipotle cheddar Jack cheese, ⅓ piece (33 g)	5
Sargento Ultra Thin	
Baby Swiss cheese slices, 3 slices (32 g)	4
Cheddar Jack cheese slices, 3 slices (32 g)	5
Colby-jack cheese slices, 3 Slices (31 g)	5
Longhorn colby cheese slices, 3 slices (32 g)	5
Mild cheddar cheese slices, 3 slices (32 g)	5
Provolone cheese slices, 3 slices (31 g)	4
Sharp cheddar cheese slices, 3 slices (32 g)	5
Schnucks	
Colby Jack cheese, ¼ cup	3
Shamrock Farms	
Low-fat cottage cheese, ½ cup	3
ShopRite	
Shredded cheese, mozzarella, part-skim, ¼ cup	3
Silver Goat Chevre	
Cheese, goat, 1 oz	0
Sonoma Jacks Sonoma Cheese	
Cheese wedges, gourmet, light, pepper Jack, 1 wedge (19 g)	1
Cheese wedges, gourmet, light, smoked gouda, 1 wedge (19 g)	1
Sorrento	
Low-fat ricotta cheese, ¼ cup	2
Sorrento Stricksters	
Cheese, reduced fat, colby Jack, 1 stick (24 g)	2

	SmartPoints® value
Stick cheese, reduced fat, colby Jack, 1 stick (24 g)	2
Mozzarella string cheese, 1 stick (28 g)	3
String cheese, mozzarella, low moisture, part skim, 1 oz	3
String cheese, reduced fat, mozzarella, 1 oz	2
Spartan	
Light mozzarella string cheese, 1 piece (24 g)	1
Specially Selected	
Aged reserve white cheddar, 1 oz	4
Brie cheese, 1 oz	4
Crumbled blue cheese, 2 Tbsp	4
Crumbled feta cheese, 1 oz	2
Sprouts Farmers Market	
Low moisture part skim mozzarella string cheese, 1 piece (28 g)	3
Stater Bros.	
Fat free shredded mozzarella and cheddar cheeses, ¼ cup	0
Finely shredded low moisture part skim mozzarella cheese, ¼ cup	3
Light string cheese, 1 piece (24 g)	1
Mozzarella light string cheese, 1 stick (24 g)	1
Reduced fat deli style Swiss cheese, 1 slice (19 g)	2
Stella Reduced Fat	
Crumbled blue cheese, ¼ cup	3
Supremo	
Quesadilla cheese queso chihuahua, ¼ cup	4
Temptee	
Cream cheese, 2 Tbsp	4
The Kryssos Co.	
Fat free feta cheese, 1 oz	1
Tillamook	
Cheese, medium cheddar, 1 oz	4
Cheese, sharp cheddar, 1 oz	4
Deli sliced cheese, medium cheddar, 1 slice (21 g)	3

	SmartPoints® value
Medium cheddar really thin natural cheese slices, 3 slices (34 g)	5
Sharp cheddar cheese, 1 oz	4
Sharp cheddar sliced cheese, 1 slice (21 g)	3
Sliced Swiss cheese, 1 slice (28 g)	4
Tnuva	
Light edam cheese, 1 slice (28 g)	1
Light edam sliced cheese, 1 oz	1
Trader Giotto's	
Traditional whole milk ricotta cheese, 2 Tbsp	2
Trader Joe's	
Chevre creamy fresh goat cheese, 1 oz	3
Crumbled blue cheese, 1 oz	4
Crumbled gorgonzola cheese, 2 Tbsp	4
Fat free crumbled feta, 1 oz	0
Fresh goat cheese medallions, 1 oz	3
Freshly shaved parmesan Romano and asiago cheese, 1 Tbsp	1
Light feta cheese, 1 oz	1
Light whipped cream cheese, 2 Tbsp	3
Lite mild cheddar cheese snack sticks, 1 stick (24 g)	1
Low-fat cottage cheese, ½ cup	2
Organic shredded mozzarella cheese, ¼ cup	2
Shaved grana padano parmesan, 1 Tbsp	1
Shaved grana padano parmesan cheese, 1 Tbsp	1
Trader Joe's Organic	
Fat free cottage cheese, ½ cup	2
Light string cheese, 1 stick (28 g)	2
Lowfat cottage cheese, ½ cup	3
String cheese, 1 stick (28 g)	2

	SmartPoints® value
Trader Joe's Refrigerated	
Fancy shredded lite Mexican blend, ¼ cup	2
Fresh mozzarella cheese sticks, 1 stick (28 g)	2
Lite havarti cheese, 1 slice (28 g)	2
Lite shredded 3 cheese blend with mozzarella, Monterey Jack, & cheddar, ¼ cup	2
Lite shredded mozzarella cheese, 1 oz	1
Mini brie bites, 1 piece (25 g)	3
Sliced lite cheddar cheese, 1 slice (28 g)	2
Sliced lite provolone cheese, 1 slice (28 g)	2
String cheese, low moisture part-skim mozzarella lite, 1 stick (28.35 g)	2
Trader Jose's	
Fancy shredded Mexican cheeses blend, ¼ cup	4
Treasure Cave	
Crumbled blue cheese, ¼ cup	4
Crumbled cheese, reduced fat, blue, ¼ cup	3
Velveeta	
Cheese product, pasteurized process, 1 oz	3
Original flavor cheese product slices, 1 slice (21 g)	1
Velveeta Shreds	
Cheddar cheese, ¼ cup	2
Original flavor shredded cheese, ¼ cup	2
Shredded mozzarella cheese, ¼ cup	2
Velveeta Slices	
Cheese product, jalapeño, 1 slice (21 g)	2
Cheese product, sharp cheddar, 1 slice (21 g)	2

Cheese, Velveeta Slices (cont'd)

	SmartPoints® value
Original cheese, 1 slice (19 g)	1
Queso blanco, 1 slice (21 g)	1
Viva	
Grade A fat free cottage cheese small curd, ½ cup	1
Wegman's	
2% reduced fat thin sliced colby cheese, 1 slice (21 g)	2
Cheese sticks, mozzarella, 1 stick (28 g)	3
Cheese sticks, reduced fat, mozzarella, 1 stick (28 g)	2
Colby Jack cheese sticks, 1 stick (24 g)	3
Singles, fat free, American cheese, yellow, 1 slice (21 g)	1
Thin sliced cheese, provolone, 2% milk, 1 slice (21 g)	2
Thin sliced cheese, Swiss, 2% milk, 1 slice (21 g)	1
Traditional fat free crumbled feta cheese, ¼ cup	1
Ultra thin sliced provolone cheese, 3 slices (32 g)	4
Wegman's Food You Feel Good About	
Ultra thin sliced Swiss cheese, 3 slices (32 g)	4
Weight Watchers Cheese Shreds	
Reduced fat Mexican style blend, ⅓ cup	3
Weight Watchers Cheese Singles	
Reduced fat cheese singles, 1 slice	2
Reduced fat pepper Jack singles, 1 slice	1
Weight Watchers Cheese Snacks	
Light jalapeño string cheese, 1 stick	1
Natural light mozzarella string cheese, 1 stick	1

	SmartPoints® value
Natural reduced fat colby Jack cheese stick, 1 stick	2
Reduced fat mild cheddar cheese sticks, 1 stick, 1 stick	2
Weight Watchers Cream Cheese	
Reduced fat cream cheese spread, 1 portion cup	3
Reduced fat whipped cream cheese spread, 2 Tbsp	3
Weis Quality	
Light mozzarella string cheese, 1 piece (24 g)	1
Wellsley Farms	
All natural sliced provolone cheese, 1 slice (21 g)	3
Colby Jack medium cheddar sliced cheese pack, 1 slice (21 g)	3
Grated parmesan cheese, 1 Tbsp	1
Low moisture part skim shredded mozzarella cheese, ¼ cup	3
Mexican blend finely shredded cheese, ¼ cup	4
Wellsley Farms All Natural	
Colby Jack and medium cheddar sliced 2 cheese pack, 1 slice (21 g)	3
Sliced pepper Jack cheese, 1 slice (21 g)	3
Sliced Swiss cheese, 1 slice (21 g)	3
Shredded parmesan cheese, 1 Tbsp	1
Western Family	
Cream cheese, 2 Tbsp	4
Whole Foods Market	
Goat cheese crumbles, 2 Tbsp	3
WinCo Foods	
Finely shredded parmesan cheese, ⅓ cup	3
Grated parmesan cheese, 2 tsp	1
Low moisture part skim mozzarella cheese, ⅓ cup	3
Low moisture part skim mozzarella string cheese, 1 piece (28 g)	3

	SmartPoints® value
Low-fat cottage cheese, ½ cup	2
Mexican style blend cheese, ⅓ cup	4
Part skim mozzarella string cheese, 1 stick (28 g)	3
Winn-Dixie	
Sharp cheddar cheese, ¼ cup	4

Cream and Creamers

	SmartPoints® value
365 Everyday Value	
Hazelnut coffee creamer, 1 Tbsp	2
365 Everyday Value Organic	
Vanilla coffee creamer, 1 Tbsp	2
Bailey's	
Chocolatini coffee creamer, 1 Tbsp	2
Coffee creamer, caramel, 1 Tbsp	2
Coffee creamer, French vanilla, 1 Tbsp	2
Coffee creamer, mudslide, 1 Tbsp	2
Coffee creamer, non-alcoholic, French vanilla, 1 Tbsp	2
Hazelnut caramel blondie coffee creamer, 1 Tbsp	1
The original Irish cream coffee creamer, 1 Tbsp	2
Beaumont Coffee	
French vanilla liquid coffee creamer, 4 tsp	3
Original coffee creamer, 1 tsp	0
Sugar free French vanilla coffee creamer, 1 Tbsp	1
Borden	
Half & half, 2 Tbsp	2
Breakstone's	
All natural sour cream, 2 Tbsp	3
Reduced fat sour cream, 2 Tbsp	1
Byrne Dairy	
Ultra pasteurized half and half, 2 Tbsp	2
Cabot	
Whipped cream, sweetened, light, 2 Tbsp	1
Califia Farms	
Hazelnut almond milk creamer, 1 Tbsp	1
Pecan caramel almond milk creamer, 1 Tbsp	1
Vanilla almond milk creamer, 1 Tbsp	1
Clover Valley	
French vanilla non dairy creamer, 1 Tbsp	2
Coffee Dream	
Fat free French vanilla coffee creamer, 1 Tbsp	1
Coffee-Mate	
Caramel macchiato liquid coffee creamer, 1 Tbsp	2
Chocolate chip cookie coffee creamer, 1 Tbsp	2
Chocolate toffee truffle coffee creamer, 1 Tbsp	2
Classic vanilla liquid coffee creamer, 1 Tbsp	2
Coconut creme liquid coffee creamer, 1 Tbsp	2
Coffee creamer, French vanilla, single serve, 1 tub (11 ml)	2
Coffee creamer, hazelnut, 1 Tbsp	2
Coffee creamer, hazelnut, single serve, 1 tub (11 ml)	2
Coffee creamer, original, lite, 1 tsp	0
Coffee creamer, peppermint mocha, 1 Tbsp	2
Coffee creamer, pumpkin spice, 1 Tbsp	2
Coffee creamer, sugar free, creamy chocolate, 2 tsp	2
Coffee creamer, sugar free, peppermint mocha, 1 Tbsp	0

	SmartPoints® value
Coffee creamer, sugar free, pumpkin spice, 1 Tbsp	0
Coffee creamer, the original, single serve, 1 tub (11 ml)	1
Creamy chocolate powder coffee creamer, 4 tsp	3
Creamy chocolate powder coffee creamer, 4 tsp	3
Fat free French vanilla powder coffee creamer, 4 tsp	2
French vanilla coffee creamer, 1 Tbsp	2
French vanilla fat free liquid coffee creamer, 1 Tbsp	1
French vanilla flavored concentrated creamer, 1 tsp	1
French vanilla liquid coffee creamer, 1 Tbsp	2
French vanilla liquid coffee creamer, 1 Tbsp	2
French vanilla single serve creamer, 1 serving (11 ml)	2
Girl scouts caramel & coconut liquid coffee creamer, 1 Tbsp	2
Girl scouts thin mints liquid coffee creamer, 1 Tbsp	2
Hazelnut creamer, 1 tub (11 ml)	2
Hazelnut liquid coffee creamer, 1 Tbsp	2
Hazelnut powder coffee creamer, 4 tsp	3
Hazelnut sugar free coffee powder creamer, 1 Tbsp	2
Natural bliss hazelnut flavor all-natural coffee creamer, 1 Tbsp	2
Non-dairy creamer, cinnamon vanilla creme, 1 Tbsp	2
Original coffee creamer, 1 container (11 ml)	1
Peppermint mocha coffee creamer, 1 serving (11 ml)	2

	SmartPoints® value
Peppermint mocha liquid coffee creamer, 1 Tbsp	2
Pumpkin spice coffee creamer, 1 tub (11 ml)	2
Pumpkin spice creamer, 1 Tbsp	2
Salted caramel coffee creamer, 1 Tbsp	2
Snickerdoodle coffee creamer, 1 Tbsp	2
Sugar free French vanilla flavored coffee creamer, 1 tub (11 ml)	1
Sugar free French vanilla powder coffee creamer, 1 Tbsp	2
Sugar free, peppermint mocha liquid coffee creamer, 1 Tbsp	0
The original coffee creamer, 1 serving (2 g)	0
The original fat free liquid coffee creamer, 1 Tbsp	0
The original fat free powder coffee creamer, 4 tsp	2
Vanilla caramel liquid coffee creamer, 1 Tbsp	2
Vanilla caramel powder coffee creamer, 4 tsp	3
Coffee-Mate 2Go	
French vanilla concentrated coffee creamer, 1 tsp	1
Hazelnut concentrated coffee creamer, 1 tsp	1
Salted caramel chocolate coffee creamer, 1 Tbsp	2
Coffee-Mate Café Collection	
Sugar free caramel macchiato liquid coffee creamer, 1 Tbsp	0
Coffee-Mate Italian Series	
Sugar free Italian sweet creme liquid coffee creamer, 1 Tbsp	0
Coffee-Mate Natural Bliss	
Caramel flavor liquid coffee creamer, 1 Tbsp	2
Cinnamon cream all-natural coffee creamer, 1 Tbsp	2

	SmartPoints® value
Sweet cream flavor coffee creamer, 1 Tbsp	2
Vanilla flavor liquid coffee creamer, 1 Tbsp	2
Cremora	
Non-dairy creamer, original, 1 tsp	1
Daily Chef	
Rich and creamy non-dairy creamer, 1 tsp	0
Daisy	
Light sour cream, 2 Tbsp	2
Sour cream, 2 Tbsp	3
Sour cream squeeze, 2 Tbsp	3
Darigold	
Creamer, French vanilla, 1 Tbsp	2
Fat free half and half, 2 Tbsp	1
Half and half, 1 fl oz	2
Darigold Pure & Simple	
Sour cream, 2 Tbsp	3
Dean's	
Half and half, 2 Tbsp	2
Dunkin' Donuts	
Caramel coffee creamer, 1 Tbsp	2
Caramel flavor single serve non-dairy creamers, 1 serving (9 ml)	1
Extra extra lquid coffee creamer, 1 Tbsp	2
Hazelnut coffee creamer, 1 Tbsp	2
Original liquid coffee creamer, 1 Tbsp	1
Vanilla non dairy liquid coffee creamer, 1 Tbsp	2
Enhance	
Fat free French vanilla coffee creamer, 1 Tbsp	1
Enjoyably Yours	
Fat free sour cream, 2 Tbsp	1
Essential Everyday	
Coffee creamer, sugar free, French vanilla, liquid, 1 Tbsp	0

	SmartPoints® value
Farmland Special Request	
Fat free half and half skim plus liquid coffee creamer, 2 Tbsp	1
Food Lion	
Fat free French vanilla coffee creamer, 1 Tbsp	1
Fat free half and half, 2 Tbsp	1
Fat free sour cream, 2 Tbsp	1
Friendly Farms	
Fat free hazelnut coffee creamer, 1 Tbsp	2
French vanilla coffee creamer, 1 Tbsp	2
Heavy whipping cream, 1 Tbsp	2
Italian sweet cream coffee creamer, 1 Tbsp	2
Light sour cream, 2 Tbsp	1
Sugar free French vanilla coffee creamer, 1 Tbsp	0
Sugar free hazelnut coffee creamer, 1 Tbsp	0
Vanilla caramel creamer, 1 Tbsp	2
Garelick Farms	
Half & half, fat free, 2 Tbsp	1
Giant	
Fat free French vanilla coffee creamer, 1 Tbsp	1
Fat free half and half, 2 Tbsp	1
French vanilla coffee creamer, 1 Tbsp	2
Hazelnut coffee creamer, 1 Tbsp	1
Giant Eagle	
Fat free half and half, 2 Tbsp	1
Fat free sour cream, 2 Tbsp	1
Great Value	
Coffee creamer, cinnamon vanilla, 1 Tbsp	2
Extra creamy whipped cream, 2 Tbsp	1
Fat free coffee creamer, 1 serving (2 g)	0

Cream and Creamers, Great Value (cont'd)

	SmartPoints® value
Fat free powder creamer, 1 tsp	0
French vanilla fat free coffee creamer, 1 Tbsp	1
French vanilla liquid coffee creamer, 1 Tbsp	2
Half & half, 2 Tbsp	2
Half & half, fat free, 2 Tbsp	1
Hazelnut coffee creamer, 1 Tbsp	3
Hazelnut liquid coffee creamer, 1 Tbsp	2
Italian sweet creme coffee creamer, 1 Tbsp	2
Non dairy extra rich powder coffee creamer, 1 tsp	0
Non-dairy powder coffee creamer, 1 tsp	0
Original coffee creamer, 1 tsp	0
Original liquid coffee creamer, 1 Tbsp	0
Sugar free French vanilla powder creamer, 1 Tbsp	1
Vanilla caramel liquid coffee creamer, 1 Tbsp	2
Whipping cream, heavy, 1 Tbsp	2
Harris Teeter	
Fat free half and half, 2 Tbsp	1
H-E-B	
Crema acidificada, 2 Tbsp	1
Fat free French vanilla coffee creamer, 1 Tbsp	2
Fat free half and half, 2 Tbsp	1
Hood	
Half and half liquid coffee creamer, 2 Tbsp	2
Light liquid cream, 1 Tbsp	1
Sour cream, low-fat, 2 Tbsp	1
Hood Country Creamer	
Fat free liquid coffee creamer, 1 Tbsp	0
Non-dairy creamer, 1 Tbsp	1

	SmartPoints® value
Hood Simply Smart	
Fat free half and liquid coffee creamer, 2 Tbsp	1
Horizon Organic	
Half & half, 2 Tbsp	2
Half & half, ultra-pasteurized, 2 Tbsp	2
Lowfat sour cream, 2 Tbsp	1
Hy-Vee	
Fat free sour cream, 2 Tbsp	1
Half and half, 2 Tbsp	2
Light sour cream, 2 Tbsp	2
International Delight	
Amaretto cafe gourmet coffee creamer, 1 Tbsp	2
Caramel coffee creamer, 1 Tbsp	2
Caramel macchiato creamer, 1 Tbsp	2
Coffee creamer, almond joy, 1 Tbsp	2
Coffee creamer, cinnabon, 1 Tbsp	2
Coffee creamer, gourmet, caramel macchiato, 1 Tbsp	2
Coffee creamer, gourmet, cinnabon, 1 Tbsp	2
Coffee creamer, gourmet, cold stone creamery sweet cream, 1 Tbsp	2
Coffee creamer, gourmet, fat free, caramel macchiato, 1 Tbsp	2
Coffee creamer, gourmet, fat free, French vanilla, 1 Tbsp	2
Coffee creamer, gourmet, hazelnut, 1 Tbsp	2
Coffee creamer, gourmet, heath, 1 Tbsp	2
Coffee creamer, gourmet, sugar free caramel macchiato, 1 Tbsp	1
Coffee creamer, gourmet, sugar free, hazelnut, 1 Tbsp	1
Coffee creamer, gourmet, vanilla caramel creme, 1 Tbsp	2

	SmartPoints® value
Coffee creamer, gourmet, white chocolate mocha, 1 Tbsp	2
Coffee creamer, southern butter pecan, 1 Tbsp	2
Coffee creamer, sugar free, French vanilla, 1 Tbsp	1
Cold stone creamery sweet cream coffee creamer, 1 Tbsp	2
Cold stone creamery sweet cream creamer, 1 Tbsp	2
French vanilla flavored non dairy creamer, 1 container (13 ml)	2
French vanilla gourmet coffee creamer, 1 Tbsp	2
French vanilla gourmet coffee creamer, 1 Tbsp	2
French vanilla sugar free single serve liquid coffee creamer, 1 creamer (13 ml)	1
Frosted sugar cookie gourmet liquid coffee creamer, 1 Tbsp	2
Gourmet coffee creamer, cold stone creamery sweet cream, 1 Tbsp	2
Hazelnut creamer, 1 Tbsp	2
Hershey's chocolate caramel gourmet coffee creamer, 1 Tbsp	2
Irish creme gourmet coffee creamer, 1 Tbsp	2
Peppermint mocha creamer, 1 Tbsp	2
Vanilla coffee creamer, 1 Tbsp	2
Vanilla macchiato coffee creamer, 1 Tbsp	2
White chocolate and raspberry flavored gourmet coffee creamer, 1 Tbsp	2
White chocolate macadamia gourmet coffee creamer, 1 Tbsp	2
International Delight Coffee House Inspirations	
Coffee creamer, caramel macchiato, 1 Tbsp	2
Vanilla caramel coffee creamer, 1 Tbsp	2

	SmartPoints® value
International Delight Creamer Singles	
Liquid, hazelnut, 1 creamer (15 ml)	2
International Delight Fat Free & Sugar Free	
Caramel creme gourmet coffee creamer, 1 Tbsp	0
Caramel marshmallow gourmet coffee creamer, 1 Tbsp	0
Chocolate almond biscotti gourmet coffee creamer, 1 Tbsp	0
Gourmet toasted hazelnut coffee creamer, 1 Tbsp	0
Pumpkin pie spice liquid coffee creamer, 1 Tbsp	0
International Delight Mini I.D.'s	
French vanilla single serve coffee creamer, 1 creamer (13 ml)	2
International Delight Seasonal Edition	
Pumpkin pie spice gourmet coffee creamer, 1 Tbsp	**2**
Salted caramel mocha gourmet coffee creamer, 1 Tbsp	2
Kemps	
Fat free half and half, 2 Tbsp	1
Kroger	
Fat free French vanilla lactose free liquid coffee creamer, 1 Tbsp	2
Fat free half and half, 2 Tbsp	1
Fat free original coffee creamer, 1 Tbsp	0
Fat free sour cream, 1 tsp	0
French vanilla coffee creamer, 1 Tbsp	1
Half and half, 2 Tbsp	2
Hazelnut coffee creamer, 1 Tbsp	0
Heavy whipping cream, 1 Tbsp	2
Sour cream, original, 2 Tbsp	3
Sugar free French vanilla coffee creamer, 1 Tbsp	0
Sugar free hazelnut flavored coffee creamer, 1 Tbsp	0

Cream and Creamers, Kroger (cont'd)

	SmartPoints® value
Vanilla caramel coffee creamer, 1 Tbsp	2
White chocolate mocha coffee creamer, 1 Tbsp	2
Kroger Sugar Free	
French vanilla liquid coffee creamer, 2 Tbsp	1
Land O Lakes	
Coffee creamer, sweetened with sugar, sweet valley creams, 2 Tbsp	3
Fat free half and half, 2 Tbsp	1
Half & half, 2 Tbsp	2
Half and half, 2 Tbsp	2
Heavy cream, whipped, extra creamy, 2 Tbsp	1
Low-fat half and half, 2 Tbsp	1
Rich and creamy light cream, 1 Tbsp	1
Whipped light cream, 2 Tbsp	1
Land O Lakes Mini Moo's	
Dairy creamers, 1 creamer (9 ml)	0
Leaner Creamer	
Coffee creamer supplement, 1 tsp	0
Lucerne	
Coffee creamer, fat free, hazelnut, 1 Tbsp	1
Coffee creamer, Italian sweet cream, 1 Tbsp	2
Coffee creamer, salted caramel, 1 Tbsp	2
Coffee creamer, sugar free, French vanilla, 1 Tbsp	0
Half-and-half, fat free, 2 Tbsp	1
Sugar free hazelnut coffee creamer (lactose free), 1 Tbsp	0
Market Basket	
Half and half, 2 Tbsp	2
Light cream, 1 Tbsp	1
Low-fat sour cream, 2 Tbsp	2

	SmartPoints® value
Market Pantry	
Fat free half and half, 2 Tbsp	1
Fat free half and half ultra pasteurized, 2 Tbsp	1
French vanilla coffee creamer, 1 Tbsp	2
Sour cream, 2 Tbsp	3
Meadow Gold Dairy Pure	
Half and half, 2 Tbsp	2
Mid-America Farms Top The Tater	
Chive and onion sour cream, 2 Tbsp	3
Mocha Mix	
Coffee creamer, non-dairy, original flavor, 1 Tbsp	1
Mountain Dairy	
Fat free half and half, 2 Tbsp	1
Half and half, 2 Tbsp	2
Nestlé	
Hazelnut coffee creamer, 1 tsp	1
Sugar free pumpkin spice coffee creamer, 1 Tbsp	0
N'Joy	
Coffee creamer, 1 tsp	0
Coffee creamer, non-dairy, 1 tsp	0
Open Nature	
Vanilla dairy creamer, 1 Tbsp	2
Organic Valley	
Half & half, organic, 2 Tbsp	2
Soy creamer, French vanilla, 1 Tbsp	1
Soy creamer, original, 1 Tbsp	1
Publix	
Coffee creamer, rich & creamy, non-dairy, 1 tsp	0
Half and half cream, 2 Tbsp	2
Light whipped cream, 2 Tbsp	1
Ultra pasteurized half and half, 2 Tbsp	2

	SmartPoints® value
Ultra pasteurized non dairy coffee creamer, 1 Tbsp	0
Whipped heavy cream, 2 Tbsp	1
Publix GreenWise Market	
Organic half and half, 2 Tbsp	2
Reddi Wip	
Original whipped cream, 2 Tbsp	1
Whipped cream, extra creamy, 2 Tbsp	1
Whipped light cream, original, 2 Tbsp	1
Rock View	
Ultra pasteurized sweetened whipped light cream, 1 Tbsp	1
Shamrock Farms	
Fat free French vanilla coffee creamer, 1 Tbsp	2
Half and half, fat free, 2 Tbsp	1
ShopRite	
Coffee creamer, fat free, French vanilla, 1 Tbsp	1
Coffee creamer, sugar free, French vanilla, 1 Tbsp	0
Half and half, fat free, 2 Tbsp	1
Whipped light cream, 2 Tbsp	1
Silk	
Almond creamer, vanilla, 1 Tbsp	1
Caramel almond creamer, 1 Tbsp	1
Caramel flavor almond creamer, 1 Tbsp	1
Creamer, French vanilla, 1 Tbsp	1
Creamer, hazelnut, 1 Tbsp	1
Creamer, original, 1 Tbsp	1
French vanilla soy creamer, 1 Tbsp	1
Hazelnut almond creamer, 1 Tbsp	1
Vanilla almond creamer, 1 Tbsp	1
Simple Truth Organic	
Half and half, 2 Tbsp	2
Simply Nature	
Organic French vanilla creamer, 1 Tbsp	2

	SmartPoints® value
So Delicious	
Coconut milk, hazelnut creamer, 1 Tbsp	1
Creamer, coconut milk, French vanilla, 1 Tbsp	1
Creamer, original, coconut milk, 1 Tbsp	0
Original almond milk creamer, 1 Tbsp	0
So Delicious Dairy Free	
Creamer, coconut milk, French vanilla, barista style, 1 Tbsp	1
French vanilla almond milk creamer, 1 Tbsp	1
Sprouts Farmers Market	
Half and half, 2 Tbsp	2
Standard Coffee	
Non dairy creamer, 1 tsp	0
Stonyfield Farm	
Organic half and half, 1 fl oz	2
Tillamook	
Sour cream, fat free, 2 Tbsp	1
Sour cream, light, 2 Tbsp	2
Trader Joe's	
Half and half, 2 Tbsp	2
Hazelnut flavor coffee creamer (lactose and gluten free), 1 Tbsp	1
Light sour cream, 2 Tbsp	2
Organic half and half, 2 Tbsp	2
Soy milk creamer, 1 Tbsp	1
Vanilla flavor lactose free coffee creamer, 1 Tbsp	1
Trader Joe's Refrigerated	
Simply fat-free sour cream, 2 Tbsp	0
Walden Farms	
Sweet cream naturally flavored coffee creamer sugar free, 1 Tbsp	0
Wawa	
Hazelnut flavor non dairy creamer, 1 Tbsp	2

Cream and Creamers (cont'd)

	SmartPoints® value
Weight Watchers In-Meeting/ Online Products: Café Creations	
Mucho mocha, 1 packet	0
Pumpkin spice, 1 packet	0
Vanilla bean, 1 packet	0
Wellsley Farms	
Non dairy creamer, 1 tsp	0
Wildwood	
Original soymilk creamer, 1 Tbsp	1
WinCo Foods	
Light sour cream, 2 Tbsp	2

Egg and Egg Substitutes

	SmartPoints® value
4 Grain	
All natural large eggs, 1 egg	2
AllWhites	
100% liquid egg whites, 3 Tbsp	0
Alma Sol	
Hard boiled eggs, 1 egg	2
Almark Foods	
Hard boiled egg, 1 egg	2
Best Choice	
Grade A large eggs, 1 egg	2
Better'n Eggs	
Real egg product, ¼ cup	0
Better'n Eggs Plus	
Real egg product, 3 Tbsp	0
Brown Marketside	
Vegetarian fed large brown eggs, 1 egg	2
Daily Chef Gourmet Foods	
100% liquid egg whites, 3 Tbsp	0
Dutch Farms	
Grade A large eggs, 1 egg	2
Egg Beaters	
100% egg whites, liquid, 3 Tbsp	0
Egg product, real, southwestern style, 3 Tbsp	0
Real egg product, original, ¼ cup	0
Southwestern flavored egg whites, ¼ cup	0
Egg Beaters SmartCups	
All natural 100% egg whites, 1 container (113 g)	1
Egg Innovations	
Eggs, antioxidant, cage free, 1 egg	2
Eggs, cage free, large, brown, 1 egg	2
Eggs, free range, brown, large, 1 egg	2
Eggland's Best	
100% liquid egg whites, 3 Tbsp	0
Cracked and ready liquid egg product, 3 Tbsp	2
Eggs, brown, organic, large, 1 egg	2
Eggs, grade A, extra large, 1 egg	2
Extra large grade A eggs, 1 egg	2
Grade A extra large brown eggs, 1 egg	2
Hard cooked peeled medium egg, 1 egg	2
Jumbo grade A egg, 1 egg	2
Large egg, 1 egg	2
Liquid egg whites, 3 Tbsp	0
Eggland's Best Organic	
Eggs, grade A brown, large, 1 egg	2
Farm Fresh	
Grade A large eggs, 1 egg	2
Large white eggs, 1 egg	6
Farmers Market	
Extra large grade A eggs, 1 egg	2
Grade A extra large eggs, 1 egg	2
Grade A large eggs, 1 egg	2
Farmhouse	
Grade A cage free large eggs, 1 egg	2
Grade A large eggs, 1 egg	2
Fit & Active	
Egg substitute, ¼ cup	0
Liquid egg whites, 3 Tbsp	0

	SmartPoints® value
Food Lion	
100% liquid egg whites, 3 Tbsp	0
Egg mates, 3 Tbsp	0
Grade A large white eggs, 1 egg	2
Large white eggs, 1 egg	2
Giant	
Egg whites, ¼ cup	0
Egg whites, liquid, ¼ cup	0
Eggs, large, grade A, 1 egg	2
Giant Eagle	
Egg whites, 3 Tbsp	0
Grade A large eggs, 1 egg	2
Great Day Farms	
Hard boiled eggs, 1 egg	2
Great Day Foods	
Farmers market large farm fresh egg, 1 egg	2
Hard boiled eggs, 1 egg	2
Great Day Foods Farmers Market	
Large grade A farm fresh egg, 1 egg	2
Great Value	
Original liquid eggs, ¼ cup	0
Hannaford	
Egg whites, 3 Tbsp	0
Harris Teeter	
100% liquid egg whites, 3 Tbsp	0
Grade A large eggs, 1 egg	2
H-E-B	
Cage free large brown eggs, 1 egg	2
Real egg, ¼ cup	0
Real egg whites, ¼ cup	0
Hickman's	
Extra large grade AA eggs, 1 egg	2
Hill Country Fare	
Extra large eggs, 1 egg	2
Hillandale Farms	
Grade A large eggs, 1 egg	2

	SmartPoints® value
Hy-Vee	
100% egg whites, 3 Tbsp	0
Grade A large eggs, 1 egg	2
Kirkland Signature	
100% liquid egg whites, 3 Tbsp	0
Kirkland Signature Organic	
Large brown eggs, 1 egg	2
Kroger	
Grade A extra large eggs, 1 egg	2
Grade A jumbo eggs, 1 egg	3
Grade A medium eggs, 1 egg	2
Real egg product, break-free, ¼ cup	0
Kroger Break-Free	
100% liquid egg whites, 3 Tbsp	0
Real egg product, ¼ cup	0
Land O Lakes	
Large brown eggs, 1 egg	2
Large grade A brown eggs, 1 egg	2
Lucerne Best of the Egg	
Original pasteurized real egg product, 3 Tbsp	0
Lucerne Best of the Egg Whites	
100% liquid egg whites, 3 Tbsp	0
Market Basket	
Grade A large eggs, 1 egg	2
Pure egg whites, 3 Tbsp	0
Market Basket Egg Starts	
Egg product, 3 Tbsp	0
Market Basket Pure Whites	
Liquid egg whites, 3 Tbsp	0
Market Pantry	
Egg substitute, 3 Tbsp	0
Grade A jumbo eggs, 1 egg	2
Marketside	
Cage free brown eggs, 1 egg	2
Organic cage free brown eggs, 1 egg	2

Egg and Egg Substitutes (cont'd)

	SmartPoints® value
Meijer	
Eggs, large, 1 egg	2
Grade A large eggs, 1 egg	2
Great egg spectations, 3 Tbsp	0
Meijer Great Eggspectations	
Real egg product, 3 Tbsp	0
Meijer Organics	
Extra large brown eggs, 1 egg	2
Member's Mark	
100% liquid egg whites, 3 Tbsp	0
Nature's Touch	
Grade A large eggs, 1 egg	2
Nellie's Nest	
Cage free grade A eggs, 1 egg	2
Nulaid ReddiEgg	
Real egg product, ¼ cup	0
O Organics	
Grade A large brown eggs, 1 egg	2
Ozark Farmers Market	
Jumbo eggs, 1 egg	3
Penrose	
Pickled eggs, beet flavored, 1 egg	2
Pete and Gerry's Organic Eggs	
Cage free liquid egg whites, 3 Tbsp	0
Publix	
Eggs, large, 1 egg	2
Sauder's Eggs	
Grade A large eggs, 1 egg	2
ShopRite	
Egg whites, ¼ cup	0
ShopRite The Great Eggscape	
99% real egg product, ¼ cup	0
Simple Truth	
Grade A large brown eggs, 1 egg	2
Natural cage free grain fed large brown egg, 1 egg	2
Simply Balanced	
Large brown eggs, 1 egg	2

	SmartPoints® value
Smith's	
Large eggs, 1 egg	2
Sprouts Farmers Market	
Omega 3 large eggs, 1 egg	2
Stater Bros.	
100% egg whites, ¼ cup	0
Sunny Meadow	
Large grade A farm fresh eggs, 1 egg	2
Sunnyside Farms	
Liquid egg whites, ¼ cup	0
Real egg, ¼ cup	0
Sunups	
Extra large grade A eggs, 1 egg	2
Grade A large eggs, 1 egg	2
Trader Joe's	
Cage free 100% liquid egg whites, 3 Tbsp	0
Cage free fresh hard-cooked peeled eggs, 1 egg	2
Grade A large brown eggs, 1 egg	2
Vital Farms	
Alfresco eggs, 1 egg	2
Wellsley Farms	
Extra large grade A eggs, 1 egg	2
Whitewater Valley	
Large eggs, 1 egg	2
Large grade A eggs, 1 egg	2
Wilcox Family Farm	
Grade AA extra large eggs, 1 egg	2
Wilcox Organic	
Hard boiled eggs, 1 egg	2

Margarine

Blue Bonnet	
46% vegetable oil spread, 1 Tbsp	2
Vegetable oil spread, 53%, 1 Tbsp	3
Blue Bonnet Light	
Vegetable oil spread, 31%, 1 Tbsp	1

	SmartPoints® value
Brummel & Brown	
Spread, 1 Tbsp	2
Spread made with yogurt, 1 Tbsp	2
Country Crock	
39% vegetable oil spread, 1 Tbsp	2
39% vegetable oil spread, plus calcium & vitamins, 1 Tbsp	2
Countryside Creamery	
Homestyle spread, country recipe, 1 Tbsp	2
Earth Balance	
Buttery spread, organic, whipped, 1 Tbsp	3
Fleischmann's	
Light margarine, 1 Tbsp	1
Vegetable oil spread, 60% whipped, 1 Tbsp	2
I Can't Believe It's Not Butter!	
45% vegetable oil spread made with olive oil, 1 Tbsp	2
Light 30% vegetable oil spread, 1 Tbsp	1
Light vegetable spread, 1 Tbsp	1
Original 45% vegetable oil spread, 1 Tbsp	2
Imperial	
Vegetable oil spread, 65%, cholesterol free, 1 Tbsp	3
Land O Lakes	
Spread, fresh buttery taste, 1 Tbsp	3
Move Over Butter	
Vegetable oil spread, whipped with sweet cream buttermilk, 1 Tbsp	2
Parkay	
60% vegetable oil spread, original, 1 Tbsp	3
Promise	
Vegetable oil spread, buttery light, 1 Tbsp	2

	SmartPoints® value
Shedd's	
39% vegetable oil spread, calcium plus vitamin D, 1 Tbsp	2
39% vegetable oil spread, light, 1 Tbsp	2
48% vegetable oil spread, 1 Tbsp	2
53% vegetable oil spread, original, 1 Tbsp	3
Shedd's Spread Country Crock	
Light vegetable oil spread, 1 Tbsp	2
Original country fresh taste margarine, 1 Tbsp	2
Original vegetable oil spread, 1 Tbsp	2
Smart Balance	
Light buttery spread, 1 Tbsp	2

Milk and Milk Based Drinks

Anderson Erickson	
1% grade A lowfat milk, 1 cup	4
Egg nog, ½ cup	12
Lite egg nog, ½ cup	6
Braum's	
1% low-fat milk, 1 cup	5
Carnation	
Milk, evaporated, 2 Tbsp	2
Club Foods	
2% reduced fat milk, 1 cup	5
Colorado	
Fat free milk, 8 fl oz	3
Cub	
Fat free milk, 1 cup	3
Daily Chef	
Fat free skim milk, 1 cup	3
Light egg nog, 4 fl oz	7
Milk, fat free, 1 cup	3
Dean's Dairy Pure	
2% reduced fat milk, 1 container (414 ml)	9
Dillon's	
Skim milk, 8 fl oz	3

Milk and Milk Based Drinks (cont'd)

	SmartPoints® value
Fairlife	
2% lactose free chocolate milk, 1 cup	5
2% low-fat chocolate milk, 11 ½ fl oz	7
Lactose free 2% milk, 1 cup	4
Lactose free skim milk, 1 cup	2
Reduced fat ultra filtered milk, 11 ½ fl oz	5
Farmland Special Request	
Milk, skim plus, 1 cup	4
Milk, skim plus, fat free, 1 cup	4
Fit & Active	
Milk chocolate flavored weight loss shake, 1 bottle (325 ml)	7
Food Lion	
Fat free milk, 1 cup	3
Fred Meyer	
1% lowfat milk, 8 fl oz	4
Skim milk, 8 fl oz	3
Friendly Farms	
1% low-fat milk, 1 cup	4
2% reduced fat milk, 1 cup	5
Fat free milk with vitamins A & D, 1 cup	3
Fat free skim milk, 1 cup	3
Lactose free fat free milk, 1 cup	3
Garelick Farms Dairy Pure	
2% reduced fat milk, 1 cup	5
Giant Eagle	
1% lowfat milk, 1 cup	4
Fat free skim milk, 1 cup	3
Skim milk, 1 cup	3
Good Karma	
Flax milk, unsweetened, 1 cup	1
Great Value	
1% low-fat chocolate milk, 1 cup	8
Evaporated fat free milk, 1 oz	1
Evaporated milk, 1 oz	2
Milk, 1% low-fat, 1% milkfat, 1 cup	4

	SmartPoints® value
Milk, 2% reduced fat, 2% milkfat, 1 cup	5
Milk, fat free, 0% milkfat, 1 cup	3
Milk, fat free, lactose free, 1 cup	3
Milk, fat free, organic, 1 cup	3
Milk, reduced fat, lactose free, 2% milkfat, 1 cup	5
Milk, vitamin D, 1 cup	6
Hannaford	
Fat free milk, 1 cup	3
Harris Teeter	
Milk, non-fat, skim, 1 cup	3
H-E-B	
1% low-fat milk, 1 cup	4
Fat free milk, 1 cup	3
Low-fat 1% milk, 1 cup	4
H-E-B Mootopia	
Fat free lactose free milk, 1 cup	2
Lactose free fat free milk, 1 cup	2
Whole milk, 1 cup	4
Hiland	
Fat free skim milk, 1 cup	3
Skim milk, 1 cup	3
Hill Country Fare	
Fat free milk, 1 cup	3
Hood	
Milk, fat free, skim, 1 cup	3
Milk, fat free, skim, vitamins a, c & d, 1 cup	3
Hood Simply Smart	
Milk, fat free, 1 cup	3
Horizon Organic	
2% reduced fat milk, 1 cup	5
Fat free milk, 1 cup	3
Milk, 2% reduced fat, 1 cup	5
Milk, lowfat, 1% milkfat, 1 cup	4
Whole milk with vitamin D, 1 cup	6
Hy-Vee	
1% lowfat milk, 1 cup	4

	SmartPoints® value
Kemps	
1% low-fat milk, 8 fl oz	4
Swiss style chocolate low-fat milk, 1 cup	8
Kirkland Signature	
2% reduced fat milk, 1 cup	5
Fat free milk, 1 cup	3
Homogenized milk, 1 cup	7
Milk, reduced fat, 2% milkfat, 1 cup	5
Organic 1% low-fat milk, 1 cup	5
Organic whole milk, 1 cup	7
Reduced fat milk, 1 cup	6
Kroger	
1% lowfat milk, 8 fl oz	4
2% reduced fat milk, 8 fl oz	5
Fat free skim milk, 8 fl oz	3
Low-fat milk, 8 fl oz	3
Reduced sugar nonfat chocolate milk, 8 fl oz	2
Vanilla carbmaster nonfat reduced sugar milk, 8 fl oz	1
Kroger Value CARBmaster	
Nonfat reduced sugar milk, 8 fl oz	1
Lactaid	
Fat free lactose free milk, 1 carton (236 ml)	3
Fat free milk, 1 cup	3
Milk, fat free, 1 cup	3
Milk, fat free, 100% lactose free, calcium enriched, 1 cup	3
Milk, lowfat, 1% milkfat, 1 cup	4
Milk, reduced fat, 2% milkfat, 1 cup	5
Land O Lakes	
Light egg nog, ½ cup	6
Land O Lakes Mini Moo's	
Half and half liquid single serve creamer, 1 serving (9 ml)	0
Lifeway	
Kefir cultured milk, nonfat, plain, unsweetened, 1 cup	3

	SmartPoints® value
Lucerne	
Milk, fat free, 1 cup	3
Milk, lowfat, 1% milkfat, 1 cup	4
Market Basket	
1% lowfat milk, 1 cup	4
Fat free skim milk, 1 cup	3
Skim fat free milk, 1 cup	3
Market Pantry	
2% reduced fat milk, 1 cup	5
Meadow Gold	
Egg nog, 4 fl oz	9
Meijer	
Milk, 1% lowfat, 1 cup	4
Mountain Dairy	
Fat free milk, 8 fl oz	3
Nature's Touch	
Fat free milk, 1 cup	3
Oak Farms Dairy	
Whole milk, 1 cup	6
Oak Farms Dairy Trumoo	
Chocolate whole milk, 1 cup	11
Organic Valley	
Milk, lowfat, 1% milkfat, organic, 1 cup	4
Over the Moon	
Milk, fat free, 1 cup	4
Prairie Farms	
Milk, skim, fat free, 1 cup	3
Price First	
2% reduced fat milk, 1 cup	5
Fat free milk, 1 cup	3
Publix	
1% lowfat milk, 1 cup	4
2% milkfat lowfat grade A egg nog, ½ cup	7
All natural fat free grade A milk, 1 cup	3
Fat free milk, 1 cup	3
Publix GreenWise Market	
Organic fat free milk, 1 cup	3

Milk and Milk Based Drinks (cont'd)

	SmartPoints® value
Ralph's	
Fat free skim milk, 8 fl oz	3
Roundy's	
1% low-fat milk, 1 cup	4
2% reduced fat milk, 1 cup	5
Skim milk, 1 cup	3
Schneider	
Super skim milk, 1 cup	3
Schnucks	
Skim milk, 1 cup	3
Shamrock Farms	
Lowfat milk, 1 carton (236 ml)	4
Simple Truth Organic	
Fat free milk, 8 fl oz	3
Spartan	
Fat free milk, 1 cup	3
Springdale	
Skim milk, 8 fl oz	3
Stater Bros.	
Fat free milk, 1 cup	3
Stonyfield Farm Organic	
Fat free milk, 1 cup	3
Lowfat milk, 1% milkfat, 1 cup	4
Trader Joe's	
Low-fat kefir, 8 fl oz	3
Trader Joe's Organic	
Ultra pasteurized half and half, 2 Tbsp	2
United	
Fat free milk, 1 cup	3
Wal-Mart	
1% low-fat milk, 1 cup	4
Wegman's Food You Feel Good About	
Milk, fat free, 1 cup	3
Weigel's	
Skim milk, 1 cup	3
Wellsley Farms	
Fat free milk, 1 cup	3
Organic 1% low-fat milk, 1 cup	4
Organic fat free milk, 1 cup	3
WinCo Foods	
1% lowfat milk, 1 cup	4
Fat free half and half, 2 Tbsp	1

Yogurt

	SmartPoints® value
365 Everyday Value	
Organic fat free vanilla yogurt, 1 container (170 g)	6
Activia	
Black cherry flavored lowfat yogurt, 1 container (113 g)	5
Blueberry flavored lowfat yogurt, 1 container (113 g)	6
Light blueberry flavored yogurt, 1 container (113 g)	2
Mixed berry flavored lowfat yogurt, 1 container (113 g)	5
Peach flavored lowfat yogurt, 1 container (113 g)	5
Strawberry flavored lowfat yogurt, 1 container (113 g)	5
Vanilla flavored lowfat yogurt, 1 container (113 g)	5
Activia Greek	
Garden blueberry fruit on the bottom nonfat yogurt, 1 container (150 g)	5
Strawberry patch fruit on the bottom nonfat yogurt, 1 container (150 g)	5
Vanilla flavored nonfat yogurt, 1 container (150 g)	6
Activia Light	
Peach favored yogurt, 1 container (113 g)	2
Raspberry flavored nonfat yogurt, 1 container (113 g)	2

Dairy & Eggs

	SmartPoints® value
Strawberry banana flavored nonfat yogurt, 1 container (113 g)	2
Strawberry flavored nonfat yogurt, 1 container (113 g)	2
Vanilla flavored nonfat yogurt, 1 container (113 g)	2
Ahold	
Nonfat plain Greek yogurt, 1 container (150 g)	2
Cabot	
Yogurt, lowfat, Greek-style, plain, 1 cup	5
Yogurt, lowfat, Greek-style, vanilla, 1 cup	9
Chobani	
Black cherry fruit on the bottom nonfat Greek yogurt, 1 container (150 g)	5
Blueberry nonfat Greek yogurt, 1 container (150 g)	5
Coconut blended 2% milkfat low-fat Greek yogurt, 1 container (150 g)	6
Coffee blended low-fat Greek yogurt, 1 container (150 g)	6
Peach nonfat Greek yogurt, 1 container (150 g)	4
Pineapple low-fat Greek yogurt, 1 container (150 g)	6
Plain Greek nonfat yogurt, 1 cup	3
Strawberry banana 2% milkfat low-fat Greek yogurt, 1 container (150 g)	6
Strawberry nonfat Greek yogurt, 1 container (150 g)	4
Vanilla blended Greek nonfat yogurt, 1 cup	6
Chobani Blended	
Coconut Greek low-fat yogurt, 1 oz	6
Key lime Greek low-fat yogurt, 1 container (150 g)	6
Lemon Greek nonfat yogurt, 1 container (150 g)	5
Raspberry Greek low-fat yogurt, 6 oz	4
Strawberry Greek nonfat yogurt, 1 cup	7
Vanilla Greek nonfat yogurt, 1 container (150 g)	4
Watermelon flavored Greek lowfat yogurt, 1 container (150 g)	5
Chobani Flip	
Almond coco loco Greek low-fat yogurt, 1 container (150 g)	10
Chipotle pineapple Greek yogurt, 1 container (150 g)	7
Chocolate haze craze flavored Greek yogurt, 1 container (150 g)	10
Key lime crumble Greek low-fat yogurt, 1 container (150 g)	8
Nutty for 'nana Greek low-fat yogurt, 1 container (150 g)	8
Pb and j Greek yogurt, 1 container (150 g)	8
Peachy pistachio Greek low-fat yogurt, 1 container (150 g)	8
Salted caramel crunch flavored Greek yogurt, 1 container (150 g)	7
Sriracha mango Greek yogurt, 1 container (150 g)	7
Strawberry summer crisp low-fat yogurt with graham crackers and white chocolate, 1 container (150 g)	7
Tropical escape Greek low-fat yogurt, 1 container (150 g)	9
Chobani Fruit on the Bottom	
Apricot Greek low-fat yogurt, 1 container (150 g)	6
Black cherry Greek nonfat yogurt, 1 container (150 g)	5
Blackberry Greek nonfat yogurt, 1 oz	4
Blood orange Greek nonfat yogurt, 1 container (150 g)	4

Yogurt, Chobani Fruit on the Bottom (cont'd)

	SmartPoints® value
Blueberry Greek nonfat yogurt, 1 container (150 g)	5
Mango Greek low-fat yogurt, 1 container (150 g)	6
Peach Greek nonfat yogurt, 1 container (150 g)	4
Pomegranate Greek nonfat yogurt, 1 container (150 g)	4
Raspberry Greek nonfat yogurt, 1 container (150 g)	5
Strawberry banana Greek low-fat yogurt, 1 container (150 g)	6
Strawberry Greek nonfat yogurt, 1 container (150 g)	4
Chobani Greek Yogurt Simply 100	
Strawberry blended Greek yogurt, 1 container (150 g)	3
Chobani Kids	
Strawberry flavored low-fat Greek yogurt, 1 tube (57 g)	2
Chobani Oats	
Apple cinnamon with steel cut oats low-fat Greek yogurt, 1 container (150 g)	6
Banana maple low-fat Greek yogurt, 1 container (150 g)	6
Chobani Simply 100	
Black cherry flavored nonfat blended Greek yogurt, 1 container (150 g)	3
Black cherry on the bottom Greek nonfat yogurt, 1 container (150 g)	3
Blueberry blended nonfat Greek yogurt, 1 container (150 g)	3
Blueberry cookie crumble yogurt, 1 container (119 g)	3
Blueberry on the bottom Greek nonfat yogurt, 1 container (150 g)	3
Key lime blended Greek nonfat yogurt, 1 container (150 g)	3
Mango passion fruit nonfat Greek yogurt, 1 container (150 g)	3
Peach on the bottom Greek nonfat yogurt, 1 container (150 g)	3

	SmartPoints® value
Pineapple coconut blended Greek nonfat yogurt, 1 container (150 g)	3
Pineapple on the bottom Greek nonfat yogurt, 1 container (150 g)	3
Raspberry lemon blended Greek nonfat yogurt, 1 container (150 g)	3
Strawberry chocolate truffle yogurt, 1 container (119 g)	3
Strawberry on the bottom Greek nonfat yogurt, 1 container (150 g)	3
Tropical citrus blended Greek yogurt, 1 container (150 g)	3
Vanilla blended Greek nonfat yogurt, 1 container (150 g)	3
Coburn Farms	
Cherry cheesecake light yogurt, 6 oz	4
Dannon	
Lemon fruit on the bottom yogurt, 1 container (170 g)	7
Dannon Activia	
Fat free blueberry yogurt, 1 container (113 g)	2
Fruit fusion lowfat yogurt, 1 container (113 g)	4
Light peach flavored nonfat yogurt, 1 container (113 g)	2
Dannon Activia Fiber	
Strawberry low-fat yogurt with cereal, 1 container (113 g)	5
Dannon Activia Fruit Frusion	
Strawberry and raspberry lowfat yogurt, 1 container (113 g)	4
Dannon Activia Light	
Blueberry fruit on the bottom nonfat Greek yogurt, 1 container (150 g)	2
Cherry on the bottom nonfat Greek yogurt, 1 container (150 g)	2
Strawberry flavored nonfat yogurt, 1 container (113 g)	2
Strawberry fruit on the bottom nonfat Greek yogurt, 1 container (150 g)	2

	SmartPoints® value
Dannon All Natural	
Plain nonfat yogurt, 1 cup	4
Plain yogurt, 1 cup	6
Vanilla flavored lowfat yogurt, 1 container (170 g)	8
Dannon Greek	
Strawberry flavored nonfat yogurt, 1 container (150 g)	2
Dannon Light & Fit	
Banana flavored nonfat yogurt, 1 container (170 g)	3
Banana flavored nonfat yogurt, 1 container (170 g)	3
Blueberry flavored nonfat yogurt, 1 container (170 g)	3
Cherry flavored nonfat yogurt, 1 container (170 g)	3
Cherry vanilla flavored nonfat yogurt, 1 container (170 g)	3
French vanilla Greek yogurt mousse, 1 container (113 g)	3
Greek crunch caramel fudge pretzel nonfat yogurt (with toppings), 1 container (141 g)	5
Greek crunch coconut chocolate bliss nonfat yogurt (with toppings), 1 container (141 g)	4
Greek crunch key lime pie nonfat yogurt (with toppings), 1 container (141 g)	5
Key lime flavored nonfat yogurt, 1 container (170 g)	3
Nonfat caramel apple yogurt, 1 container (170 g)	3
Peach flavored nonfat yogurt, 1 container (170 g)	3
Raspberry flavored nonfat yogurt, 1 container (170 g)	3
Raspberry white chocolate Greek mousse, 1 container (113 g)	3
Strawberry banana flavored nonfat yogurt, 1 container (170 g)	3
Strawberry cheesecake flavored nonfat yogurt, 1 container (170 g)	3

	SmartPoints® value
Strawberry flavored nonfat yogurt, 1 container (170 g)	3
Strawberry shortcake Greek mousse, 1 container (113 g)	3
Vanilla flavored nonfat yogurt, 1 cup	4
Vanilla flavored nonfat yogurt, 1 container (170 g)	3
Dannon Light & Fit 50 Calorie Packs	
Strawberry flavored nonfat yogurt, 1 container (113 g)	2
Dannon Light & Fit Greek	
Blueberry flavored nonfat yogurt, 1 container (150 g)	2
Peach flavored nonfat yogurt, 1 container (150 g)	2
Raspberry chocolate flavored nonfat yogurt, 1 container (150 g)	2
Salted caramel flavored nonfat yogurt, 1 container (150 g)	2
Salted caramel nonfat yogurt mousse, 1 container (113 g)	3
Strawberry banana flavored nonfat yogurt, 1 container (150 g)	2
Strawberry cheesecake flavored nonfat yogurt, 1 container (150 g)	2
Tiramisu flavored nonfat yogurt, 1 container (150 g)	2
Toasted coconut vanilla flavored nonfat yogurt, 1 container (150 g)	2
Dannon Light & Fit Greek Blends	
Caramel macchiato flavored nonfat yogurt, 1 container (150 g)	2
Caramel macchiato/banana cream flavored nonfat yogurt, 1 container (150 g)	2
Cherry chocolate flavored nonfat yogurt, 1 container (150 g)	2
Raspberry chocolate flavored nonfat yogurt, 1 container (150 g)	2
Strawberry cheesecake flavored nonfat yogurt (variety pack), 1 container (150 g)	2

Yogurt (cont'd)

	SmartPoints® value
Dannon Oikos	
Banana peanut butter crunch yogurt, 1 container (141 g)	7
Blueberry flavored Greek nonfat yogurt (variety pack), 1 container (150 g)	5
Coconut chocolate crunch Greek nonfat yogurt, 1 container (141 g)	7
Greek nonfat coffee yogurt, 1 container (150 g)	3
Greek nonfat yogurt variety pack, 1 container (150 g)	5
Key lime crumble crunch yogurt, 1 container (141 g)	7
Plain blended Greek nonfat yogurt, 1 container (150 g)	3
Plain Greek nonfat yogurt, 1 container (150 g)	2
Triple zero banana cream yogurt, 1 container (150 g)	3
Triple zero chocolate Greek nonfat yogurt, 1 container (150 g)	3
Triple zero plain Greek nonfat yogurt, 1 cup	4
Vanilla almond crunch yogurt, 1 container (141 g)	6
Vanilla flavored Greek nonfat yogurt, 1 container (150 g)	5
Vanilla flavored Greek nonfat yogurt, 1 container (150 g)	5
Vanilla flavored Greek nonfat yogurt, 1 cup	7
Dannon Oikos Fruit on the Bottom	
Black cherry Greek nonfat yogurt, 1 container (150 g)	5
Blueberry Greek nonfat yogurt, 1 container (150 g)	5
Peach Greek nonfat yogurt, 1 container (150 g)	5
Strawberry Greek nonfat yogurt, 1 container (150 g)	5

	SmartPoints® value
Dannon Oikos Traditional	
Key lime flavored Greek yogurt, 1 container (150 g)	7
Raspberry flavored Greek yogurt, 1 container (150 g)	7
Strawberry flavored Greek yogurt, 1 container (150 g)	6
Dannon Oikos Triple Zero	
Banana creme nonfat yogurt, 1 container (150 g)	3
Mixed berry flavored nonfat Greek yogurt, 1 container (150 g)	3
Vanilla flavored blended Greek nonfat yogurt, 1 cup	5
FAGE Total 0%	
Greek strained cherry yogurt, 1 container (150 g)	4
Nonfat Greek strained yogurt, 1 container (170 g)	2
Nonfat Greek strained yogurt, 1 cup	3
Nonfat Greek strained yogurt with blueberry acai, 1 container (150 g)	4
Nonfat Greek strained yogurt with cherry pomegranate, 1 container (150 g)	4
Nonfat Greek strained yogurt with honey, 1 container (150 g)	7
Nonfat Greek yogurt with peach, 1 container (150 g)	4
Yogurt, Greek strained, with blueberry, 1 container (150 g)	4
Yogurt, Greek strained, with strawberry, 1 container (150 g)	4
Yogurt, Greek, nonfat, strained, with raspberry, 1 container (150 g)	4
FAGE Total 2%	
Greek strained lowfat yogurt, 1 cup	5
Greek yogurt with pineapple, 1 container (150 g)	5
Lowfat Greek strained yogurt, 1 cup	5

	SmartPoints® value
Lowfat Greek strained yogurt with blueberry, 1 container (150 g)	5
Lowfat Greek strained yogurt with honey, 1 container (150 g)	9
Lowfat Greek strained yogurt with strawberry, 1 container (150 g)	5
Nonfat Greek strained yogurt with cherry, 1 container (150 g)	5
Yogurt, Greek, lowfat, strained, with blood orange, 1 container (150 g)	5
Yogurt, Greek, lowfat, strained, with key lime, 1 container (150 g)	5
Yogurt, Greek, lowfat, strained, with raspberry pomegranate, 1 container (150 g)	5
Fit & Active	
Vanilla nonfat yogurt, 1 cup	5
Fred Meyer	
Lite vanilla Greek yogurt, 1 container (150 g)	2
Plain Greek nonfat yogurt, 1 cup	3
Friendly Farms	
Blueberry Greek yogurt, 1 container (150 g)	3
Caramel macchiato Greek light yogurt, 1 container (150 g)	2
Light strawberry cheesecake Greek yogurt, 1 container (150 g)	2
Friendly Farms 100 Calorie	
Blackberry flavored nonfat strained Greek yogurt, 1 container (150 g)	3
Mixed berries Greek nonfat strained yogurt, 1 container (150 g)	3
Strawberry flavored Greek nonfat yogurt, 1 container (150 g)	3
Tropical fruit Greek nonfat strained yogurt, 1 container (150 g)	3
Giant	
Blueberry Greek 100 calorie nonfat yogurt, 1 container (150 g)	3

	SmartPoints® value
Great Value	
Banana cream light Greek nonfat yogurt, 1 container (150 g)	2
Black cherry flavored light Greek nonfat yogurt, 1 container (150 g)	3
Light Greek nonfat yogurt, 1 container (150 g)	2
Light peach flavor Greek nonfat yogurt, 1 container (150 g)	2
Light vanilla nonfat yogurt, 1 cup	5
Plain nonfat yogurt, 1 cup	4
Toasted coconut vanilla flavored nonfat Greek yogurt, 1 container (150 g)	2
Vanilla Greek nonfat yogurt, 1 cup	7
Yogurt, nonfat, light, blueberry, 6 oz	3
Yogurt, nonfat, light, cherry, 6 oz	3
Yogurt, nonfat, light, peach, 6 oz	3
Yogurt, nonfat, light, strawberry, 6 oz	3
Yogurt, nonfat, light, strawberry banana, 6 oz	3
Yogurt, nonfat, light, vanilla, 6 oz	3
Great Value Light	
Pina colada flavored nonfat yogurt, 1 container (170 g)	3
Greek Gods	
Yogurt, Greek style, traditional, honey flavored, 4 oz	8
Yogurt, Greek, nonfat, plain, 4 oz	2
Yogurt, Greek, vanilla honey, 1 cup	14
Green Mountain Creamery	
Blueberry strained Greek nonfat yogurt, 1 container (150 g)	4
Greek yogurt strawberry, 1 container (150 g)	4
Maple flavored nonfat Greek yogurt, 1 container (150 g)	3
Plain Greek yogurt, 1 cup	3
Vanilla Greek yogurt, 1 cup	5

Yogurt (cont'd)

	SmartPoints® value
Green Mountain Farms	
Whipped Greek cream cheese and Greek yogurt, 2 Tbsp	2
Healthy Choice	
Frozen yogurt, Greek, vanilla bean, 1 container (67 g)	4
H-E-B	
Plain Greek yogurt, 1 cup	3
Vanilla bean Greek yogurt, 1 container (150 g)	3
Vanilla Greek yogurt, 1 cup	7
Hy-Vee	
Plain Greek strained nonfat yogurt, 1 cup	3
Kirkland Signature	
Plain nonfat Greek yogurt, 1 cup	3
Kroger	
Apple and oats Greek nonfat yogurt, 1 container (150 g)	2
Lemon zucchini nonfat Greek yogurt, 1 container (150 g)	4
Pineapple spinach kiwi Greek yogurt, 1 container (150 g)	4
Toasted coconut lowfat yogurt, 1 container (150 g)	4
Yogurt, nonfat, lite, strawberry, 1 container (170 g)	3
Kroger CARBmaster	
Banana cream pie cultured dairy blend yogurt, 1 container (170 g)	2
Black forest cake flavored cultured dairy blend yogurt, 1 container (170 g)	2
Blackberry cultured dairy blend yogurt, 1 container (170 g)	2
Blueberry muffin flavored cultured dairy blend yogurt, 1 container (170 g)	2
Cherry cultured dairy blend yogurt, 1 container (170 g)	2
Cinnamon roll cultured dairy blend yogurt, 1 container (170 g)	2

	SmartPoints® value
Key lime cultured dairy blend yogurt, 1 container (170 g)	2
Peach cultured dairy blend yogurt, 1 container (170 g)	2
Strawberry banana cultured dairy blend yogurt, 1 container (170 g)	2
Strawberry yogurt, 1 container (170 g)	2
Vanilla cultured dairy blend yogurt, 1 container (170 g)	2
White chocolate flavored raspberry cultured dairy blend yogurt, 1 container (170 g)	2
Kroger Greek	
Blended vanilla nonfat yogurt, 1 container (150 g)	2
Lite blueberry nonfat yogurt, 1 container (150 g)	2
Lite peach nonfat yogurt, 1 container (150 g)	2
Lite raspberry nonfat yogurt, 1 container (150 g)	2
Lite strawberry nonfat yogurt, 1 container (150 g)	2
Lite vanilla nonfat yogurt, 1 container (150 g)	2
Original plain nonfat yogurt, 1 container (150 g)	2
Light & Fit Greek	
Banana cream flavored nonfat yogurt, 1 Container (150 g)	2
Blackberry flavored nonfat yogurt, 1 container (150 g)	2
Boston cream pie nonfat yogurt, 1 container (150 g)	2
Cherry chocolate flavored nonfat yogurt, 1 container (150 g)	2
Cherry flavored nonfat yogurt, 1 container (150 g)	2
Key lime flavored nonfat yogurt, 1 container (150 g)	2
Peach flavored nonfat yogurt, 1 container (150 g)	2

	SmartPoints® value
Strawberry banana flavored nonfat yogurt, 1 container (150 g)	2
Strawberry cheesecake nonfat yogurt, 1 container (150 g)	2
Strawberry flavored nonfat yogurt, 1 container (150 g)	2
Toasted coconut flavored nonfat yogurt, 1 container (150 g)	2
Vanilla flavored nonfat yogurt, 1 container (150 g)	2
Market Pantry	
Honey almond blended light nonfat yogurt, 1 container (170 g)	3
Meijer	
Greek strained nonfat yogurt, 1 container (150 g)	2
Plain Greek yogurt, 1 cup	3
Mountain High	
Yoghurt, all natural, fat free, plain, 1 cup	4
Nancy's	
Yogurt, nonfat, plain, 1 cup	5
Noosa	
Blueberry aussie style yogurt, 1 container (113 g)	6
Blueberry yoghurt, 4 oz	6
Tart cherry aussie style yogurt, 1 container (113 g)	6
Yoghurt, finest, honey, 4 oz	6
Yoghurt, lemon, 4 oz	8
Yoghurt, raspberry, 4 oz	5
Yoghurt, strawberry rhubarb, 8 oz	13
Oikos	
Black cherry fruit on the bottom Greek nonfat yogurt, 1 container (150 g)	5
Plain nonfat Greek yogurt, 1 cup	3
Vanilla flavored Greek nonfat yogurt, 1 container (150 g)	5
Oikos Greek	
Strawberry fruit on the bottom nonfat yogurt, 1 container (150 g)	5

	SmartPoints® value
Oikos Traditional	
Banana cream flavor Greek yogurt, 1 container (150 g)	7
Lemon meringue flavored Greek yogurt, 1 container (150 g)	7
Orange cream flavored Greek yogurt, 1 container (150 g)	7
Oikos Triple Zero	
Yogurt, Greek, nonfat, blended, coconut creme flavor, 1 container (150 g)	3
Yogurt, Greek, nonfat, blended, mixed berry flavor, 1 container (150 g)	3
Yogurt, Greek, nonfat, blended, strawberry flavor, 1 container (150 g)	3
Yogurt, Greek, nonfat, blended, vanilla, 1 container (150 g)	3
Open Nature Greek	
Nonfat plain yogurt, 8 oz	2
Yogurt, Greek, nonfat, strained, plain, 1 container (170 g)	2
Prairie Farms	
Vanilla Greek strained nonfat yogurt, 1 container (150 g)	4
ShopRite	
Plain Greek nonfat yogurt, 1 cup	3
Siggi's	
Acai and mixed berries Icelandic style skyr strained non-fat yogurt, 1 container (150 g)	3
Blueberry Icelandic style skyr strained non-fat yogurt, 1 container (150 g)	3
Coconut Icelandic style skyr strained low-fat yogurt, 1 container (150 g)	6
Orange and ginger Icelandic style skyr strained non-fat yogurt, 1 container (150 g)	3
Peach Icelandic style skyr strained non-fat yogurt, 1 container (150 g)	3

Yogurt, Siggi's (cont'd)

	SmartPoints® value
Plain Icelandic style skyr strained non-fat yogurt, 1 container (150 g)	1
Plain Icelandic style skyr strained non-fat yogurt, 1 cup	2
Pomegranate and passion fruit Icelandic style skyr strained non-fat yogurt, 1 container (150 g)	3
Pumpkin and spice Icelandic style cream skyr low-fat strained yogurt, 1 container (150 g)	4
Raspberry nonfat strained yogurt, 1 container (150 g)	3
Strawberry & rhubarb Icelandic style 4% milkfat strained yogurt, 1 container (125 g)	4
Strawberry flavored Icelandic style skyr strained nonfat yogurt, 1 container (150 g)	3
Vanilla flavor Icelandic style strained nonfat yogurt, 1 container (150 g)	3
Vanilla flavor strained whole milk yogurt, 1 container (125 g)	4
Vanilla Icelandic style skyr strained non-fat yogurt, 1 container (150 g)	3
Simple Truth Organic	
Nonfat plain Greek yogurt, 1 container (150 g)	3
Plain Greek nonfat yogurt, 1 cup	2
Simply Nature Organic	
Vanilla whole milk yogurt, 1 cup	11
Smari	
Vanilla flavor nonfat organic Icelandic yogurt, 1 container (142 g)	3
Stonyfield Farm	
Plain organic nonfat Greek yogurt, 1 container (150 g)	2
Vanilla organic nonfat Greek yogurt, 1 container (150 g)	5

	SmartPoints® value
Stonyfield Farm Organic	
Smooth and creamy plain nonfat yogurt, 1 cup	4
Yogurt, nonfat, Greek, plain, 1 cup	3
Stonyfield Organic	
Yogurt, low-fat, French vanilla, 1 container (170 g)	6
Stonyfield Smooth & Creamy	
French vanilla fat free organic yogurt, 1 cup	7
Taste of Inspirations	
Nonfat Greek yogurt, 1 container (150 g)	5
Peach nonfat Greek yogurt, 1 container (150 g)	5
Plain Greek nonfat yogurt, 1 cup	3
The Greek Gods	
Traditional plain Greek yogurt, 1 cup	10
Yogurt, Greek style, traditional plain, 4 oz	6
Tillamook	
Spiced chai Greek yogurt, 1 serving (150 g)	4
Tillamook Farmstyle Greek	
Old fashioned vanilla flavored strained yogurt, 1 container (150 g)	5
Oregon marionberry strained yogurt, 1 container (150 g)	4
Plain and simple strained nonfat yogurt, 8 oz	2
Trader Joe's	
Chocolate mousse whole milk Greek yogurt, 1 container (227 g)	14
French village vanilla nonfat yogurt, 1 cup	9
Greek strawberry vanilla yogurt, 1 container (227 g)	15
Greek style nonfat vanilla bean yogurt, 1 container (150 g)	5

	SmartPoints® value
Organic Greek style nonfat yogurt 0% milkfat plain, 1 cup	3
Pomegranate flavored Greek style nonfat yogurt, 1 container (150 g)	3
Trader Joe's Refrigerated	
Greek style nonfat plain yogurt, 1 oz	0
Organic Greek style nonfat yogurt - plain, 1 container (150 g)	2
Upstate Farms	
Vanilla Greek nonfat yogurt, 8 oz	6
Wallaby	
Organic vanilla bean yogurt, 1 container (170 g)	7
Plain low-fat organic Greek yogurt, 1 cup	4
Plain organic Greek yogurt, 1 cup	7
Wallaby Organic	
Greek plain nonfat yogurt, 1 container (170 g)	2
Wawa Grocery	
Apple and yogurt parfait, 1 package (206 g)	13
Wegman's Food You Feel Good About	
Yogurt, Greek, plain, 1 container (170 g)	2
Yogurt, Greek, plain, 1 cup	3
Wellsley Farms	
Plain organic Greek yogurt, 1 container (150 g)	1
Whole Foods Market Organic	
Plain nonfat yogurt, 1 cup	2
Yasso	
Chocolate chip cookie dough frozen Greek yogurt bar, 1 bar (62 g)	5
Vanilla bean frozen Greek yogurt, 1 bar (70 g)	3
Yoplait	
Apple pie blended Greek 100 calorie fat free yogurt, 1 container (150 g)	3
Blueberry patch light fat free yogurt, 1 container (170 g)	3
Lemon meringue Greek yogurt, 1 container (150 g)	6
Light chai latte yogurt, 1 container (170 g)	3
Light vanilla yogurt, 1 container (170 g)	3
Strawberries 'n bananas light fat free yogurt, 1 container (170 g)	3
Strawberry low-fat yogurt, 1 container (170 g)	6
Yoplait 100 Calorie	
Vanilla flavor Greek nonfat yogurt, 1 container (150 g)	3
Yoplait Go-Gurt	
Berry blue blast flavored portable low-fat yogurt, 1 tube (64 g)	3
Yoplait Go-Gurt Simply	
Strawberry flavored portable low-fat yogurt, 1 tube (64 g)	3
Yoplait Greek	
Vanilla fat free yogurt, 1 container (150 g)	5
Yoplait Greek 100	
Banana caramel fat free yogurt, 1 container (150 g)	3
Blended blueberry fat free yogurt, 1 container (150 g)	3
Caramel apple flavored nonfat yogurt, 1 container (150 g)	3
Coconut flavor fat free yogurt, 1 container (150 g)	3
Fat free yogurt, blended strawberry banana, 1 container (150 g)	3
Mixed berry fat free yogurt fruit on the bottom, 1 container (150 g)	3

Yogurt, Yoplait Greek 100 (cont'd)

	SmartPoints® value
Orange creme fat free yogurt, 1 container (150 g)	3
Plain nonfat yogurt, 1 cup	3
Tropical fruit fat free yogurt, 1 container (150 g)	3
Yogurt, fat free, apple pie, 1 container (150 g)	3
Yoplait Greek 100 Calorie Whips!	
Blackberry fat free yogurt mousse, 1 container (113 g)	4
Blueberry fat free yogurt mousse, 1 container (113 g)	4
Key lime pie fat free yogurt, 1 container (113 g)	4
Lemon meringue fat free yogurt, 1 container (113 g)	4
Raspberry fat free yogurt mousse, 1 container (113 g)	4
Strawberry cheesecake fat free yogurt mousse, 1 container (113 g)	4
Strawberry fat free yogurt, 1 container (113 g)	4
Vanilla cupcake fat free yogurt mousse, 1 container (113 g)	4
Yoplait Greek 100 Calories	
Black cherry fat free yogurt, 1 container (150 g)	3
Blackberry pie fat free yogurt, 1 container (150 g)	3
Blended blueberry fat free yogurt, 1 container (150 g)	3
Blended strawberry cheesecake fat free yogurt, 1 container (150 g)	3
Boston cream pie fat free yogurt, 1 container (150 g)	3
Key lime fat free yogurt, 1 container (150 g)	3
Lemon fat free yogurt, 1 container (150 g)	3
Mango fat free yogurt, 1 container (150 g)	3

	SmartPoints® value
Mixed berry fat free yogurt, 1 container (150 g)	3
Peach fat free yogurt, 1 container (150 g)	3
Pineapple fat free yogurt, 1 container (150 g)	3
Raspberry fat free yogurt, 1 container (150 g)	3
Strawberry banana blended fat free yogurt, 1 container (150 g)	3
Strawberry fat free yogurt, 1 container (150 g)	3
Vanilla fat free yogurt, 1 container (150 g)	3
Vanilla fat free yogurt, 1 cup	4
Yoplait Greek 100 Calories Whips!	
Chocolate cherry fat free yogurt, 1 container (113 g)	4
Coconut macaroon fat free yogurt, 1 container (113 g)	4
Yoplait Light	
Banana cream pie flavored fat free yogurt, 1 container (170 g)	3
Blackberry flavored fat free yogurt, 1 container (170 g)	3
Blueberry patch fat free yogurt (variety pack), 1 container (170 g)	3
Boston cream pie flavored fat free yogurt, 1 container (170 g)	3
Harvest peach (variety pack), 1 container (170 g)	3
Harvest peach flavored fat free yogurt, 1 container (170 g)	3
Key lime pie flavored fat free yogurt, 1 container (170 g)	3
Lemon cream pie flavored fat free yogurt, 1 container (170 g)	3
Orange creme flavored fat free yogurt, 1 container (170 g)	3
Raspberry cheesecake flavored fat free yogurt, 1 container (170 g)	3

	SmartPoints® value
Red raspberry flavored fat free yogurt, 1 container (170 g)	3
Strawberries'n bananas flavored fat free yogurt, 1 container (170 g)	3
Strawberry flavored yogurt with nature valley granola, 1 container (170 g)	8
Strawberry or blueberry patch flavored fat free yogurt, 1 container (170 g)	3
Strawberry shortcake fat free yogurt, 1 container (170 g)	3
Very cherry flavored fat free yogurt, 1 container (170 g)	3
Very vanilla flavored fat free yogurt, 1 container (170 g)	3
Yoplait Original	
French vanilla low-fat yogurt, 1 container (170 g)	8
Harvest peach flavor low-fat yogurt, 1 container (150 g)	10
Harvest peach low-fat yogurt, 1 container (170 g)	8
Strawberry banana low-fat yogurt, 1 container (170 g)	8
Strawberry flavored low-fat yogurt, 1 container (170 g)	8
Yoplait Plenti	
Apple cinnamon oatmeal and Greek yogurt, 1 container (155 g)	6
Blueberry oatmeal Greek yogurt, 1 container (155 g)	6
Blueberry with whole grain oats flax and pumpkin seeds Greek yogurt, 1 container (155 g)	5
Maple brown sugar oatmeal and Greek yogurt, 1 container (155 g)	6
Oatmeal meets Greek yogurt vanilla flavor, 1 container (155 g)	6
Peach oatmeal Greek yogurt, 1 container (155 g)	6

	SmartPoints® value
Strawberry oatmeal Greek yogurt, 1 container (155 g)	6
Strawberry with whole grain oats flax and pumpkin seeds Greek yogurt, 1 container (155 g)	5
Vanilla with whole grain oats flax and pumpkin seeds Greek yogurt, 1 container (155 g)	5
Yoplait Whips!	
Chocolate yogurt mousse, 1 container (113 g)	8
Greek 100 cafe latte yogurt, 1 container (113 g)	4
Greek 100 cinnamon swirl Greek yogurt, 1 container (150 g)	3
Greek 100 peaches n cream yogurt, 1 container (113 g)	4
Greek 100 salted caramel yogurt, 1 container (113 g)	4
Yoplait® 100 Calorie	
Blended blueberry fat free Greek yogurt, 1 container (150 g)	3
Zoi	
Yogurt, Greek, nonfat, plain, 8 oz	4

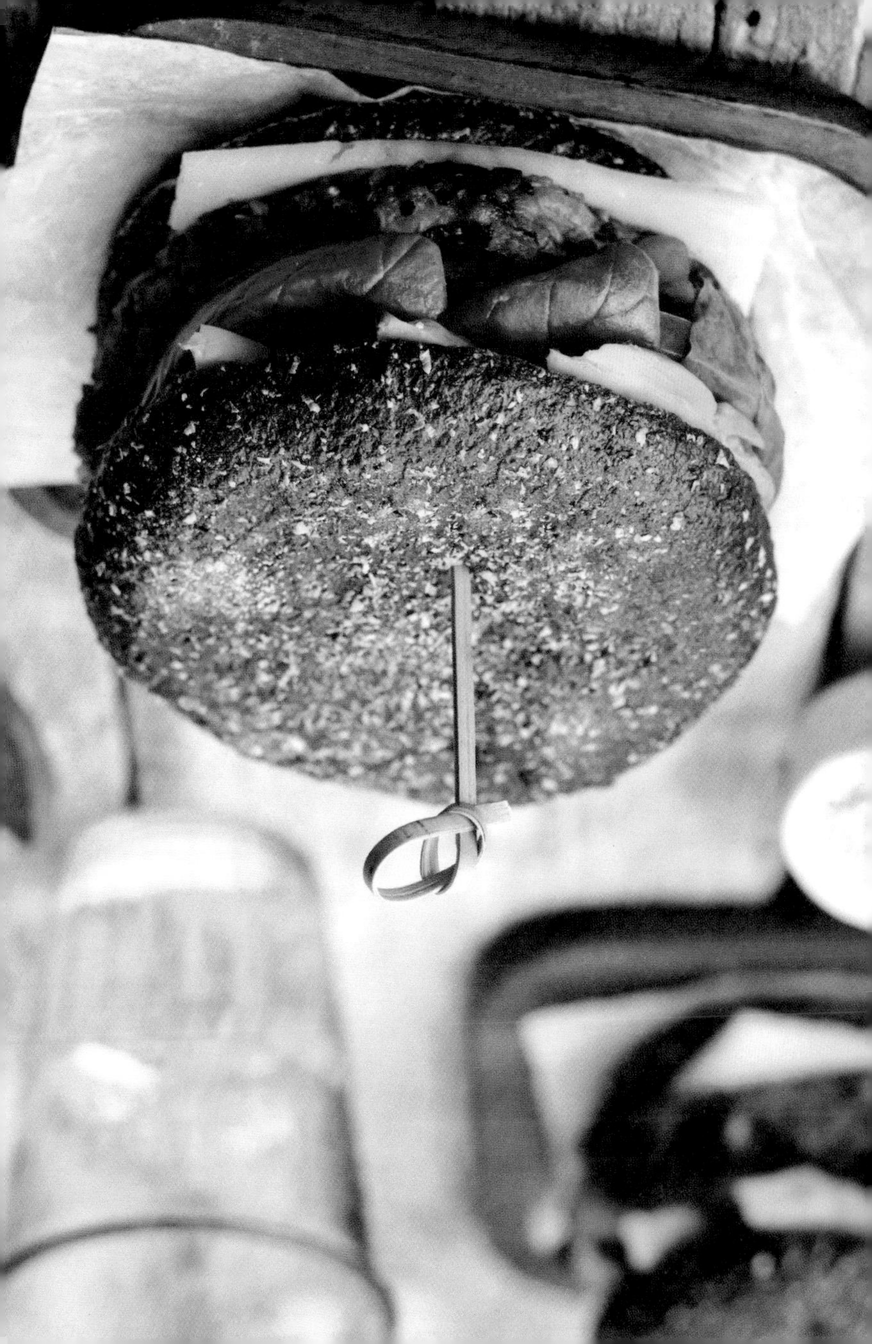

dairy substitutes & meat substitutes

	SmartPoints® value
Bacon Substitutes	
Lightlife Smart Bacon	
Veggie protein strips, bacon style, 1 slice (10 g)	0
Cheese Substitutes	
Daiya	
Shreds, cheddar style, ¼ cup	3
Shreds, mozzarella style, ¼ cup	3
Galaxy	
Veggie slices, American flavor, 1 slice (17 g)	1
Veggie slices, cheddar flavor, 1 slice (17 g)	1
Veggie slices, pepper Jack flavor, 1 slice (17 g)	1
Smart Beat	
Healthy fat free non-dairy slices, American flavor, 1 slice (19 g)	0
Tofutti Better Than Cream Cheese	
Imitation cream cheese, plain, 2 Tbsp	2
Trader Joe's	
Almond mozzarella style shreds cheese alternative, ¼ cup	1
Plain classic vegan cream cheese alternative, 2 Tbsp	4
Chicken Substitutes	
Beyond Meat	
Beyond chicken grilled strips, 6 strips (85 g)	2
Morningstar Farms	
Buffalo chik patties, 1 patty (71 g)	5
Veggie chik'n nuggets, 4 nuggets (86 g)	5

	SmartPoints® value
Luncheon Meat Substitutes	
Tofurky	
Bologna style deli slices, 3 slices (52 g)	2
Deli slices, hickory smoked, 5 slices (52 g)	2
Deli slices, oven roasted, 5 slices (52 g)	2
Sausage Substitutes	
Lightlife Gimme Lean	
Veggie protein, ground sausage style, 2 oz	1
Lightlife Smart Dogs	
Veggie protein links, 1 link (42 g)	1
Veggie protein links, jumbo, 1 link (76 g)	1
Lightlife Smart Sausages	
Veggie protein sausages, Italian style, 1 link (85 g)	3
Morningstar Farms	
Breakfast maple flavored sausage patties, 1 patty (38 g)	2
Hot and spicy sausage patties, 1 patty (38 g)	1
Original sausage patties, 1 patty (38 g)	1
Original veggie sausage patty, 1 patty (38 g)	2
Sausage patties, 1 patty (38 g)	1
Sausage patties, veggie, breakfast, original, value pack, 1 patty (38 g)	2
Veggie sausage pattie, maple flavored, 1 patty (38 g)	2
Veggie sausage patties, hot & spicy, 1 patty (38 g)	1
Veggie sausage patties, original, 1 patty (38 g)	2
Morningstar Farms Breakfast	
Sausage links, veggie, 2 links (45 g)	2

	SmartPoints® value
Tofu	
House Foods	
Tofu, shirataki, spaghetti, 4 oz	1
Trader Joe's Organic	
Sprouted tofu extra firm, 3 oz	2
Veggie Burgers	
Boca	
All American classic veggie burger, 1 burger (71 g)	1
Spicy chik'n veggie patty, 1 patty (71 g)	4
Vegan veggie burger, 1 burger (71 g)	1
Veggie ground crumbles, ½ cup	1
Bubba Burger	
Veggie burger, 1 burger (85 g)	3
Don Lee Farms	
Veggie patty, 1 patty (85 g)	5
Dr. Praeger's Sensible Foods	
Kale veggie burgers, 1 burger (71 g)	4

	SmartPoints® value
Gardenburger	
Original veggie burgers, 1 patty (29 g)	4
Morningstar Farms	
Mediterranean chickpea veggie burger, 1 burger (67 g)	3
Veggie burgers, grillers original, 1 burger (64 g)	3
Veggie burgers, roasted garlic & quinoa, 1 burger (67 g)	4
Season's Choice	
Veggie burger, 1 patty (71 g)	3
Trader Joe's	
Pizza veggie burgers with tomato basil and mozzarella cheese, 1 patty (67 g)	4
Yogurt Substitutes	
So Delicious Dairy Free	
Coconut milk yogurt, 1 container (150 g)	7

desserts, cakes, candy & cookies

	SmartPoints® value
Brownies	
Duncan Hines Oven Ready!	
Homestyle brownies, chocolate fudge, 1 serving (40 g)	7
Fiber One	
Chocolate chip cookie brownies, 1 brownie (25 g)	4
Mint fudge brownies, 1 brownie (25 g)	4
Kellogg's Special K Brownies	
Divine fudge, 1 brownie (20 g)	3
Heavenly caramel, 1 brownie (20 g)	3
Kroger	
High fiber lemon brownie, 1 brownie (25 g)	3
Medifast	
Soft bake brownie, 1 packet (31.4 g)	4
Nature's Bakery	
Double chocolate brownie, 1 oz	4
Sheila G's	
Salted caramel brownie brittle, 1 oz	7
Special K	
Fudge brownie bites, 1 package (21 g)	4
Special K Brownie Bites	
Blondie made with real chocolate, 1 package (21 g)	4
Cakes	
Aldi	
Triple chocolate creme cake, 1 slice (57 g)	9
Drake's	
Devil dogs, 1 cake (47 g)	8
Hill & Valley	
Angel food cake, sugar free, 1 slice (43 g)	2
Hostess	
Cup cakes, 1 cake (45 g)	8

	SmartPoints® value
Frosted yellow cake with creamy filling, 1 cake (45 g)	8
Twinkies, 1 cake (42 g)	7
Hostess Snack Classics	
Cupcakes, chocolate, 2 cakes (90 g)	16
Hostess Zingers	
Raspberry flavor iced cake, 2 cakes (76 g)	14
Little Debbie	
Swiss rolls, 2 cakes (61 g)	13
McVities	
Jaffa cake, 1 cake (12 g)	2
Meijer Fresh	
Pound cake, sliced lemon, 1 slice (45 g)	6
Mila's European Bakery	
Birthday cake, 5", yellow, white buttercream, 2 oz	8
Pepperidge Farm	
3-layer cake, coconut, ⅛ cake (69 g)	11
Publix	
Shortcake dessert shells, 1 shell (31 g)	4
Safeway	
Cake, red velvet, 1 layer, 1 slice (71 g)	11
Cupcakes, red velvet, cream cheese iced, 1 cupcake (48 g)	8
Safeway Select	
Flourless cake, dark chocolate truffle, 1 serving (59 g)	12
Sara Lee	
Pound cake slice, 1 slice (45 g)	7
The Bakery at Walmart	
Sponge sugar free cakes, 2 cakes (47 g)	4
The Cheesecake Factory	
Original cheesecake, 1 piece (151 g)	24
The Father's Table	
Pumpkin cake roll with cream cheese filling, 1 slice (73 g)	13

	SmartPoints® value
Trader Jacques'	
Macarons des fetes (a festive rainbow of French macarons), 3 pieces (30 g)	5
Trader Joe's	
Blueberry fiber mini cakes, 1 cake (57 g)	2
Vitalicious Mini VitaCakes	
Fudgy chocolate, 1 cake (32 g)	3
YoGo	
Blueberry Greek yogurt cake, 1 cake (43 g)	4

Candy, Chocolate

	SmartPoints® value
3 Musketeers	
Candy bar, 1 bar (54 g)	13
Candy bar, fun size, 3 bars (45 g)	10
Minis whipped fluffy chocolate candy, 7 pieces (41 g)	10
3 Musketeers Minis	
Milk chocolate candy, 7 pieces (40 g)	9
Almond Joy	
Candy bars, 1 bar (17 g)	4
Miniatures, fall, 3 pieces (40.89 g)	10
Andes	
Creme de menthe thins, 6 pieces (42 g)	13
Creme de menthe thins, 8 pieces (38 g)	12
Archer Farms	
Dark chocolate almonds, ¼ cup	9
Atkins Endulge	
Chocolate candies treat, 1 package (28 g)	4
Chocolate peanut candies treat, 1 package (34 g)	5
Milk chocolate caramel squares, 3 pieces (35 g)	6
Baby Ruth	
Fun size peanut caramel nougat bars, 2 bars (37 g)	9
Bark Thins	
Dark chocolate almond with sea salt snacking chocolate, 1½ oz	9
Blue Diamond Almonds	
Oven roasted dark chocolate almonds, 24 almonds (28 g)	5
Brookside	
Cherry and Tahitian vanilla dark chocolate, 16 pieces (40 g)	9
Dark chocolate acai & blueberry flavors, 1 package (19 g)	5
Dark chocolate acai and blueberry, 16 pieces (40 g)	9
Dark chocolate crunchy clusters, 22 pieces (40 g)	10
Dark chocolate pomegranate, 16 pieces (40 g)	9
Butterfinger	
Bars, minis, 1 bar (9.8 g)	2
Candy bar, 1 bar (60 g)	13
Fun size crunchy peanut bars, 2 bars (37 g)	8
Cadbury	
Caramel egg, 1 egg	8
Chocolate creme egg, 1 piece (34 g)	9
Creme egg, 1 egg	8
Creme egg, mini, 4 pieces (36 g)	9
Royal dark chocolate mini eggs, 12 pieces (40 g)	10
Cadbury Dairy Milk	
Fine milk chocolate, 7 blocks (39.6 g)	10
Cadbury Mini Eggs	
Milk chocolate mini eggs, 12 pieces (40.43 g)	10
Mini eggs, 12 pieces (39.23 g)	10
Cadbury Royal Dark	
Dark chocolate, indulgent, semi-sweet, 10 blocks (42 g)	11
Cella's	
Milk chocolate, 3 pieces (43 g)	9

Candy, Chocolate (cont'd)

	SmartPoints® value
Charleston Chew	
Chewy flavored nougat with chocolate coating, ⅓ bar (38 g)	8
Choceur	
Cocoa dusted truffles, 4 pieces (40 g)	13
Dark chocolate covered almonds, ⅓ cup	9
Creative Snacks Co.	
Dark chocolate peppermint pretzels, 9 pretzels (40 g)	8
Daily Chef	
Milk chocolate covered almonds, 9 pieces (40 g)	10
DeMet's Turtles	
Original chocolates with pecans and caramel, 2 pieces (33 g)	8
Dole Dippers	
Strawberry halves coated in dark chocolate, 4 pieces (35 g)	3
Dove	
Chocolate promises, dark, peppermint bark, 5 pieces (40.17 g)	11
Dark chocolate promises, silky smooth, 5 pieces (38.47 g)	11
Dark chocolate snowflakes, 5 pieces (38 g)	10
Dark chocolate, hearts, 6 hearts (44.6 g)	11
Milk chocolate promises, 5 pieces (38.99 g)	11
Milk chocolate snowflakes, 5 pieces (38 g)	11
Milk chocolate, hearts, 6 hearts (44.6 g)	12
Peanut butter and dark chocolate, 5 pieces (39 g)	10
Dove Promises	
Dark chocolate, 5 pieces (40 g)	11
Dark chocolate, silky smooth, 6 hearts (42 g)	11

	SmartPoints® value
Milk chocolate and red velvet swirl heart shaped chocolates, 6 pieces (42 g)	12
Milk chocolate, hearts, 6 hearts (42 g)	12
Mint & dark chocolate swirl, 5 pieces (40 g)	11
Silky smooth almond & dark chocolate, 5 pieces (39 g)	10
Silky smooth sea salt caramel & dark chocolate, 5 pieces (40 g)	10
Durham's	
Chocolate pecans, ¼ cup	8
Emerald Cocoa Roast	
Dark chocolate almonds 100 calorie pack, 1 pack (18 g)	3
Fannie May	
Mint meltaways, 5 pieces (40.89 g)	11
Ferrero Rocher	
Fine hazelnut chocolates, 3 pieces (38 g)	10
Fralinger's	
Chocolate walnut boardwalk fudge, 1 serving (38 g)	7
Ghirardelli Chocolate	
Chocolate squares with strawberry filling, 1 square (15 g)	4
Chocolate, intense dark, sea salt soiree, 3 sections (38 g)	9
Dark 60% cacao chocolate squares, 4 squares (43 g)	11
Dark and sea salt caramel chocolate, 3 sections (38 g)	9
Dark chocolate square, with white mint filling, 3 squares (45 g)	11
Dark melting wafers, 18 wafers (41 g)	13
Milk and caramel chocolate square, 1 square (15 g)	4
Milk and dark chocolate, 1 square (13 g)	4
Milk and white chocolate, 1 square (13 g)	4

	SmartPoints® value
Milk chocolate brownie squares, 3 pieces (37 g)	11
Peppermint bark chocolate, 3 pieces (38 g)	11
Peppermint bark chocolate minis, 6 pieces (43 g)	12
Peppermint bark minis, 6 pieces (43 g)	12
Peppermint bark squares, 3 squares (35 g)	10
Ghirardelli Chocolate Intense Dark	
Chocolate, sea salt soiree, 4 pieces (43 g)	10
Ghirardelli Chocolate Squares	
Chocolate, dark & mint, 3 squares (51.6 g)	11
Dark & sea salt caramel, 3 squares (45 g)	11
Dark chocolate with raspberry filling, 1 piece (15 g)	4
Dark chocolate, 60% cacao, 4 squares (43 g)	11
Milk chocolate, with caramel filling, 3 squares (44 g)	11
Peppermint bark, 1 square (12 g)	3
Peppermint bark flavoured chocolate, 2 pieces (24 g)	7
Ghirardelli Chocolate Twilight Delight	
Dark chocolate, 4 pieces (43 g)	11
Intense dark 72% cacao chocolate, 1 square (11 g)	3
Ghirardelli Intense Dark	
Chocolate, midnight reverie, 86% cacao, 4 sections (45 g)	12
Chocolate, twilight delight, 72% cacao, 3 sections (40 g)	10
Sea salt soiree chocolate candy, 4 pieces (43 g)	10
Ghirardelli Minis	
Dark chocolate candy, 5 pieces (38 g)	10
Milk chocolate caramel filling, 5 pieces (39 g)	10

	SmartPoints® value
Godiva	
Dark chocolate, 4 blocks (40 g)	11
Layered assorted dessert truffles, 4 pieces (41 g)	10
Truffles, dark chocolate, 4 pieces (41 g)	10
Truffles, milk chocolate, 4 pieces (42 g)	11
Green & Black's Organic	
Dark chocolate, 85% cocoa, 12 pieces (40 g)	12
Gudrun	
Belgian chocolate box bag assorted chocolates, 3 pieces (42 g)	12
Hawaiian Host Aloha Gems	
Creamy milk chocolate covered macadamias, 2 pieces (32 g)	9
Heath	
Candy bar, snack size, 3 pieces (43 g)	12
English toffee bar, milk chocolate, 1 bar (39 g)	11
Hershey's	
Candy bar, cookies 'n' creme, 1 bar (43 g)	11
Dark chocolate nuggets with toffee and almonds, 4 nuggets (38 g)	10
Hugs, kisses hugged by white chocolate, 9 pieces (37.78 g)	11
Kisses milk chocolates, 9 pieces (41 g)	10
Kisses milk chocolates filled with caramel, 9 pieces (42 g)	10
Milk chocolate, 1 bar (43 g)	11
Milk chocolate bars, snack size, 3 pieces (38 g)	10
Milk chocolate eggs, candy coated, 8 pieces (40.43 g)	10
Milk chocolate kisses, 9 pieces (41 g)	10
Milk chocolate, extra creamy, hearts, 5 pieces (40.43 g)	11

	SmartPoints® value
Milk chocolate, large bars, 7 blocks (42 g)	12
Milk chocolate, with almonds, 1 bar (41 g)	10
Miniatures, 5 pieces (43 g)	11
Miniatures assortment, 5 pieces (43 g)	11
Nuggets chocolates with toffee and almonds, 4 pieces (38 g)	10
Nuggets, dark chocolate with almonds, 4 pieces (41.2 g)	10
Nuggets, milk chocolate, 4 pieces (41.2 g)	11
Nuggets, milk chocolate with almonds, 4 pieces (41.2 g)	10
Reese's peanut butter cup, 1 piece (15 g)	4
Hershey's Bliss	
Dark chocolate, rich & creamy, 6 pieces (41.5 g)	11
Hershey's Eggs	
Milk chocolate, 7 pieces (40 g)	10
Hershey's Kisses	
Candy cane, 9 pieces (42 g)	11
Dark chocolate truffle, 9 pieces (42 g)	11
Dark chocolate, filled with mint truffle, 9 pieces (40.43 g)	11
Deluxe whole roasted hazelnut center, 5 pieces (41 g)	10
Mildly sweet chocolate, special dark, 9 pieces (40 g)	10
Milk chocolate, 9 pieces (41 g)	10
Milk chocolate, with almonds, 9 pieces (40 g)	10
Milk chocolates filled with cherry cordial crème, 9 pieces (42 g)	10
Special dark mildly sweet chocolate, 9 pieces (41 g)	10
Hershey's Kisses Deluxe	
Chocolate kisses with hazelnut center, 1 package (25 g)	6

	SmartPoints® value
Hershey's Miniatures	
Chocolate variety pack, 5 pieces (43 g)	11
Hershey's Special Dark	
Candy bar, 1 bar (41 g)	10
Chocolate bar, mildly sweet, 5 blocks (38 g)	9
Miniatures, 5 pieces (40 g)	11
Hershey's Sugar Free Bars	
Dark chocolate, 5 pieces (40 g)	7
Junior Mints	
Creamy mints, 16 pieces (37.67 g)	10
Justin's	
Milk chocolate peanut butter cups, 3 pieces (40 g)	10
Peanut butter cups, organic, dark chocolate, 1 package (40 g)	10
Kirkland Signature	
Chocolate covered raisins, 20 pieces (40 g)	10
Dark chocolate covered almonds, ¼ cup	9
Milk and dark chocolates, 3 pieces (40 g)	11
Milk chocolate almonds, 11 pieces (30 g)	7
Kit Kat	
Bar, 1 four-piece bar (42 g)	12
Candy bars, minis, 5 pieces (40.43 g)	11
Crisp wafers, in milk chocolate, snack size, 3 wafers (42 g)	11
Mint mini crisp wafers in dark chocolate, 5 pieces (43 g)	11
Kit Kat Minis	
Crisp wafers in milk chocolate, 9 pieces (42 g)	11
Kit Kat Snack Size	
Triple chocolate crisp wafers, 3 pieces (42 g)	10

	SmartPoints® value
Lake Champlain Chocolates	
Crunchy praline & roasted hazelnuts milk chocolate, 1 bar (51 g)	13
Lindt Excellence	
70% cocoa smooth dark chocolate, 4 squares (40 g)	12
85% cocoa extra dark chocolate, 4 squares (40 g)	9
90% cocoa supreme dark chocolate, 4 squares (40 g)	11
Chili dark chocolate, 4 squares (40 g)	10
Intense orange dark chocolate, 4 squares (40 g)	9
Pomegranate dark chocolate, 4 pieces (40 g)	10
Touch of sea salt dark chocolate, 4 squares (40 g)	10
Lindt Lindor	
Assorted chocolate truffles, 3 pieces (36 g)	11
Chocolate truffles, 3 pieces (36 g)	12
Dark chocolate truffles, 3 truffles (36 g)	12
Extra dark peppermint chocolate truffles, 3 truffles (36 g)	12
Milk and white chocolate truffles, 3 truffles (36 g)	12
Milk and white milk chocolate truffle, 3 pieces (36 g)	12
Milk chocolate truffles, 2 truffles (24 g)	8
Milk chocolate truffles, 3 pieces (36 g)	11
White chocolate truffles, 3 truffles (36 g)	12
M&M's	
Café mocha chocolate candies, ¼ cup	11
Chocolate candies with peanut, ¼ cup	10
Chocolate candies with peanuts, ½ pack (40 g)	9

	SmartPoints® value
Chocolate candies, milk chocolate, 1 pack (48 g)	12
Crispy chocolate candies, ⅓ cup	10
Crispy chocolate candies, ⅓ cup	10
Dark chocolate candies, 1½ oz	11
Milk chocolate candies, ¼ cup	11
Milk chocolate candies, 6 packs (79.4 g)	20
Mint dark chocolate candies, ¼ cup	11
Peanut butter chocolate candies, ¼ cup	11
Peanut chocolate candies, 1 pack (49 g)	11
Peanut chocolate candies, ¼ cup	11
Peanut filled chocolate candy, ¼ cup	11
Pretzel chocolate candies, 17 pieces (39 g)	9
M&M's Fun Size	
Milk chocolate candies, 3 packs (45 g)	12
Peanut butter chocolate candies, 2 packs (36 g)	9
Peanut chocolate candies, 2 packs (36 g)	8
M&M's Minis	
Milk chocolate candies, 2 packs (33 g)	8
Mars	
Hot chocolate candies made with dark chocolate, ¼ cup	11
Mini mix, twix, milky way,	
3 musketeers, snickers, milky way midnight, 5 pieces (41 g)	10
Mighty Malts	
Malted milk balls, 16 pieces (39 g)	9
Milk Duds	
Candy, 13 pieces (39 g)	8
Milky Way	
Candy bar, 1 bar (52 g)	13
Candy bars, fun size, 2 bars (34 g)	9
Chocolate bar, 1 bar (22 g)	5

	SmartPoints® value
Milky Way Midnight Midnight	
Dark chocolate golden caramel vanilla nougat minis, 5 pieces (43 g)	10
Mounds	
Bars, dark chocolate, snack size, 1 bar (17 g)	4
Mr. Goodbar	
Candy, snack size, 3 pieces (38 g)	9
Nestlé Crunch	
Fun size chocolate bar, 3 bars (38 g)	9
Milk chocolate with crisped rice, 1 piece (34 g)	9
Nips	
Hard candy, rich & creamy, chocolate parfait, 2 pieces (14.16 g)	3
Orchard Valley Harvest	
Dark chocolate covered almonds, 1 package (28 g)	7
Palmer	
Peppermint bark bar, ⅓ piece (43 g)	14
Pearson's	
Original mint patties, 5 pieces (38 g)	8
Quality Confections	
Dark chocolate sea salt caramels, 2 pieces (38 g)	7
Reese's	
Milk chocolate peanut butter cups, 1 package (42 g)	10
Milk chocolate peanut butter eggs, 1 piece (17 g)	4
Milk chocolate, peanut butter filled hearts, 5 pieces (40.43 g)	10
Peanut butter candy, 51 pieces (40 g)	10
Peanut butter candy pieces, 51 pieces (40 g)	10
Peanut butter cups, 1 package (45 g)	10
Peanut butter cups, milk chocolate, 1 package (42 g)	10

	SmartPoints® value
Peanut butter cups, milk chocolate, miniatures, 5 pieces (44 g)	10
Peanut butter eggs, milk chocolate bite size foiled eggs, 5 pieces (38 g)	10
Peanut butter footballs, 1 piece (38 g)	10
Peanut butter hearts, 1 package (68 g)	15
Peanut butter trees, milk chocolate, 1 piece (17 g)	4
Snack size milk chocolate peanut butter cup, 1 piece (15 g)	4
White chocolate peanut butter egg, 1 package (34 g)	8
Reese's Hearts	
Peanut butter filled milk chocolate candy, 5 pieces (41 g)	10
Reese's Miniatures	
Peanut butter cups, 5 pieces (39 g)	10
Reese's Minis	
Milk chocolate peanut butter cups, 11 pieces (39 g)	10
Reese's Pieces	
Candy, peanut butter, 51 pieces (40 g)	10
Ritter Sport	
Fine extra dark chocolate, 1 bar (100 g)	28
Rolo	
Chewy caramels in milk chocolate, 7 pieces (42 g)	10
Russell Stover	
Dark chocolate and coconut cream santa candy, 1 piece (28 g)	7
Fine assorted chocolates, 2 pieces (33 g)	8
Peanut butter cups, sugar free, 2 pieces (34 g)	6
Pecan delights, 2 pieces (34 g)	8
Peppermint cream flavored santa covered in dark chocolate, 1 piece (28 g)	6

	SmartPoints® value
Sugar free dark chocolate assortment, 3 pieces (43 g)	7
Russell Stover Sugar Free	
Mint patties, chocolate, 3 pieces (43 g)	7
Pecan delights, 4 pieces (57 g)	10
Toffee squares, 2 pieces (28 g)	4
Schogetten	
Dark chocolate bar, 7 pieces (39 g)	10
See's	
Chocolates, assorted, 2 pieces (32.73 g)	8
Mint krispys, 5 pieces (41 g)	10
Nuts & chews, 3 pieces (44.43 g)	10
Simply Lite	
Sugar free dark chocolate, 1 square (25 g)	4
Sixlets	
Candy coated chocolate flavored candy, 1 tube (7 g)	2
Skinny Cow	
Candy bar, heavenly crisp, milk chocolate flavor, 1 bar (22 g)	5
Candy bar, peanut butter flavor, heavenly crisp, 1 bar (22 g)	5
Candy, dreamy clusters, milk chocolate, 1 pouch (28.3 g)	6
Chocolate truffle luscious filled bites, 1 pouch (28 g)	6
Dark chocolate blissful truffle candy bar, 1 bar (22 g)	6
Dreamy clusters candy, milk chocolate, 1 pouch (28 g)	6
Mochaccino candy bar, 1 bar (47 g)	7
Peanut butter and chocolate candy bar, 1 bar (22 gs)	5
Skinny Cow Dreamy Clusters	
Dark chocolate candy, 1 pouch (28 g)	6
Snickers	
Candy bar, fun size, 2 bars (34 g)	7

	SmartPoints® value
Candy bars, 1 bar (53 g)	12
Crisper milk chocolate bar, 1 bar (40 g)	9
Milk chocolate with creamy caramel and peanuts tree, 1 candy (31 g)	8
Minis, 4 pieces (36 g)	8
Snickers Bites	
Candy bar, unwrapped, 8 pieces (41 g)	9
Snickers Fun Size	
Almond bar, 2 bars (39 g)	9
Snickers Minis	
Caramel & peanut chocolates, 4 pieces (36 g)	8
Snickers Snack Time Pack	
Fun size chocolate bars, 2 bars (32 g)	7
Starbucks Coffee	
Salted almond chocolate bites, 1 tube (57 g)	13
Sweet's	
Chocolate cinnamon bears, 3 pieces (38 g)	8
Take 5	
Candy bar, 1 package (42 g)	9
Theo	
Organic sea salt 70% dark chocolate, ½ bar (42 g)	10
Toblerone Tobelle	
Milk chocolate, Swiss, with honey and almond nougat, 5 pieces (40 g)	11
Tootsie Roll	
Chocolate flavor candy, 1 piece (14 g)	2
Chocolate flavored candy, 6 pieces (40 g)	7
Tootsie Roll Midgees	
Chewy candies, 6 pieces (40 g)	7
Trader Joe's	
72% cacao dark chocolate baton, 1 bar (35 g)	9

	SmartPoints® value
Dark chocolate caramel wedges 70% cacao, 2 pieces (13 g)	3
Dark chocolate covered almonds, ¼ cup	10
Dark chocolate minty mallows, 2 pieces (40 g)	8
Dark chocolate nibs, 1 Tbsp	3
Dark chocolate salted caramels, 1 box (60 g)	16
Organic dark chocolate bar, 12 squares (40 g)	11
Uncured bacon ganache bar, ½ bar (43 g)	10
Trader Joe's Grocery	
Dark chocolate covered espresso beans, ¼ cup	8
Dark chocolate peanut butter cups, 3 pieces (36 g)	9
Sea salt & turbinado sugar dark chocolate almonds, 13 pieces (40 g)	9
Twix	
Caramel milk chocolate cookie bars, 2 cookies (51 g)	12
Cookie bars, fun size, 1 cookie (16 g)	4
Twix Minis	
Caramel and milk chocolate cookie bars, 3 pieces (30 g)	7
Virginia Diner	
Peanut butter buckeyes, gourmet, 2 pieces (35 g)	8
Wegman's	
Chocolate covered strawberries, dark chocolate, 6 pieces (40.43 g)	9
Chocolate covered strawberries, milk chocolate, 6 pieces (40.43 g)	9
Weight Watchers by Whitman's	
Bite size dark chocolates, 1 pouch	5
Bite size red velvet chocolates, 1 pouch	5
Caramel bite size covered in milk chocolate, 1 pouch	6

	SmartPoints® value
Caramel chocolates, 3 pieces	8
Caramel with crispies chocolates, 3 pieces	7
Chocolate mousse dark chocolates, 3 pieces	6
Coconut chocolates, 3 pieces	7
English toffee chocolate candies, 3 pieces	6
Mint patties dark chocolate candies, 3 pieces	6
Pecan crown bite size chocolates, 1 pouch	6
Pecan crowns chocolates, 3 pieces	7
Werther's Original Sugar Free	
Chocolate flavored chewy caramels, 6 pieces (37 g)	4
Whitman's Sampler	
Assorted chocolates, 3 pieces (35 g)	8
Whoppers	
Malted milk balls, original, 18 pieces (39.6 g)	10
Malted milk candy, robin eggs, 8 pieces (40.43 g)	10
York	
Chocolate covered peppermint patties, 3 patties (40.9 g)	8
Minis peppermint patties, 1 package (34 g)	7
Peppermint pattie hearts, dark chocolate covered, 3 patties (41 g)	8
Peppermint pattie, dark chocolate covered, 1 piece (39 g)	8
Peppermint patties, 3 pieces (41 g)	8
Peppermint patties, Christmas, 3 patties (40.4 g)	8
Peppermint patties, dark chocolate covered, 3 patties (41 g)	8
Peppermint patties, dark chocolate covered, party bag, 3 pieces (41 g)	8

	SmartPoints® value
York Minis	
Dark chocolate covered peppermint patties unwrapped, 10 pieces (40 g)	8
Zachary	
Chocolate covered marshmallow eggs, 4 pieces (47 g)	9

Candy, Non-chocolate

	SmartPoints® value
AirHeads Xtremes Bites	
Rainbow berry soft and chewy candy, 1 bag (57 g)	10
Albanese	
Gummi bears, 12 pieces (40 g)	6
Altoids	
Mints, peppermint, 3 pieces (2 g)	1
Bit O Honey	
Taffy flavored candy bites with real honey, 6 pieces (40 g)	7
Black Forest	
Gummy bears, 15 pieces (39 g)	5
Bobs Sweet Stripes	
Soft mint candy, 3 pieces (15 g)	4
Brach's	
Cinnamon jelly hearts, 5 candies (39 g)	7
Conversation hearts candy, small, 12 pieces (15 g)	4
Jube jel cherry hearts, 5 candies (37 g)	6
Brach's Classic	
Jelly bird eggs, 14 pieces (41 g)	8
Brach's Heart Lines	
Conversational hearts candy, 1 box (21 g)	5
Brown & Haley	
Almond roca, 3 pieces (36 g)	10
Charms	
Blow pops, assorted flavors, 1 piece (18.4 g)	4
Coffee Rio	
Original roast premium caramel coffee candy, 4 pieces (15 g)	3
CVS	
Mini candy canes, peppermint flavor, 3 canes (11.76 g)	2
Dots	
Gumdrops, assorted fruit flavored, 11 dots (40 g)	6
Dum Dum	
Dum dum pops, 1 pop (5 g)	1
Fluff	
Marshmallow, 2 Tbsp	2
Frosty Nerds	
Crunchy candy, 1 Tbsp	4
Gobstopper	
Jawbreakers, everlasting, 9 pieces (15 g)	4
Goetze's Caramel Creams®	
Chewy caramel candies, 3 pieces (34 g)	6
Good & Plenty	
Licorice candy, 33 pieces (40 g)	7
Great Value	
Peppermint starlight mints hard candy, 3 pieces (15 g)	3
Haribo Gold-Bears	
Original gummi candy, 17 pieces (39 g)	7
Sour gummi candy, 16 pieces (41 g)	7
Harris Teeter	
Mini marshmallows, ½ cup	4
Hot Tamales	
Candies, flavored chewy, fierce cinnamon, 20 pieces (40 g)	7
Candy, hot tamales, chewy cinnamon flavored candies, 20 pieces (38 g)	7
Jelly Belly	
Gourmet jelly bean, 49 flavors, 35 pieces (39.43 g)	8
Jelly bean, 35 pieces (40 g)	8
Jelly belly, 50 individual flavors, 35 pieces (39.67 g)	8

Candy, Non-chocolate (cont'd)

	SmartPoints® value
Jet Puffed	
Marshmallow creme, 2 Tbsp	2
Jolly Rancher	
Hard candy, assorted flavors, 3 pieces (16.5 g)	3
Hard candy, cinnamon fire, 3 pieces (17 g)	3
Juicy Twists	
Green apple candy, 6 candies (40 g)	6
Kirkland Signature Jelly Belly	
Gourmet jelly beans, 35 pieces (40 g)	8
Kraft	
Caramels, traditional, 5 pieces (41 g)	8
Kraft Jet-Puffed	
Miniature marshmallows, ⅔ cup	5
Laffy Taffy	
Candy, assorted flavors, 5 pieces (43 g)	9
Life Savers	
Candy, 5 flavors, 2 pieces (5 g)	1
Candy, pep o mint, 3 mints (5 g)	1
Candy, sugar free, wint o green, 4 mints (14 g)	1
Life Savers Gummies	
Candy, 5 flavors, 10 pieces (40 g)	7
Luden's	
Wild cherry throat drops, 1 piece (3.5 g)	1
Mentos	
Mints, chewy, fruit, 1 piece (3 g)	1
Mike and Ike	
Candies, chewy, assorted fruit flavored, original fruits, 23 pieces (40 g)	7
Nips	
Hard candy, rich & creamy, coffee, 2 pieces (14 g)	2
Rich and creamy caramel hard candy, 2 pieces (14 g)	3

	SmartPoints® value
Old Dominion	
Old fashioned peanut brittle, 1 oz	5
PayDay	
Peanut caramel bar, 1 bar (52 g)	10
Peeps	
Marshmallow bunnies, yellow, 4 bunnies (31.67 g)	7
Marshmallow chicks, 5 peeps (42 g)	8
Marshmallow snowmen, 3 peeps (32 g)	6
Red velvet flavored marshmallow, 3 peeps (42 g)	9
Red Vines	
Candy twists, original red, 6 twists (40 g)	6
Licorice twist, 5 vines (40.31 g)	6
Vines, sugar free, strawberry, 7 twists (40 g)	3
Riesen	
Caramel, chewy, chocolate covered, 4 pieces (36 g)	8
Sanders	
Sea salt caramels, 1 serving (40 g)	7
See's	
Little pops assorted hard candy treats, 4 pieces (14 g)	3
Lollypops, gourmet, 1 lollipop (20 g)	4
Skinny Cow	
Divine filled chocolates candy, caramel, 1 pouch (28.3 g)	7
Skinny Cow Divine Filled Chocolates	
Caramel, 1 pouch (28 g)	7
Skittles Fun Size	
Original skittles, 3 packages (46 g)	10
Skittles Original	
Fruit flavored bite size chewy candies, ¼ cup	9
Original bite size candies, 1 package (45 g)	10

	SmartPoints® value
Smarties	
Assorted flavors candy rolls, 1 roll (7 g)	1
Sour Patch Kids	
Candy, soft & chewy, 16 pieces (40 g)	7
Starburst	
Fruit chews, 8 pieces (40 g)	8
Jelly beans, original, ¼ cup	8
Original jelly beans, ¼ cup	8
Strawberry and green apple candy canes, 1 candy cane (14 g)	3
Swedish Fish	
Candy, soft & chewy, 19 pieces (40 g)	8
Candy, soft & chewy, red, 7 pieces (42 g)	8
SweeTarts	
Cherry punch candy ropes, 3 candies (42 g)	7
Sweethearts	
Candy hearts, 1 box (26 g)	6
Sweethearts candies, 40 pieces (40 g)	9
Sweet's	
Salt water taffy, 7 pieces (42 g)	8
Target	
Mini peppermint candy canes, 3 pieces (13 g)	3
The Ginger People Ginger Chews	
Sweet hot ginger candy, 2 pieces (12 g)	2
Tic Tac	
Mints, orange, big pack, 1 piece (0.5 g)	0
Tootsie	
Tootsie pops, assorted, 1 pop (17 g)	3
Tootsie Roll	
Mini chews, 30 pieces (41 g)	8
Tootsie pop lollipops assortment, 1 lollipop (17 g)	3

	SmartPoints® value
Trader Joe's	
Scandinavian swimmers soft and chewy gummy candy, 9 pieces (42 g)	8
Twizzlers	
Cherry bites candy, 17 pieces (40 g)	6
Low-fat strawberry twists, 6 pieces (40 g)	7
Strawberry twists, 3 pieces (36 g)	5
Twizzlers Bites	
Cherry bites, 17 pieces (40 g)	6
Twizzlers Twist	
Strawberry licorice, 6 pieces (43 g)	7
Blackberry sugar free candies, 8 candies	1
Cherry & grapefruit drops sugar free candies, 11 candies	1
Citrus drops sugar free candies, 11 candies	1
Strawberry sugar free candies, 8 candies	1
Weight Watchers In-Meeting/ Online Products: Candies	
Blackberry sugar free candies, 8 candies	1
Cherry & grapefruit drops sugar free candies, 11 candies	1
Citrus drops sugar free candies, 11 candies	1
Strawberry sugar free candies, 8 candies	1
Werther's	
Hard candies, caramel apple, sugar free, 5 pieces (16 g)	1
Hard candies, minis, sugar free, 5 pieces (16 g)	1
Werther's Original	
Hard candies, 3 pieces (16 g)	4
Soft caramels, 6 pieces (38 g)	7
Sugar free chewy caramels, 6 pieces (37 g)	4

	SmartPoints® value
Cookie Dough	
GFS	
Holiday cookie dough, 1 cookie (37.8 g)	8
Otis Spunkmeyer	
Cookie dough, chocolate chip, 1 cookie (38 g)	8
Pillsbury	
Chocolate chip cookie dough, 1 rounded tsp	6
Cookie dough, sugar cookies, 2 cookies (32 g)	6
Toll House	
Cookie dough, double chocolate chip, 1 cookie (28 g)	6
Cookie dough, peanut butter chocolate chip, 1 cookie (19 g)	3
Toll House Mini	
Chocolate chip cookie dough, prepared, 3 cookies (35 g)	7
Cookies	
365 Everyday Value	
Ginger snap cookies, 5 cookies (30 g)	5
Albertsons	
Chocolate chip cookies, 1 cookie (26 g)	6
Alyssa's	
Healthy oatmeal bites, 2 bites (42 g)	2
Anna's	
Ginger thins, 6 cookies (28 g)	6
Annie's Homegrown	
Chocolate chunk cookies, 1 cookie (17 g)	4
Archer Farms	
Milk chocolate salted caramel biscotti, 1 biscotti (24 g)	5
Austin Lemon OHs!	
Lemon creme cookies, 1 package (51 g)	10

	SmartPoints® value
Bakery Fresh	
Oatmeal raisin cookies, 1 cookie (25.2 g)	4
Bakery Fresh Goodness	
Mini chocolate chip cookies, 2 cookies (24 g)	6
Barry's Bakery	
French twists, original, 2 twists (15 g)	2
Benton's Best	
Fudge marshmallow cookies, 1 cookie (29 g)	7
Berger Cookies	
Chocolate cremes cookies, 1 cookie (34 g)	7
Best Express Foods	
Traditional Aussie bites biscuits with omega-3, 1 cookie (27 g)	5
Bud's Best Cookies	
Vanilla wafers, 11 cookies (31 g)	6
Cadbury	
Creme egg cookies, 2 cookies (35 g)	8
Café Bistro	
Pfeffernusse iced gingerbread cookies, 3 pieces (30 g)	5
Chips Ahoy	
Cookies, chocolate chip, original, 3 cookies (33 g)	7
Cookies, real chocolate chip, original, 3 cookies (33 g)	7
Cookies, real chocolate chunk, chunky, 1 cookie (16 g)	3
Cookies, reduced fat, real chocolate chip, 3 cookies (33 g)	6
Chips Ahoy Chewy	
Cookies, chocolate chip, 2 cookies (31 g)	6
Creme de Pirouline	
Dark chocolate wafer sticks, 3 cookies (30 g)	7
Famous Amos	
Bite size chocolate chip cookies (snack packs), 1 pouch (34 g)	7

	SmartPoints® value
Cookies, bite size, chocolate chip, 4 cookies (29 g)	6
Fiber One	
Chocolate chip crunchy cookies, 1 cookie (26 g)	5
Double chocolate soft-baked cookie, 1 cookie (31 g)	5
Oatmeal raisin soft baked cookie, 1 cookie (31 g)	5
Peanut butter soft baked cookies, 1 cookie (31 g)	5
Soft baked chocolate chunk cookie, 1 cookie (31 g)	5
Sugar crunchy cookies, 1 cookie (26 g)	5
Fig Newtons	
Cookies, 2 cookies (30.46 g)	5
Fruit chewy cookies, 1 cookie (30 g)	4
Fit & Active	
S'mores drizzled mini crisps, 1 package (21 g)	4
Fit & Active 100 Calorie	
Baked chocolate wafer snacks, 1 package (23 g)	4
Ginger Snaps	
Cookies, 4 cookies (28 g)	5
Girl Scout Cookies	
Caramel delites®, 1 cookie (14 g)	3
Cranberry citrus crisps, 1 serving (34 g)	6
Cranberry citrus crisps, 4 cookies (34 g)	6
Do-si-dos®, 1 cookie (11.33 g)	2
Lemonades, 1 cookie (15.5 g)	3
Peanut butter patties®, 1 cookie (12.5 g)	3
Peanut butter sandwich, 1 cookie (11.67 g)	2
Peanut butter sandwich, 3 cookies (35 g)	6
Rah-rah raisins™, 1 serving (25 g)	5
Samoas®, 1 cookie (14.5 g)	3

	SmartPoints® value
Savannah smiles, 1 cookie (6 g)	1
Shortbread, 1 cookie (6.5 g)	1
Shortbread cookies with lemon icing, 2 cookies (31 g)	7
Shortbread with tangy lemon flavored icing, 2 cookies (31 g)	7
Tagalongs®, 1 cookie (12.5 g)	3
Thanks a lot shortbread cookies, 2 cookies (31 g)	7
Thanks-a-lot, 1 cookie (15.5 g)	4
Thin mints®, 2 cookies (16 g)	4
Toffee-tastic™ (gluten free), 1 serving (28 g)	6
Traditional shortbread cookies, 4 cookies (26 g)	5
Trefoils™, 1 cookie (6.4 g)	1
Trios oatmeal cookies, 3 cookies (34 g)	7
Goldfish Flavor Blasted	
Grahams, vanilla cupcake, 35 pieces (31.17 g)	5
Goldfish Grahams	
Vanilla cupcake baked graham snacks, 35 pieces (30 g)	5
Goya	
Maria cookies, 5 cookies (33 g)	5
Grandma's Homestyle	
Peanut butter cookies, 1 cookie (40 g)	7
Grasshopper	
Cookies, fudge mint, 4 cookies (29 g)	7
Great Value	
Fudge marshmallow cookies, 1 cookie (29 g)	7
HannahMax Baking	
Chocolate chip crunchy cookie chips, 5 cookies (28 g)	6
Hershey's	
Triple chocolate cookies, 1 cookie (35 g)	7

	SmartPoints® value
Honey Maid	
Chocolate grahams, 8 crackers (31 g)	5
Cinnamon grahams, 8 crackers (31 g)	5
Grahams, low-fat, honey, 8 crackers (34 g)	5
Low-fat cinnamon grahams, 8 crackers (31 g)	5
Kashi Cookies	
Oatmeal dark chocolate, 1 cookie (30 g)	5
Kedem	
Tea biscuits, 2 biscuits (8 g)	1
Keebler	
Crispy lemon delight cookie thins, 5 cookies (28 g)	6
Original fudge stripes cookies, 2 cookies (27 g)	6
Wafers, vanilla, 8 cookies (30.91 g)	6
Keebler 100 Calorie Right Bites Fudge Shoppe	
Cookies, mini fudge stripes, 1 pouch (21 g)	5
Keebler Chips Deluxe	
Rainbow chocolate chip cookies, 2 cookies (31 g)	7
Keebler Fudge Stripes	
Cookies, original, 2 cookies (27 g)	6
Keebler Sandies	
Pecan shortbread cookies, 2 cookies (31 g)	7
Keebler Scooby-Doo!	
Baked graham cracker sticks, cinnamon, 10 crackers (31.2 g)	5
Keebler Simply Made	
Crispy chocolate chip cookie thins, 5 cookies (28 g)	6
Kirkland Signature	
Organic animal crackers, 11 crackers (28 g)	4
Kroger	
Graham crackers, honey, 4 crackers (27 g)	4

	SmartPoints® value
Graham crackers, original, 4 crackers (26.65 g)	4
Lacey's	
Almond and dark chocolate toffee wafers, 1 cookie (28 g)	7
Lance Nekot	
Peanut butter cookies, 1 package (50 g)	9
Leclerc Praeventia	
Dark chocolate chip cookies, 1 pouch (30 g)	5
Lenny & Larry's The Complete Cookie	
Chocolate chip cookie, ½ package (56.5 g)	7
Oatmeal raisin cookie, 2 oz	7
Lil' Dutch Maid	
Butter ring cookies, 5 cookies (29 g)	5
Little Debbie Nutty Bars	
North Pole wafers with peanut butter, 1 bar (21 g)	5
Wafers with extra peanut butter, 2 cookies (60 g)	14
Lofthouse	
Delicious cookies, frosted sugar cookies, 1 cookie (42.5 g)	6
Frosted sugar cookies, 1 cookie (38 g)	7
Lorna Doone	
Cookies, shortbread, 4 cookies (28 g)	5
Lotus Biscoff	
Cookies, 2 cookies (25 g)	5
Cookies, 4 biscuits (31 g)	7
Mallomars	
Cookies, pure chocolate, 2 cookies (25.11 g)	6
Market Pantry	
Vanilla wafer cookies, 8 wafers (30 g)	6
McVities Digestive	
Biscuits, the original, 2 cookies (30 g)	5

	SmartPoints® value
Metamucil	
Cinnamon spice multigrain wafers, 2 wafers (22 g)	4
Mini Fudge Stripes 100 Calorie Right Bites	
Fudge striped shortbread cookies, 1 pouch (21 gs)	5
Mrs. Fields	
Cookies, snickerdoodle, 1 cookie (28 g)	5
Mrs. Thinsters	
Chocolate chip cookie thins, 5 cookies (28 g)	6
Maple syrup waffle crisps, 15 crisps (28 g)	5
Toasted coconut cookie thin, 5 cookies (28 g)	8
Murray	
Cookies, ginger snaps, 5 cookies (30.2 g)	6
Murray Sugar Free	
Cookies, shortbread, 8 cookies (34 g)	4
Wafers, vanilla, 4 cookies (28.33 g)	5
Nabisco	
Cinnamon bun oreo sandwich cookies, 2 cookies (29 g)	7
Oreo chocolate sandwich cookies thins, 1 package (29 g)	6
Oreo thins sandwich cookies, 4 cookies (29 g)	6
Nabisco 100 Calorie Packs	
Cookie crisps, shortbread, Lorna Doone, 1 package (21 g)	4
Oreo thin crisps, 1 pack (23 g)	4
Thin crisps, chips ahoy!, 1 package (23 g)	4
Nabisco Classics	
Cookies, snickerdoodle, 1 cookie (18.87 g)	4
Nature Valley	
Biscuits with almond butter filling, 1 biscuit (38 g)	7

	SmartPoints® value
Biscuits with peanut butter filling, 1 biscuit (38 g)	7
Newtons	
Cookies, fig, fat free, 2 cookies (28.33 g)	4
Nilla	
Wafers, 8 wafers (30 g)	6
Wafers, mini, 1 package (28 g)	5
Wafers, mini, 20 wafers (30 g)	6
Wafers, reduced fat, 8 wafers (28.27 g)	5
Nonni's	
Almond thins, cranberry, 1 package (21 g)	4
Almond thins, pistachio, 1 package (21 g)	3
Biscotti, cioccolati, 1 biscotti (24.13 g)	5
Biscotti, decadence, 1 biscotti (24.13 g)	4
Biscotti, originali, 1 biscotti (19.5 g)	4
Biscotti, salted caramel, 1 biscotti (24 g)	5
Originali mini biscotti, 1 biscotti (15 g)	3
Salted caramel mini biscotti, 1 biscotti (17 g)	3
Nutrisystem Snack	
Chocolate chip cookies, 1 package (36 g)	6
Nutter Butter	
Cookies, peanut butter sandwich, 2 cookies (24.5 g)	5
Cookies, peanut butter sandwich, bites, go-paks!, 10 cookies (30 g)	6
Oreo	
Brownie batter flavor crème sandwich cookies, 2 cookies (29 g)	6
Chocolate sandwich cookies, 3 cookies (34 g)	7
Chocolate sandwich cookies, double stuff, 2 cookies (29 g)	6

	SmartPoints® value
Chocolate sandwich cookies, milk chocolate covered, 1 cookie (17.67 g)	4
Cookies, sandwich, birthday cake flavor creme, 2 cookies (28 g)	6
Cookies, sandwich, chocolate, 3 cookies (34 g)	7
Cookies, sandwich, golden, 3 cookies (34 g)	7
Cookies, sandwich, red velvet, 2 cookies (29 g)	6
Double stuf chocolate sandwich cookies, 2 cookies (29 g)	6
Filled cupcake chocolate sandwich cookies, 2 cookies (29 g)	6
Golden sandwich cookies, 3 cookies (34 g)	7
Lemon twist flavor creme chocolate sandwich cookies, 2 cookies (29 g)	6
Mint chocolate sandwich thins cookies, 4 cookies (29 g)	6
Peppermint creme chocolate sandwich cookies, 2 cookies (29 g)	6
Red velvet cream cheese sandwich cookies, 2 cookies (29 g)	6
Reduced fat chocolate sandwich cookies, 3 cookies (34 g)	7
Oreo Mini	
Chocolate sandwich cookie, 9 cookies (29 g)	6
Cookies, sandwich, chocolate, bite size, go-paks!, 9 cookies (29 g)	6
Mint creme flavored chocolate sandwich cookies, 9 cookies (29 g)	6
Pepperidge Farm	
Cookies, distinctive, chessmen, 3 cookies (25.75 g)	5
Cookies, distinctive, milano mint, 2 cookies (25 g)	6

	SmartPoints® value
Cookies, distinctive, milano, double chocolate, 2 cookies (27 g)	6
Ginger family cookie collection, 4 cookies (34 g)	7
Pepperidge Farm Milano	
Cookies, dark chocolate, 3 cookies (34 g)	8
Pillsbury Ready To Bake!	
Cookies, chocolate chip, 2 cookies (38 g)	7
Poppies	
Coconut chocolate macaroon, 1 cookie (40 g)	10
Priano Pizzelle	
Pizzelle vanilla flavored Italian style cookies, 6 cookies (30 g)	5
Reko	
Vanilla pizzelle, 6 cookies (30 g)	5
Reko Pizzelle	
Anise Italian waffle cookie, 6 cookies (30 g)	5
Rip van Wafels	
Cocoa filled Amsterdam wafel, 1 piece (33 g)	7
Royal Dansk	
Danish butter cookies, 4 cookies (30 g)	7
Danish butter cookies, 4 pieces (34 g)	7
Sheila G's	
Chocolate chip brownie brittle, 6 pieces (28 g)	6
Slimfast	
Smores drizzled crisps, 1 bag (28 g)	4
SnackWell's	
Cookies, creme sandwich, 2 cookies (24 g)	5
Creme sandwich cookie, 1 pack (48 g)	9
Devil's food cookie cakes, 1 cookie (16 g)	2

	SmartPoints® value
Mini chocolate chip cookies, 1 pack (30 g)	5
Special K	
Chocolatey caramel pastry crisps, 2 crisps (25 g)	4
Cookies and creme pastry crisps, 2 crisps (25 g)	4
Specially Selected	
Anise flavored pizzelle Italian waffle cookies, 6 cookies (30 g)	5
Specially Selected Laceys	
Dark chocolate almond cookies, 1 cookie (28 g)	7
Starbucks Coffee	
Petite French madeleines, 3 cakes (51 g)	10
Stauffer's	
Animal crackers, chocolate, 16 crackers (29.36 g)	5
Animal crackers, original, 16 crackers (30.27 g)	4
Stella Doro Breakfast Treats	
Cookies, original, 1 cookie (21.25 g)	4
Stella Doro Coffee Treats	
Cookies, anisette toast, 3 cookies (32.4 g)	5
Sugar Bowl Bakery	
Madeleines, 1 cookie (28 g)	6
Tate's Bake Shop	
Cookies, chocolate chip, 1 cookie (14 g)	4
Cookies, gluten free, chocolate chip, 1 cookie (15 g)	4
Teddy Grahams	
Graham snacks, 13 pieces (29.89 g)	5
The Bakery	
Soft chocolate chip cookie, 1 cookie (26 g)	5
The Bakery at Walmart	
Peanut butter fudge no bake cookies, 1 cookie (43 g)	7

	SmartPoints® value
THINaddictives	
Pistachio almond thins, 1 package (23 g)	4
Toll House	
Cookies, chocolate chip, 1 cookie (19.5 g)	5
Milk chocolate peanut butter blondie kit, 1 package (29 g)	6
Trader Jacques'	
Chocolate and vanilla French macarons, 3 pieces (30 g)	5
Trader Joe's	
Cocoa batons, 2 pieces (24 g)	5
Dark chocolate mini heart cookies, 5 cookies (28 g)	4
Speculoos cookies, 4 cookies (32 g)	6
Trader Joe's Grocery	
Chocolate cats cookies, 15 cookies (30 g)	5
Cinnamon schoolbook cookies, 15 cookies (30 g)	5
Cookie thins - meyer lemon, 9 cookies (28 g)	7
Cookie thins - toasted coconut, 9 cookies (28 g)	6
Cookie thins - triple ginger, 9 cookies (28 g)	6
Dress circle crispy crunchy chocolate chip cookies, 12 cookies (30 g)	7
Organic animal crackers, 17 cookies (30 g)	4
Soft bite mini almond biscotti, 3 pieces (27 g)	5
Triple ginger snaps, 6 cookies (30 g)	6
Twix	
Cookie bars, minis, 3 pieces (30 g)	7
Two-Bite	
Blueberry scones, 3 scones (60 g)	10

	SmartPoints® value
Voortman	
Wafer cookies, sugar free, vanilla, 3 cookies (27 g)	4
Walker's	
Shortbread, pure butter, 1 piece (19 g)	4
Wal-Mart	
Chocolate chip cookies, 1 cookie (25 g)	5
Wegman's	
Organic animal cookies, 10 cookies (30 g)	5
Weissella Grocery	
Sugar glazed soft gingerbread cookies, 1 cookie (29 g)	5

Dessert Toppings

Ahold	
Fat free dairy whipped topping, 2 Tbsp	0
Cool Whip	
Whipped topping, extra creamy, with real cream, 2 Tbsp	2
Whipped topping, fat free, 2 Tbsp	1
Whipped topping, lite, 2 Tbsp	1
Whipped topping, original, 2 Tbsp	1
Whipped topping, sugar free, 2 Tbsp	1
Cool Whip Lite	
Whipped topping, 2 Tbsp	1
Fit & Active	
Fat free whipped topping, 2 Tbsp	1
Hershey's	
Topping, hot fudge, 2 Tbsp	7
Kroger	
Lite whipped topping, 2 Tbsp	1
Original dairy whipped topping, 2 Tbsp	1
Whipped topping, fat free, 2 Tbsp	1
Whipped topping, lite, 2 Tbsp	1
Lucerne	
Whipped topping, fat free, 2 Tbsp	0
Meijer	
Fat free whipped topping, 2 Tbsp	1
Publix	
Lite whipped topping, 2 Tbsp	1
Small and fluffy marshmallows, ⅔ cup	5
Whipped fat free topping, 2 Tbsp	0
Whipped light cream, 2 Tbsp	1
Reddi Wip	
Dairy whipped topping, extra creamy, 2 Tbsp	1
Dairy whipped topping, original, 2 Tbsp	1
Original whipped topping, 2 Tbsp	1
Smucker's	
Topping, caramel, sugar free, 2 Tbsp	3
Smucker's Sugar Free	
Topping, hot fudge, 2 Tbsp	3
Truwhip	
Skinny whipped topping, 2 Tbsp	1

Eclairs

Delizza	
Belgian double chocolate mini eclairs, 6 eclairs (84 g)	12
Private Selection	
Miniature eclairs, 6 eclairs (87 g)	14

Frozen Fruit Bars

Diana's	
Banana babies, dark chocolate, 1 piece (60 g)	5
Edys Outshine	
Creamy coconut fruit bar, 1 bar (87 g)	6
Lime fruit bar, 1 bar (46 g)	2
Strawberry fruit bar, 1 bar (85 g)	4
Edy's Outshine No Sugar Added	
Assorted fruit bar, 1 bar (43 g)	1
Strawberry fruit bar, 1 bar (43 g)	1

	SmartPoints® value
Popsicle Sugar Free	
Ice pops, orange, cherry, grape, 1 pop (50 g)	0
Ice pops, tropicals, 1 piece (48.75 ml)	0

Frozen Ices

Luigi's	
Real Italian ice, lemon, 1 cup	5

Frozen Yogurt

Kemps	
Frozen yogurt, vanilla, ½ cup	2
Ruby Rocket's	
Beam me up berry non dairy frozen yogurt, 1 tube (57 g)	3
Stellar strawberry non dairy yogurt, 1 tube (57 g)	3
Telescopic tropic non dairy frozen yogurt, 1 tube (57 g)	3
Yasso	
Chocolate fudge frozen Greek yogurt bar, 1 bar (65 g)	3
Coffee chocolate chip frozen Greek yogurt bar, 1 bar (65 g)	4
Frozen Greek yogurt bar strawberry flavored, 1 bar (70 g)	3
Sea salt caramel frozen Greek yogurt, 1 bar (70 g)	4
Sea salt caramel Greek frozen yogurt, 1 bar (65 g)	4

Gelatins

	SmartPoints® value
Jell-O	
Black cherry low calorie sugar free gelatin snack, 1 snack (89 g)	0
Gelatin and pudding, sugar free, variety pack (gelatin flavors), 1 snack (89 g)	0
Gelatin dessert, low calorie, sugar free, orange, ⅛ package (2.5 g)	0
Gelatin dessert, low calorie, sugar free, raspberry, ¼ package (2.1 g)	0
Gelatin snacks, low calorie, orange, 1 snack (89 g)	0
Gelatin snacks, low calorie, strawberry, 1 snack (89 g)	0
Gelatin snacks, low calorie, sugar free, black cherry, 1 snack (89 g)	0
Gelatin snacks, low calorie, sugar free, cherry, 1 snack (89 g)	0
Gelatin snacks, low calorie, sugar free, raspberry, 1 snack (89 g)	0
Gelatin snacks, low calorie, sugar free, strawberry, 1 snack (92 g)	0
Gelatin snacks, low calorie, sugar free, strawberry, 8 pack, 1 container (89 g)	0
Gelatin snacks, original, strawberry, 1 snack (96 g)	4
Lemon lime low calorie sugar free gelatin snack, 1 snack (89 g)	0
Low calorie gelatin dessert, sugar free, black cherry, ¼ package (2.1 g)	0
Low calorie gelatin dessert, sugar free, orange, ¼ package (2.1 g)	0
Original strawberry gelatin snack, 1 snack (96 g)	4
Sugar free lemon-lime gelatin snacks, 1 snack (89 g)	0
Sugar free low calorie gelatin dessert, cranberry, ⅛ package (2.1 g)	0
Snack Pack	
Cherry juicy gels, sugar free, 1 container (92 g)	0
Juicy gels, strawberry & orange, sugar free, 1 gel snack (92 g)	0
Winky Brand	
Jilly's gelatin sugar free, 1 container (92 g)	0
Winky Sugar Free	
Parfait assorted gelatin, 1 container (99 g)	1

	SmartPoints® value
Ice Cream	
Almond Dream	
Cappuccino swirl non dairy frozen dessert, ½ cup	6
Arctic Zero	
Chunky cookie dough chip fit frozen dessert, ½ cup	3
Gluten free lactose free chocolate frozen dessert, ½ cup	1
Gluten free lactose free chocolate peanut butter frozen dessert, ½ cup	1
Gluten free lactose free creamy cookies and cream frozen dessert, ½ cup	1
Gluten free lactose free creamy salted caramel frozen dessert, ½ cup	1
Gluten free lactose free hint of mint creamy frozen dessert, ½ cup	1
Gluten free lactose free vanilla maple frozen dessert, ½ cup	1
Belmont	
Caramel pretzel crunch ice cream, ½ cup	7
Vanilla light ice cream, ½ cup	5
Ben & Jerry's Core	
Chocolate and peanut butter fudge flavored ice cream, ½ cup	14
Blue Bell	
Ice cream, cookies 'n cream, ½ cup	8
Ice cream, homemade vanilla flavored, ½ cup	8
Blue Bunny Blue Ribbon Classics	
Fudge bars, freezer pack, 1 bar (61 g)	4
Blue Bunny Mini Swirls	
Vanilla cone, 1 cone (43 g)	6
Blue Bunny Sweet Freedom	
Fudge no sugar added ice cream bars, 2 bars (88 g)	3
Ice cream cones, no sugar added, vanilla, snack size, 1 cone (43 g)	4

	SmartPoints® value
Ice cream sandwiches, no sugar added, vanilla, 1 sandwich (69 g)	4
Ice cream, light, no sugar added, vanilla, ½ cup	4
Breyers	
Homemade vanilla ice cream, ½ cup	7
Ice cream, butter pecan, ½ cup	7
Ice cream, chocolate, ½ cup	7
Ice cream, mint chocolate chip, ½ cup	8
Ice cream, vanilla, ½ cup	6
Breyers Carb Smart	
Frozen dairy dessert, chocolate, ½ cup	4
Frozen dairy dessert, vanilla, ½ cup	4
Fudge bar, 1 bar (56 g)	4
Breyers No Sugar Added	
Light vanilla ice cream, ½ cup	3
Breyers Smooth & Dreamy	
Ice cream, extra creamy, no sugar added, butter pecan, ½ cup	4
Ice cream, fat free, creamy vanilla, ½ cup	4
Carvel	
Ice cream cake, celebration, 1 serving (118 ml)	9
Dreyer's	
Butterfinger ice cream, ½ cup	8
Dreyer's Slow Churned	
Cookies 'n cream light ice cream, ½ cup	5
Drumstick Lil' Drums	
Frozen dairy dessert cones, assorted, snack size, 1 cone (45 g)	6
Edy's Slow Churned	
Butter pecan light ice cream, ½ cup	5
Caramel delight light ice cream, ½ cup	5
Chocolate light ice cream, ½ cup	5
Coffee light ice cream, ½ cup	5

	SmartPoints® value
Cookie dough light ice cream, ½ cup	6
French silk light ice cream, ½ cup	7
Mint chocolate chip light ice cream, ½ cup	6
Vanilla bean light ice cream, ½ cup	5
Edy's Slow Churned No Sugar Added	
Fudge tracks light ice cream, ½ cup	4
Triple chocolate light ice cream, ½ cup	4
Vanilla light ice cream, ½ cup	4
Enlightened	
Chocolate peanut butter swirl low-fat ice cream bar, 1 bar (68 g)	3
Cinnamon caramel swirl ice cream bar, 1 bar (70 g)	3
Ice cream bars, low-fat, fudge, 1 bar (74 g)	2
Enlightened The Good-For-You Ice Cream	
Peanut butter low-fat ice cream bars, 1 bar (73 g)	2
Toasted almond low-fat ice cream bars, 1 bar (74 g)	2
Vanilla bean low-fat ice cream sandwiches, 1 sandwich (69 g)	3
Fit & Active	
Chocolate fudge ice cream bar, 1 bar (76 g)	5
Friendly's	
Chocolate marshmallow swirl ice cream, ½ cup	8
Fudgsicle	
Fudge bars, original, 1 pop (43 g)	3
Fudge pops, low-fat, the original, 1 bar (43 g)	3
Original fudge bar, fat free, 1 piece (52 ml)	3
Giant	
Inside out ice cream sandwiches, 1 sandwich (59 g)	7

	SmartPoints® value
Great Value	
Ice cream cups, chocolate & vanilla, 1 cup	5
Ice cream sandwich, no sugar added, vanilla, 1 sandwich (64 g)	4
Häagen-Dazs	
Ice cream, vanilla, ½ cup	12
Peppermint bark ice cream bar, 1 bar (84 g)	14
Tres leches brigadeiro ice cream, 1 container (94 g)	12
Halo Top Creamery	
All natural light lemon cake ice cream, ½ cup	2
Ice cream, light, all natural, chocolate, ½ cup	3
Light strawberry ice cream, ½ cup	2
Healthy Choice	
Fudge bars, 1 bar (64 g)	3
Fudge bars, premium, 1 bar (74 ml)	3
Klondike	
Ice cream bars, no sugar added, vanilla, 1 bar (78 g)	8
Ice cream bars, the original, 1 bar (86 g)	13
Klondike 100 Calorie	
Ice cream sandwiches, vanilla, 1 sandwich (46 g)	4
Kroger	
No sugar added low-fat fudge bar, 1 bar (64 g)	3
Lactaid	
Vanilla ice cream, ½ cup	7
Polar Treats	
Vanilla flavored low-fat ice cream, ½ cup	5
Publix	
Fudge bars, 1 bar (61 g)	4
Skinny Cow	
Double caramel swirl ice cream bars, 1 bar (67 g)	8
Fudge bars, low-fat, 1 bar (69 g)	5

	SmartPoints® value
Ice cream bars, caramel truffle, 1 bar (63 g)	5
Ice cream bars, chocolate truffle, 1 bar (64 g)	5
Ice cream cone, low-fat, chocolate with fudge, 1 cone (75 g)	7
Ice cream cone, low-fat, vanilla with caramel, 1 cone (75 g)	7
Ice cream cones, chocolate mint ganache, 1 cone (72 g)	7
Ice cream cones, chocolate mousse ganache, 1 cone (72 g)	7
Ice cream sandwiches, low-fat, chocolate peanut butter, 1 sandwich (71 g)	6
Ice cream sandwiches, low-fat, cookies 'n cream, 1 sandwich (72 g)	6
Ice cream sandwiches, low-fat, mint, 1 sandwich (71 g)	6
Ice cream sandwiches, low-fat, no sugar added, vanilla, 1 sandwich (71 g)	4
Ice cream sandwiches, low-fat, vanilla and cookies 'n cream, 1 sandwich (71 g)	6
Low-fat vanilla and chocolate ice cream sandwich (variety pack), 1 sandwich (71 g)	6
Low-fat vanilla ice cream sandwich, 1 sandwich (71 g)	6
Salted caramel pretzel ice cream bars, 1 bar (50 g)	8
Triple chocolate ripple ice cream bars, 1 bar (68 g)	8
Vanilla almond crunch ice cream bars, 1 bar (66 g)	8
Skinny Cow Limited Editions	
Snickerdoodle ice cream sandwiches, 1 sandwich (71 g)	6
Smooth Churned	
Smooth churned fudge swirl light ice cream, ½ cup	6
Snickers	
Ice cream bars, 1 bar (50 g)	9

	SmartPoints® value
So Delicious	
Dark chocolate truffle cashew milk non dairy frozen dessert, ½ cup	8
Mini coconut sandwich ice cream, 1 sandwich (37 ml)	4
Sundae Shoppe	
Chocolate fudge pops, 1 pop (49 g)	4
TCBY Grocery	
Chocolate chip cookie dough frozen yogurt, ½ cup	7
Trader Joe's	
Peppermint joe-joe's ice cream, ½ cup	10
Trader Joe's Frozen	
Hold the cone! Mini ice cream cones, chocolate, 1 cone (21 g)	3
Hold the cone! Mini ice cream cones, vanilla, 1 cone (29 g)	3
Turkey Hill	
Ice cream, fat free, Dutch chocolate, ½ cup	2
Ice cream, fat free, vanilla bean, ½ cup	3
Ice cream, light, denali original, moose tracks, ½ cup	4
Weight Watchers Frozen Novelties	
Dark chocolate mint bars, 1 bar	3
Dark chocolate raspberry bars, 1 bar	3
Giant chocolate fudge bars, 1 bar	4
Snack size chocolate fudge bars, 1 bar	2
Snack size cookies & cream bars, 1 bar	4
Snack size divine triple chocolate bars, 1 bar	4
Snack size double caramel swirl cones, 1 cone	4
Snack size English toffee crunch bars, 1 bar	4
Snack size mocha latte bars, 1 bar	2
Snack size peanut butter caramel candy bars, 1 bar	4

	SmartPoints® value
Snack size salted caramel bars, 1 bar	4
Snack size vanilla fudge swirl cones, 1 cone	4
Weight Watchers Smart Ones Smart Delights	
Chocolate chip cookie dough sundae, 1 dessert	6
Peanut butter cup sundae, 1 dessert	6

Mousses

	SmartPoints® value
Jell-O Temptations	
Mousse snacks, chocolate indulgence flavor, 1 container (63 g)	2
Mousse snacks, dark chocolate decadence flavor, 1 snack (63 g)	2
Mousse snacks, lemon meringue pie, 1 snack (95 g)	4
Mousse snacks, sugar free, chocolate indulgence flavor, 1 snack (65 g)	2

Pies

	SmartPoints® value
Bakery Fresh	
Sweet potato pie, 1 serving (125 g)	14
Daily Chef	
Pumpkin pie, 1 serving (137 g)	16
Field's	
Pecan pie, ⅛ pie (113 g)	18
Good Life	
Sweet potato pie, 1 slice (119 g)	19
H-E-B	
Pumpkin pie (serves 5), 1 slice (122 g)	13
Marie Callender's	
Cherry crunch pie, 1 slice (126 g)	17
Pumpkin pecan streusel pie, 1 slice (119 g)	16
Sara Lee	
Southern sweet potato pie, 1 slice (121 g)	12
Tastykake	
Blueberry pie, 1 pie (113 g)	13
Trader Joe's	
Mini pie medley variety pack (blueberry), 1 pie (43 g)	7

Puddings

	SmartPoints® value
Baker's Corner	
Sugar free fat free chocolate pudding and pie filling, ¼ package (11 g)	1
Great Value	
Chocolate instant pudding and pie filling, ¼ package (28 g)	5
Hunt's	
Pudding, sugar free, chocolate, 1 pudding cup (99 g)	3
Jell-O	
Fat free chocolate pudding snacks, 1 snack (110 g)	5
Fat free chocolate vanilla swirls pudding snacks, 1 snack (110 g)	5
Instant reduced calorie pudding & pie filling, sugar free/fat free, banana cream, ¼ package (6.3 g)	1
Pudding & pie filling, instant, fat free, sugar free, disney pixar toy story, unprepared, 1 serving (8 g)	1
Pudding & pie filling, instant, reduced calorie, vanilla, ¼ package (8 g)	1
Pudding snacks, original, chocolate flavor, 1 snack (110 g)	6
Pudding snacks, reduced calorie, rice, creme brulee, 1 container (103 g)	2
Pudding snacks, reduced calorie, rice, original, 1 container (103 g)	2
Pudding snacks, reduced calorie, sugar free, chocolate flavor, 8 pack, 1 snack (103 g)	2
Pudding snacks, reduced calorie, sugar free, chocolate vanilla swirl, 8 pack, 1 snack (103 g)	2

Puddings, Jell-O (cont'd)

	SmartPoints® value
Pudding snacks, reduced calorie, sugar free, double chocolate flavor, 1 snack (106 g)	2
Pudding snacks, reduced calorie, sugar free, rice pudding, cinnamon, 1 snack (106 g)	2
Reduced calorie sugar free chocolate vanilla swirls pudding, 1 pudding cup (103 g)	2
Sugar free dark chocolate pudding snacks, 1 snack (103 g)	2
Sugar free double chocolate pudding snack, 1 snack (103 g)	2
Jell-O 60 Calorie, Sugar Free	
Boston cream pie pudding snacks, 1 snack (103 g)	2
Jell-O Cook & Serve	
Reduced calorie pudding & pie filling, sugar free/fat free, chocolate, unprepared, 1 serving (9 g)	1
Reduced calorie pudding & pie filling, sugar free/fat free, vanilla, ¼ package (5.5 g)	1
Jell-O Reduced Calorie	
Pudding snacks, chocolate flavor, 1 snack (103 g)	2
Pudding snacks, dulce de leche, 1 snack (103 g)	2
Pudding snacks, vanilla, 1 snack (103 g)	2

	SmartPoints® value
Kozy Shack	
All natural pudding, original rice, 1 snack cup (113 g)	6
Pudding, tapioca, 1 cup	6
Tapioca pudding, 1 serving (113 g)	6
Kozy Shack Simply Well	
Rice pudding no sugar added (gluten free), 4 oz	3
Tapioca pudding no suagr added (gluten free), 4 oz	3
Lunch Buddies	
Sugar free chocolate pudding, 1 serving (99 g)	3
Snack Pack	
Chocolate pudding, 1 snack cup (92 g)	5
Pudding cups, chocolate, sugar free, 1 pudding cup (92 g)	2
Pudding cups, vanilla, sugar free, 1 pudding cup (92 g)	2
Pudding, sugar free, caramel, 1 pudding cup (92 g)	2
Sugar free chocolate pudding cup, 1 pudding cup (92 g)	2
Wegman's	
Pudding, sugar free, chocolate vanilla swirl, 1 snack (106 g)	2

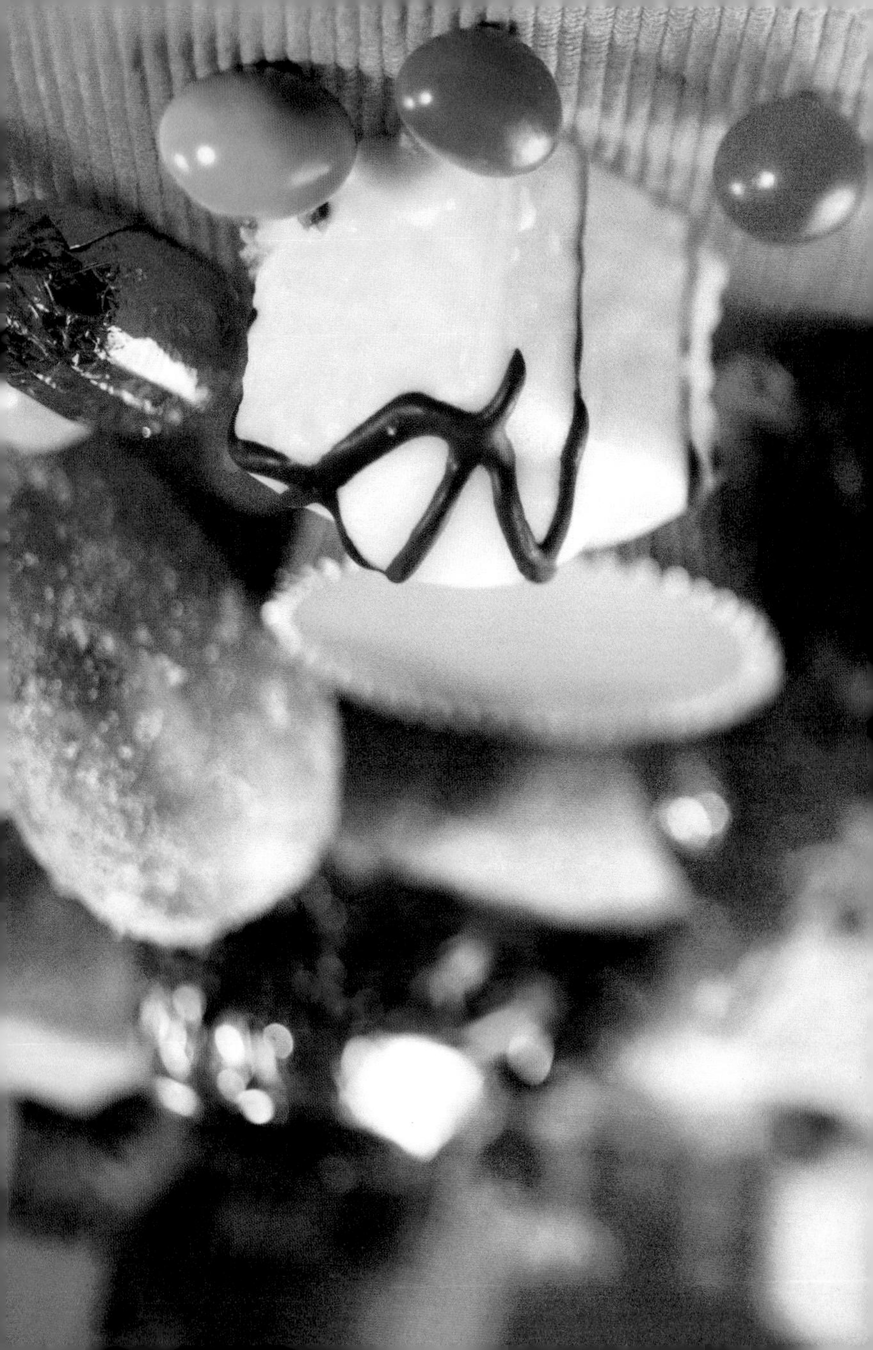

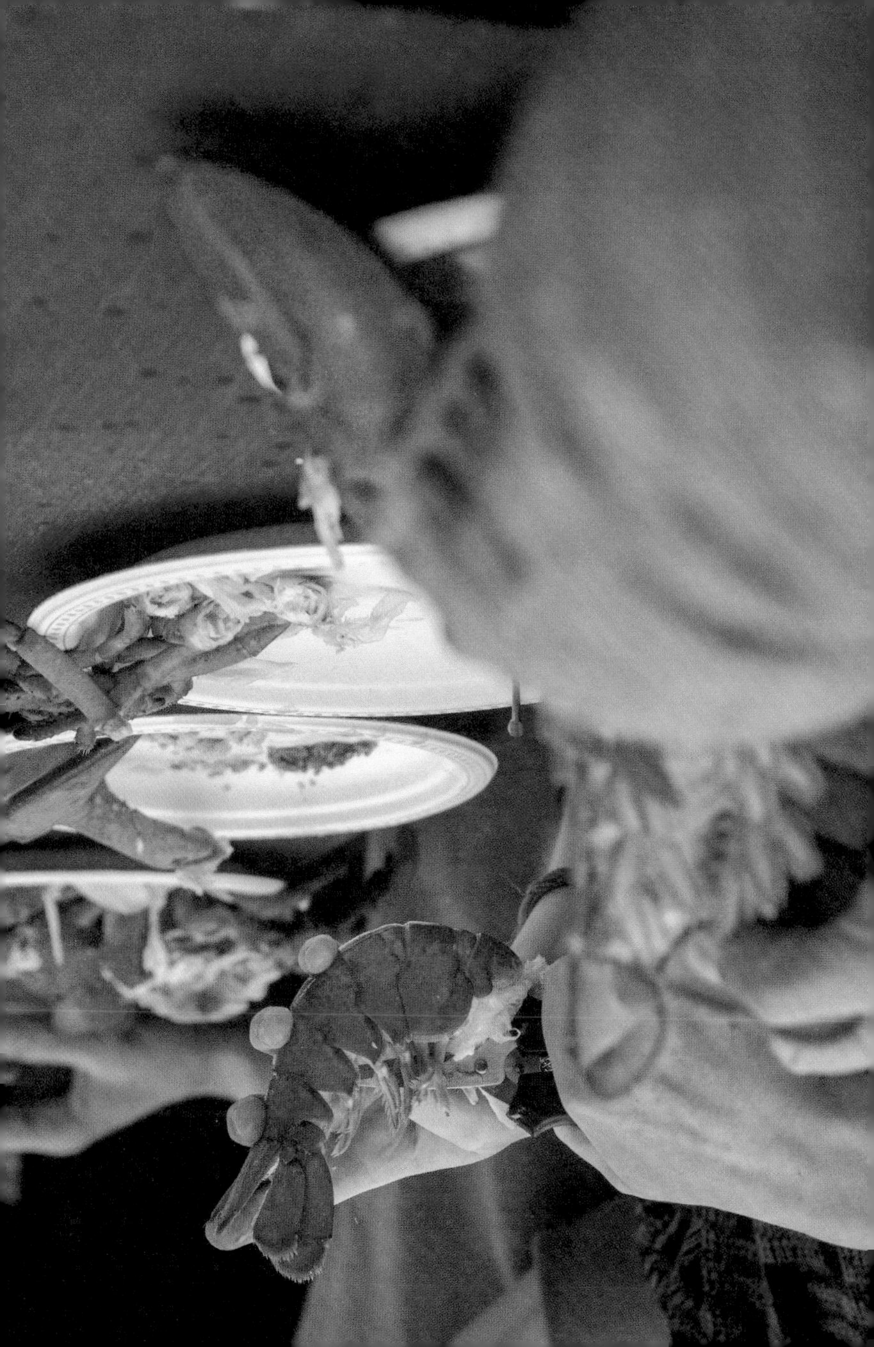

fish & seafood

	SmartPoints® value
Cod	
High Liner Atlantic Cod	
Premium cod loins, 3 oz	1
Icelandic	
Beer battered cod fillets, 2 fillets (112 g)	7
Ocean Beauty	
Pacific cod, 4 oz	0
Sea Cuisine	
Cod, potato crusted, 1 fillet (140 g)	6
Trader Joe's	
Oven ready breaded cod fillets, 2 pieces (149 g)	7
Trident Seafoods	
Panko breaded cod, 2 pieces (85 g)	4
Crab	
Kanimi	
Imitation crab flakes, ½ cup	2
Kroger Crab Select	
Flake style imitation crab meat, ½ cup	2
Louis Kemp Crab Delights	
Crab delights, flake style, ½ cup	3
Crab delights, leg style, 3 legs (91 g)	2
Louis Kemp Seafood Co. Crab Delights	
Imitation king crabmeat, flake style, ½ cup	2
Leg style imitation crab, 3 oz	2
Phillips	
Crab cakes, Maryland style, 1 cake (85 g)	4
Seafest	
Imitation crab meat, salad style, ½ cup	3

	SmartPoints® value
Trans Ocean	
Crab classic, chunk style, ½ cup	2
Crab classic, leg style, 3 pieces (90 g)	3
Trans Ocean Crab Classic	
Imitation crab meat, flake style, ½ cup	3
Crawfish	
Baby Lobster	
Crawfish tail meat, 3 oz	1
Fish Fillets	
Gorton's	
Fish fillets, beer battered, 2 fillets (103 g)	8
Fish fillets, crunchy breaded, 2 fillets (108 g)	8
Fish sandwich fillets, 1 fillet (65 g)	5
Grilled fillets, garlic butter, 1 fillet (107 g)	1
Gorton's Smart & Crunchy	
Breaded fish fillets, 2 fillets (108 g)	6
Sea Queen	
Crunchy fish fillets, 2 fillets (105 g)	7
Van de Kamp's	
Fish fillets, beer battered, 2 fillets (108 g)	7
Fish Sticks	
Gorton's	
Fish sticks, value pack, 6 sticks (91 g)	7
Gorton's Smart & Crunchy	
Breaded fish sticks, 5 sticks (86 g)	6
Trident Seafoods	
The ultimate fish stick, 3 pieces (85 g)	4

	SmartPoints® value

Herring

Blue Hill Bay

Herring in wine sauce, 5 pieces (55 g)	3

Lobster

Louis Kemp Seafood Co. Lobster Delights

Imitation lobster meat, chunk style, fat free, ½ cup	2

Mahi Mahi

Inland Market

Sea salt and roasted garlic mahi, 5 oz	3

Kirkland Signature

Pacific wild mahi mahi, 4 oz	1

Trader Joe's

Mahi mahi burgers, 1 patty (91 g)	2

Wellsley Farms

Mahi mahi loin, 4 oz	1

Salmon

Acme

Salmon, smoked nova, 2 slices (57 g)	1

C. Wirthy

Blackened salmon, 1 fillet (170 g)	8
Salmon, Atlantic, 1 fillet (170 g)	6

Chicken of the Sea

Pink salmon, skinless & boneless, 1 pouch (74 g)	1

Daily Chef

Wild Alaskan salmon burgers, 1 burger (113 g)	2
Wild Alaskan sockeye salmon, 1 portion (170 g)	5

Gorton's

Grilled salmon, classic grilled, 1 fillet (89 g)	2
Signature seasoned salmon, 1 fillet (100 g)	1

	SmartPoints® value

Gorton's Simply Bake

Salmon, roasted garlic & butter, 1 fillet (126 g)	2

Great Value

Skinless salmon fillets, 4 oz	1

High Liner Sea Cuisine

Salmon, Mediterranean crusted, 1 fillet (120 g)	6

Kirkland Signature

Atlantic salmon, 1 portion (196 g)	9
Wild Alaskan pink salmon, ¼ cup	1
Wild Alaskan smoked sockeye salmon, 2 oz	1
Wild Alaskan sockeye salmon, 1 piece (170 g)	6

Kroger

Wild caught Alaskan salmon burger, 1 burger (85 g)	3

Lasc Co.

Wild caught smoked nova salmon, 2 oz	1

Morey's

Marinated wild Alaskan salmon, 1 fillet (170 g)	5

Phillips Seafood Restaurants

Salmon cakes, 1 cake (85 g)	5

Salmolux

Smoked salmon, nova lox, 3 oz	3

Sea Cuisine

Honey chipotle salmon, 1 fillet (119 g)	7

Sea Queen

Pink salmon fillets, 4 oz	1
Wild caught pink salmon fillet, 4 oz	1

SeaPak Daily Chef

Wild Alaskan salmon burgers, 1 burger (113 g)	2

StarKist

Skinless boneless pink salmon in water, 1 pouch (74 g)	1

Salmon (cont'd)

	SmartPoints® value
StarKist Salmon Creations	
Lemon dill seasoned wild caught pink salmon, 1 pouch (74 g)	2
Mango chipotle marinated salmon, 1 pouch (74 g)	2
Trader Joe's	
Nova salmon pieces, 2 oz	1
Pastrami style smoked Atlantic salmon, 2 oz	3
Premium salmon burgers, 1 patty (91 g)	2
Trident Seafoods	
Alaskan salmon burgers, 1 burger (79 g)	3

Shrimp

	SmartPoints® value
Aquastar	
Cocktail shrimp, 8 shrimp (113 g)	2
Arctic Shores	
Peeled and deveined tail on frozen cooked shrimp, 13 shrimp (85 g)	1
Barilla	
Medium large shrimp, 3 oz	1
Daily Chef	
Cooked medium shrimp, 3 oz	1
Uncooked jumbo shrimp, 4 oz	0
Gorton's	
Shrimp, grilled, classic grilled, 8 shrimp (113 g)	2
Kirkland Signature	
Cooked tail on shrimp, 3 oz	1
Raw tail on shrimp, 4 oz	1
Kroger	
Cooked shrimp, 5 shrimp (85 g)	1
Medium cooked shrimp, 11 shrimp (85 g)	1
Shrimp, cocktail, peeled & deveined, with sauce, 9 shrimp (85 g)	2
Sea Pak Shrimp Company	
Popcorn shrimp, 14 shrimp (70 g)	6
Sea Queen	
Jumbo cooked shrimp, 4 oz	1
Medium raw shrimp, 4 oz	1
Trader Joe's	
Medium cooked shrimp, 3 oz	1
Trader Joe's Frozen	
Shrimp stir fry, 1¾ cups	2
Wellsley Farms	
Extra jumbo cooked shrimp, 4 shrimp (85 g)	1

Swai

	SmartPoints® value
Safeway Kitchens	
Boneless and skinless swai fillets, ¼ pound (113.5 g)	1
Simply Balanced	
Swai fillets, 4 oz	1
Valu Time	
Swai fillets, 4 oz	1

Tilapia

	SmartPoints® value
Cape Gourmet	
Tilapia fillets, 4 oz	1
Daily Chef	
Parmesan encrusted tilapia, 3½ oz	6
Fishin'	
Tilapia fillets, 4 oz	1
Gorton's	
Battered, skillet crisp tilapia, 1 fillet (99 g)	6
Tilapia with signature seasoning, 1 fillet (128 g)	2
Tilapia, grilled, roasted garlic & butter, 1 fillet (89 g)	1
Tilapia, grilled, signature grilled, 1 fillet (89 g)	1
High Liner	
Basil pesto tilapia, 1 fillet (101 g)	2
Tortilla crusted tilapia, 1 fillet (105 g)	4

	SmartPoints® value
Morey's	
Cajun tilapia, 5 oz	5
Publix	
Tilapia fillets, 3 oz	1
Sea Cuisine	
Mango habanero tilapia, 1 fillet (126 g)	2
Pan sear garlic and herb tilapia, 1 fillet (126 g)	5
Parmesan crusted tilapia, 1 fillet (140 g)	7
Tilapia, 1 piece (112 g)	2
Tortilla crusted tilapia, 1 fillet (140 g)	6
Sea Queen	
Tilapia fillets, 4 oz	1
Trident	
Panko breaded tilapia, 4 oz	6
Trident Seafoods	
Tilapia burgers, 1 burger (79 g)	1
Van de Kamp's	
Parmesan and roasted garlic tilapia, 1 fillet (141 g)	7

Trout

Trader Joe's	
Smoked rainbow trout fillets, 2 oz	2

Tuna

	SmartPoints® value
365 Everyday Value	
Chunk white albacore tuna in water (no salt added), 2 oz	1
Bumble Bee	
Chunk light tuna in water, ¼ cup	0
Chunk white albacore tuna in water, 2 oz drained	1
Jalapeño seasoned tuna, 1 pouch (71 g)	1
Solid white albacore tuna in water, ¼ cup	1
Spicy Thai chili seasoned tuna, 1 pouch (71 g)	2
Sun-dried tomato & basil seasoned tuna, 1 pouch (71 g)	1
Tuna, chunk light, in water, 2 oz	0
Tuna, premium albacore, in water, ¼ cup	1
Chicken of the Sea	
Chunk light tuna in water, ¼ cup	0
Tuna, albacore, solid white, in water, ¼ cup	1
Chicken of the Sea Chunk Light	
Albacore tuna in water, ¼ cup drained	0
Tuna, in water, ¼ cup	0
Daily Chef	
Center cut ahi tuna steak, 4 oz	1
Solid white albacore tuna in water, ¼ cup	1
Genova Tonno	
Solid light tuna in olive oil, ¼ cup	2
Hawaiian Select	
Ahi tuna steak, 1 piece (113 g)	1
Kirkland	
Signature solid white albacore tuna packed in water, ¼ cup	1
Kroger	
Ranch flavor tuna, 1 pouch (70 g)	2
Sweet and spicy tuna, 1 package (70 g)	1
Tuna, chunk light, in water, 2 oz	1
Northern Catch	
Premium original chunk light tuna in water, 2½ oz	1
Zesty lemon pepper chunk light tuna in water, 1 pouch (71 g)	1
Omaha Steaks	
Ahi tuna steaks, 6 oz	2
Orca Bay	
Ahi tuna, wild caught, 4 oz	1

Tuna (cont'd)

	SmartPoints® value
StarKist	
Albacore white tuna in water single serve, 1 pouch (74 g)	1
Chunk white albacore in water, ¼ cup drained	0
Low sodium chunk white tuna in water, 1 pouch (74 g)	0
Solid white albacore tuna in water, 1 can (85 g)	1
Solid white albacore tuna in water, 2 oz	1
Tuna, chunk light, in water, 1 pouch (74 g)	0
Tuna, chunk light, in water, ¼ cup	0
Tuna, chunk light, in water, 2 oz	1
Tuna, premium chunk light, in water, flavor fresh pouch, 1 pouch (85 g)	1
Tuna, solid white albacore, in water, ¼ cup	1
Tuna, white albacore, white, 2 oz	1
Tuna, white, albacore, low sodium, in water, 1 pouch (74 g)	1
Starkist Flavor Fresh Pouch	
Chunk light tuna in water, ¼ cup	1
StarKist Gourmet Selects	
Mexican style tuna, 1 pouch (74 g)	2
Thai style tuna, 1 pouch (74 g)	4
StarKist Kid's Creations	
Bacon ranch lightly marinated chunk light tuna, 1 pouch (74 g)	2
Honey bbq lightly marinated chunk light tuna, 1 pouch (74 g)	2
StarKist Lunch-To-Go	
Tuna kit, chunk light, in water, 1 kit (116 g)	7

	SmartPoints® value
StarKist Tuna Creations	
Hot buffalo style chunk light tuna, 1 pouch (74 g)	1
Ranch flavor chunk light tuna, 1 pouch (74 g)	1
Tuna, chunk light, herb & garlic, single serve, 1 pouch (74 g)	2
Tuna, chunk light, hickory smoked, single serve, 1 pouch (74 g)	2
Tuna, chunk light, sweet & spicy, single serve, 1 pouch (74 g)	2
Tuna, chunk light, zesty lemon pepper, single serve, 1 pouch (74 g)	1
Trader Joe's	
Half salt albacore solid white tuna in water, 2 oz drained	1
No salt added albacore tuna in water, ¼ cup	1
Tuna burgers, 1 burger (91 g)	4
Wegman's	
Tuna, solid white albacore, in water, ¼ cup	1
Wild Planet	
Tuna, wild albacore, 2 oz	2
WinCo Foods	
Chunk light tuna, ¼ cup	0

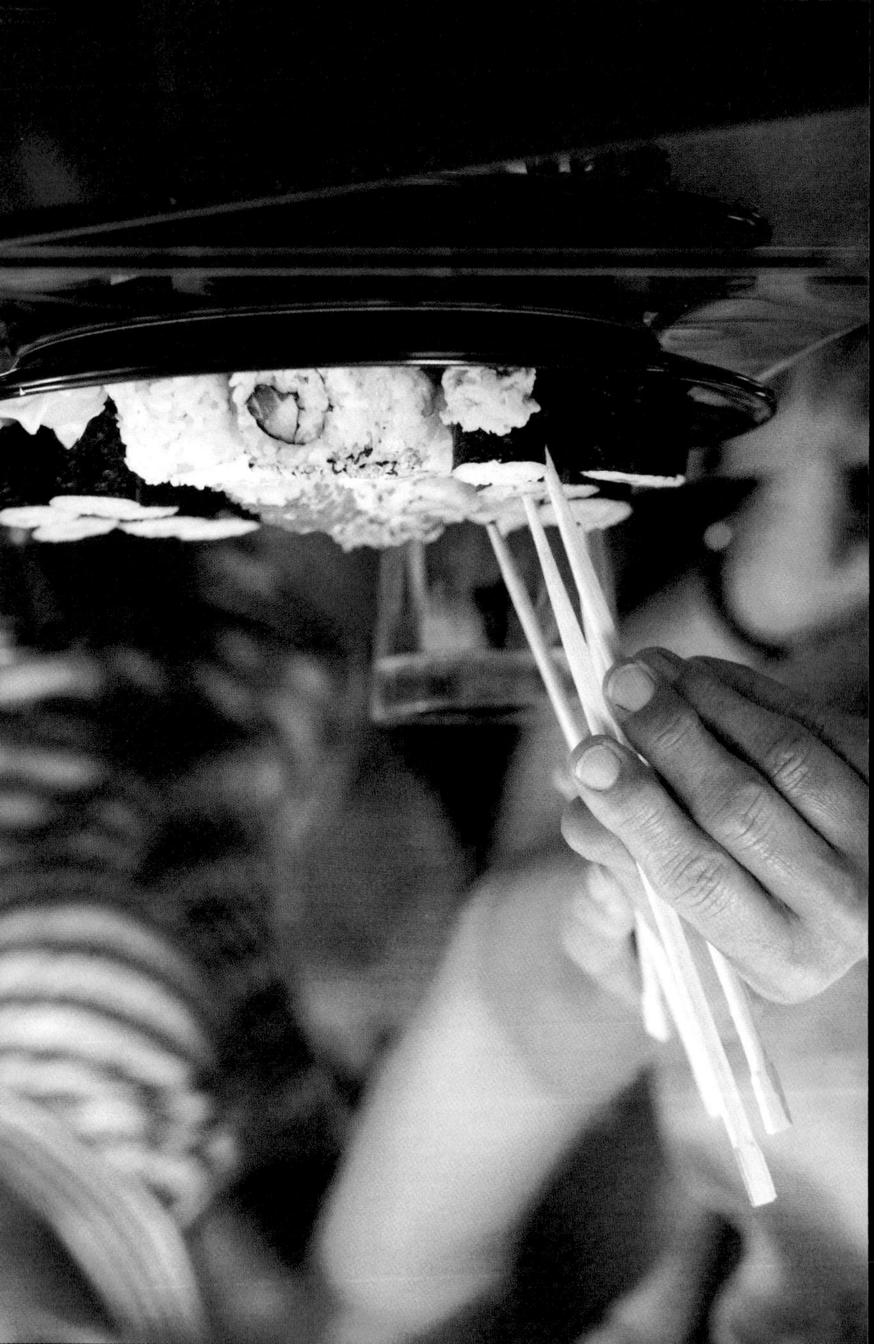

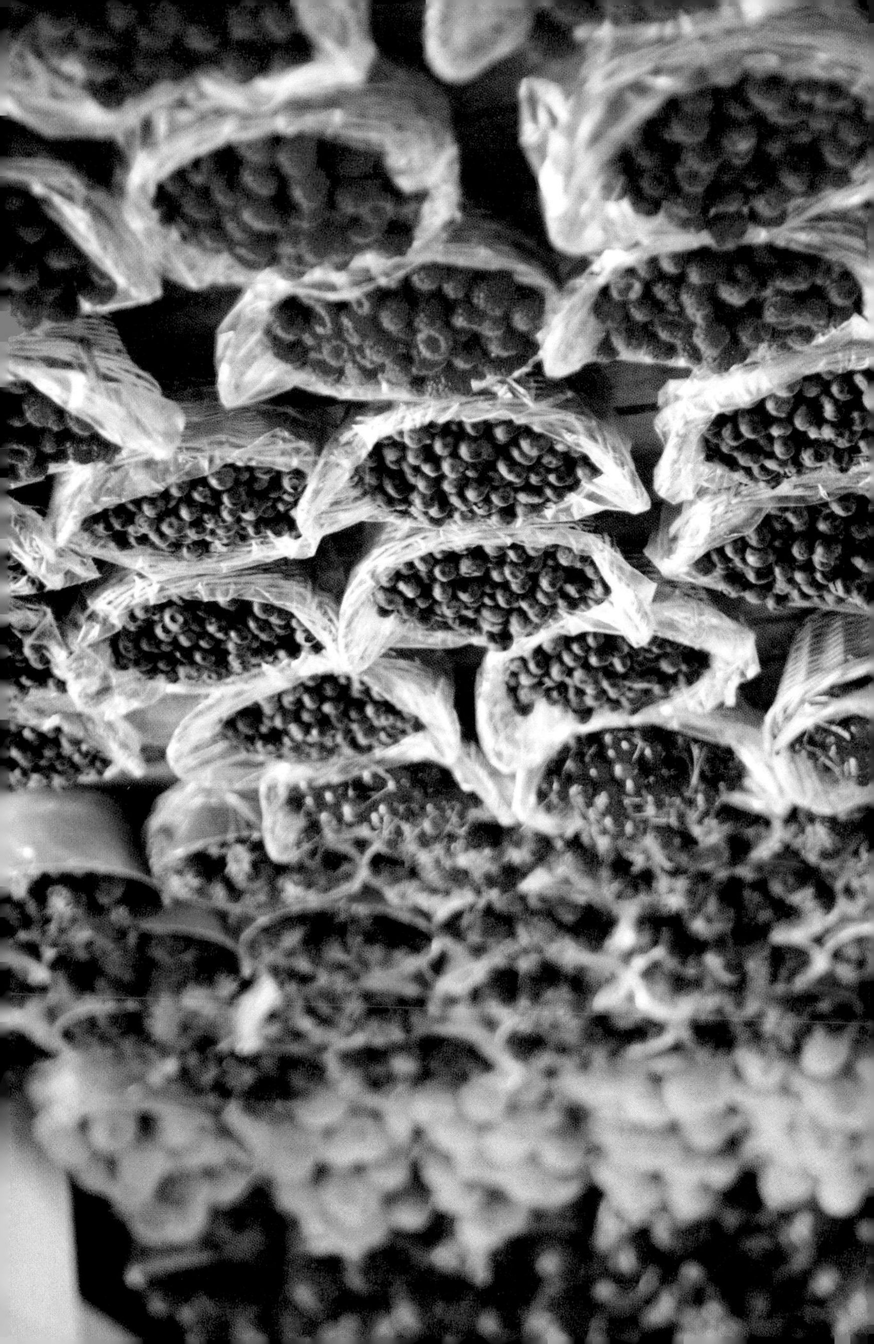

fruits

	SmartPoints® value
Acai	
Sambazon	
Acai superfruit packs, 1 pack (100 g)	5
Applesauce	
Great Value	
Natural unsweetened applesauce, 1 container (113 g)	0
Unsweetened apple sauce, 1 container (113 g)	0
Unsweetened apple sauce, ½ cup	0
Kirkland Signature	
Apple sauce no sugar added (gluten free), 1 pouch (90 g)	0
Kroger	
Cinnamon applesauce, ½ cup	5
Market Pantry	
Applesauce, 4 oz	2
Materne Gogo Squeez	
Apple cinnamon applesauce, 1 pouch (90 g)	3
Mott's	
Apple sauce, cinnamon, ½ cup	7
Apple sauce, original, ½ cup	6
Applesauce, original, 1 container (113 g)	6
Natural applesauce, ½ cup	0
Natural applesauce (individual containers), 1 container (111 g)	0
Mott's Healthy Harvest	
Blueberry delight naturally flavored applesauce, 1 container (111 g)	0
Granny smith flavored applesauce no sugar added, 1 container (111 g)	0
Summer strawberry applesauce, 1 container (111 g)	0
Mott's Organic	
Applesauce no sugar added, 1 container (111 g)	0

	SmartPoints® value
Musselman's	
Apple sauce, lite, cinnamon, 4 oz	0
Apple sauce, natural, unsweetened, big cup, 1 container (170 g)	0
Apple sauce, unsweetened, natural, 4 oz	0
Simply Balanced	
Organic unsweetened applesauce, 1 serving (113 g)	0
Tree Top	
Apple sauce, no sugar added, ½ cup	0
Bananas	
Dole	
Banana dippers, dark chocolate, 4 slices (44 g)	5
Berries	
Daily Chef	
Antioxidant berry blend, 1 cup	4
Dole Wildly Nutritious Signature Blends	
Cherry berry blend frozen fruit, 1 cup	0
Driscoll's	
Raspberries, 1 cup	0
Great Value	
Berry medley, no sugar added, 1 cup	0
Kirkland Signature	
Frozen strawberries, 1 cup	0
Organic blueberries, 1 cup	0
Kirkland Signature Rader Farms	
Nature's three berries raspberries, blueberries and blackberries, 1 cup	0
Market Pantry	
Triple berry fruit blend (fresh frozen), 1 cup	0
Private Selection	
Triple berry medley, 1 cup	0

	SmartPoints® value
Publix	
Blackberries, lush & plump, 1 cup	0
Triple berry, 1 cup	0
Starbucks Coffee	
Fresh blueberries, 1 cup	0
Trader Joe's Frozen	
Organic mixed berry blend, ¾ cup	0
Very cherry berry blend, 1 cup	0
Welch's	
Four berry frozen fruit mix, 1 cup	0
Wyman's	
Fresh frozen mixed berries, ¾ cup	0
Wild blueberries, fresh frozen, 1 cup	0
Wyman's of Maine	
Fresh frozen strawberries blueberries cherries with kale, 1 cup	0

Cherries

Dole	
Dark sweet pitted cheeries, 1 cup	0
Giant	
Dark sweet cherries, 1 cup	0
Trader Joe's	
Pitted dark sweet cherries (fresh frozen), ⅔ cup	0

Clementines

Cuties	
California clementines, 1 clementine (74 g)	0
Produce Partners	
Clementines, 2 clementines (148 g)	0

Cranberries

Paradise Meadow	
Fresh cranberries, ½ cup	0

Fruit Cocktail and Salad

	SmartPoints® value
Del Monte	
Cherry mixed fruit cups, 1 cup	4
Fruit cocktail, no sugar added, ½ cup	0
Lite mixed fruit, ½ cup	3
Mixed fruit, no sugar added, 1 cup	0
Del Monte No Sugar Added	
Very cherry mixed fruit, ½ cup	0
Dole	
Cherry mixed fruit no sugar added, 1 container (113 g)	0
Mixed fruit, ¾ cup	0
Mixed fruit, in cherry gel, sugar free gel, 1 container (123 g)	2
Dole Fruit & Veggie Blends	
Fruit n greens (mangos bananas apples pineapples and spinach), ¾ cup	0
Orange medley frozen fruit and vegetables, ¾ cup	0
Dole Wildly Nutritious	
Mixed fruit, 1 cup	0
Giant	
Tropical fruit medley, 1¼ cups	4
Great Value	
Lite fruit cocktail, 4½ oz	3
Tropical fruit mix pineapple mango strawberries and papaya (no sugar added), 1 cup	0
Great Value Fruit selections	
Mixed fruit, 1 bowl (108 g)	0
Market Pantry	
Mango fruit blend, 1 cup	0
Our Family Fresh Frozen	
Mixed fruit, 1 cup	0
Private Selection	
Fruit blend, for smoothies, ¾ cup	0
Publix	
Mixed fruit, ¾ cup	0

Fruit Cocktail and Salad (cont'd)

	SmartPoints® value
Signature Café	
Fresh mixed fruit, 1½ cups	0
Simple Truth Organic	
Frozen mixed fruit medley, 1 cup	0
Wawona Frozen Foods	
Daybreak blend organic mixed fruit, 1 cup	4
Festival blend frozen fruit, 1 cup	0

Fruit, Dried

	SmartPoints® value
Craisins	
Original dried cranberries, 1 oz	5
Fresh Gourmet	
Cranberries, 1 Tbsp	1
Great Value	
Dried apples, ½ cup	6
Happy Valley Farms	
Dried mangoes, 1½ oz	8
Kirkland Signature Sunsweet	
Dried plums, 5 dried plums (40 g)	5
Market Pantry	
California raisins, 1 oz	5
Navitas Naturals	
Goji berries, sun-dried, organic, 1 oz	4
Ocean Spray Craisins	
Cranberries, sweetened dried, original, ⅓ cup	7
Dried cranberries, original, ⅓ cup	7
Dried cranberries, sweetened, reduced sugar, ¼ cup	5
Reduced sugar dried cranberries, ¼ cup	5
Sweetened dried cranberries, ⅓ cup	7
Paradise Meadow	
Organic plump whole dried cranberries, ⅓ cup	7
Publix	
Sweetened dried cranberries, ¼ cup	7
Southern Grove	
Pitted prunes, 1 oz	3
Sun Date	
California medjool dates, 3 pieces (40 g)	7
Sun-Maid	
Raisins, natural California, 1 box (28 g)	5
Sun-Maid Mini-Snacks	
Natural California raisins, 1 box (14 g)	3
Sunsweet	
Pitted prunes, 5 prunes (40 g)	5
Prunes, pitted, bite size, petite, 7 prunes (40 g)	5
Sunsweet Gold Label	
Prunes, pitted dried plums, ones, 4 prunes (40 g)	4
Sunsweet Ones	
California prunes, 4 prunes (40 g)	5
Tropical Fields	
Mixed fruit chips, 1 serving (30 g)	7

Grapefruit

Del Monte Fruit Naturals	
Red grapefruit, no sugar added, 1 container (184 g)	0
Del Monte Sun Fresh	
No sugar added red grapefruit, ½ cup	0
Kirkland Signature	
Red grapefruit pieces, ½ cup	3

Grapes

Columbine Vineyards	
Black seedless grapes, ¾ cup	0

Mangoes

Great Value	
Frozen mango chunks, 1 cup	0

	SmartPoints® value
Oranges	
Del Monte No Sugar Added	
Mandarin oranges, in water, no sugar added, 1 container (113 g)	0
Dole	
Mandarin oranges, no sugar added, 1 container (113 g)	0
Peaches	
Del Monte	
No sugar added California sliced peaches, ½ cup	0
Peaches diced in light syrup, 1 cup	4
Del Monte Fruit Naturals	
Peach, yellow cling, chunks, no sugar added, 1 container (184 g)	0
Del Monte No Sugar Added	
Peaches, California, diced, no sugar added, 1 container (106 g)	0
Dole	
Peaches, diced, yellow cling, no sugar added, 1 container (113 g)	0
Pears	
Del Monte	
Pears, diced, in water, no sugar added, 1 cup	0
Del Monte No Sugar Added	
Pears, northwest, sliced, no sugar added, ½ cup	0

	SmartPoints® value
Pineapple	
Dole	
Pineapple tidbits, 1 container (113 g)	2
Pineapple tidbits, in 100% pineapple juice, 1 container (113 g)	3
Dole Dippers	
Pineapple covered in dark chocolate, 1 pouch (30 g)	4
Dole Tropical Gold	
Pineapple chunks, ¾ cup	0
Kirkland Signature	
Frozen golden sweet pineapple chunks, ¾ cup	0
Libby's Skinny Fruits	
Pineapple, chunk, ½ cup	0
Sweet Harvest	
Crushed pineapple, ½ cup	0
Trader Joe's Frozen	
Pineapple tidbits, 1 cup	0
Tangerines	
Halos	
California mandarins, 1 small (76 g)	0

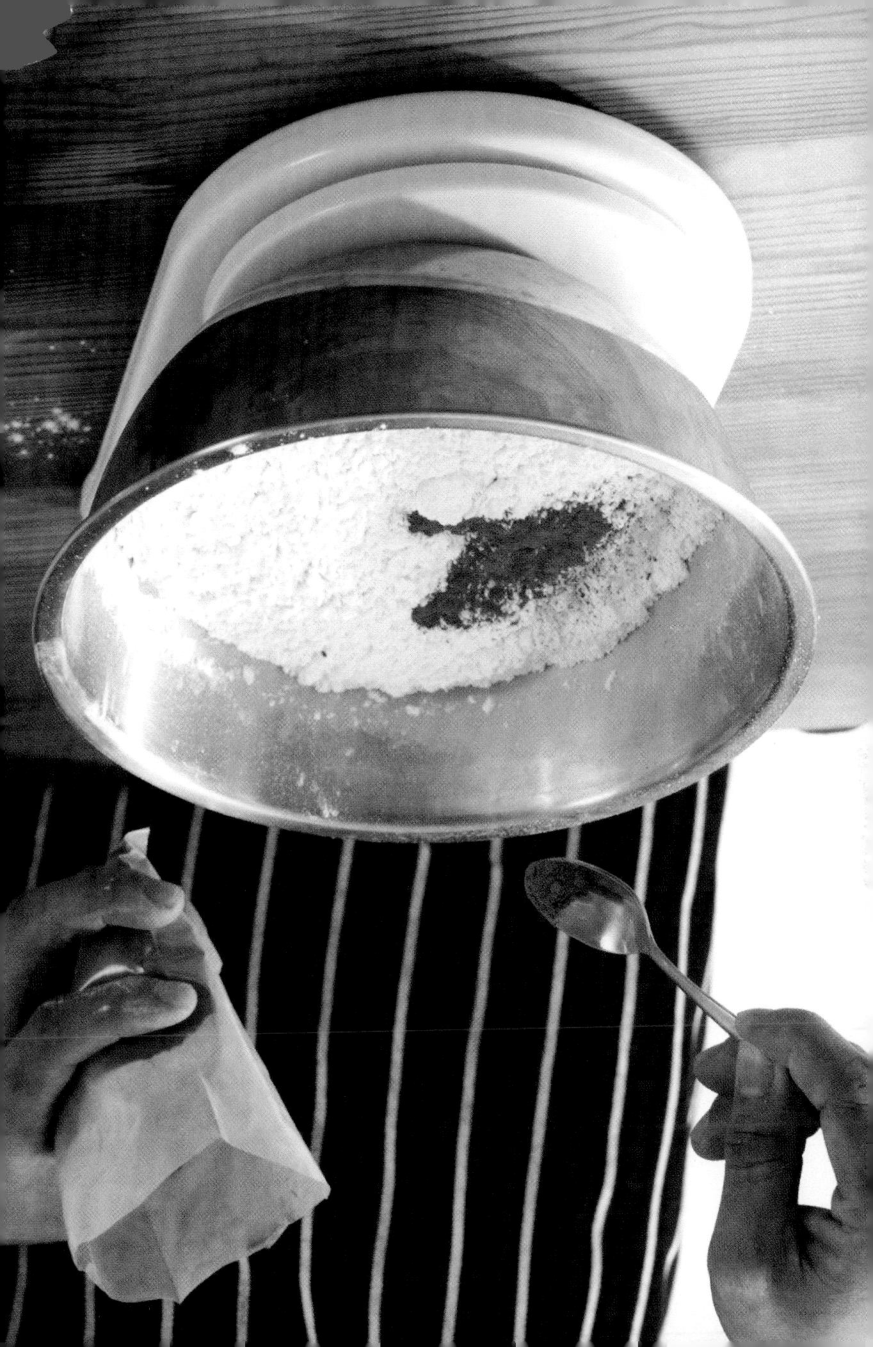

ingredients

	SmartPoints® value
Almond Meal/Flour	
Bob's Red Mill	
Almond meal/flour, finely ground, ¼ cup	5
Baking Mixes	
Baker's Corner	
Extra moist classic white cake mix (unprepared), ⅓ cup	7
Pumpkin quick bread and muffin mix (unprepared), ¼ cup	6
Betty Crocker	
Angel food cake mix (serves 12), 1 serving (38 g)	7
Brownie mix, fudge brownies, unprepared, 1 serving (26 g)	5
Chocolate chip cookie mix, 3 Tbsp	6
Betty Crocker Super Moist	
Cake mix, spice, 1 serving (43 g)	7
Strawberry cake mix (serves 10), 1 serving (43 g)	7
Bisquick	
Baking mix, original all-purpose, ⅓ cup	5
Pancake and baking mix, ⅓ cup	4
Pancake and baking mix, heart smart, ⅓ cup	4
CB Old Country Store	
Buttermilk baking and pancake mix (unprepared), ⅓ cup	6
Duncan Hines Decadent	
German chocolate cake mix (serves 12), 1 serving (50 g)	10
Fleischmann's Simply Homemade	
Raspberry muffin and bread mix specially for Greek yogurt (unprepared), 3 Tbsp	5

	SmartPoints® value
Ghirardelli	
Brownie mix, triple fudge, 3 Tbsp dry	7
Ghirardelli Chocolate	
Triple chocolate brownie mix, ¼ cup	7
Jiffy	
Corn muffin mix, ¼ cup	6
Kroger	
White cake mix (unprepared), ⅓ cup	7
Krusteaz	
Pumpkin spice bread mix with latte glaze (unprepared), ¼ cup	7
Mam Papaul's	
Cake mix, mardi gras king, 3 ½ oz	14
Marie Callender's	
Cranberry orange muffin mix (unprepared), 1 cup	5
Martha White	
Cinnamon biscuit mix (unprepared), ⅓ cup	8
Cornbread mix (unprepared), 1 oz	3
Pumpkin spice muffin mix (unprepared), ¼ cup	6
Medifast	
Chocolate chip pancakes, 1 packet (31 g)	3
Morrison's	
Texas style honey sweet cornbread mix (unprepared), ¼ cup	5
Pillsbury	
Chocolate fudge brownie mix family size(serves 20), 1 serving (26 g)	5

	SmartPoints® value
Pillsbury Funfetti	
Cake & cupcake mix, premium, with candy bits, happy birthday!, unprepared, 1 serving (43 g)	8
Pillsbury Moist Supreme	
Cake mix, premium, sugar free, classic yellow (serves 12), 1 serving (38 g)	3
Pillsbury Purely Simple	
Chocolate chunk brownie mix (unprepared), 1 oz	6
Planters	
Oatmeal raisin cookie mix, 3 Tbsp	6

Chocolate and Candy, Baking

	SmartPoints® value
Baker's Corner	
Milk chocolate morsels, 1 Tbsp	4
Mini real semi sweet chocolate morsels, 132 morsels (15 g)	4
Enjoy Life	
Chocolate chips, semi-sweet, ½ oz	4
Ghirardelli	
60% cacao bittersweet chocolate premium baking chips, 16 chips (15 g)	4
Baking chips, premium, bittersweet chocolate, 16 chips (15 g)	4
Baking chips, premium, milk chocolate, 16 chips (15 g)	4
Baking chips, premium, mini, semi-sweet chocolate, 115 chips (15 g)	4
Baking chips, premium, semi-sweet chocolate, 32 chips (15 g)	4
Bittersweet chocolate premium baking chips, 16 chips (15 g)	4
Great Value	
Semi sweet chocolate chips, 1 Tbsp	4
Guittard	
Chocolate chips, 63% cacao, extra dark, 30 pieces (15 g)	4
Hershey's	
Cocoa, 100% cacao, special dark, 1 Tbsp	0
Natural unsweetened cocoa, 1 Tbsp	0
Hershey's Special Dark	
Mildly sweet chocolate chips, 1 Tbsp	4
Lily's	
Dark chocolate premium baking chips, 60 chips (14 g)	2
M&M's Minis	
Chocolate candy baking bits, 1 Tbsp	4
Navitas Naturals	
Cacao powder, 2 ½ Tbsp	2
Toll House	
Morsels, dark chocolate, 53% cacao, 1 Tbsp	4
Morsels, milk chocolate, 1 Tbsp	4
Original semi-sweet morsels, 1 Tbsp	4
Semi sweet chocolate morsels, 1 Tbsp	4
Toll House Mini	
Semi-sweet chocolate morsels, 1 Tbsp	4

Coconut

Great Value	
Sweetened coconut flakes, 2 Tbsp	4

	SmartPoints® value
Crumb and Coating Mixes	
Great Value	
Plain panko bread crumbs, ½ cup	3
Kraft Shake 'N Bake	
Original chicken seasoned coating mix, ⅛ packet (8 g)	1
Progresso	
Italian style bread crumbs, ¼ cup	3
Publix	
Original style bread crumbs, ¼ cup	3
Shake N Bake	
Coating mix, seasoned, extra crispy, ⅛ packet (9 g)	1
Ranch and herb seasoned coating mix, ⅛ packet (8 g)	1
Flaxseed Meal	
Bob's Red Mill	
Flaxseed meal, whole ground, 2 Tbsp	2
Whole ground golden flaxseed meal, 2 Tbsp	2
Bob's Red Mill Organic	
Flaxseed meal, golden, 100% whole ground, 2 Tbsp	2
Flour	
Great Value	
All purpose flour, ¼ cup	3
Honey	
Really Raw	
Honey, 1 Tbsp	4
Thrifty Bee	
Dark and robust honey, 1 Tbsp	4
Trader Joe's Grocery	
Organic raw honey, 1 Tbsp	4

	SmartPoints® value
Pie Filling	
Great Value	
Cherry pie filling, ⅓ cup	5
Pie/Pastry Dough and Crusts	
Boboli	
Pizza crust, mini 8", ½ shell (71 g)	6
Pizza crust, thin, 1 serving (47 g)	4
Brooklyn Bred	
Ancient grains pizza crust, ¼ crust (57 g)	4
Goya	
Para empanadas dough, 1 serving (40 g)	4
Great Value	
Pizza crust dough (serves 6), 1 piece (65 g)	5
Hospitality	
Ready to eat graham cracker pie crust, ⅛ crust (21 g)	4
Mama Mary's	
Pizza crusts, thin & crispy, 7", ½ pizza crust (43 g)	4
Pillsbury	
Pizza crust, classic, 1 serving (65 g)	5
Pizza crust, thin (serves 5), 1 serving (62 g)	5
Wholly Wholesome	
9 pie shells, ⅛ crust (25 g)	3
Seasonings, Herbs, and Spices, Dried	
Kraft Shake 'N Bake	
Pork seasoned coating mix, ⅛ packet (9 g)	1
McCormick Original	
Taco seasoning mix, 2 tsp	1

	SmartPoints® value
Old El Paso	
Seasoning mix, taco, 2 tsp	0
Seasoning mix, taco, original, 2 tsp	0
Ortega	
Taco seasoning mix (serves 6), 1 serving (6 g)	1
Tajin	
Seasoning, clasico, with lime, ¼ tsp	0

Sugar and Sugar Substitutes

Agave in the Raw	
Agave nectar, organic, 1 Tbsp	4
Born Sweet	
Stevia and cane sugar baking blend, ½ tsp	0
Born Sweet Zing	
Zero calorie stevia sweetener, 1 packet (1 g)	0
C&H	
Pure cane sugar cubes, 1 cube (4 g)	1
Pure cane sugar, individual packets, 1 packet (4 g)	1
Domino	
Brown sugar, light, 1 tsp	1
Sugar, premium, granulated, pure cane, 1 tsp	1
Domino Dots	
Sugar cubes, premium pure cane sugar, 1 cube (2 g)	1
Equal	
Artificial sweetener, 1 tsp	0
Original zero calorie sweetener, 1 packet (1 g)	0
Sweetener, 0 calorie, 1 packet (1 g)	0

	SmartPoints® value
Florida Crystals	
Demerara sugar, 1 tsp	1
Organic cane sugar, 1 tsp	1
Great Value	
Confectioner's powdered sugar, ¼ cup	7
No calorie stevia, 1 tsp	0
No calorie sweetener, 1 packet (1 g)	0
Pure sugar, 1 tsp	1
Stevia, ¾ tsp	0
Kirkland Signature	
Fine granulated organic sugar, 1 tsp	1
Madhava	
Agave nectar, light, 1 Tbsp	4
Coconut sugar, organic, 1 tsp	1
McCormick	
Cinnamon sugar, 1 tsp	1
Monk Fruit In The Raw	
All natural sugar substitute, 1 packet (0.8 g)	0
PureVia	
Stevia, 1 packet (1 g)	0
Pyure	
Organic stevia sweetener, 1 packet (1 g)	0
Splenda	
Brown sugar blend, ½ tsp	1
Granulated no calorie sweetener, 1 tsp	0
No calorie sweetener, granulated, 1 tsp	0
Splenda 1 Gram of Fiber	
No calorie sweetener, granulated, 1 tsp	0
Splenda Packets	
No calorie sweetener, 1 packet (1 g)	0

Sugar and Sugar Substitutes (cont'd)

	SmartPoints® value
Splenda Sugar Blend	
Mixed sweetener, ½ tsp	1
Stevia in the Raw	
Sweetener, zero calorie, 1 packet (1 g)	0
Sweetener, zero calorie, granulated, 1 tsp	0
Zero calorie sweetener, 1 packet (1 g)	0
Sugar in the Raw	
Natural cane turbinado sugar, 1 tsp	1
Organic white cane sugar, 1 tsp	1
Sugar in the raw, liquid, turbinado cane, 1 tsp	1
Turbinado cane sugar, 1 tsp	1
Turbinado sugar, natural cane, 1 tsp	1
Sweet Additions	
0 calorie sucralose sweetener, 1 packet (1 g)	0
Sweet 'N Low	
Granulated sugar substitute, 1 packet (1 g)	0
Sweetener, zero calorie, 1 packet (1 g)	0
Sweet'n low, 1 pack (1 g)	0
Trader Joe's	
Fair trade turbinado raw cane sugar, 1 tsp	1
Organic brown sugar, 1 tsp	1
Organic sugar (evaporated cane juice), 1 tsp	1
Truvia	
Baking blend, ½ tsp	0
Natural sweetener with brown sugar blend, ½ tsp	0
Sweetener, calorie-free, ¾ tsp	0
Sweetener, calorie-free, 1 packet (4 g)	0

	SmartPoints® value
Wholesome Sweeteners	
Coconut palm sugar, organic, 1 tsp	1
Organic blue agave nectar, 1 Tbsp	4

Syrup

Aunt Jemima	
Original lite syrup, ¼ cup	6
Original syrup, ¼ cup	10
Syrup, butter lite, ¼ cup	6
Aunt Maple's	
Lite syrup, ¼ cup	7
Cary's	
Syrup, sugar free, artificial maple flavor, ¼ cup	1
Great Value	
Syrup, sugar free, chocolate flavored, 2 Tbsp	0
Hershey's	
Lite chocolate syrup, 2 Tbsp	3
Syrup, caramel, 2 Tbsp	6
Syrup, chocolate flavor, 2 Tbsp	5
Syrup, sugar free, chocolate, 2 Tbsp	0
Hungry Jack Sugar Free	
Butter breakfast syrup, ¼ cup	1
IHOP At Home	
Sugar free syrup, ¼ cup	1
Kirkland Signature	
Grade A dark amber organic maple syrup, ¼ cup	12
Kroger	
Cinnamon maple pancake syrup, ¼ cup	11
Syrup, sugar free, ¼ cup	1

	SmartPoints® value
Log Cabin	
Lite syrup no high fructose corn syrup, ¼ cup	6
Original syrup, ¼ cup	9
Original syrup no high fructose corn syrup, ¼ cup	9
Syrup, sugar free, ¼ cup	1
Maple Grove Farms of Vermont	
Maple syrup, pure, ¼ cup	6
Syrup, sugar free, butter flavor, ¼ cup	1
Syrup, sugar free, maple flavor, ¼ cup	1
Market Pantry	
Sugar-free syrup in original flavour, ¼ cup	1
Mrs. Butterworth	
Original syrup, ¼ cup	11
Syrup, lite, ¼ cup	6
Syrup, sugar free, ¼ cup	1
Publix	
Sugar free syrup, ¼ cup	1
ShopRite	
Sugar free syrup, ¼ cup	1
Smucker's	
Syrup, breakfast, sugar free, ¼ cup	1
Smucker's Sugar Free	
Sundae syrup, caramel, 2 Tbsp	3
Starbucks	
Starbucks syrup, vanilla, 2 Tbsp	4
Starbucks Grocery	
Sugar free vanilla syrup, 2 Tbsp	0

	SmartPoints® value
Torani	
Caramel sauce, 2 Tbsp	6
Chocolate sauce, 2 Tbsp	5
Flavoring syrup, sugar free, classic caramel, 2 Tbsp	0
Flavoring syrup, sugar free, classic hazelnut, 2 Tbsp	0
Flavoring syrup, sugar free, vanilla, 2 Tbsp	0
Sugar free French vanilla syrup, 2 Tbsp	0
Syrup, vanilla, 1 oz	4
Syrup, vanilla, sugar free, 1 oz	0
Vermont	
Low calorie syrup, sugar free, ¼ cup	0
Walden Farms	
Flavored chocolate syrup, 2 Tbsp	0
Syrup, pancake, ¼ cup	0
Wellsley Farms	
Organic 100% pure maple syrup, ¼ cup	12

Yeast

Bragg	
Premium nutritional yeast seasoning, 1 Tbsp	0
Red Star	
Nutritional yeast, 1½ Tbsp	1

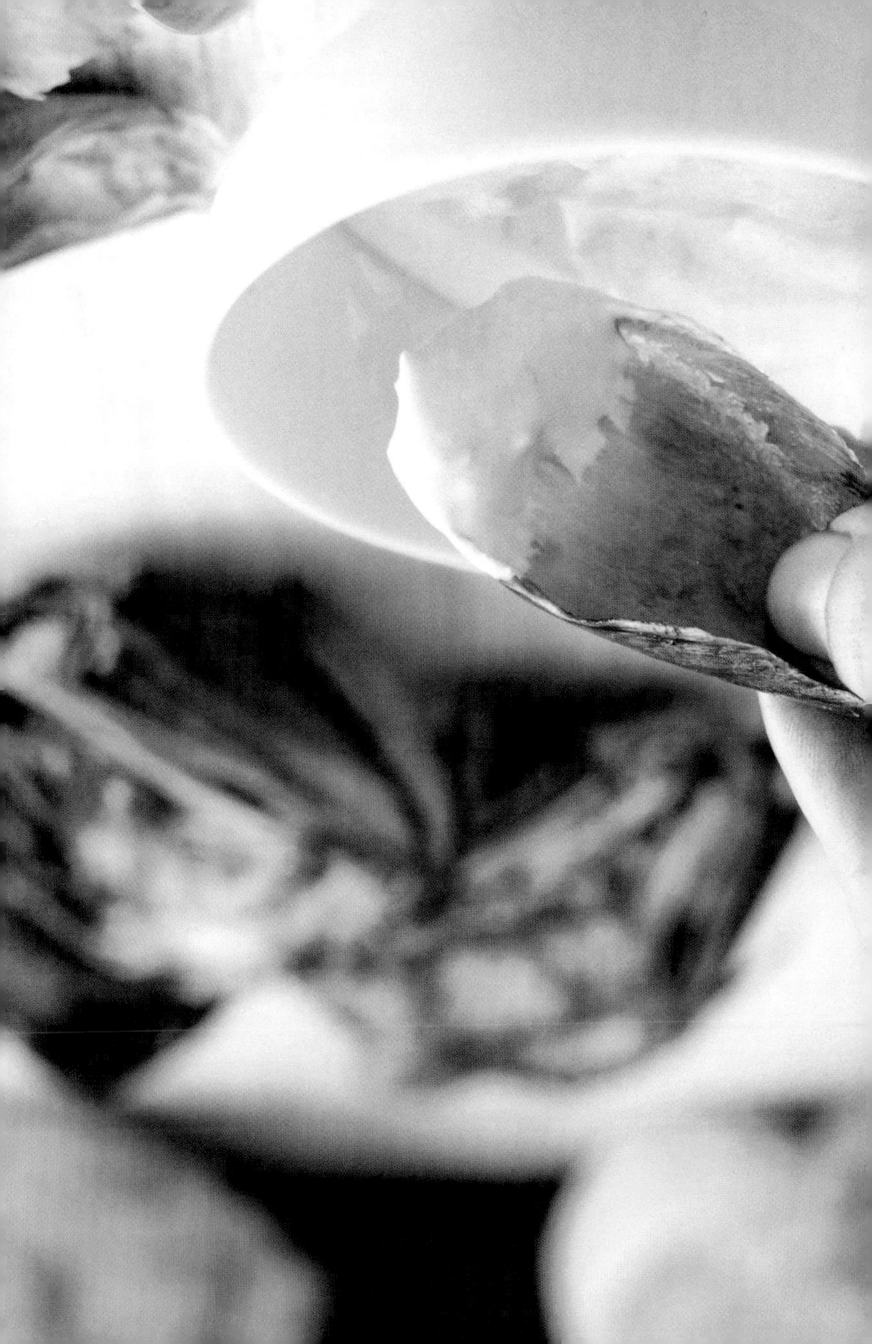

jams, spreads, salsa & dips

Dips

	SmartPoints® value
Bubba's Back 9 Dips	
Chicken dip, buffalo blue cheese, 2 oz	3
Cedar's	
Cucumber garlic tzatziki, 2 Tbsp	1
Cheez Whiz	
Dip, cheese, original, 2 Tbsp	3
Daily Chef	
Raspberry chipotle dip, 2 Tbsp	4
Dean's	
French onion dip, 2 Tbsp	3
Fountain of Health	
Baba gannouj, 2 Tbsp	2
Friendly Farms	
Dill and cucumber Greek yogurt dip, 2 Tbsp	2
Jalapeño Greek yogurt dip, 2 Tbsp	2
Fritos	
Original flavor bean dip, 2 Tbsp	1
Good Foods	
Feta cucumber dip with Greek yogurt, 2 Tbsp	2
Hannah	
Tzatziki yogurt dip with Greek yogurt, 1 Tbsp	1
Hannah Organic	
Tzatziki Greek style yogurt dip, 2 Tbsp	2
Heluva Good!	
French onion sour cream dip, 2 Tbsp	2
Hidden Valley	
Dips mix, the original ranch, 1 serving (2 g)	0
Hy-Vee	
Ranch dip, 2 Tbsp	5
Kraft	
Dip, creamy ranch, 2 Tbsp	3

	SmartPoints® value
Kroger	
Medium Monterey Jack queso cheese dip, 2 Tbsp	2
La Terra Fina	
Spinach, artichoke and parmesan dip, 2 Tbsp	3
Lay's	
French onion dip, 2 Tbsp	2
Lipton Recipe Secrets	
Onion recipe soup and dip mix, 1 Tbsp	1
Marketside	
Spinach dip, 2 Tbsp	3
Marzetti	
Caramel apple-dip, light, 2 Tbsp	5
Dill veggie dip, 2 Tbsp	4
Fruit-dip, cream cheese, 2 Tbsp	4
Light dill veggie dip, 2 Tbsp	2
Light ranch veggie dip, 2 Tbsp	2
Ranch veggie dip, 2 Tbsp	4
Veggie-dip, fat free, ranch, 2 Tbsp	1
Opaa!	
Tzatziki Greek yogurt dip, 2 Tbsp	0
Opadipity by Litehouse	
Chipotle ranch Greek yogurt dip, 2 Tbsp	2
Cucumber dill Greek yogurt dip, 2 Tbsp	1
Otria	
Veggie dip, Greek yogurt, cucumber dill feta, 2 Tbsp	2
Veggie dip, Greek yogurt, garden herb ranch, 2 Tbsp	2
Pancho's	
White cheese dip, 1 oz	3
Publix Deli	
Buffalo style chicken breast dip, 2 Tbsp	1

	SmartPoints® value
Rojo's	
Black bean and cotija cheese 6 layer dip, 2 Tbsp	2
Sabra	
Babaganoush, 2 Tbsp	3
Cucumber dill tzatziki Greek yogurt dip, 2 Tbsp	2
Tzatziki cucumber dill Greek yogurt dip, 2 Tbsp	2
Skotidakis	
Jalapeño yogurt dip, 2 Tbsp	2
Mild jalapeño Greek yogurt dip, 2 Tbsp	2
Stonemill Kitchens	
Spinach & artichoke parmesan dip, 2 Tbsp	4
Spinach and artichoke parmesan dip, 2 Tbsp	2
Tostitos	
Dip, nacho cheese, medium, 1 cup	6
Queso blanco dip, 2 Tbsp	2
Salsa con queso, medium, 2 Tbsp	2
Trader Joe's	
Chunky artichoke and jalapeño dip, 2 Tbsp	2
Jalapeño Greek yogurt dip, 2 Tbsp	2
Muhammara dip, 2 Tbsp	4
Spinach and artichoke dip, 2 Tbsp	2
Trader Joe's Grocery	
Fat free spicy black bean dip, 2 Tbsp	1
Trader Joe's Refrigerated	
Cilantro & chive yogurt dip, 1 oz	2
Reduced guilt spinach and kale Greek yogurt dip, 1 oz	2
Velveeta	
Salsa con queso cheese dip, 2 Tbsp	3

Fruit butter

	SmartPoints® value
Musselman's	
Apple butter, 1 Tbsp	2

Guacamole

	SmartPoints® value
Cabo Fresh	
Classic mild guacamole, 1 cup	3
Guacamole, 2 Tbsp	2
Guacamole snack pack, 1 pack (57 g)	3
Calavo	
Guacamole, 2 Tbsp	1
GoodFoods Tableside	
Chunky guacamole with garlic onions and tomatoes, 2 Tbsp	1
Little Salad Bar	
Spicy guacamole, 2 Tbsp	2
Sabra	
Guacamole, 2 oz	3
Guacamole, classic, 2 Tbsp	2
Sabra Classic Singles	
Chunky guacamole, 2 oz	3
Trader Joe's	
Reduced guilt chunky guacamole with Greek yogurt, 2 Tbsp	1
Trader Joe's Reduced Guilt	
Chunky guacamole, 2 Tbsp	1
Wholly 100 Calorie Cups	
Guacamole, classic, minis, 1 cup	3
Guacamole, spicy, minis, 1 cup	3
Wholly 100 Calorie Snack Packs	
Classic flavor guacamole, 1 pouch (57 g)	3
Wholly Guacamole	
Guacamole dip, 2 Tbsp	2
Spicy homestyle minis guacamole dip, 1 serving (57 g)	3
Wholly Guacamole 100 Calories	
Spicy guacamole snack packs, 1 pouch (57 g)	3

Guacamole (cont'd)

	SmartPoints® value
Wholly Guacamole Minis	
100 calorie classic guacamole, 1 container (57 g)	3
Classic guacamole, 1 container (57 g)	3
Organic classic guacamole, 1 container (57 g)	3
Spicy guacamole, 1 container (57 g)	3
Yucatan	
Authentic guacamole, 2 Tbsp	2
Guacamole (gluten free), 1 container (57 g)	3

Hummus

	SmartPoints® value
Boar's Head	
Roasted chipotle pepper hummus, 2 Tbsp	2
Roasted red pepper hummus, 2 Tbsp	2
Cedar's	
Balsamic caramelized onion hommus, 2 Tbsp	2
Chipotle hommus, 2 Tbsp	1
Hommus, 2 Tbsp	2
Hommus, garlic lovers, 2 Tbsp	1
Hommus, red pepper, roasted, party size, 2 Tbsp	2
Original organic hummus, 2 Tbsp	2
Roasted red pepper hummus, 2 Tbsp	1
Cedar's All Natural	
Gluten free everything hommus, 2 Tbsp	2
Gluten free roasted red pepper hommus, 2 Tbsp	1
Eat Well Embrace Life	
Beet hummus, 2 Tbsp	2
Eat Well Enjoy Life	
Hummus, black bean, sweet & spicy, with spicy roasted corn relish topping, medium, 2 Tbsp	1
Hummus, edamame (baby soybean), with roasted red peppers and toasted sesame, 2 Tbsp	3
Hummus, spicy yellow lentil, with sunflower seeds and apricot, medium, 2 Tbsp	2
Hummus, tuscan white bean, with roasted pine nuts & herbs, 2 Tbsp	3
Garden Fresh Gourmet	
Original hummus, 2 Tbsp	2
Hannah	
Original hommus trio, 2 Tbsp	2
Hannah Organic Classic	
Hommus, 1 container (68 g)	5
Hannah Organic Singles	
Hommus, 2 Tbsp	2
Hope Foods Organic	
Spicy avocado hummus, 2 Tbsp	2
Joseph's	
Roasted red pepper hommus, 2 Tbsp	2
Little Salad Bar	
Roasted garlic hummus, 2 Tbsp	1
Three layer hummus, 2 Tbsp	1
Tomato & basil hummus, 2 Tbsp	2
Sabra	
Basil pesto hummus, 2 Tbsp	3
Classic hummus, 2 Tbsp	2
Classic hummus singles, 1 container (57 g)	5
Hummus with roasted pine nuts, 2 Tbsp	3
Hummus, luscious lemon, 2 Tbsp	2
Hummus, roasted garlic, 2 Tbsp	2

	SmartPoints® value
Hummus, roasted red pepper, 2 Tbsp	2
Olive tapenade hummus, 2 Tbsp	3
Roasted pine nut hummus, 2 Tbsp	3
Roasted red pepper hummus (single serve container), 1 container (57 g)	5
Spinach and artichoke hummus, 2 Tbsp	2
Sun dried tomatoes hummus, 2 Tbsp	2
Supremely spicy hummus, 2 Tbsp	2
Simple Enjoy	
Gluten free original hummus, 2 Tbsp	2
Simple Truth Organic	
Garlic hummus, 2 Tbsp	2
Roasted red pepper hummus, 2 Tbsp	2
Simply Balanced	
Organic roasted red pepper hummus, 2 Tbsp	2
Simply Enjoy	
Kalamata olive hummus, 2 Tbsp	2
Roasted garlic hummus, 2 Tbsp	1
Roasted red pepper hummus, 2 Tbsp	1
Spinach & artichoke hummus, 2 Tbsp	2
Taste of Inspirations	
All natural roasted red pepper hummus, 2 Tbsp	2
Roasted garlic hummus, 2 Tbsp	1
Trader Joe's	
Beet hummus, 2 Tbsp	2
Freshly made eggplant hummus, 2 Tbsp	1
Hummus dip, 2 Tbsp	2
Roasted garlic hummus dip, 2 Tbsp	1
Sriracha hummus, 2 Tbsp	2

	SmartPoints® value
Trader Joe's Refrigerated	
Mediterranean hummus, 1 oz	2
Tribe	
Everything hummus, 2 Tbsp	2
Hummus, roasted garlic, 2 Tbsp	1
Hummus, spicy red pepper, 2 Tbsp	2
Mediterranean style hummus, 2 Tbsp	2
Sweet roasted red pepper hummus, 2 Tbsp	1
Tribe Swirl	
Fiery sriracha hummus (gluten free), 2 Tbsp	2
Garlic and herb hummus, 2 Tbsp	2
Sweet red pepper hummus, 2 Tbsp	2
Wegman's	
Roasted red pepper hummus, 2 Tbsp	2

Jams, Jellies, and Preserves

365 Everyday Value	
Mixed berry conserve, 1 Tbsp	2
Berryhill	
Red raspberry preserves, 1 Tbsp	3
Bonne Maman	
Preserves, cherry, 1 Tbsp	3
Preserves, raspberry, 1 Tbsp	3
Preserves, strawberry, 1 Tbsp	3
Preserves, wild blueberry, 1 Tbsp	3
Bonnie's Jams	
Fig preserves jam, 1 Tbsp	1
E.D. Smith	
Black cherry raspberry blood orange spread, 1 Tbsp	1
Fit & Active	
Strawberry preserves, 1 Tbsp	0
Sugar free apricot preserves, 1 Tbsp	0

Jams, Jellies, and Preserves (cont'd)

	SmartPoints® value
Fit & Active Sugar Free	
Red raspberry preserves, 1 Tbsp	0
Great Value	
Concord grape jelly, 1 Tbsp	2
Red raspberry preserves, 1 Tbsp	2
Strawberry preserves, 1 Tbsp	2
Sugar free strawberry preserves, 1 Tbsp	0
Kirkland Signature	
Strawberry spread, 1 Tbsp	2
Kirkland Signature Organic	
Strawberry spread, 1 Tbsp	2
Kroger	
Strawberry jelly, 1 Tbsp	2
Market Pantry	
Sugar free red raspberry preserves, 1 Tbsp	0
Sugar free strawberry preserves, 1 Tbsp	0
Polaner	
Preserves, apricot, with fiber, sugar free, 1 Tbsp	0
Preserves, with fiber, seedless blackberry, sugar free, 1 Tbsp	0
Preserves, with fiber, sugar free, seedless raspberry, 1 Tbsp	0
Preserves, with fiber, sugar free, strawberry, 1 Tbsp	0
Polaner All Fruit	
Spreadable fruit, raspberry, 1 Tbsp	2
Strawberry spreadable fruit, 1 Tbsp	2
Polaner Sugar Free with Fiber	
Concord grape jam, 1 Tbsp	0
Smucker's	
Blackberry jam, 1 Tbsp	3
Concord grape jelly, 1 Tbsp	3
Jam, red raspberry, 1 Tbsp	3
Jam, sugar free, seedless, blackberry, 1 Tbsp	0
Jelly, strawberry, 1 Tbsp	3
Preserves, strawberry, 1 Tbsp	3

	SmartPoints® value
Preserves, strawberry, sugar free, 1 Tbsp	0
Red tart cherry fruit spread, 1 Tbsp	2
Seedless strawberry jam, 1 Tbsp	3
Strawberry fruit & honey spread, 1 Tbsp	2
Strawberry jam, 1 Tbsp	3
Smucker's Fruit & Honey	
Tropical fruit spread, 1 Tbsp	2
Smucker's Low Sugar	
Jelly, reduced sugar, concord grape, 1 Tbsp	1
Preserves, strawberry, reduced sugar, 1 Tbsp	1
Smucker's Natural	
Strawberry fruit spread, 1 Tbsp	2
Smucker's Simply 100% Fruit	
Spreadable fruit, seedless, strawberry, ⅔ oz	2
Smucker's Simply Fruit	
Spreadable fruit, apricot, 1 Tbsp	2
Spreadable fruit, black raspberry, 1 Tbsp	2
Spreadable fruit, strawberry, 1 Tbsp	2
Smucker's Squeeze	
Fruit spread, reduced sugar, strawberry, 1 Tbsp	1
Fruit spread, strawberry, 1 Tbsp	3
Jelly, grape, 1 Tbsp	3
Smucker's Sugar Free	
Concord grape jam, 1 Tbsp	0
Preserves, apricot, 1 Tbsp	0
Preserves, peach, 1 Tbsp	0
Red raspberry preserves, 1 Tbsp	0
Seedless blackberry jam, 1 Tbsp	0
Seedless strawberry jam, 1 Tbsp	0
Strawberry preserves, 1 Tbsp	0
Welch's Natural	
Spread, concord grape, 1 Tbsp	2
Spread, strawberry, 1 Tbsp	2

	SmartPoints® value
Welch's Reduced Sugar	
Concord grape jelly, 1 Tbsp	1

Marmalade

Polaner	
Marmalade, orange, with fiber, sugar free, 1 Tbsp	0
Smucker's	
Marmalade, sweet orange, 1 Tbsp	3
Smucker's Sugar Free	
Marmalade, orange, 1 Tbsp	0

Nut Butters

365 Everyday Value	
Creamy almond butter, 2 Tbsp	6
Crunchy almond butter, 2 Tbsp	6
Barney Butter	
Almond butter, smooth, 2 Tbsp	6
Jif	
Almond butter, creamy, 2 Tbsp	6
Justin's	
Almond butter, honey, 2 Tbsp	6
Almond butter, vanilla, 2 Tbsp	7
Classic almond butter, 2 Tbsp	6
Hazelnut butter, chocolate, 2 Tbsp	7
Maple almond butter, 2 Tbsp	6
MaraNatha	
All natural no stir creamy almond butter, 2 Tbsp	6
Almond butter, crunchy, no stir, 2 Tbsp	6
Nutella Mini Cups	
Hazelnut spread, 1 mini cup (15 g)	4
SimplyNature	
Coconut spread, 1 Tbsp	3
Sunbutter	
Sunbutter, creamy, 2 Tbsp	6
Trader Joe's	
Creamy salted cashew butter, 2 Tbsp	6
Crunchy almond butter, 2 Tbsp	6

	SmartPoints® value
Trader Joe's Grocery	
Almond butter, raw, creamy, unsalted, 2 Tbsp	6
Almond butter, raw, crunchy, unsalted, 2 Tbsp	6

Peanut Butter

365 Everyday Value	
Creamy unsweetened organic peanut butter, 2 Tbsp	6
365 Everyday Value Organic	
Unsweetened and no salt creamy peanut butter, 2 Tbsp	6
Adams	
Peanut butter, creamy, 2 Tbsp	6
Adams 100% Natural	
Creamy peanut butter, 2 Tbsp	6
Crunchy peanut butter, 2 Tbsp	6
Algood Food	
Creamy peanut butter, 2 Tbsp	6
Better Body Foods PB Fit	
Chocolate peanut butter powder, 2 Tbsp	1
Peanut butter powder, 2 Tbsp	1
Better'n Peanut Butter	
Low sodium, 2 Tbsp	3
Original peanut spread, 2 Tbsp	3
Betty Lou's Just Great Stuff	
Organic powdered chocolate peanut butter, 2 Tbsp	1
Crazy Richard's	
Peanut butter, creamy, 2 Tbsp	6
Pure pb (pure pressed peanuts), 2 Tbsp	1
Earth Balance	
Creamy coconut and peanut spread, 2 Tbsp	7
Peanut butter, natural, and flaxseed, creamy, 2 Tbsp	6
Giant	
Creamy peanut butter, 2 Tbsp	6
Creamy peanut butter (duplicate), 2 Tbsp	6

Peanut Butter (cont'd)

	SmartPoints® value
Great Value	
No stir creamy natural peanut butter spread, 2 Tbsp	6
Hy-Vee	
Chocolate powdered peanut butter, 2 Tbsp	1
Jif	
Extra crunchy peanut butter, 2 Tbsp	6
Honey crunch natural peanut butter, 2 Tbsp	6
Omega-3 creamy peanut butter, 2 Tbsp	6
Peanut butter spread, creamy, reduced fat, 2 Tbsp	6
Peanut butter spread, natural, creamy, 2 Tbsp	6
Peanut butter, creamy, 2 Tbsp	6
Reduced fat creamy peanut butter, 2 Tbsp	6
To go, creamy natural peanut butter spread, 1 container (43 g)	8
Jif Natural	
Peanut butter spread & honey, creamy, 2 Tbsp	6
Peanut butter spread, creamy, 2 Tbsp	6
Peanut butter spread, creamy, low sodium, 2 Tbsp	6
Peanut butter spread, crunchy, 2 Tbsp	6
Peanut butter, crunchy, 2 Tbsp	6
Jif Simply	
Peanut butter, creamy, 2 Tbsp	6
Jif To Go	
Creamy peanut butter, 1 snack cup (43 g)	8
Peanut butter, crunchy, 1 cup	8
Reduced fat creamy peanut butter spread, 1 container (48 g)	8

	SmartPoints® value
Jif Whips	
Peanut butter, whipped, & chocolate flavored spread, 2 Tbsp	6
Peanut butter, whipped, creamy, 2 Tbsp	5
Just Great Stuff	
Peanut butter, organic, powdered, 2 Tbsp	1
Powdered natural peanut butter, 2 Tbsp	1
Justin's	
Peanut butter blend, honey, 2 Tbsp	6
Peanut butter, classic, 2 Tbsp	6
Kellogg's Jif	
Creamy peanut butter, 2 Tbsp	6
Peanut powder, 3 Tbsp	1
Kellogg's Jif Reduced Fat	
Crunchy peanut butter spread, 2 Tbsp	6
Kellogg's Jif Whips	
Whipped peanut butter and salty caramel spread, 2 Tbsp	5
Kirkland Signature	
Creamy almond butter, 2 Tbsp	6
Krema	
Peanut butter, natural, smooth & creamy, 2 Tbsp	6
Kroger	
Crunchy peanut butter, 2 Tbsp	6
Natural creamy peanut butter, 2 Tbsp	6
Natural crunchy peanut butter, 2 Tbsp	6
Laura Scudder's	
Old fashioned peanut butter, smooth, 2 Tbsp	6
Peanut butter, old fashioned, nutty, 2 Tbsp	6

	SmartPoints® value
Market Pantry	
Reduced fat creamy peanut butter spread, 2 Tbsp	6
My Essentials	
Creamy peanut butter, 2 Tbsp	7
Nature's Promise Organics	
Peanut butter, organic smooth, salted, 2 Tbsp	6
Old Home	
100% all natural creamy peanut butter no sugar added (gluten free), 2 Tbsp	6
Old Home 100% All Natural	
Creamy peanut butter (sugar and gluten free), 2 Tbsp	6
Honey creamy peanut butter spread (gluten free), 2 Tbsp	6
Olde Style	
Fresh ground peanut butter, unsalted, 2 Tbsp	6
PB2	
Powdered peanut butter, 2 Tbsp	1
Powdered peanut butter with premium chocolate, 2 Tbsp	1
Peanut Butter & Co.	
Chocolate powdered peanut butter, 2 Tbsp	1
Original powdered peanut butter, 2 Tbsp	1
Peanut Delight	
Peanut butter, creamy, 2 Tbsp	6
Peter Pan	
Honey roast creamy peanut and natural honey spread, 2 Tbsp	7
Peanut & natural honey spread, honey roast, creamy, 2 Tbsp	7
Peanut butter, creamy, 2 Tbsp	7
Peanut butter, crunchy, 2 Tbsp	6
Peanut butter, whipped creamy, ⅓ less sugar, 2 Tbsp	5
Peanut spread, reduced fat, creamy, 2 Tbsp	6

	SmartPoints® value
Peter Pan Creamy	
Honey roast peanut butter, 2 Tbsp	7
Peter Pan Natural	
Peanut butter spread, creamy, 2 Tbsp	7
Peter Pan Simply Ground	
Peanut butter, 2 Tbsp	7
Simple Truth Organic	
Creamy peanut butter, 2 Tbsp	6
Crunchy peanut butter, 2 Tbsp	6
Simply Balanced	
Organic creamy peanut butter, 2 Tbsp	6
Simply Nature	
Creamy peanut butter with honey, 2 Tbsp	6
Creamy peanut butter, 2 Tbsp	6
Skippy	
Creamy peanut butter, 2 Tbsp	6
Natural peanut butter spread, creamy, 2 Tbsp	6
Peanut butter spread, reduced fat, creamy, 2 Tbsp	6
Peanut butter spread, reduced fat, super chunk, 2 Tbsp	6
Peanut butter spread, super chunk, reduced fat, 2 Tbsp	6
Peanut butter, creamy, 2 Tbsp	6
Peanut butter, extra crunchy, super chunk, 2 Tbsp	6
Skippy Natural	
Peanut butter spread, creamy, ⅓ less sodium & sugar, 2 Tbsp	7
Peanut butter spread, creamy, with honey, 2 Tbsp	7
Peanut butter spread, extra crunchy, super chunk, 2 Tbsp	6
Skippy Natural Super Chunk	
Extra crunchy peanut butter, 2 Tbsp	6

Peanut Butter (cont'd)

	SmartPoints® value
Smart Balance	
Peanut butter, real, chunky, 2 Tbsp	6
Smart Balance Natural	
Creamy peanut butter, 2 Tbsp	6
Smucker's Natural	
Chunky peanut butter, 2 Tbsp	6
Creamy peanut butter, 2 Tbsp	6
Smucker's Natural	
Peanut butter, chunky, 2 Tbsp	6
Smucker's Organic	
Peanut butter, creamy, 2 Tbsp	6
Teddie	
Peanut butter, all natural, smooth, 2 Tbsp	6
Peanut butter, old fashioned, unsalted, smooth, 2 Tbsp	6
Peanut butter, unsalted, super chunky, 2 Tbsp	6
Peanut butter, with flaxseed, smooth, 2 Tbsp	5
Trader Joe's	
Creamy no stir peanut butter spread, 2 Tbsp	6
Crunchy no stir peanut butter spread, 2 Tbsp	6
Crunchy salted peanut butter with flax & chia seeds, 1 oz	5
Trader Joe's Grocery	
Peanut butter, creamy salted, 2 Tbsp	6
Peanut butter, creamy unsalted, 2 Tbsp	6
Peanut butter, crunchy salted, 2 Tbsp	6
Trader Joe's Organic	
Valencia creamy salted peanut butter, 2 Tbsp	6

	SmartPoints® value
Tru-Nut Butter	
Chocolate powdered peanut butter, 2 Tbsp	1
Powdered peanut butter, 2 Tbsp	1
Wegman's	
Peanut butter, creamy, 2 Tbsp	7
Whole Foods 365 Organic	
Creamy peanut butter, 2 Tbsp	6
Wonder Natural Foods	
Better'n peanut butter, original, 2 Tbsp	3

Salsa

Aldi	
Mango peach salsa, 2 Tbsp	1
Casa Mamita	
Salsa, thick & chunky, medium, 2 Tbsp	0
Salsa, thick & chunky, mild, 2 Tbsp	0
Chi-Chi's	
Medium salsa, 2 Tbsp	0
Garden Fresh Gourmet	
Salsa, Jack's special, medium, 2 Tbsp	1
Salsa, Jack's special, mild, 2 Tbsp	0
Golden Sun Organic	
Fresh organic salsa, 2 Tbsp	0
Great Value	
Medium cantina style salsa, 2 Tbsp	0
Herdez	
Medium guacamole salsa, 2 Tbsp	2
Salsa, medium, 2 Tbsp	0
Salsa, verde, 2 Tbsp	0
Italian Rose	
Fresh salsa with cilantro, 2 Tbsp	0

	SmartPoints® value
Kirkland Signature Organic	
Salsa, 2 Tbsp	0
Nature's Kitchen	
Mild fresh salsa, 2 Tbsp	0
Newman's Own	
Salsa, all natural chunky, mild, 2 Tbsp	0
Salsa, medium chunky, 2 Tbsp	0
Newman's Own All Natural	
Salsa, pineapple, medium, chunky, 2 Tbsp	1
On the Border	
Medium salsa, 2 Tbsp	0
Salsa, mild, 2 Tbsp	0
Pace	
Chunky medium salsa, 2 Tbsp	0
Chunky mild salsa, 2 Tbsp	0
Medium chunky salsa, 2 Tbsp	0
Salsa, restaurant style, medium, 2 Tbsp	0
The original picante sauce, mild flavor, 2 Tbsp	1
Private Selection	
Mild mellow black bean and corn salsa, 2 Tbsp	0
Santa Barbara	
Mango with peach salsa, 2 Tbsp	1
Tostitos	
Salsa, chunky, mild, 2 Tbsp	0
Salsa, medium, 2 Tbsp	1
Trader Joe's	
Fire roasted tomato salsa no salt added, 2 Tbsp	1
Trader Joe's Grocery	
Corn and chile tomato-less salsa, 2 Tbsp	1
Salsa autentica, 2 Tbsp	0

Spreads

	SmartPoints® value
Challenge	
Spreadable butter, lite, 1 Tbsp	2
Dalmatia	
Original fig spread, 1 Tbsp	4
Follow Your Heart Original	
Dressing and sandwich spread, 1 Tbsp	3
Follow Your Heart Reduced Fat	
Dressing and sandwich spread, 1 Tbsp	1
Full Circle Organic	
European strawberry fruit spread, 1 Tbsp	2
Inland Market	
Blue crab spread, 2 oz	4
Land O Lakes	
Butter spread, honey, 1 Tbsp	3
Lotus	
Creamy biscoff spread, 1 Tbsp	4
Nutella	
Hazelnut spread with cocoa, 2 Tbsp	10
Hazelnut spread with skim milk and cocoa, 2 Tbsp	10
Olivio	
Light vegetable oil spread, 1 Tbsp	2
Original vegetable oil spread, 1 Tbsp	3
Something Special	
Red chili pepper spread, 1 tsp	1
Sunbutter	
Sunflower seed spread, natural, 2 Tbsp	6
Trader Joe's	
Feta cheese spread, 1 oz	2
Pumpkin butter, 1 Tbsp	2
Trader Joe's Grocery	
Bruschetta, 2 Tbsp	1
Speculoos cookie butter, 1 Tbsp	4

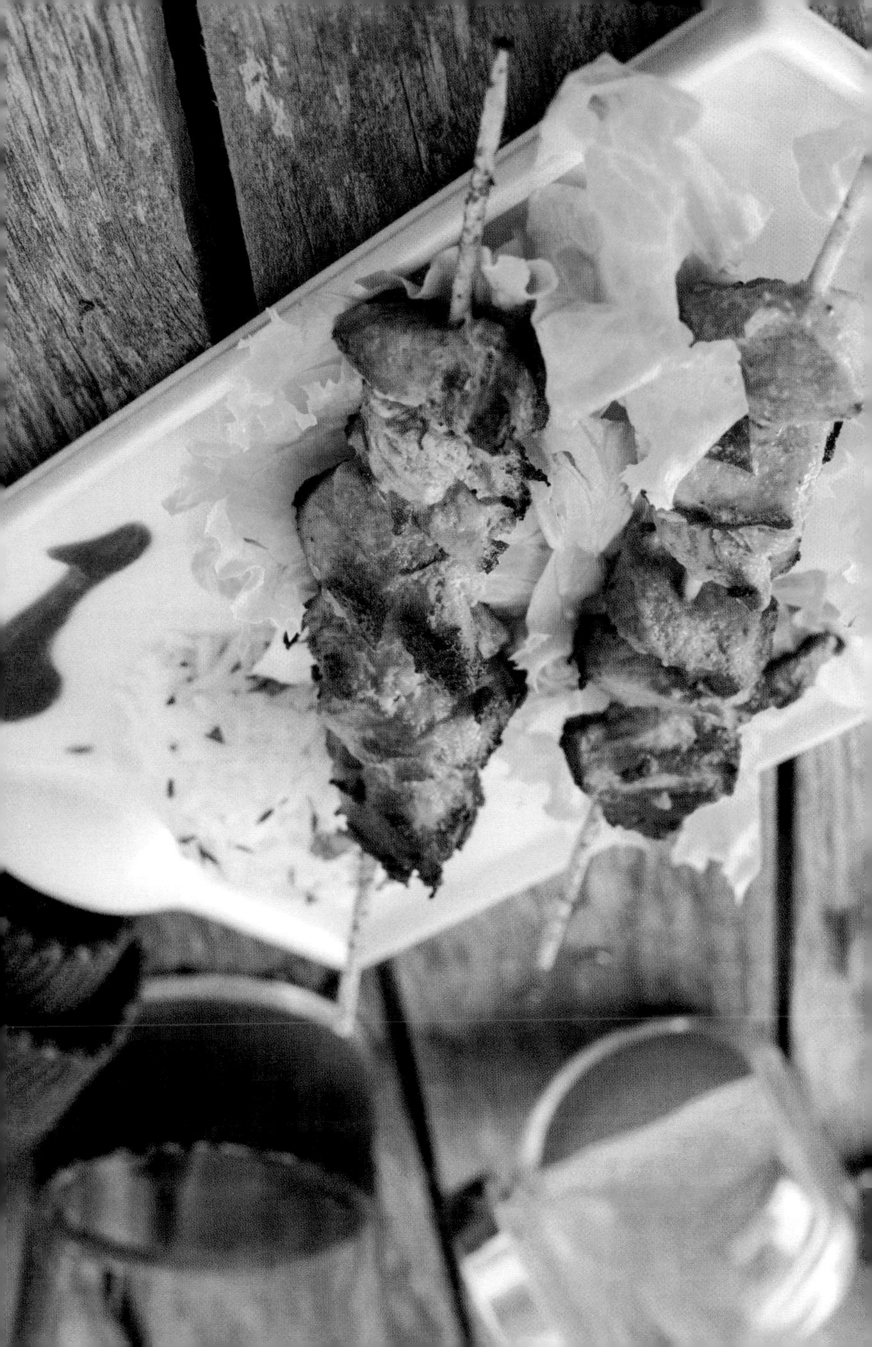

meat & poultry

Bacon and Canadian Bacon

	SmartPoints® value
Al Fresco	
Uncured chicken bacon, 2 slices (12 g)	1
Applegate	
Turkey bacon, uncured, 1 slice (28 g)	0
Applegate Naturals	
Bacon, Sunday, uncured, 2 slices (14 g)	2
Appleton Farms	
Fully cooked bacon, 3 slices (15 g)	2
Hickory smoked uncured bacon, 2 slices (11 g)	2
Betty Crocker Bac-Os	
Bacon flavor bits, 1½ Tbsp	1
Boar's Head	
Bacon, imported, naturally smoked, fully cooked (gluten free), 3 slices (14 g)	2
Butterball Everyday	
Lower sodium turkey bacon, 1 slice (14 g)	1
Original turkey bacon, 1 slice (14 g)	1
Thin and crispy turkey bacon, 2 slices (18 g)	1
Columbus	
Uncured hickory smoked turkey bacon, 1 slice (28 g)	1
Farmland	
Bacon, hickory smoked, 2 slices (45 g)	3
Honey and maple flavored naturally hickory smoked bacon, 2 slices (16 g)	3
Fit & Active	
Turkey bacon, 1 slice (14 g)	1
Godshall's	
Turkey bacon, smoked sliced, 1 slice (28 g)	1
Uncured turkey bacon (gluten free), 1 slice (28 g)	1

	SmartPoints® value
Greenfield Natural Meat Co.	
Natural apple wood smoked uncured bacon, 2 slices (12 g)	1
H-E-B	
Center cut bacon, 3 slices (15 g)	2
Family pack fully cooked bacon, 4 slices (17 g)	2
Hardwood smoked turkey bacon, 2 slices (12 g)	1
Hickory smoked bacon, 4 slices (17 g)	2
Hormel	
Bacon pieces, real, 1 Tbsp	1
Bacon, crumbled, real, original, 1 Tbsp	1
Bacon, fully cooked, 2 slices (14 g)	2
Bacon, microwave ready, original, 2 slices (15 g)	3
Black label bacon, center cut, regular, 2 slices (49 g)	2
Black label bacon, thick slice, 2 slices (65 g)	4
Canadian bacon thick slices, 2 slices (56 g)	1
Crumbled bacon, 1 Tbsp	1
Pizza style Canadian bacon, 22 slices (56 g)	2
Real bacon bits, 1 Tbsp	1
Hormel Black Label	
Bacon, 4 slices (15 g)	2
Bacon, original, 2 fried slices (15 g)	3
Hormel Natural Choice	
Bacon, uncured, original, sliced, 2 slices (15 g)	3
Canadian bacon, sliced, 2 slices (56 g)	1
Jennie-O	
Turkey bacon, 1 slice (15 g)	1
Jennie-O Lower Sodium	
Turkey bacon made with sea salt, 1 slice (15 g)	1

	SmartPoints® value
Jennie-O Turkey Store	
Turkey bacon, 1 slice (15 g)	1
Jones Dairy Farm	
Canadian bacon, naturally hickory smoked, 3 slices (51 g)	1
Cherrywood smoked uncured turkey bacon, 1 slice (15 g)	1
Jones Dairy Farm All Natural	
97% fat free uncured Canadian bacon, 3 slices (51 g)	1
Kirkland Signature	
Crumbled bacon, 1 Tbsp	1
Fully cooked thick sliced bacon, 2 slices (18 g)	3
Sliced bacon, 2 slices (15 g)	2
Thick sliced bacon hickory smoked center cut, 1 slice (13 g)	2
Kroger	
Bacon, turkey, 1 slice (14 g)	1
Canadian bacon, sliced, 4 slices (57 g)	1
Original roasted bacon, 2 slices (14 g)	2
Real bacon bits, hickory smoke flavor, 1 Tbsp	1
Kroger Meals Made Simple	
Bacon, fully cooked, 3 slices (15 g)	2
Land O Frost Breakfast Cuts	
Canadian bacon, thick sliced, natural hickory smoked, 3 slices (60 g)	1
Land O'Frost	
Natural hickory smoked Canadian bacon, 5 pieces (61 g)	1
McCormick	
Bits bac'n pieces, 1 Tbsp	1
Nature's Promise	
Uncured turkey bacon, 1 slice (28 g)	1
Oscar Mayer	
Bacon, center cut, 2 slices (34 g)	2
Bacon, fully cooked, family size, 3 slices (18 g)	2

	SmartPoints® value
Bacon, fully cooked, original, 3 slices (18 g)	2
Bacon, fully cooked, thick cut, 2 slices (14 g)	2
Bacon, thick cut, 1 slice (38 g)	2
Bacon, turkey, 1 slice (15 g)	1
Lower sodium bacon, 2 slices (14 g)	2
Real bacon, bits, 1 Tbsp	1
Real bacon, bits, value size, 1 Tbsp	1
Real bacon, recipe pieces, 1 Tbsp	1
Turkey bacon bits, 1 Tbsp	0
Oscar Mayer Selects	
Bacon, uncured, smoked, 2 slices (15 g)	3
Uncured turkey bacon, 1 slice (15 g)	1
Private Selection	
Bacon, center cut, 2 slices (15 g)	1
Publix	
Fully cooked bacon, 3 slices (12 g)	2
Rose	
Fully cooked hardwood smoked uncured Canadian bacon, 3 slices (51 g)	1
Uncured Canadian bacon, 3 slices (51 g)	1
Sam's Choice	
Fully cooked turkey bacon slices, 2 slices (12 g)	1
Wood smoked original turkey bacon, 1 slice (24 g)	1
Shady Brook Farms	
Smoked turkey bacon, 1 slice (14 g)	1
Smithfield	
Bacon, naturally hickory smoked, thick sliced, 1 slice (12 g)	2
Fully cooked applewood bacon, 3 slices (18 g)	3
Hometown original bacon, 2 slices (17 g)	3

Bacon and Canadian Bacon (cont'd)

	SmartPoints® value
Smithfield Bacon	
Applewood thick cut bacon, 1 slice (14 g)	3
Specially Selected	
Center cut bacon, 3 slices (15 g)	2
Sweet Earth	
Bacon, 2 slices (38 g)	2
Trader Joe's	
Applewood smoked peppered uncured turkey bacon, 1 slice (28 g)	1
Uncured turkey bacon, 1 slice (28 g)	0
Trader Joe's Refrigerated	
Apple smoked fully cooked uncured bacon, 3 slices (18 g)	3
Tyson	
Applewood smoked bacon, 2 slices (15 g)	3
W Brand All Natural	
Classic sliced dry rubbed uncured bacon, 2 slices (12 g)	2
Wellshire	
94% fat free turkey peppered bacon, 1 slice (28 g)	1
Wright	
Bacon, applewood, 2 slices (15 g)	3
Bacon, naturally hickory smoked, 2 slices (15 g)	3

Beef

	SmartPoints® value
Birds Eye	
Asiago beef, 2⅓ cups	7
Boar's Head	
Prime rib of beef, seasoned, 3 oz	9
Cargill Meat Solutions	
Lean ground beef burger, 1 patty (112 g)	4
Century Farm	
Extra lean ground beef, 96% lean, 4 oz	2
Certified Angus Beef	
Ground beef chuck, 80/20, 4 oz	9
FarmRich	
Original meatballs, 6 meatballs (85 g)	10
Full Circle Organic	
Beef, grass-fed, free range, ribeye steak, 3½ oz	3
Giant	
100% ground beef, 80/20, quarter pound hamburgers, 1 patty (113 g)	9
Gold & Masters	
The original skinny burger, 1 burger (112 g)	6
The original skinny ground, 1 burger (112 g)	6
Great American Hamburgers	
Hamburgers, 1 patty (63 g)	6
H-E-B	
100% pure extra lean ground beef, 4 oz	3
Hormel	
Beef crumbles pizza toppings, 2 oz	3
Beef roast, au jus, 5 oz	5
Slow simmered beef tips & gravy, ½ cup	5
Hormel Taco Meats	
Fully cooked seasoned beef crumbles, ⅓ cup	4
Kirkland Signature	
Ground sirloin and loin of beef patty, 1 patty (151 g)	10
Organic ground beef, 4 oz	7
Kroger	
Beef patties, ground, 4 oz	3
Ground beef burgers, 1 patty (112 g)	5
Italian style meatballs, 6 meatballs (85 g)	9
Landis	
Lean sirloin tip beef steak, 4 oz	4
Laura's Lean Beef	
Ground beef, 4 oz	4
Ground round beef, 4 oz	2

	SmartPoints® value
Market Pantry	
93% lean ground beef patties, 4 oz	4
Meal Mart	
Cooked corn beef, 2 oz	3
Old Neighborhood	
Beef shaved steak, 2 oz	3
Omaha Steaks	
4 oz beef tenderloin steak (filet mignon), 4 oz	9
4 oz beef top sirloin steaks, 4 oz	7
4 oz ground beef burgers, 4 oz	9
Beef sirloin tips, 3 oz	5
Chicken fried steak, 1 steak (126 g)	9
Hamburger steak, 8 oz	14
London broil top sirloin steak, 10 oz	7
Sirloin supreme top sirloin steak, 4 oz	2
Oscar Mayer Selects	
Roast beef, slow roasted, 6 slices (51 g)	1
Quick 'N Eat!	
Fully cooked choice angus beef patties, 1 patty (113 g)	8
Ranchers Reserve	
Petite beef sirloin steak, 4 oz	6
Rancher's Reserve Tender Beef	
Beef round roast, bottom, 4 oz	4
Beef top round, London broil, 4 oz	4
Beef, burger, 90% lean, seasoned, 4 oz	4
Boneless chuck eye beef steak, 4 oz	5
Boneless, beef loin ny strip steak, 4 oz	6
Boneless, ribeye steak, 4 oz	13
Boneless, thin New York strip beef steaks, 4 oz	6
Top round, london broil, 4 oz	4

	SmartPoints® value
Simple Truth Organic	
Ground beef, 4 oz	5
Sommers Organic	
Organic beef prime rib, 3 oz	7
Steak-umm	
Sliced steak, 1 cooked portion (32 g)	4
Trader Joe's	
Extra lean ground beef patties (96% lean 4% fat), 1 patty (113 g)	2
Grass fed ground angus beef, 85% lean, 4 oz	6
Trader Joe's Butcher Shop	
Extra lean ground beef, 4 oz	2
Trader Joe's Refrigerated	
Carne asada autentica, 4 oz	4
TSD Sales & Distribution	
Ground beef sirloin, 4 oz	5
Wal-Mart	
Lean ground beef, 4 oz	4

Chicken

Aidells	
Meatballs, chicken, caramelized onion, 3 meatballs (64 g)	4
Organic chicken & apple smoked sausage, 1 link (85 g)	4
Archer Farms	
Natural shredded chicken, 3 oz	2
Birds Eye Voila!	
Garlic chicken, 1⅔ cups	7
Garlic chicken, family size, 1⅔ cups (170 g)	8
Boar's Head	
Roasted chicken breast, boneless, skinless, maple glazed, 2 oz	1
Brookdale	
Premium white chunk chicken breast in water, 2 oz	1
Bumble Bee	
Premium white chicken chunk in water, 2 oz	1

Chicken (cont'd)

	SmartPoints® value
Butterfield Farms	
White chicken, 2 oz	1
Columbus	
Rotisserie style chicken breast, 2 oz	1
Daily Chef	
Boneless skinless chicken breast, 4 oz	1
Buffalo style chicken breast, 2 oz	1
Chicken breast in water, ⅓ cup	1
Daily Chef All Natural	
Boneless skinless chicken breast tenderloins, 4 oz	1
Delia's	
Gluten free chicken sausage patties, 2 patties (85 g)	3
Foster Farms	
99% fat free chicken breasts, 4 oz	1
Chicken breast grilled strips, 3 oz	1
Chicken breast strips, grilled, 3 oz	1
Chicken breast strips, southwestern seasoned, 3 oz	1
Chicken breast tenders, boneless & skinless, 4 oz	1
Fajita marinated raw chicken breast strips, 4 oz	1
Gardein	
Crispy tenders, seven grain, 1 tender (51 g)	2
Giant	
Chicken legs, boneless, skinless, with lemon pepper rub, 5 oz	5
Great Value	
Boneless skinless chicken breasts, 4 oz	1
Chicken breast tenderloins, 4 oz	1
Chunk chicken breast, 2 oz	1
Hannaford	
Chicken breast, premium chunk, in water, canned, 2 oz	1
Harvest Creek	
White chicken in buffalo sauce, 2 oz	1

	SmartPoints® value
Harvestland	
Chicken breasts, 1 breast (136 g)	1
Grilled chicken breast strips, 3 oz	1
Roasted chicken breast strips, 3 oz	1
Hillshire Farms Naturals	
Rotisserie chicken breast (99% fat free gluten free), 3 slices (49 g)	0
Hormel	
Premium chicken breast in water, 2 oz drained	0
Isernio's	
Premium ground chicken, 4 oz	2
John Soules Foods	
Chicken breast fajitas, 3 oz	2
Chicken fajitas breast strips, 3 oz	1
Grilled chicken breast strips, 3 oz	1
Kirkland Signature	
Chicken breast boneless and skinless (uncooked), 4 oz	1
Chicken tenderloins, 4 oz	1
Grilled chicken breast strips, 3 oz	0
Premium chunk chicken breast, 2 oz drained	1
Premium chunk chicken breast packed in water, 2 oz	1
Kirkwood	
Fully cooked grilled southwestern flavor chicken breast strips, 3 oz	1
Kirkwood Original	
Grilled chicken breast strips, 3 oz	2
Kroger	
Boneless skinless chicken breast, 4 oz	2
Grilled diced chicken breast, 3 oz	1
Teriyaki grilled and glazed chicken breast fillets, 1 fillet (112 g)	3
Market Basket	
Premium chunk white chicken in water, 2 oz	1
Market Pantry	
Chicken breast tenderloins, 4 oz	1

	SmartPoints® value
Marketside	
Lemon pepper rotisserie chicken, 3 oz	5
Maya Kaimal	
Butter chicken, 5 oz	6
Nature's Place	
Chicken breast, 4 oz	1
Nature's Promise	
Buffalo style glazed chicken wings, 4 pieces (85 g)	4
Nature's Promise Naturals	
Chicken, boneless skinless breast with rib meat., 1 fillet (113 g)	1
Oberto	
Smokey sweet bbq chicken strips, 1 oz	3
Oscar Mayer Carving Board	
Rotisserie seasoned chicken breast, 2 oz	1
Perdue	
Boneless skinless chicken breasts, 4 oz	2
Bourbon chicken, 3 oz	5
Carved chicken breast, ½ cup	1
Chicken breast cutlets, homestyle, 1 cutlet (85 g)	4
Chicken breast cutlets, original, 1 cutlet (85 g)	6
Chicken leg quarters, 3 oz	6
Chicken roast, boneless, 4 oz	2
Chicken tenderloins, 4 oz	1
Fresh ground chicken patties, 1 patty (112 g)	4
Olive oil & rosemary chicken strips, ½ cup	1
Original chicken breast nuggets, 5 nuggets (85 g)	5
Original chicken breast tenderloin, 3 oz	5
Sweet chili glazed chicken, 3 oz	5
Perdue Baked	
Chicken breast strips, 2 pieces (74 g)	5

	SmartPoints® value
Chicken breast tenderloins, original, 3 oz	4
Perdue Original	
Breaded chicken breast cutlets, 1 piece (84 g)	6
Perdue Oven Ready	
Chicken breast, roaster, bone-in, whole seasoned, 4 oz	3
Perdue Perfect Portions	
Chicken breasts, boneless skinless, 1 fillet (136 g)	1
Chicken breasts, boneless skinless, Italian style, 1 fillet (136 g)	2
Fresh boneless skinless chicken breasts, 1 breast (136 g)	2
Perdue Short Cuts	
Carved chicken breast, grilled Italian style, ½ cup	2
Carved, original roasted chicken breast, ½ cup	1
Carved, southwestern style chicken breast, ½ cup	2
Chicken breast, carved, grilled, ½ cup	1
Curved chicken breast, honey roasted, ½ cup	2
Grilled fajita style carved chicken breast, ½ cup	1
Original carved chicken breast, ½ cup	1
Rotisserie seasoned carved chicken breast, ½ cup	1
Perdue Simply Smart	
Chicken breast cutlets, lightly breaded, 1 piece (90 g)	4
Chicken breast tenders, breaded, gluten-free, 3 pieces (87 g)	5
Chicken strips, original grilled, 3 oz	1
Lightly breaded chicken filets, 1 fillet (115 g)	5
Lightly breaded chicken strips, 1 serving (84 g)	3

Chicken (cont'd)

	SmartPoints® value
Psst...	
Breaded chicken patties, 1 piece (75 g)	6
Safeway Farms	
Chicken leg quarters, fresh, 4 oz	6
ShopRite Kitchen Perdue	
Oven roasted rotisserie chicken, 3 oz	4
Simple Truth	
Sliced chicken fajita strips, 3 oz	1
Springer Mountain Farms	
Boneless skinless chicken breasts, 4 oz	1
Stouffer's Classics	
Baked chicken breast, 1 package (251 g)	5
Stouffer's Fit Kitchen	
Oven roasted chicken, 1 package (375 g)	6
Swanson	
Chicken breast, white, premium chunk, 1 can (85 g)	1
White premium chunk chicken breast, 2 oz	1
White premium chunk chicken breast with rib meat in water, 2 oz	1
T.G.I. Friday's	
Boneless chicken bites, 6 pieces (80 g)	4
Chicken wings, buffalo, 3 pieces (96 g)	5
Trader Joe's	
All natural chicken breasts fully cooked, 4 oz	2
Fully cooked grilled chicken burger patties, 1 burger (113 g)	3
Grilled chicken strips, 3 oz	1
Grilled lemon pepper chicken breasts, 3 oz	2
Just chicken, 3 oz	1
Marinated chicken breasts, 3 oz	3
Roasted chicken patties, 1 patty (112 g)	4

	SmartPoints® value
Trader Joe's Frozen	
Breaded chicken tenderloin breasts, 1 oz	1
Chicken breast tenderloins, 4 oz	1
Chile lime chicken burgers, 1 burger (114 g)	3
Mandarin orange chicken, 1 cup	9
Trader Joe's Refrigerated	
Grilled balsamic vinegar & rosemary chicken, 3 oz	2
Trader Joe's Simply	
Sliced roast chicken breast, 3 slices (84 g)	2
Tyson	
All natural chicken breast tenderloin, 4 oz	1
Boneless chicken wings, buffalo style, 3 wings (78 g)	3
Boneless chicken wings, honey bbq, 3 pieces (98 g)	6
Breaded chicken breast tenderloins, 4 oz	5
Breaded white meat chicken patties, 1 piece (76 g)	5
Breast patties, 1 piece (74 g)	5
Chicken breast strips, 3 oz	1
Chicken breast tenderloins, 4 oz	1
Chicken breast tenderloins, 4 oz	1
Chicken breast tenderloins, southern style, 3 oz	5
Chicken breast tenders, 5 pieces (85 g)	7
Chicken breasts, boneless, skinless, 4 oz	1
Chicken nuggets, 5 pieces (90 g)	8
Chicken strips, buffalo style, 2 pieces (101 g)	6
Chicken strips, crispy, 3 oz	5
Chicken wings, 4 pieces (120 g)	7
Chicken, white, premium chunk, in water, 2 oz	1
Fully cooked and breaded chicken patties, 1 piece (76 g)	6

	SmartPoints® value
Fully cooked lightly breaded chicken breast strips, 3 oz	4
Fully cooked spicy chicken breast patties, 1 piece (74 g)	5
Hot wings, buffalo style, 3 pieces (100 g)	6
Panko breaded chicken breast patties, 1 piece (76 g)	5
Panko breaded chicken breast tenderloins, 4 oz	5
Panko chicken nuggets, 5 pieces (85 g)	6
Teriyaki chicken breast fillet, 1 piece (139 g)	3
Tyson All Natural	
Boneless skinless chicken breast portions, 4 oz	2
Tyson Any'tizers	
Boneless chicken bites, buffalo style, 3 pieces (84 g)	4
Chicken fries, homestyle, 7 pieces (90 g)	6
Chicken wings, boneless, honey bbq, 3 pieces (80 g)	6
Chicken wyngs, boneless, buffalo style, 3 pieces (84 g)	4
Homestyle chicken fries, 7 pieces (90 g)	6
Popcorn chicken, 3 oz	4
Tyson Grilled	
Chicken breast fillets, with rib meat, 1 piece (98 g)	1
Tyson Grilled & Ready	
Chicken breast strips, 3 oz	1
Chicken breast strips, 3 oz	1
Chicken breast strips, fajita, 3 oz	1
Chicken fillets, teriyaki flavored, 3 oz	3
Diced chicken breast, oven roasted, 3 oz	2
Fajita chicken breast strips, 3 oz	1
Fully cooked pulled chicken breast, 2 oz	1

	SmartPoints® value
Oven roasted diced chicken breast, 3 oz	1
Tyson Teriyaki Grills	
Flavored chicken breasts, 1 piece (89 g)	4
Valley Fresh	
Chicken, breast, in water, 2 oz	0
Wegman's Food You Feel Good About	
Premium chunk chicken breast in water, 2 oz	1
Wellsley Farms	
Premium chunk chicken breast in water, 2 oz	1
Yummy Dino Buddies	
Chicken breast nuggets, dinosaur-shaped, 5 pieces (93 g)	6

Frankfurters/Hot Dogs

Applegate	
Hot dog, the great organic uncured beef, 1 hot dog (57 g)	3
Hot dogs, uncured turkey, 1 hot dog (42 g)	1
Ball Park	
Beef franks, 1 frank (53 g)	7
Classic corn dogs, 1 corn dog (76 g)	8
Franks, beef, lean, bun size, 1 frank (50 g)	2
Franks, smoked white turkey, fat free, bun size, 1 frank (50 g)	1
Original angus beef franks, 1 frank (50 g)	6
Fit & Active	
Hardwood smoked turkey franks, 1 frank (34 g)	2
Foster Farms	
Honey crunch jumbo corn dogs, 1 corn dog (112 g)	10
Grillman's	
Black angus beef franks, 1 frank (56 g)	6

	SmartPoints® value
Hebrew National	
Franks, beef, 1 frank (49 g)	6
Franks, beef, 97% fat free, 1 frank (45 g)	1
Franks, beef, reduced fat, 1 frank (45 g)	4
Hofmann	
German brand franks, 1 frank (75 g)	8
Jennie-O	
Turkey franks, 1 frank (34 g)	2
Kirkland Signature	
Beef hot dogs, 1 link (57 g)	6
Nathan's	
Beef frank, 1 link (57 g)	6
Oscar Mayer	
95% fat free wieners, 1 link (50 g)	1
Franks, beef, premium, 1 link (42 g)	5
Franks, turkey, classic, 1 link (45 g)	3
Hot dogs, turkey, 1 link (45 g)	3
Lean beef franks, 1 link (50 g)	2
Wieners, 1 link (45 g)	4
Oscar Mayer Selects	
Turkey franks, hardwood smoked, 1 link (57 g)	4
State Fair	
Corn dogs, 1 corn dog (76 g)	8
Trader Joe's	
Turkey corn dog, 1 corn dog (71 g)	5
Uncured turkey hot dog no nitrates, 1 hot dog (57 g)	2

Lamb

Trader Joe's	
Seasoned rack of lamb, 3 oz	9

Luncheon and Deli Meats

	SmartPoints® value
Aldi Lunch Mate	
Premium black forest deli ham, 2 oz	2
Applegate	
Chicken breast, roasted, 2 oz	1
Ham, black forest, uncured, 2 oz	1
Ham, slow cooked, uncured, 2 oz	1
Turkey breast, roasted, 2 oz	0
Applegate Farms	
Organic smoked turkey breast, 2 oz	0
Applegate Farms Organic	
Turkey breast, roasted, 2 oz	1
Applegate Naturals	
Pepperoni, turkey, uncured, 1 oz	1
Armour	
Pepperoni slices, 16 slices (30 g)	5
Turkey pepperoni, 14 slices (28 g)	1
Artisan Preferred	
Slow roasted turkey breast, 2 oz	1
Bar-S	
Deli shaved black forest ham, 7 slices (56 g)	1
Smoked deli shaved ham, 7 slices (56 g)	1
Best Kosher	
Sliced cooked corn beef, lean, 2 oz	2
Black Bear of the Black Forest	
Oven roasted turkey breast, 1 slice (28 g)	0
Boar's Head	
Bold blackened oven roasted turkey breast (gluten free), 2 oz	1
Bold Cajun style smoked oven roasted turkey breast (gluten free), 2 oz	1
Bold jerk turkey breast (gluten free), 2 oz	1
Bold salsalito roasted turkey breast (gluten free), 2 oz	1
Boneless smoked ham with natural juices, sweet slice, 3 oz	2
Cracked pepper mill smoked turkey breast (gluten free), 2 oz	1
Genoa salami, 8 slices (56 g)	6

	SmartPoints® value
Golden catering style oven roasted turkey breast - 43% lower sodium (gluten free), 2 oz	1
Ham, cooked, 2 oz	1
Hard salami, 5 slices (28 g)	4
Honey smoked turkey breast, 2 oz	1
Lemon pepper roasted chicken breast, 2 oz	1
London broil, 2 oz	1
Maple glazed honey coat cured turkey breast (gluten free), 2 oz	1
Mesquite wood smoked roasted turkey breast (gluten free), 2 oz	1
No salt added oven roasted turkey breast (gluten free), 2 oz	1
Oven roasted seasoned beef, Italian style, 2 oz	1
Oven roasted turkey breast, 2 oz	0
Ovengold roasted breast of turkey (gluten free), 2 oz	1
Pastrami seasoned turkey breast (gluten free), 2 oz	1
Pork shoulder butt roast, 3 oz	5
Premium 46% lower sodium oven roasted turkey breast - skinless (gluten free), 2 oz	1
Smoked ham, 2 oz	1
Turkey breast, black forest, hickory smoked, 2 oz	1
Turkey pepperoni, 1 oz	1
Virginia ham, 2 oz	1
Boar's Head Deli Dinners	
Ovengold roast breast of turkey, coated with seasoning, 3 oz	1
Bridgford	
Pepperoni, turkey, sliced, 12 slices (30 g)	2
Buddig	
Beef, original, 1 package (56 g)	2
Chicken lunch meat, ⅛ package (56 g)	2
Chicken, original, 1 package (56 g)	2

	SmartPoints® value
Corned beef, original, 1 package (56 g)	2
Ham, 1 package (56 g)	2
Ham, honey, original, 1 package (56 g)	3
Original turkey deli meat, 2 oz	2
Oven roasted turkey breast deli meat, 6 slices (50 g)	2
Premium deli black forest ham, 4 slices (50 g)	1
Premium deli smoked honey ham, 6 slices (50 g)	2
Rotisserie flavored chicken breast, 6 slices (50 g)	2
Turkey, honey roasted, 1 package (56 g)	3
Turkey, original, 1 package (56 g)	2
Buddig Original	
Original oven roasted turkey, 2 oz	3
Buddig Premium Deli	
Smoked honey turkey breast, 6 slices (50 g)	3
Butterball	
Oven roasted turkey breast deli meat, 1 slice (28 g)	0
Turkey breast, Cajun style, regular sliced, 2 oz	1
Butterball Natural Inspirations	
Oven roasted turkey breast, 1 oz	1
CB Old Country Store	
97% fat free gluten free black forest ham, 2 oz	1
Celebrity	
Black forest healthy smoked ham (99% fat free), 1 slice (28 g)	0
Columbus	
Applewood smoked ham, 2 oz	2
Honey cured turkey breast, 2 oz	1
Reduced sodium turkey breast, 2 oz	
Roasted turkey breast, 2 oz	1
Rotisserie seasoned chicken breast, 2 oz	1
Salame, Italian dry, 1 oz	3

Luncheon and Deli Meats (cont'd)

	SmartPoints® value
Columbus Salame Company	
Calabrese salame, 1 oz	3
Columbus Salumeria San Francisco	
Peppered turkey breast, 2 oz	1
Daily Chef	
Applewood smoked ham, 2 oz	1
Black forest ham, 2 oz	2
Black forest ham thinly shaved deli meat (gluten free), 2 oz	1
Herb roasted and sliced turkey breast, 2 oz	1
Hickory smoked and sliced turkey breast, 2 oz	1
Honey turkey breast, 2 oz	1
Oven roasted and sliced four pepper turkey breast, 2 oz	1
Oven roasted and sliced turkey breast, 2 oz	1
Sliced turkey pastrami, 2 oz	1
Thinly shaved honey ham, 2 oz	1
Thinly sliced honey ham, 2 oz	2
Turkey pastrami, 2 oz	1
Deli Select	
Chicken breast, rotisserie seasoned, ultra thin, 2 oz	1
Hard salami, ultra thin, 5 slices (28 g)	4
Dietz & Watson	
Breast of turkey, gourmet lite, 3 slices (54 g)	1
Chicken breast, buffalo style, 2 oz	1
Ham, tavern, 2 oz	1
Roast beef, London broil, 2 oz	1
Turkey breast, maple & honey, 2 oz	1
Turkey breast, oven classic, 2 oz	1
Dietz & Watson Gourmet Lite	
Ham, cooked, 2 oz	1
Eckrich	
Deli style thin sliced black forest ham, 7 slices (56 g)	1
Ham, off the bone, 2 oz	2

	SmartPoints® value
Oven roasted turkey breast, 1 slice (28 g)	0
Smoked deli style thin sliced turkey breast, 2 oz	1
Essential Everyday	
Ham, baked honey, shaved, 2 oz	2
Fit & Active	
Smoked honey ham, 2 oz	2
Foster Farms	
Turkey breast, oven roasted, premium, thin sliced, 4 slices (56 g)	1
Gallo	
Light Italian dry salame deli thin sliced, 6 slices (28 g)	2
Giant	
Turkey breast, deli, thin sliced, oven roasted, 4 slices (56 g)	1
Giant Eagle	
Turkey pepperoni, 14 slices (28 g)	2
Great Value	
97% fat free cooked ham, 1 slice (28 g)	0
98% fat free thin sliced smoked turkey breast, 4 slices (51 g)	1
Deli sliced black forest smoked ham, 5 slices (53 g)	1
Deli sliced rotisserie seasoned chicken breast, 4 slices (51 g)	1
Premium honey smoked turkey breast, 4 slices (50 g)	3
Rotisserie flavor chicken breast, 1 slice (28 g)	1
Thin sliced oven roasted turkey breast, 4 slices (51 g)	1
Thin sliced premium black forest ham, 4 slices (50 g)	1
Thin sliced smoked turkey breast (98% fat free), 4 slices (51 g)	1
Thinly sliced roast beef, 6 slices (56 g)	2
Hannaford	
Turkey pepperoni, 15 slices (30 g)	2

	SmartPoints® value
Healthy Ones	
Deli thin sliced black forest ham, 6 slices (54 g)	1
Honey ham, deli thin-sliced, 6 slices (54 g)	2
Honey smoked turkey breast, 6 slices (54 g)	1
Turkey breast, oven roasted, deli thin-sliced, 4 slices (52 g)	1
H-E-B	
97% fat free black forest ham, 2 oz	1
Oven roasted turkey breast, 2 oz	1
Heritage Farm	
Cooked ham, 1 slice (28 g)	1
Hillshire Farm	
Deli meat, turkey breast honey ham variety pack, thin sliced, 2 oz	1
Fresh pack chipotle chicken breast, 3 slices (49 g)	1
Ham, honey, thin sliced, family size, 2 oz	2
Oven roasted turkey breast, 2 oz	1
Ultra thin honey ham, 2 oz	2
Ultra thin lower sodium oven roasted turkey breast, 2 oz	1
Hillshire Farm Deli Select	
Ham, baked, ultra thin, brown sugar, family size, 2 oz	1
Ham, baked, Virginia brand, hearty slices, 1 slice (28 g)	1
Ham, smoked, ultra thin, family size, 2 oz	1
Honey ham, ultra thin, 2 oz	2
Honey ham, ultra thin, lower sodium, 2 oz	2
Honey roasted ultra thin turkey breast, 2 oz	1
Mesquite smoked ultra thin turkey breast, 2 oz	1
Oven roasted chicken breast, 2 oz	1
Oven roasted turkey breast, 5 slices (54 g)	1

	SmartPoints® value
Roast beef, ultra thin, 2 oz	1
Rotisserie seasoned ultra thin chicken breast (family size), 2 oz	1
Smoked ham, water added, ultra thin, 2 oz	1
Turkey breast, oven roasted, lower sodium, 2 oz	1
Turkey breast, oven roasted, ultra thin, 2 oz	1
Ultra thin black forest ham, 2 oz	1
Ultra thin brown sugar ham, 2 oz	2
Ultra thin oven roasted turkey breast, 2 oz	1
Ultra thin pastrami, 2 oz	1
Ultra thin roast beef, 2 oz	1
Hillshire Farm Farm Classics	
97% fat free oven roasted turkey breast deli meat, 4 slices (50 g)	1
Hillshire Farm Naturals	
Black forest ham deli meat, 3 slices (49 g)	1
Hardwood smoked turkey breast deli meat, 3 slices (52 g)	1
Honey roasted ham deli meat, 3 slices (49 g)	2
Rotisserie seasoned sliced chicken breast deli meat (99% fat free/ gluten free), 3 slices (49 g)	0
Slow roasted turkey breast deli meat, 3 slices (52 g)	0
Hillshire Farm Thin Sliced	
Honey roasted turkey breast, 2 oz	1
Hormel	
Pepperoni, 15 slices (30 g)	4
Pepperoni, minis, 1 oz	5
Pepperoni, original, 14 slices (28 g)	5
Pepperoni, turkey, 17 slices (30 g)	2
Pepperoni, turkey, minis, 1 oz	2
Spam, lite, 2 oz	3
Turkey pepperoni, 17 slices (30 g)	2
Turkey pepperoni stix, 1 stick (21 g)	1

	SmartPoints® value
Hormel Natural Choice	
Cherrywood smoked deli ham, 4 slices (56 g)	1
Chicken breast, deli, rotisserie style, 3 slices (56 g)	0
Ham, deli, honey, 4 slices (56 g)	2
Ham, deli, smoked, 4 slices (56 g)	1
Hard uncured salami, 6 slices (28 g)	4
Honey deli ham, 4 slices (56 g)	2
Oven roasted deli turkey, 3 slices (56 g)	1
Roast beef, deli, 4 slices (56 g)	1
Smoked deli turkey, 3 slices (56 g)	1
Turkey, deli, oven roasted, 3 slices (56 g)	1
Turkey pepperoni, 17 slices (30 g)	2
Hy-Vee	
Turkey pepperoni, 15 slices (30 g)	2
Jennie-O	
Extra lean turkey breast 97% fat free, 2 oz	1
Turkey ham, lean, 2 oz	2
Jennie-O Turkey Store Premium Seasoned	
Turkey breast, sun dried tomato, 2 oz	0
Jones	
Ham, 3 slices (51 g)	1
Kirkland Signature	
Extra lean ham sliced 98% fat free, 1 slice (28 g)	0
Rotisserie seasoned chicken breast, 2 oz	1
Turkey breast slices, 2 slices (56 g)	1
Kraft Deli Fresh	
Honey ham water added, 2 oz	1
Krakus	
Ham, polish, 2 oz	1
Polish ham, sliced, 2 slices (56 g)	1

	SmartPoints® value
Kroger	
Deli thin sliced mesquite smoked turkey breast, 2 oz	1
Deli thin sliced oven roasted turkey breast, 2 oz	1
Deli thin sliced turkey pastrami, 2 oz	1
Ham, diced, ½ cup	1
Ham, honey, deli thin sliced, 2 oz	2
Ham, smoked, deli thin sliced, 2 oz	2
Roast beef, deli thin sliced, 2 oz	1
Turkey breast, honey, deli thin sliced, 2 oz	1
Kroger Deli Style	
Chicken breast, oven roasted, value pack, 6 slices (56 g)	2
Turkey breast, oven roasted, value pack, 6 slices (57 g)	2
Kroger Private Selection	
Oven roasted breast of turkey, 1 oz	0
Land O Frost Simply Delicious	
Black forest ham, 5 slices (51 g)	1
Honey cured ham, 5 slices (51 g)	1
Honey roasted turkey breast, 5 slices (51 g)	1
Slow roasted turkey breast, 5 slices (51 g)	1
Land O'Frost Premium	
Brown sugar ham, 4 slices (50 g)	2
Chicken breast, oven roasted, 6 slices (57 g)	2
Hickory smoked lean turkey breast, 4 slices (50 g)	3
Honey smoked lean turkey breast, 4 slices (50 g)	2
Lean honey ham, 4 slices (50 g)	1
Natural hickory lean smoked ham, 4 slices (57 g)	1
Oven roasted lean turkey breast, 4 slices (52 g)	2

	SmartPoints® value
Lunch Mate	
97% fat free cooked ham, 1 slice (28 g)	1
97% fat free honey ham, 1 slice (28 g)	1
Finely sliced honey ham water added deli meat, 2 oz	1
Ham, 1 slice (28 g)	1
Honey smoked turkey breast, 2 oz	1
Premium hickory smoked turkey breast, 2 oz	2
Rotisserie seasoned chicken breast, 2 oz	1
Smoked ham, 2 oz	1
Smoked turkey breast, 1 slice (28 g)	1
Uncured black forest ham deli meat, 2 oz	1
Lunch Mate Deli Style	
Mesquite smoked turkey breast, 2 oz	1
Oven roasted turkey breast, 2 oz	1
Thin sliced oven roasted turkey breast, 2 oz	1
Lunch Mate Premium	
Lean oven roasted cured turkey breast deli meat, 2 oz	2
Lunch Mate Premium Deli Slices	
Oven roasted cured chicken breast, 2 oz	2
Mama Cozzi's	
Turkey pepperoni, 16 slices (28 g)	2
Margherita	
Hard salami, 6 slices (28 g)	4
Snack size hard salami, 6 slices (28 g)	4
Turkey pepperoni, 16 slices (28 g)	2
Market Pantry	
97% fat free honey ham deli slices, 2 oz	2
Turkey breast, oven-roasted, ultra-thin deli slices, 2 oz	1

	SmartPoints® value
Ultra thin deli slices honey ham, 2 oz	1
Meijer	
Hickory smoked honey ham steaks water added, 2 oz	2
Neese's	
Liver pudding, 2 oz	2
Oscar Mayer	
98% fat free bologna, 1 slice (28 g)	0
Bologna, 1 slice (28 g)	3
Bologna, beef, light, 1 slice (28 g)	2
Bologna, light, 1 slice (28 g)	2
Bologna, turkey, 1 slice (32 g)	2
Combos, oven roasted turkey breast, smoked ham, 2 oz	1
Ham, baked, cooked, 3 slices (63 g)	1
Ham, boiled, 3 slices (63 g)	1
Ham, honey, 3 slices (57 g)	1
Honey ham and smoked turkey sandwich meat, 4 slices (57 g)	1
Oven roasted shaved white turkey 95% fat free, 2 oz	1
Oven roasted, extra lean turkey breast and white turkey, 3 slices (62 g)	2
Premium shaved oven roasted turkey breast & white turkey, 2 oz	1
Salami, cotto, Louis Rich turkey, 1 slice (28 g)	1
Salami, hard, 3 slices (27 g)	3
Slow roasted roast beef cured extra lean, 1 slice (28 g)	1
Smoked shaved ham 97% fat free, 2 oz	1
Turkey breast, & white turkey, oven roasted, 1 slice (28 g)	1
Turkey breast, & white turkey, smoked, 1 slice (28 g)	1

	SmartPoints® value
Oscar Mayer Carving Board	
Oven roasted turkey breast, 2 oz	1
Roast beef, cured, slow roasted, 2 oz	1
Oscar Mayer Deli Fresh	
Black forest ham water added, 2 oz	1
Bold chipotle seasoned chicken breast, 2 oz	1
Bold honey maple ham, 2 oz	1
Chicken breast, buffalo style, 3 oz	1
Chicken breast, chipotle seasoned, bold, 2 oz	1
Chicken breast, grilled, strips, 3 oz	1
Chicken breast, shaved, rotisserie style, 6 slices (51 g)	1
Chicken breast, southwestern seasoned, strips, 3 oz	1
Classic combo oven roasted turkey breast & smoked ham, 2 oz	1
Cracked black pepper turkey breast, 2 oz	1
Ham, black forest, 2 oz	1
Ham, smoked, shaved, family size, 6 slices (56 g)	1
Ham, Virginia brand, shaved, 6 slices (51 g)	1
Honey ham water added, 2 oz	1
Honey ham water added, 2 oz	1
Honey ham water added deli meat, 2 oz	1
Honey smoked turkey breast, 2 oz	1
Mesquite seasoned smoked chicken breast, 2 oz	1
Mesquite turkey breast (family size), 2 oz	1
Oven roasted turkey breast, 2 oz	1
Oven roasted turkey breast deli meat, 2 oz	1
Rotisserie seasoned chicken breast, 2 oz	1
Rotisserie seasoned chicken breast, 2 oz	1

	SmartPoints® value
Slow roasted cured roasted beef, 2 oz	1
Smoked chicken breast, 2 oz	1
Smoked ham water added, 2 oz	1
Smoked turkey breast, 2 oz	1
Smoked turkey breast, 2 oz	1
Turkey breast, cracked black pepper, shaved, 6 slices (51 g)	1
Turkey breast, smoked, 6 slices (51 g)	1
Oscar Mayer Natural	
Turkey breast, oven roasted, 3 slices (63 g)	1
Oscar Mayer Premium Deli Meat	
Ham, smoked, shaved, 4 slices (56 g)	1
Oscar Mayer Selects	
Slow roasted turkey breast, 2 oz	1
Plainville Farms Organic	
Oven roasted turkey breast (gluten free), 2 oz	0
Premium	
Hickory smoked ham, 2 oz	2
Prima Della	
Sliced oven roasted chicken breast, 2 oz	1
Primo Taglio	
Turkey breast, oven roasted, 2 slices (56 g)	1
Publix	
98% fat free roasted turkey breast, 2 oz	1
Hard salami, 4 slices (28 g)	2
Roasted turkey breast deli meat, 1 slice (28 g)	0
Sliced reduced fat genoa salami, 8 slices (57 g)	3
Thin sliced cooked ham water added, 2 oz	1
Thin sliced roasted turkey breast, 2 oz	1
Thin sliced rotisserie seasoned chicken, 2 oz	1

	SmartPoints® value
Publix Deli	
Hickory smoked turkey breast, 1 oz	1
Oven roasted turkey breast, 2 oz	0
Sam's West	
Sliced angus seasoned roast beef, 2 oz	1
Sara Lee Fresh Ideas	
Honey roasted turkey breast deli meat, 2 oz	1
Oven roasted turkey breast, 2 oz	1
Sara Lee Premium Meats	
Honey ham deli meat, 2 slices (47 g)	2
Oven roasted chicken breast deli meat, 2 slices (57 g)	1
Shady Brook Farms	
Extra lean ground white turkey, 4 oz	2
Simple Truth	
Oven roasted turkey, 2 oz	1
Peppered turkey, 2 oz	1
Smithfield Anytime	
Hickory smoked lean sliced ham, 3 oz	2
Spam	
Spam, classic, 2 oz	6
Thin 'n Trim	
Honey mesquite chicken breast, 2 slices (50 g)	1
Trader Joe's	
Oven roasted turkey breast, 4 slices (56 g)	1
Smoked turkey breast, 4 slices (56 g)	1
Trader Joe's Refrigerated	
Sliced rosemary ham, 2 slices (56 g)	1
True Story	
Organic oven roasted turkey breast, 1 pouch (35 g)	0

	SmartPoints® value
Wegman's	
Sliced turkey pepperoni, 16 slices (28 g)	2
Wegman's Delicatessen	
Turkey breast, 2 oz	1
Wellshire	
Classic sliced turkey, 1 slice (28 g)	1
Wilson	
Turkey pepperoni, sliced, 15 slices (30 g)	2

Pork and Ham

Boar's Head	
Ham, 2 oz	1
Bob Evans	
Ham steaks, 1 steak (112 g)	2
Carolina Pride	
Honey ham, 1 slice (28 g)	1
Claim Jumper	
Pork ribs, baby back, 3 ribs and sauce (140 g)	7
Cooks	
Ham steak, 4 oz	4
Curly's	
Baby back pork ribs, 3 oz	7
DAK	
Premium sliced ham, 1 slice (28 g)	0
Del Real	
Pork in green sauce, chile verde, 5 oz	3
Double G Brands	
Hickory smoked ham, 3 oz	3
Farmland	
Ham, fully cooked, cubed, 2 oz	2
Hickory smoked ham, 3 oz	4
Hickory smoked ham steaks, 1 slice (65 g)	1
Spiral sliced ham, hickory smoked, 3 oz	4

	SmartPoints® value
Giant	
Pork ribs, baby back, original, 5 oz	8
Hatfield	
Ham steak, traditional, 3 oz	2
Hillshire Farm	
Pulled pork, barbeque, 2 oz	2
Hormel	
Pork chops, smoked, thick cut, bone-in, 3 oz	4
Pork loin filet, center cut, extra lean, lemon garlic, 4 oz	3
Pork tenderloin, extra lean, teriyaki, 4 oz	3
Hormel Cure 81	
Ham, 3 oz	2
Hormel Taco Meats	
Fully cooked shredded and seasoned pork, ½ cup	1
John Morrell	
Diced ham, 2 oz	2
Ham, mini cubed, 2 oz	2
Jones Dairy Farm	
Ham slices, naturally hickory smoked, 2 slices (45 g)	1
Kentucky Legend	
Hickory smoked ham steak, 3 oz	1
King Cheese Spirella Minis	
Proscuitto and soupressata with sliced mozzarella, 3 servings (54 g)	5
Kirkland Signature	
Smoked pulled pork, 2 oz	4
Land O'Frost Bistro Favorites	
Ham, black forest, 6 slices (57 g)	1
Land O'Frost Premium	
Black forest ham, old world style, 4 slices (50 g)	1
Lloyd's Barbeque Company	
Original bbq sauce with seasoned shredded pork, ¼ cup	3
Meijer	
Diced ham, 2 oz	1

	SmartPoints® value
Oscar Mayer Carving Board	
Slow cooked ham with natural juices, 2 oz	1
Oscar Mayer Selects	
Ham, applewood smoked, 6 slices (51 g)	1
PrimoTaglio	
Ham off the bone, with natural juices, hickory smoked, 4 slices (57 g)	2
Rose Premium	
Canadian bacon 97% fat free, 3 slices (60 g)	1
Safeway	
Pork chops, loin, center cut, bone in, 4 oz	6
Pork shoulder, blade steak, 4 oz	7
Sahlens	
Ham, smokehouse, 2 oz	1
Smithfield	
Ham steak, boneless, hickory smoked, 3 oz	2
Smithfield Anytime Favorites	
Ham, diced, 97% fat free, 2 oz	2
Smithfield Pork Lean Generations	
Boneless center cut pork loin chops, thin sliced, 4 oz	2
Spartan Fresh Selections	
Ham, honey, spiral sliced, hickory smoked, 3 oz	3
Specially Selected	
Prosciutto dry cured ham, 1 oz	1
Stubbs	
Pork, pulled, ½ cup	8
Sugardale	
Diced ham, 2 oz	2
Taylor	
Pork roll, 1 slice (56 g)	5
Trader Joe's	
Bbq shredded pork with barbeque sauce, ¼ cup	2
Fully cooked pork belly, 3 oz	8

Sausage

	SmartPoints® value
Aidells	
Sausage, smoked chicken & turkey, Italian style with mozzarella cheese, 1 link (85 g)	5
Aidells Chef Bruce	
Chicken & apple smoked chicken sausage, 1 link (85 g)	5
Smoked pork sausage, Cajun style, 1 link (85 g)	5
Al Fresco	
Chicken sausage with jalapeños and roasted red peppers, 1 link (85 g)	3
Chicken sausage, roasted garlic, 1 link (85 g)	3
Hot Italian style chicken sausage, 1 link (78 g)	3
Sausage, sweet apple chicken, 1 link (85 g)	5
Sweet Italian style chicken sausage, 1 link (85 g)	3
Wild blueberry chicken sausage, 1 link (32 g)	2
Al Fresco All Natural	
Country style chicken sausage, 1 link (32 g)	1
Roasted pepper and asiago chicken sausage, 1 link (85 g)	3
Smoked andouille chicken sausage, 1 link (85 g)	3
Spinach and feta chicken sausage, 1 link (85 g)	3
Sweet apple chicken sausage, 1 link (80 g)	3
Sweet Italian style chicken sausage, 1 link (80 g)	2
Al Fresco Country Style	
Chicken sausage breakfast patties, 1 patty (50 g)	2
Applegate Naturals	
Breakfast sausage, chicken & apple, 3 links (59 g)	3

	SmartPoints® value
Breakfast sausage, chicken & maple, 3 links (59 g)	3
Breakfast sausage, savory turkey, 3 links (59 g)	3
Chicken and apple breakfast sausage patty, 1 patty (33 g)	2
Chicken and maple breakfast sausage patty, 1 patty (33 g)	2
Savory turkey breakfast sausage patty, 1 patty (33 g)	2
Banquet Brown 'N Serve	
Country recipe sausage links, 3 links (54 g)	6
Lite original fully cooked sausage links, 3 links (54 g)	3
Original fully cooked sausage links, 3 links (62 g)	7
Sausage links, fully cooked, lite original, 3 links (54 g)	3
Sausage links, fully cooked, maple, 3 links (54 g)	6
Sausage links, fully cooked, original, 3 links (54 g)	6
Sausage links, turkey, 3 links (60 g)	3
Sausage patties, fully cooked, original, 2 patties (45 g)	5
Sausage patties, turkey, 2 patties (45 g)	3
Maple fully cooked sausage links, 3 links (54 g)	6
Bilinski's	
Organic mild Italian chicken sausage, 1 link (68 g)	1
Bob Evans	
Fully cooked turkey sausage links, 2 links (45 g)	1
Fully cooked turkey sausage patties, 2 patties (68 g)	2
Pork sausage links, original, 3 links (51 g)	5
Pork sausage patties, original, 2 patties (59 g)	5
Turkey sausage patties, 2 patties (56 g)	2

Sausage (cont'd)

	SmartPoints® value
Bob Evans Grocery	
Pork sausage patties, 2 patties (52 g)	8
Brat Hans	
Spicy Italian chicken sausage, 1 link (85 g)	3
Breakfast Best Heat-n-Serve	
Turkey sausage links, 3 links (54 g)	3
Brown 'N Serve	
Fully cooked turkey sausage links, 2 links (45 g)	3
Butterball Everyday	
Hardwood smoked turkey sausage, 2 oz	3
Turkey breakfast sausage patties, 2 patties (71 g)	3
Turkey sausage polska kielbasa, 2 oz	3
Butterball Natural Inspirations	
Turkey breakfast sausage links, 3 links (57 g)	2
Casual Gourmet	
Sweet Italian style chicken sausage, 1 link (91 g)	3
Daily Chef	
Mozzarella and roasted garlic chicken sausage (serves 15), 1 serving (91 g)	4
Spinach and asiago chicken sausage (serves 15), 1 serving (91 g)	4
Dietz & Watson	
Chicken sausage, 1 sausage (85 g)	3
Duke's	
Hot and spicy shorty smoked sausages, 2 links (25 g)	2
Original shorty smoked sausages, 2 links (25 g)	2
Eckrich	
Li'l smokies cocktail smoked sausages, 5 links (76 g)	6
Skinless smoked sausage, 2 oz	7

	SmartPoints® value
Skinless smoked turkey sausage, 2 oz	4
Farmer John	
Quick serve sausage links, 3 links (64 g)	8
Fit & Active	
Fresh sweet Italian turkey sausage, 1 link (112 g)	4
Lean turkey Polish kielbasa, 2 oz	2
Fusia Asian Inspirations	
Spicy chicken sausage, 1 link (85 g)	4
Giant	
Turkey sausage patties, 1 patty (28 g)	1
Gilbert's	
Chicken bratwurst sausages with sauteed onions, 1 link (71 g)	3
Great Value	
Original pork sausage links, 2 links (45 g)	7
Harvestland	
Italian chicken sausage with peppers and onions, 1 link (75 g)	3
Hillshire Farm	
Beef lit'l smokies, 5 links (50 g)	6
Lite polska kielbasa, 2 oz	3
Lit'l smokies sausage (pork, turkey, beef), 5 links (50 g)	6
Polska kielbasa, 2 oz	6
Polska kielbasa, turkey, 2 oz	2
Sausage, smoked, 2 oz	6
Smoked beef sausage, 2 oz	6
Smoked sausage, turkey, 2 oz	2
Summer sausage, 2 oz	7
Hillshire Farm Lit'l Smokies	
Turkey smoked sausage, 5 links (50 g)	2
Jennie-O	
Breakfast sausage, turkey, mild, lean, 2 oz	2
Hardwood smoked turkey kielbasa, 2 oz	2

	SmartPoints® value
Italian turkey sausage, hot, lean, 1 link (109 g)	4
Italian turkey sausage, sweet, lean, 1 link (109 g)	4
Lean mild turkey breakfast sausage, 2 oz	2
Jennie-O Lean	
Turkey breakfast sausage links, 2 links (48 g)	1
Jimmy Dean	
Breakfast sausage, regular flavor, 2½ oz	2
Fully cooked turkey sausage crumbles, ½ cup	2
Fully cooked turkey sausage links, 3 links (68 g)	3
Fully cooked turkey sausage patties, 2 patties (68 g)	3
Maple turkey sausage links, 3 links (68 g)	3
Original pork sausage patties, 2 patties (68 g)	9
Pork sausage links, original, 3 links (68 g)	9
Pork sausage, premium, hot, 2 oz cooked	6
Regular premium pork sausage, 2 oz	6
Sausage patties, maple turkey, 2 patties (68 g)	3
Sausage, pork, regular, 2 oz cooked	6
Jimmy Dean Delights	
Applewood smoke chicken sausage links, 3 links (64 g)	3
Applewood smoke chicken sausage patties, 2 patties (64 g)	3
Jimmy Dean Fully Cooked Sausage	
Turkey sausage links, 3 links (68 gs)	3
Jimmy Dean Heat 'N Serve	
Sausage patties, turkey, 2 patties (52 g)	3

	SmartPoints® value
Johnsonville	
Brats, beef, 1 link (57 g)	7
Breakfast sausage, patties, original recipe, 1 patty (32 g)	3
Fully cooked turkey breakfast sausage, 2 links (45 g)	2
Fully cooked turkey breakfast sausages, 2 links (45 g)	2
Italian sausage, hot, 1 grilled link (85 g)	9
Original recipe fully cooked breakfast sausage, 2 links (45 g)	5
Sausage, chicken, 3 cheese Italian style, 1 link (85 g)	4
Sausage, chicken, apple, 1 link (85 g)	5
Sausage, chicken, chipotle Monterey Jack cheese, 1 link (85 g)	4
Sausage, Italian, mild, 1 link (85 g)	9
Sausage, Italian, sweet, 1 grilled link (85 g)	9
Smoked sausage, beddar with cheddar, 1 link (66 g)	7
Summer sausage, beef, 2 oz	6
Turkey breakfast sausage, 2 patties (68 g)	3
Turkey sausage with cheddar, 1 link (64 g)	3
Turkey sausage, smoked, 1 link (64 g)	3
Vermont maple syrup breakfast sausage, 2 links (45 g)	5
Johnsonville Brats	
Original bratwurst, 1 link (85 g)	9
Jones All Natural	
Golden brown fully cooked chicken sausage links, 4 links (56 g)	2
Golden brown fully cooked chicken sausage patty, 1 patty (35 g)	1

Sausage (cont'd)

	SmartPoints® value
Jones Dairy Farm	
Sausage links, turkey, golden brown, 4 links (56 g)	2
Turkey sausage links, 4 links (56 g)	2
Jones Dairy Farm All Natural	
Golden brown turkey sausage patties, 1 patty (35 g)	2
Kirkwood	
Fully cooked spinach and feta chicken sausage, 1 link (85 g)	4
Mild Italian chicken sausage, 1 link (85 g)	4
Kroger	
Fully cooked turkey sausage patties, 2 patties (56 g)	3
Nature's Promise Organics	
Organic spinach and cheese chicken sausage, 1 link (68 g)	2
New York Style Sausage	
Pork sausage, breakfast links, 2 links (57 g)	4
O Organics	
Spinach and feta organic chicken sausage, 1 link (57 g)	1
Odom's Tennessee Pride	
Turkey sausage patties, 2 patties (62 g)	3
Old Wisconsin	
Snack bites, turkey sausage, 6 pieces (30 g)	2
Snack sticks, turkey sausage, 1 stick (16 g)	1
Oscar Mayer	
Sausages, little smokies, 6 links (57 g)	6
Oscar Mayer Selects	
Hardwood smoked uncured turkey sausage, 2 oz	3
Parkview	
Beef smoked sausage, 2 oz	7
Cheddar brats, 1 link (66 g)	7
Premio	

	SmartPoints® value
Italian sausage, hot, 1 link (70 g)	7
Sausage, chicken, Italian, sweet, 1 link (60 g)	3
Publix	
Apple and gouda smoked chicken sausage, 2 oz	2
Spinach and feta smoked chicken sausage, 2 oz	2
Publix Premium	
Italian style and cheese smoked chicken sausage, 1 link (68 g)	3
Purnell's Old Folks	
Medium country sausage patties, 2 patties (56 g)	8
Sausages by Amylu	
Apple & gouda cheese chicken sausage, 1 link (76 g)	3
Apple and gouda chicken sausage, 1 link (76 g)	3
Sausage, chicken, apple & gouda cheese, smoked, 1 link (63 g)	3
Shady Brook Farms	
Italian turkey sausage, lean, sweet, 1 link (119 g)	3
Simms	
Fully cooked summer sausage, 2 oz	7
Simple Truth Traditional	
Breakfast sausage links, 3 links (55 g)	3
Simply Nature	
Country style chicken breakfast sausage with sage and thyme, 1 link (32 g)	1
Tennessee Pride	
Sausage patties, original, 2 patties (51 g)	6
Tennessee Pride Homestyle	
Sausage balls, 4 balls (72 g)	10
Thin 'n Trim	
Chicken sausage, 1 link (56 g)	1
Chipotle and peach salsa chicken sausage, 1 link (56 g)	1

	SmartPoints® value
Thin 'n Trim All Natural	
Sweet Italian chicken sausage with red bell peppers, 1 link (56 g)	1
Tofurky	
Sausage, Italian, with sun-dried tomatoes and basil, 3 ½ oz	6
Trader Joe's	
All natural fully cooked maple chicken breakfast sausage, 2 links (57 g)	2
Roasted garlic chicken sausage, 1 link (68 g)	3
Spicy Italian chicken sausage, 1 link (85 g)	3
Turkey summer sausage, 2 oz	2
Uncooked chicken breakfast sausage, 1 link (69 g)	3
Trader Joe's Refrigerated	
Spicy jalapeño chicken sausage, 1 link (68 g)	3
Sun-dried tomato basil chicken sausage, 1 link (68 g)	3
Sweet apple with pure Vermont maple syrup chicken sausage, 1 link (68 g)	4
Sweet Italian style red & green pepper chicken sausage, 1 link (68 g)	3
Wegman's All Natural	
Breakfast with sage chicken sausage, 1 link (32 g)	1

Turkey

	SmartPoints® value
Ball Park	
Flame grilled turkey patty, 1 patty (85 g)	2
Bubba Burger	
Turkey burger, 1 burger (112 g)	4
Butterball	
Herb roasted turkey breast, 1 oz	1
Lean ground turkey, 4 oz	3
Seasoned turkey burger patties, 1 patty (112 g)	4
Turkey breast roast, boneless, 4 oz	2
Turkey burger patties with natural flavoring, 1 patty (114 g)	2
Butterball Everyday	
97% extra lean ground turkey, 4 oz	2
All natural fresh ground turkey, 4 oz	3
Sweet onion seasoned turkey burgers, 1 patty (151 g)	5
Turkey burgers, 1 patty (151 g)	5
Turkey, ground, 93/7, lean, 4 oz	3
Butterball Natural Inspirations	
All natural turkey burgers, 1 patty (112 g)	4
Castle Wood Reserve	
Four pepper oven roasted turkey breast, 2 oz	1
Farmer John	
Savory turkey sausage patties, 2 patties (70 g)	3
Fit & Active	
Cracked pepper turkey breast tenderloins, 4 oz	2
Lean ground turkey, 4 oz	3
Oven roasted turkey breast, 2 oz	1
Foster Farms	
Fresh ground turkey, 4 oz	3
Turkey breast cutlets, boneless & skinless, 4 oz	1
Foster Farms Fresh & Natural	
99% fat free ground turkey breast, 4 oz	1
Great Value	
Breakfast patties, turkey, 1 patty (50 g)	2
Harvestland	
Fresh ground turkey burgers, 1 burger (112 g)	4
Honeysuckle White	
Breast of turkey, 4 oz	1

Turkey (cont'd)

	SmartPoints® value
Jennie-O	
90%/10% fat lean turkey burger patties, 1 patty (112 g)	4
93% lean/7% fat all white meat turkey burgers, 1 burger (149 g)	4
Cracked pepper turkey breast sticks, 1 stick (21 g)	0
Ground turkey breast, with natural flavorings, extra lean, 4 oz	1
Ground turkey, lean, 4 oz	4
Ground turkey, taco seasoning, 4 oz	4
Lean taco seasoned ground turkey, 4 oz	4
Seasoned turkey burger patties with onion and garlic seasoning, lean, 1 patty (114 g)	4
Smoke house turkey sticks, 1 stick (21 g)	0
Turkey breast stick, 1 stick (21 g)	0
Turkey breast tenderloins, roast turkey, 4 oz	1
Turkey burgers, 1 burger (112 g)	6
Turkey burgers, lean, original, 1 burger (112 g)	4
Jennie-O All Natural	
Oven roasted turkey breast stick, 1 stick (21 g)	0
Smoke house turkey breast sticks, 1 stick (21 g)	0
Sweet bbq turkey breast stick, 1 stick (21 g)	0
Jennie-O So Easy	
Turkey meatloaf, lean, 5 oz	4
Jennie-O Turkey	
Ground turkey (90% lean 10% fat), 4 oz	3
Jennie-O Turkey Store	
Seasoned turkey burger, 4 oz	6
Turkey burger, 4 oz	6
Jones Dairy Farm	
Turkey sausage patties, 1 patty (35 g)	2

	SmartPoints® value
Kirkland Signature	
Turkey burgers, 1 burger (151 g)	3
Kirkwood	
Ground turkey, 4 oz	6
Kroger	
Fresh extra lean ground turkey breast, 4 oz	1
Lunch Mate	
Cured roasted turkey breast, 1 slice (28 g)	1
Perdue	
Ground turkey, lean, 4 oz	4
Plainville Farms	
94% lean 6% fat ground turkey, 4 oz	3
Organic ground turkey, 4 oz	4
Turkey burgers, 4 oz	4
Quick 'N Eat!	
Fully cooked turkey breakfast patties, 1 patty (50 g)	1
Sara Lee Premium Meats	
Honey roasted turkey breast deli meat, 2 slices (45 g)	1
Oven roasted turkey breast deli meat, 2 slices (57 g)	1
Shady Brook Farms	
Ground turkey, 4 oz	3
Simple Truth	
Ground turkey patties, 1 patty (112 g)	3
Natural ground turkey patties, 1 patty (112 g)	3
Simple Truth Natural	
Extra lean ground turkey breast, 4 oz	1
Trader Joe's	
Turkey burger, 1 patty (113 g)	4
Trader Joe's Simply	
Turkey breast roasted and sliced, 3 oz	1

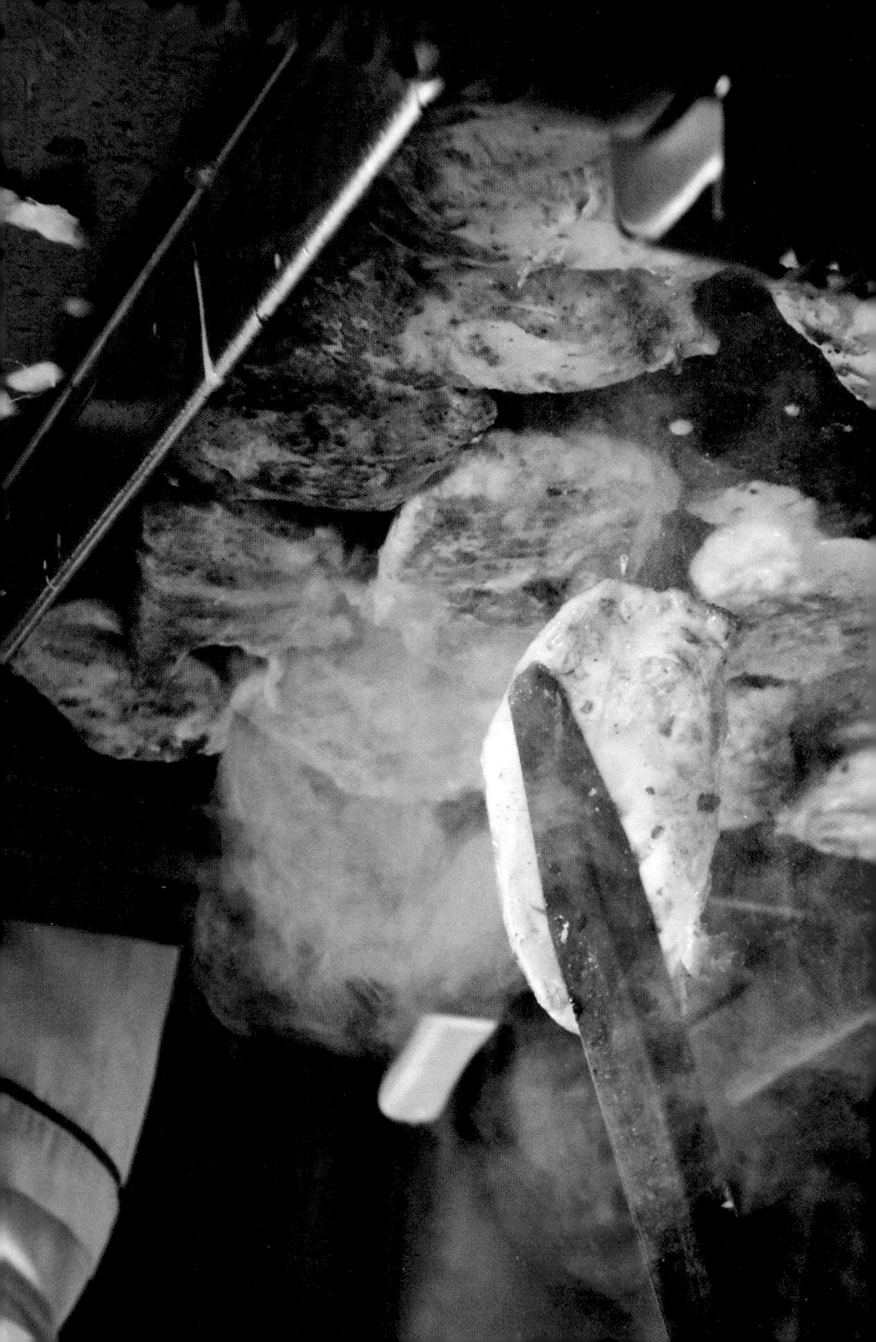

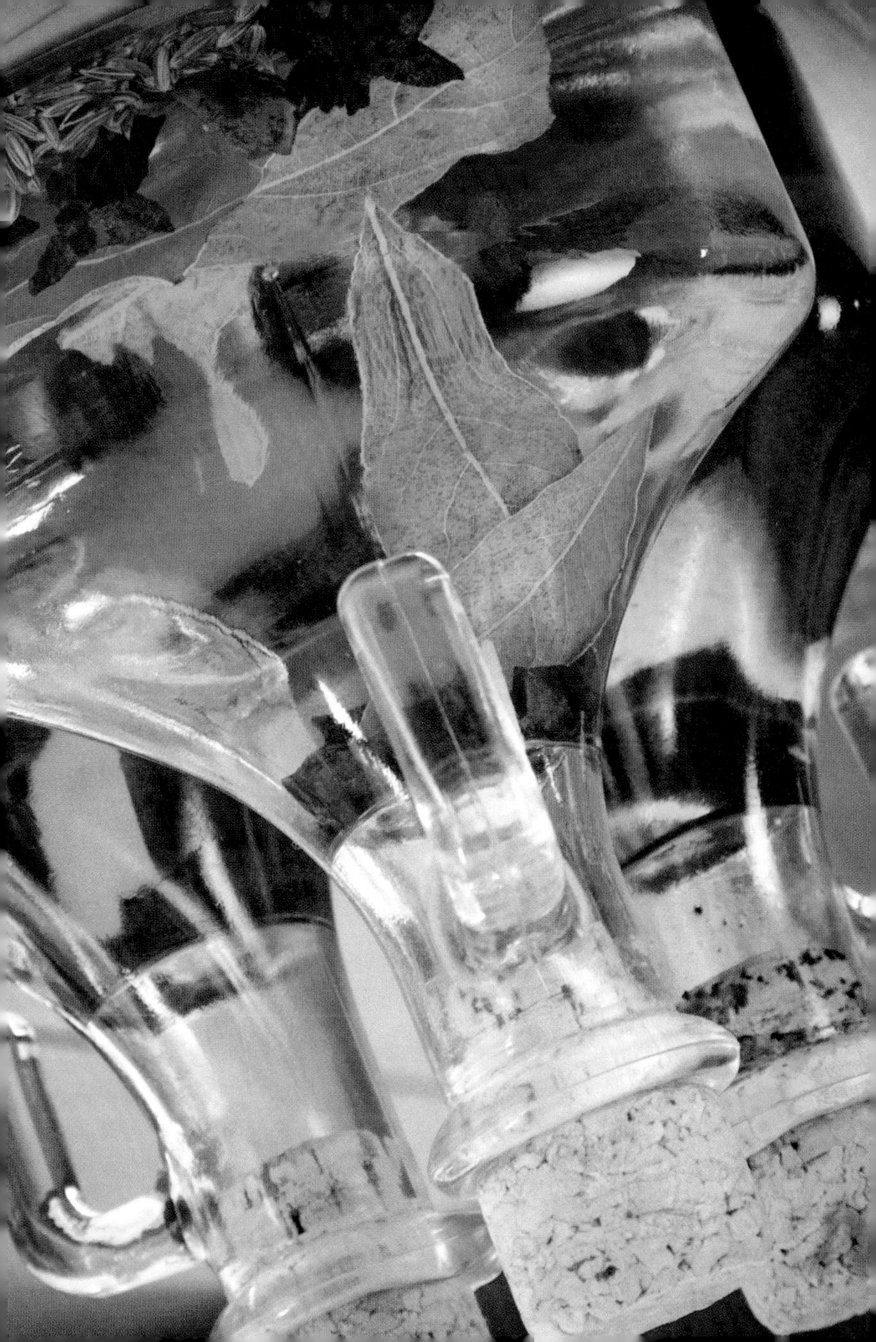

oils & dressings

Cooking and Baking Sprays

	SmartPoints® value
I Can't Believe It's Not Butter!	
Original spray, 1 spray (0.2 g)	0
Spray with extra virgin olive oil, 1 spray (0.2 g)	0
Olivio	
Buttery spray, 5 sprays (1 g)	0
Pam	
Cooking spray, no-stick, butter flavor, ¼ second spray	0
Cooking spray, no-stick, olive oil, ¼ second spray	0
Cooking spray, no-stick, original, ¼ second spray	0

Oils

Bertolli	
Extra light tasting olive oil, 1 Tbsp	4
Olive oil, extra light tasting, 1 Tbsp	4
Olive oil, extra virgin, 1 Tbsp	4
Olive oil, tasting, extra light, 1 Tbsp	4
Carlini	
All natural pure canola oil, 1 Tbsp	4
Daily Chef	
Organic extra virgin olive oil, 1 Tbsp	4
EvooRoo	
Olive oil, extra virgin, 1 Tbsp	4
Gold'n Soft	
60% vegetable oil spread, 1 Tbsp	3
Kirkland Signature	
Extra virgin Greek olive oil, 1 Tbsp	4
Organic extra virgin olive oil, 1 Tbsp	4
Pure olive oil, 1 Tbsp	4
Simply Nature Organic	
Coconut oil, 1 Tbsp	7
Trader Joe's Grocery	
Organic extra virgin coconut oil, 1 Tbsp	7
Tropical Life	
Extra virgin organic coconut oil, 1 Tbsp	7

Salad Dressings

	SmartPoints® value
365 Everyday Value	
Organic balsamic vinaigrette dressing, 2 Tbsp	1
365 Everyday Value Organic	
Balsamic vinaigrette, 2 Tbsp	2
Annie's	
Dressing, Asian sesame, 2 Tbsp	4
Dressing, goddess, lite, 2 Tbsp	2
Dressing, goddess, natural, 2 Tbsp	4
Dressing, poppy seed, lite, 2 Tbsp	3
Honey mustard vinaigrette, 2 Tbsp	2
Annie's Lite	
Raspberry vinaigrette, 2 Tbsp	2
Bolthouse Farms	
Bold blue cheese Greek yogurt dressing, 2 Tbsp	1
Caesar parmigiano yogurt dressing, 2 Tbsp	2
Caramelized onion yogurt dressing, 2 Tbsp	1
Chunky blue cheese yogurt dressing, 2 Tbsp	1
Cilantro avocado yogurt dressing, 2 Tbsp	2
Classic ranch yogurt dressing, 2 Tbsp	2
Creamy balsamic yogurt dressing, 2 Tbsp	2
Creamy roasted garlic yogurt dressing, 2 Tbsp	1
Cucumber dill Greek yogurt dressing, 2 Tbsp	1
Dressing, yogurt, salsa ranch, 2 Tbsp	2
Honey mustard yogurt dressing, 2 Tbsp	2
Italian vinaigrette dressing (serves 14), 2 Tbsp	1
Mango chipotle yogurt dressing, 2 Tbsp	2

	SmartPoints® value
Peppercorn ranch Greek yogurt dressing, 2 Tbsp	1
Salsa verde avocado yogurt dressing, 2 Tbsp	2
Vinaigrette, extra virgin olive oil, classic balsamic, 2 Tbsp	2
Vinaigrette, extra virgin olive oil, raspberry merlot, 2 Tbsp	2
Bragg	
Salad dressing, ginger & sesame, 2 Tbsp	1
Briannas	
Dressing, home style, blush wine vinaigrette, 2 Tbsp	5
Dressing, home style, creamy balsamic, 2 Tbsp	6
Dressing, home style, real French, vinaigrette, 2 Tbsp	4
Dressing, home style, rich poppy seed, 2 Tbsp	6
Cardinis	
Dressing, Caesar, 2 Tbsp	5
Dressing, Caesar, light, 2 Tbsp	3
Dressing, Greek vinaigrette, light, 2 Tbsp	2
Cindy's Kitchen	
Fresh avocado vinaigrette dressing, 2 Tbsp	2
Real bleu cheese dressing, 2 Tbsp	4
Cookwell	
Salad dressing, Asian ginger vinaigrette, 2 Tbsp	2
Dorothy Lynch	
Fat free home style dressing, 2 Tbsp	4
Home style dressing, 2 Tbsp	5
Edelweiss	
Dressing, creamy cesar, 2 Tbsp	4
Emerils	
Dressing, bleu cheese, 2 Tbsp	3
Fanny's Lite	
Italian dressing, 2 Tbsp	3

	SmartPoints® value
Fit & Active	
Buffalo ranch light dressing, 2 Tbsp	3
Fat free zesty Italian dressing, 2 Tbsp	1
Reduced fat light balsamic vinaigrette, 2 Tbsp	2
Reduced fat light ranch dressing, 2 Tbsp	3
Food Lion	
Light ranch dressing, 2 Tbsp	3
Light raspberry vinaigrette dressing, 2 Tbsp	2
Giant Eagle	
Light balsamic vinaigrette, 2 Tbsp	1
Girard's	
Dressing, Caesar, light, 2 Tbsp	3
Dressing, champagne, 2 Tbsp	5
Dressing, champagne, light, 2 Tbsp	2
Dressing, white balsamic vinaigrette, 2 Tbsp	4
Good Seasons	
Italian all natural salad dressing and recipe mix, ⅛ packet dry (2.5 g)	0
Great Value	
Chipotle ranch dressing, 2 Tbsp	4
Fat free Italian dressing, 2 Tbsp	1
House Caesar dressing, 2 Tbsp	4
Zesty Italian dressing and marinade, 2 Tbsp	2
Great Value Classic	
Light ranch dressing, 2 Tbsp	3
Great Value Light	
Raspberry vinaigrette dressing, 2 Tbsp	2
Heinz	
Light Italian dressing, 1 packet (42 g)	1
Hellmann's	
Light ranch dressing, 1 packet (43 g)	3

Salad Dressings (cont'd)

	SmartPoints® value
Hendrickson's	
Dressing, marinade & seasoning, original, sweet vinegar & olive oil, 2 Tbsp	4
Hidden Valley	
Cucumber dill Greek yogurt dressing, 2 Tbsp	2
Dressing, light, ranch, 2 Tbsp	3
Dressing, ranch, 2 Tbsp	5
Dressing, ranch, spicy, 2 Tbsp	5
Dressing, the original ranch, fat free, 2 Tbsp	1
Dressing, the original ranch, fat free, 2 Tbsp	1
Light ranch dressing, 2 Tbsp	3
Old fashioned ranch buttermilk dressing, 2 Tbsp	5
Original ranch salad dressing and seasoning mix, ½ tsp	0
Ranch dressing, 2 Tbsp	5
Ranch dressing, light, buttermilk, 2 Tbsp	3
Ranch Greek yogurt dressing, 2 Tbsp	2
Hidden Valley Farmhouse Originals	
Southwest chipotle dressing and dip, 2 Tbsp	4
Hidden Valley The Original Ranch	
Avocado dressing, 2 Tbsp	3
Cucumber dressing, 2 Tbsp	3
Fiesta salsa light dressing, 2 Tbsp	2
Light cucumber dressing, 2 Tbsp	2
Hidden Valley The Original Ranch Light	
Dressing, 2 Tbsp	3
Hidden Valley To Go	
Dressing, light, thick & creamy, single cups, 1 container (44 ml)	4
John the Greek	
Salad dressing, original, 1 Tbsp	3
Ken's	
Country French dressing, 1½ oz	8
Dressing, olive oil vinaigrette with balsamic vinegar, lite, 1½ oz	3
Ranch dressing, 1½ oz	7
Thousand Island dressing, 1½ oz	7
Ken's Light Options	
Balsamic vinaigrette dressing, 2 Tbsp	2
Parmesan & peppercorn dressing, 2 Tbsp	3
Ken's Steak House	
Balsamic with honey dressing, 2 Tbsp	4
Dressing & marinade, Italian, 2 Tbsp	5
Dressing & marinade, lite Italian, 1 oz	2
Dressing & marinade, lite, Caesar, 2 Tbsp	3
Dressing, balsamic & basil vinaigrette, 2 Tbsp	4
Dressing, buttermilk ranch, 2 Tbsp	6
Dressing, Caesar, lite, 2 Tbsp	2
Dressing, chunky blue cheese, 2 Tbsp	5
Dressing, chunky blue cheese, lite, 2 Tbsp	3
Dressing, country French with Vermont honey, lite, 2 Tbsp	5
Dressing, creamy Caesar, 2 Tbsp	6
Dressing, fat free, raspberry pecan, 2 Tbsp	3
Dressing, lite, balsamic vinaigrette, 2 Tbsp	2
Dressing, lite, Italian, 2 Tbsp	2
Dressing, lite, northern Italian with basil & Romano, 2 Tbsp	2
Dressing, lite, olive oil vinaigrette, 2 Tbsp	2
Dressing, lite, poppy seed, 2 Tbsp	4
Dressing, lite, ranch, 2 Tbsp	3
Dressing, lite, raspberry walnut vinaigrette, 2 Tbsp	4
Dressing, lite, raspberry walnut vinaigrette, 2 Tbsp	4
Dressing, lite, sweet vidalia onion, 2 Tbsp	4

	SmartPoints® value
Dressing, ranch, 2 Tbsp	5
Dressing, red wine vinegar & olive oil, lite, 2 Tbsp	2
Dressing, Thousand Island, 2 Tbsp	5
Dressing, topping & spread, lite, creamy Caesar, 2 Tbsp	3
Dressing, topping & spread, squeezable, honey mustard, 2 Tbsp	5
Dressing, zesty Italian, 2 Tbsp	3
Fat free ranch dressing, 1 packet (42.52 g)	2
Fat free raspberry pecan dressing, 2 Tbsp	3
Greek dressing, 2 Tbsp	4
Honey mustard dressing, 2 Tbsp	5
Lite Asian sesame with ginger & soy dressing, 2 Tbsp	3
Lite balsamic vinaigrette dressing, 2 Tbsp	2
Lite creamy Caesar dressing, 2 Tbsp	3
Lite honey mustard dressing, 2 Tbsp	4
Lite honey mustard dressing, topping & spread, 2 Tbsp	4
Lite strawberry vinaigrette dressing, 2 Tbsp	3
Lite Thousand Island dressing, 2 Tbsp	3
Ken's Steak House Fat Free	
Italian dressing pounch, 1 packet (42.5 g)	1
Ken's Steak House Healthy Options	
Dressing, Caesar vinaigrette, 2 Tbsp	3
Dressing, honey dijon, 2 Tbsp	3
Dressing, olive oil & vinegar, 2 Tbsp	2
Dressing, raspberry walnut, 2 Tbsp	3
Dressing, vinaigrette, sweet vidalia onion, 2 Tbsp	3

	SmartPoints® value
Ken's Steak House Light Options	
Dressing, Italian, 2 Tbsp	2
Ken's Steak House Lite	
Apple cider vinaigrette dressing, 2 Tbsp	3
Buttermilk ranch dressing, 2 Tbsp	3
Sun-dried tomato dressing, 2 Tbsp	2
Kraft	
Anything dressing, balsamic vinaigrette, 2 Tbsp	3
Anything dressing, classic ranch, 2 Tbsp	4
Anything dressing, creamy Italian, 2 Tbsp	3
Anything dressing, fat free, ranch, 2 Tbsp	2
Anything dressing, fat free, Thousand Island, 2 Tbsp	2
Anything dressing, lite, balsamic vinaigrette, 2 Tbsp	1
Anything dressing, lite, French style, 2 Tbsp	3
Anything dressing, lite, zesty Italian, 2 Tbsp	1
Anything dressing, Tuscan house Italian, 2 Tbsp	2
Balsamic vinaigrette dressing, 2 Tbsp	2
Catalina fat free dressing, 1 pouch (42.5 g)	3
Dressing & marinade, zesty Italian, 2 Tbsp	2
Dressing, Asian toasted sesame, 2 Tbsp	3
Dressing, buttermilk ranch, 2 Tbsp	4
Dressing, Caesar vinaigrette with parmesan, 2 Tbsp	2
Dressing, classic Caesar, 2 Tbsp	4
Dressing, classic, Catalina, 2 Tbsp	4
Dressing, creamy Italian, 2 Tbsp	4
Dressing, creamy poppyseed, 2 Tbsp	5

Salad Dressings, Kraft (cont'd)

	SmartPoints® value
Dressing, fat free, Catalina, 2 Tbsp	2
Dressing, Greek vinaigrette, 2 Tbsp	2
Dressing, Italian roasted red pepper with parmesan, 2 Tbsp	2
Dressing, lite, ranch, 2 Tbsp	2
Dressing, peppercorn ranch, 2 Tbsp	4
Dressing, roka blue cheese, 2 Tbsp	4
Dressing, sun dried tomato vinaigrette, 2 Tbsp	2
Dressing, Thousand Island, 2 Tbsp	5
Fat free, anything dressing, zesty Italian, 2 Tbsp	1
Strawberry vinagrette dressing, 2 Tbsp	2
Zesty lime vinaigrette dressing, 2 Tbsp	2
Kraft Free	
Anything dressing, fat free, French style, 2 Tbsp	2
Dressing, fat free, Italian, 2 Tbsp	1
Fat free dressing, ranch, 1 pouch (42 g)	2
Fat free dressing, raspberry vinaigrette, 1 pouch (43 g)	2
Kraft Light	
Dressing, Catalina, lite, 2 Tbsp	3
Dressing, lite, Asian toasted sesame, 2 Tbsp	2
Dressing, lite, creamy Caesar, 2 Tbsp	1
Dressing, lite, house Italian, 2 Tbsp	2
Dressing, lite, parmesan asiago balsamic vinaigrette, 2 Tbsp	2
Dressing, lite, Thousand Island, 2 Tbsp	3
Dressing, lite, three cheese ranch, 2 Tbsp	2
Lite raspberry vinaigrette dressing, 2 Tbsp	2

	SmartPoints® value
Kroger	
Dressing, balsamic vinaigrette, lite, 2 Tbsp	2
Dressing, creamy ranch, 2 Tbsp	5
Dressing, lite creamy ranch, 2 Tbsp	3
Dressing, lite, southwest ranch, 2 Tbsp	3
Dressing, ranch, creamy, fat free, 2 Tbsp	1
Dressing, zesty Italian, fat free, 2 Tbsp	1
Litehouse	
Blue cheese Greek style yogurt dressing, 2 Tbsp	2
Chunky bleu cheese, 2 Tbsp	5
Dressing & dip, jalapeño ranch, 2 Tbsp	4
Dressing & dip, lite ranch, 2 Tbsp	2
Dressing & dip, lite salsa ranch, 2 Tbsp	2
Dressing, sauce & marinade, toasted sesame ginger, 2 Tbsp	2
Homestyle ranch, 2 Tbsp	4
Organic balsamic vinaigrette dressing, 2 Tbsp	5
Sweet onion dressing and marinade, 2 Tbsp	3
Vinaigrette dressing, pear gorgonzola, 2 Tbsp	2
Vinaigrette dressing, pomegranate blueberry, 2 Tbsp	1
Litehouse OPA	
Jalapeño ranch Greek yogurt dressing, 2 Tbsp	1
Makoto	
Ginger dressing, 2 Tbsp	3
Maple Grove Farms of Vermont	
Dressing, balsamic vinaigrette, fat free, 2 Tbsp	0
Dressing, Caesar, fat free, 2 Tbsp	0
Dressing, citrus vinaigrette, 2 Tbsp	3

	SmartPoints® value
Dressing, cranberry balsamic vinaigrette, fat free, 2 Tbsp	2
Dressing, fat free, raspberry vinaigrette, 2 Tbsp	2
Dressing, fat free, vidalia onion, 2 Tbsp	1
Fat free honey dijon dressing, 2 Tbsp	2
Fat free poppyseed dressing, 2 Tbsp	2
Fat free wasabi dijon dressing, 2 Tbsp	2
Vinaigrette, balsamic, sugar free, 2 Tbsp	0
Vinaigrette, raspberry, sugar free, 2 Tbsp	0
Marie's	
Coleslaw yogurt dressing, 2 Tbsp	4
Dressing, balsamic vinaigrette, 2 Tbsp	2
Dressing, blue cheese vinaigrette, 2 Tbsp	5
Dressing, Caesar, 2 Tbsp	6
Dressing, chunky blue cheese, 2 Tbsp	6
Dressing, coleslaw, 2 Tbsp	6
Dressing, raspberry vinaigrette, 2 Tbsp	2
Dressing, yogurt, ranch, 2 Tbsp	2
Marzetti	
Dressing, chunky blue cheese, 2 Tbsp	5
Dressing, fat free, ranch, 1½ oz	2
Dressing, light honey French, 2 Tbsp	4
Dressing, light, classic ranch, 2 Tbsp	3
Fat free California French style dressing, 1½ oz	2
Ranch dressing, 1 oz	4
Sriracha ranch dressing, 2 Tbsp	3
Marzetti Light	
Dressing, chunky blue cheese, 2 Tbsp	3

	SmartPoints® value
Italian dressing, 1½ oz	1
Vinaigrette, balsamic, 2 Tbsp	2
Marzetti Simply Dressed	
Dressing, Caesar, 2 Tbsp	4
Dressing, ranch, 2 Tbsp	4
Lemon vinaigrette dressing, 2 Tbsp	3
Light balsamic vinaigrette dressing, 2 Tbsp	2
Light roasted tomato vinaigrette dressing, 2 Tbsp	1
Light veggie ranch dressing, 2 Tbsp	2
Vinaigrette, balsamic, 2 Tbsp	3
Vinaigrette, pomegranate, 2 Tbsp	3
Marzetti Simply Dressed & Light	
Red wine Italian vinaigrette, 2 Tbsp	1
Miracle Whip	
Dressing, 1 Tbsp	1
Dressing, nonfat, fat free, 1 Tbsp	1
Dressing, original, 1 Tbsp	1
Light dressing, 1 Tbsp	1
Naturally Fresh	
Dressing, lite, ranch, 2 Tbsp	3
Newman's Own	
Balsamic vinaigrette, 2 Tbsp	3
Dressing, creamy balsamic, 2 Tbsp	4
Dressing, family recipe Italian, 2 Tbsp	4
Dressing, light Caesar, 2 Tbsp	3
Dressing, ranch, 2 Tbsp	5
Dressing, red wine vinegar & olive oil, lite, 2 Tbsp	2
Light Italian dressing, 2 Tbsp	2
Olive oil & vinegar dressing, 2 Tbsp	5
Newman's Own Lighten Up!	
Dressing, light balsamic vinaigrette, 2 Tbsp	2
Dressing, light honey mustard, 2 Tbsp	3

Salad Dressings, Newman's Own Lighten Up! (cont'd)

	SmartPoints® value
Dressing, light raspberry & walnut, 2 Tbsp	3
Dressing, low-fat sesame ginger, 2 Tbsp	2
Light balsamic vinaigrette, 2 Tbsp	2
Light Italian dressing, 2 Tbsp	2
Vinaigrette, light lime, 2 Tbsp	2
Newman's Own Organic	
Light balsamic vinaigrette, 2 Tbsp	2
Olive Garden	
Italian dressing, 2 Tbsp	3
Light Italian dressing, 2 Tbsp	1
Signature Italian dressing, 2 Tbsp	3
OPA	
Feta dill Greek style yogurt dressing, 2 Tbsp	1
Ranch Greek style yogurt dressing, 2 Tbsp	2
OPA by Litehouse	
Caesar dressing, 2 Tbsp	2
Kalamata feta flavor Greek yogurt dressing, 2 Tbsp	2
Organic Girl	
White cheddar vinaigrette, 2 Tbsp	2
Panera Bread	
Dressing, Asian sesame vinaigrette, 2 Tbsp	2
Dressing, balsamic vinaigrette, low sodium, 2 Tbsp	4
Dressing, fuji apple vinaigrette, 2 Tbsp	4
Dressing, poppyseed, fat free, low calorie, low sodium, 2 Tbsp	2
Raspberry vinaigrette fat free salad dressing, 2 Tbsp	1
Panera Bread Grocery	
Caesar dressing, 2 Tbsp	4
Pepper Mill	
Raspberry vinaigrette dressing, 1 packet (59 ml)	3
Private Selection	
Dressing, creamy cesar, 2 Tbsp	5

	SmartPoints® value
Publix	
Lite mayonnaise dressing, 1 Tbsp	1
Lite raspberry walnut vinaigrette dressing, 2 Tbsp	3
Tangy balsamic vinaigrette dressing, 2 Tbsp	2
Sam's Choice	
Ginger sesame vinaigrette dressing, 2 Tbsp	2
Simple Nature Organic	
Chipotle ranch dressing, 2 Tbsp	4
Simply Nature	
Organic tahini goddess dressing, 2 Tbsp	4
Roasted red pepper dressing, 2 Tbsp	3
Skinnygirl	
Fat free sugar free balsamic vinaigrette dressing, 2 Tbsp	0
Fat free sugar free honey dijon dressing, 2 Tbsp	0
Smart Balance Omega Plus	
Dressing, light mayonnaise, 1 Tbsp	2
Trader Giotto's	
Balsamic vinaigrette, 2 Tbsp	3
Trader Joe's	
Asian style spicy peanut vinaigrette, 2 Tbsp	3
Champagne pear vinaigrette, 2 Tbsp	2
Cilantro salad dressing, 2 Tbsp	2
Light champagne vinaigrette, 2 Tbsp	2
Organic sriracha ranch dressing, 2 Tbsp	3
Sweet onion and bacon vinaigrette, 2 Tbsp	3
Tuscan Italian with balsamic vinegar dressing, 2 Tbsp	3
Trader Joe's Grocery	
Cranberry walnut & gorgonzola salad dressing, 2 Tbsp	3

	SmartPoints® value
Fat free balsamic vinaigrette, 2 Tbsp	1
Goddess dressing, 2 Tbsp	4
Greek style feta dressing, 2 Tbsp	4
Low-fat parmesan ranch dressing, 2 Tbsp	1
Trader Joe's Organic	
Ranch dressing, 2 Tbsp	4
Trader Ming's	
Fat free sesame soy ginger vinaigrette, 2 Tbsp	2
Tuscan Garden	
Balsamic vinaigrette dressing, 2 Tbsp	2
Honey mustard dressing, 2 Tbsp	5
Italian dressing, 2 Tbsp	3
Village ranch salad dressing, 2 Tbsp	5
Virginia Brand	
Salad dressing, vidalia onion vinegarette, 2 Tbsp	4
Vidalia onion vinegarette salad dressing, 2 Tbsp	4
Walden Farms	
Dressing, bacon ranch, 2 Tbsp	0
Dressing, balsamic vinaigrette, 2 Tbsp	0
Dressing, bleu cheese, calorie free, 2 Tbsp	0
Dressing, honey dijon, 1 packet (30 ml)	0
Vinaigrette, raspberry, 2 Tbsp	0
Western	
Dressing, lite, wish-bone, 2 Tbsp	4
Dressing, sweet & smooth, 2 Tbsp	7
Fat free sweet and smooth dressing, 2 Tbsp	3
Wild Oats Marketplace Organic	
Balsamic vinaigrette, 2 Tbsp	2
Wish-Bone	
Chipotle ranch dressing, 2 Tbsp	5
Dressing, balsamic vinaigrette, 2 Tbsp	2

	SmartPoints® value
Dressing, fat free, chunky blue cheese, 2 Tbsp	1
Dressing, Italian, 2 Tbsp	3
Dressing, Italian, fat free, 2 Tbsp	1
Dressing, Italian, light, 2 Tbsp	1
Dressing, light balsamic & basil vinaigrette, 2 Tbsp	2
Dressing, light, deluxe French, 2 Tbsp	2
Dressing, light, honey dijon, 2 Tbsp	3
Dressing, ranch, light, 2 Tbsp	3
Dressing, red wine vinaigrette, 2 Tbsp	3
Greek vinaigrette dressing, 2 Tbsp	2
Light buffalo ranch salad dressing, 2 Tbsp	3
Olive oil vinaigrette dressing, 2 Tbsp	2
Robusto Italian, 2 Tbsp	3
Robusto Italian dressing, 2 Tbsp	3
Thousand Island dressing, 2 Tbsp	5
Wish-Bone Just 2 Good!	
Low-fat dressing, ranch, 2 Tbsp	2
Wish-Bone Light!	
Parmesan peppercorn ranch dressing, 2 Tbsp	2
Raspberry walnut vinaigrette, 2 Tbsp	3
Sweet and spicy French dressing, 2 Tbsp	2
Thousand Island dressing, 2 Tbsp	2
Zia's	
Fat free sweet Italian dressing, 2 Tbsp	2

Vinegars

Bragg	
Apple cider vinegar, raw, unfiltered, organic, 1 Tbsp	0
Nakano	
Vinegar, rice, seasoned, 1 Tbsp	1

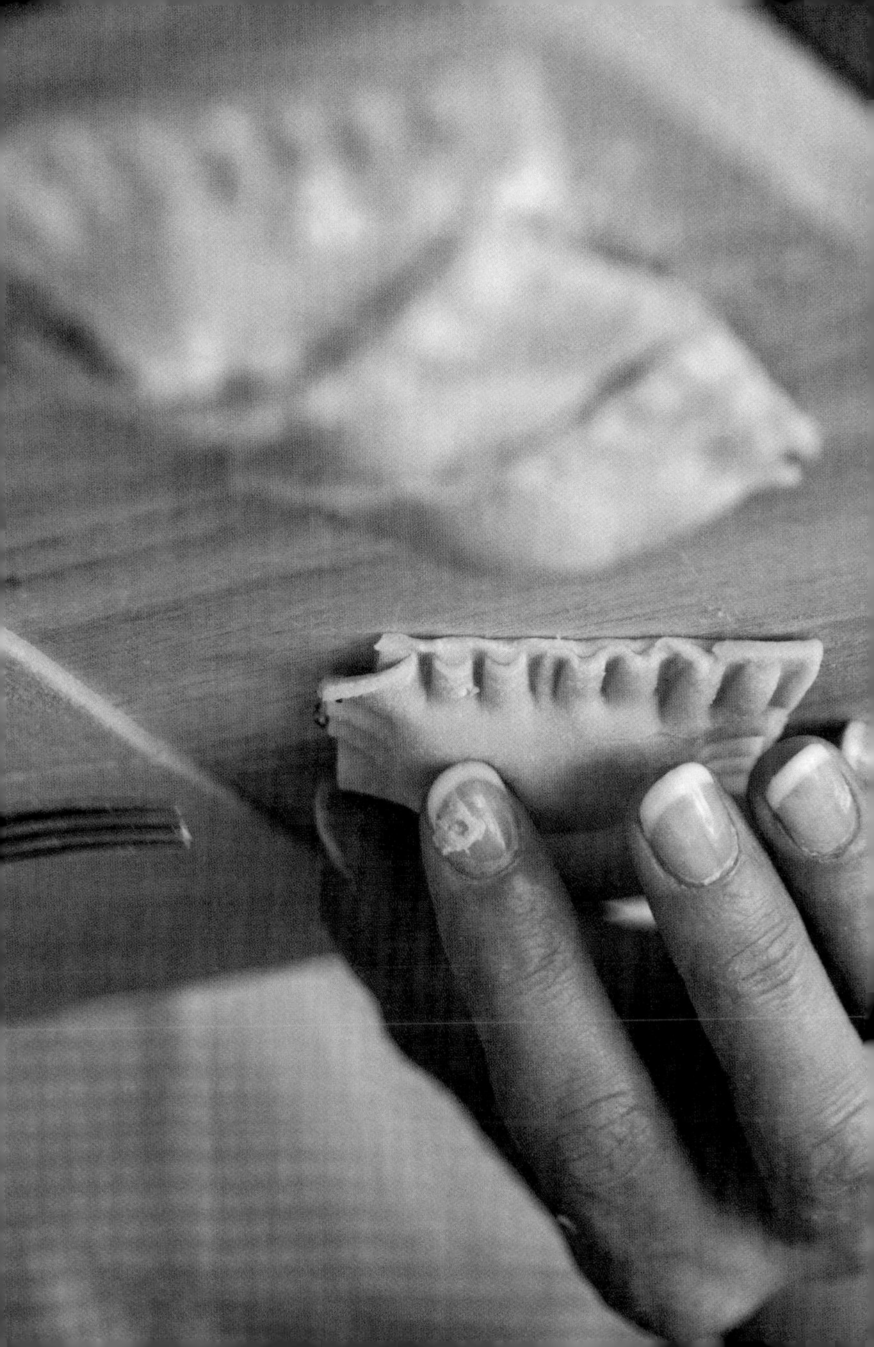

pasta & rice

	SmartPoints® value
Noodles	
Asian Gourmet	
Chinese noodles, ½ cup	6
Chinese noodles, extra crispy, 1 oz	4
Chinese wide lo mein noodles, ½ cup	6
Great Value	
Extra wide egg noodles, 2 oz	6
Kroger	
Medium egg noodles, 1 cup	6
La Choy	
Noodles, chow mein, ½ cup	4
Rice noodles, ½ cup	4
Lotus Foods	
Millet and brown rice ramen, ½ piece (35 g)	4
No Yolks	
Whole grain extra broad egg white pasta, 1½ cups	6
Reames	
Homestyle egg noodles, ½ cup	5
Pasta	
Ancient Harvest Supergrain Pasta	
Gluten free lentil and quinoa penne, 2 oz	5
Barilla	
100% whole wheat angel hair pasta, 2 oz	5
Angel hair, no. 1, 2 oz	6
Elbows, no. 41, 2 oz	6
Farfalle, no. 65, 2 oz	6
Linguine, no. 13, 2 oz	6
Penne, no. 72, 2 oz	6

	SmartPoints® value
Rotini, n. 81, 2 oz	6
Spaghetti, no. 5, 2 oz	6
Thin spaghetti, no. 3, 2 oz	6
Whole grain penne, 2 oz	5
Whole grain spaghetti, 2 oz	5
Barilla Gluten Free	
Penne, 2 oz	6
Spaghetti, 2 oz	6
Barilla Plus	
Penne, 2 oz	6
Spaghetti, 2 oz	6
Barilla Veggie	
Pasta, penne, 2 oz	6
Barilla Whole Grain	
100% whole wheat penne, 1 serving (56 g)	5
100% whole wheat rotini pasta, 1 serving (56 g)	5
100% whole wheat spaghetti, 1 serving (56 g)	5
100% whole wheat thin spaghetti, 1 serving (56 g)	5
100% whole wheat linguine pasta, 2 oz dry	5
Buitoni	
Ravioli, four cheese, 1¼ cups	10
Tortellini, three cheese, 1 cup	10
Creamette	
Vermicelli, 2 oz	6
Dreamfields	
Penne rigate, ¾ cup dry	5
Rotini, ¾ cup	5
Spaghetti, ½" circle dry (56 g)	5

	SmartPoints® value
Food Lion	
Fettuccine, 2 oz	6
Golden Grain	
100% whole grain spaghetti pasta, 2 oz	5
Great Value	
Rigatoni pasta, ¾ cup	6
Small shell pasta, 1 serving (56 g)	6
Hodgson Mill Ultragrain	
Thin spaghetti with quinoa, 2 oz	5
Hy-Vee	
Thin spaghetti, 2 oz	4
Kraft	
Macaroni & cheese dinner, spirals (unprepared), ½ box (70 g)	8
Mueller's	
Elbow macaroni, ½ cup	6
Whole grain elbow macaroni, ½ cup	5
Nasoya	
Pasta zero plus, shirataki spaghetti, ⅔ cup	1
No Yolks	
Egg white pasta, cholesterol free, extra broad, 2 oz	6
Pasta Roni	
Angel hair pasta with herbs, 2 oz	6
Ronzoni	
100% whole grain rotini, ¾ cup	5
Rotini, garden delight, ¾ cup	5
Spaghetti pasta, 1 serving (56 g)	5
Ronzoni Gluten Free	
Rotini pasta, ¾ cup	6

	SmartPoints® value
Ronzoni Healthy Harvest	
100% whole grain penne rigate, ¾ cup	5
100% whole grain thin spaghetti (serves 6), 1 serving (56 g)	5
All natural 100% whole grain linguine, 2 oz	5
Whole wheat blend pasta, penne rigate, 2 oz	5
Ronzoni Smart Taste	
Rotini, 2 oz	5
Ronzoni Smart Taste	
Spaghetti, ⅙ package (56 g)	5
Thin spaghetti, 2 oz	5
Simple Truth Organic	
Whole wheat spaghetti, 2 oz	5
Simply Natural	
Spaghetti, 2 oz	6
Trader Joe's	
Organic whole wheat penne pasta, ¾ cup	6

Rice

Bombay	
Basmati rice, ¼ cup	5
Casa Fiesta	
Mexican style rice, mild, ⅔ cup	4
Fit & Active	
Instant brown rice, ½ cup	4
Food Club	
Spanish rice, Mexican style, ¾ cup	3
Go Go Rice	
Steamed rice bowl, organic brown rice, ½ container (105 g)	4

Rice (cont'd)

	SmartPoints® value
Golden Star	
Brown jasmine rice, ¼ cup	5
Goya	
Spanish style yellow rice, ¼ cup	5
Minute® Rice	
Brown rice, ½ cup	4
White rice, ½ cup	6
Minute® Rice Ready to Serve	
Brown rice, 1 container (125 g)	5
Long grain white rice, 1 container (125 g)	6
Natural whole grain brown rice, 1 container (125 g)	7
White jasmine rice, 1 container (125 g)	7
Nature's Truth	
Organic long grain brown rice, ¼ cup	5
Organic Ecolife	
Brown basmati rice, ¼ cup	4
Rice a Roni	
Chicken flavor rice, 1 cup	5
Rice Bowl	
White rice, 1 serving (54 g)	6
Royal	
Basmati rice, ¼ cup	4
Success	
White rice, ¼ cup	4
Success Boil-in-Bag	
Brown rice, whole grain, precooked, ½ cup	4
Precooked whole grain brown rice, ½ cup dry	4
Rice, white, jasmine, ¼ cup dry	4
White rice, enriched, precooked, ½ cup dry	5

	SmartPoints® value
Trader Joe's	
Brown rice, 1 cup	7
Frozen cooked organic brown rice, 1 cup	4
Japanese style fried rice, 1 cup	8
Organic jasmine rice, 1 cup	5
Trader Joe's Frozen	
Rice medley, 1 cup	6
Uncle Ben's	
Long grain & wild rice original recipe, 1 cup	6
Natural whole grain brown rice, ¼ cup dry	5
Natural whole grain instant brown rice, ¼ cup dry	5
Uncle Ben's Boil-in-Bag	
Natural whole grain brown rice, ¼ cup dry	5
Uncle Ben's Ready Rice	
Basmati rice, 1 cup	6
Jasmine, 1 cup	7
Natural whole grain brown, 1 cup	5
Original enriched long grain white rice, 1 cup	6

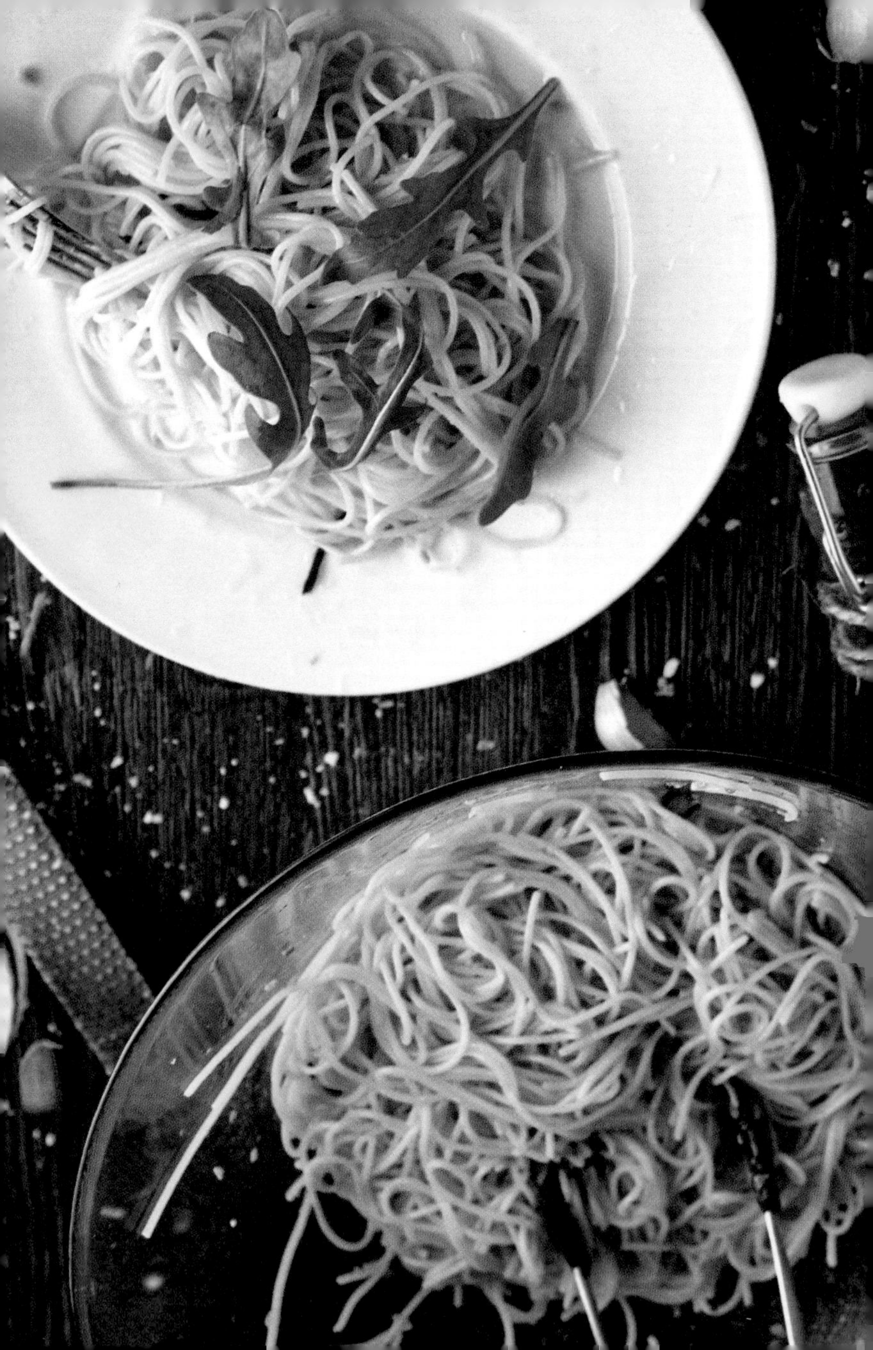

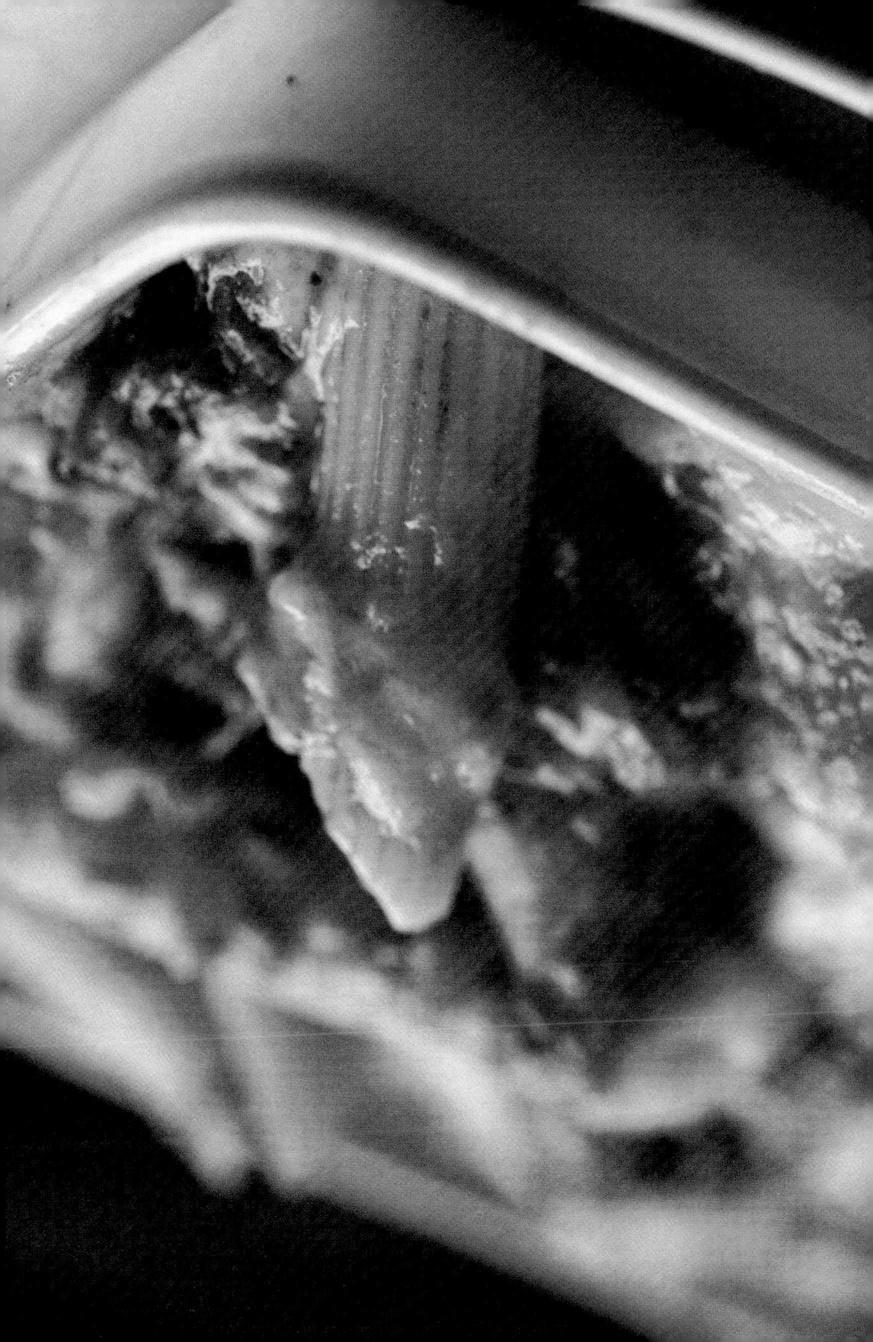

prepared foods, salads & sides

	SmartPoints® value
Appetizers	
Bibigo	
Fully cooked chicken and cilantro mini wontons, 4 pieces (36 g)	1
Pork and vegetable fully cooked mini wontons, 9 pieces (81 g)	5
FarmRich	
Mozzarella sticks, 2 pieces (65 g)	5
Foster Farms	
Buffalo breast bites, 3 oz	5
Frankly Fresh	
Stuffed grape leaves, 1 piece (42 g)	2
Golden Platter	
Gluten free buffalo style bites, 5 pieces (85 g)	4
Kroger	
Applewood smoked bacon mini quiche, 5 pieces (75 g)	7
Ling Ling	
Potstickers, chicken & vegetable dumplings, 5 pieces (148 g)	9
Potstickers, pork & vegetable dumplings, 5 pieces (145 g)	8
Michelina's Lean Gourmet	
Chicken snackers, buffalo-style, 11 snacks (85 g)	6
Sam's Choice	
Cheese franks in a blanket, 4 pieces (102 g)	9
T.G.I. Friday's	
Green bean fries, crispy, with dipping sauce, 12 pieces (84 g)	6
Mozzarella sticks, with marinara sauce, 1 piece (32 g)	3
Potato skins, cheddar & bacon, 3 pieces (96 g)	7
Trader Joe's	
Sriracha seafood potstickers, 4 potstickers (72 g)	4
Trader Joe's Frozen	
Chicken cilantro mini wontons, 4 pieces (36 g)	1

	SmartPoints® value
Chicken gyoza potstickers, 7 potstickers (140 g)	6
Pork gyoza potstickers, 7 potstickers (140 g)	7
Spanakopita-filled with spinach, ricotta & feta cheese, 3 pieces (85 g)	5
Thai vegetable gyoza, 5 pieces (140 g)	9
Van's	
Chicken egg rolls, 1 roll (76 g)	4
Yves	
Kale and quinoa bites, 4 pieces (56 g)	3
Egg Entrées	
Amy's Indian	
Paneer, mattar, 1 entrée	10
Breakfast Best	
Egg, Canadian style bacon, and cheese muffin sandwiches, 1 sandwich (121 g)	6
CedarLane	
Omelette, egg white, garden vegetable & mozzarella, 8 oz	7
Omelette, egg white, spinach and mushroom, 1 omelet (227 g)	8
El Monterey	
Egg, sausage, cheese burritos, 1 burrito (128 g)	8
Maple flavored egg and sausage roll ups, 2 pieces (142 g)	10
El Monterey Signature	
Egg, sausage, cheese, and potato burritos, 1 burrito (128 g)	8
Evol.	
Chicken, apple, sausage, scramble cup, 1 package (142 g)	5
Egg white, veggies, and cheese (gluten free), 1 container (142 g)	4
Good Food Made Simple	
Egg white patties, 1 patty (57 g)	1

	SmartPoints® value
Home Made Brand	
Spinach quiche, crustless, ¼ quiche (114 g)	11
Jimmy Dean	
Casserole, country breakfast, sausage, family size, 1 cup	12
Jimmy Dean Delights	
Bacon and spinach frittatas, 2 frittatas (113 g)	9
Turkey sausage and bacon frittatas, 2 frittatas (113 g)	10
Turkey sausage and bacon frittatas, 2 frittatas (113 g)	10
Turkey sausage and veggies frittatas, 2 frittatas (113 g)	8
Turkey sausage breakfast bowl, 1 bowl (198 g)	6
José Olé	
Egg and sausage breakfast burrito, 1 burrito (113 g)	8
Kellogg's Special K Flatbread	
Egg, bacon, and cheese medley, 1 sandwich (95 g)	7
Egg, spinach, and cheese medley, 1 sandwich (95 g)	6
Lean Cuisine Morning Collection	
Turkey sausage scramble, 1 package (198 g)	5
Veggie scramble, 1 package (198 g)	5
Nutrisystem Breakfast	
Canadian style turkey, bacon, egg, and cheese muffin, 1 package (102 g)	4
Sandwich Bros.	
Egg white and turkey sausage flatbread, 1 sandwich (84 g)	4
Timber Ridge Farms	
Scrambled egg patties, 1 patty (43 g)	2

	SmartPoints® value
Weight Watchers Smart Ones Smart Beginnings	
Cheesy scramble with hashbrowns, 1 entrée	6
Three cheese omelet, 1 entrée	6

Ethnic Entrées

Ajinomoto	
Yakitori chicken with Japanese-style fried rice, cooked, 1 cup	10
Ajinomoto Yakisoba	
Japanese style stir fried noodles with vegetables and sauce, ½ pack (128 g)	8
Amy's	
Burrito, black bean, 1 burrito (170 g)	8
Cheddar cheese burrito, 1 burrito (170 g)	9
Enchilada, black bean vegetable, 1 enchilada (135 g)	5
Enchilada, cheese, 1 enchilada (127 g)	8
Amy's Bowls	
Mexican casserole, 1 entrée	12
Amy's Gluten Free	
Burrito, cheddar cheese, 1 burrito (156 g)	8
Burrito, non-dairy, 1 burrito (156 g)	7
Amy's Light & Lean	
Enchilada, black bean & cheese, 1 entrée	8
Asian Rhythms	
Steamed dim sum, shrimp shumai, 4 pieces (72 g)	3
Bibigo	
Chicken and vegetable steamed dumplings, 1 tray (170 g)	7
CedarLane	
Burrito, beans, rice & cheese style, 1 burrito (170 g)	7

Ethnic Entrées (cont'd)

	SmartPoints® value
CedarLane	
Roasted vegetable tamales, 1 tamale (142 g)	7
Delimex	
Beef taquitos, 3 taquitos (85 g)	7
Chicken chipotle burrito bowl, 1 bowl (354 g)	15
Shredded beef taquitos, 3 taquitoa (94 g)	6
Don Miguel	
Chicken, cheese, and bean burritos, 1 burrito (198 g)	11
El Monterey	
Burritos, bean & cheese, family pack, 1 burrito (113 g)	7
Supreme egg, sausage & cheese burrito, 1 burrito (128 g)	8
Taquitos, chicken & cheese, 2 taquitos (85 g)	6
Evol. Street Tacos	
Shredded chicken and caramelized onion tacos, 1 package (181 g)	6
Full Circle	
Thai red curry chicken, 9 oz	9
Fusia Asian Inspirations	
Oriental stir fry, 1 cup	2
Healthy Choice Café Steamers	
Asian beef teriyaki, 1 entrée	9
Asian pineapple chicken, 1 entrée	10
Asian potstickers, 1 entrée	12
Asian sweet and spicy orange zest chicken, 1 entrée	8
Kung pao chicken, 1 entrée	8
Simply chicken fried rice, 1 entrée	9
John Soules Foods	
Beef fajitas, 3 oz	2
Chicken fajitas, 3 oz	1
Chicken fajitas fully cooked chicken breast strips, 3 oz	1

	SmartPoints® value
José Olé	
Chicken and cheese taquitos, 2 taquitos (85 g)	7
Kahiki	
Beef and broccoli, ½ package (312 g)	11
Kroger	
Kalbi Korean beef, 5 oz	8
Lean Cuisine	
Sesame chicken, 1 entrée	7
Sweet & spicy Korean-style beef, 1 package (248 g)	11
Lean Cuisine Culinary Collection	
Fajita style chicken spring rolls, 3 spring rolls (113 g)	5
Fiesta grilled chicken, 1 package (240 g)	7
Garlic chicken spring rolls, 3 spring rolls (113 g)	6
Orange chicken, 1 package (255 g)	10
Sesame chicken, 1 package (255 g)	10
Sweet and sour chicken, 1 package (283 g)	9
Thai style chicken spring rolls, 3 spring rolls (113 g)	6
Lean Cuisine Simple Favorites	
Asian style pot stickers, 1 package (255 g)	9
Chicken fried rice, 1 package (255 g)	7
Chicken teriyaki stir fry, 1 package (255 g)	7
Lean Cuisine Spa Collection	
Thai style noodles with chicken, 1 package (276 g)	9
Lilly B's	
Organic burritos, 1 burrito (170 g)	9
Maya Kaimal	
Coconut chicken curry, 5 oz	4

	SmartPoints® value
Mrs. T's	
Pierogies, mini, potato & cheddar, 7 pierogies (91 g)	4
Pierogies, potato & cheddar, 3 pierogies (117.6 g)	5
Pierogies, potato & cheddar, low-fat, 3 pierogies (114 g)	5
Pierogies, potato & onion, low-fat, 3 pierogies (114 g)	4
P.F. Chang's Grocery	
Signature spicy chicken, ½ package (312 g)	18
P.F. Chang's Home Menu	
Chicken fried rice, meal for two, ½ package (312 g)	11
Red's	
Steak burrito bowl, 1 bowl (240 g)	9
Saffron Road	
Chicken tikka masala, 10 oz	9
Chicken tikka masala with basmati rice, 1 entrée	8
Palak paneer with basmati rice, 10 oz	16
Supreme	
Chipotle chicken tamale, 1 tamale (113 g)	4
Sweet Earth Natural Foods Protein Lover's	
Functional breakfast burrito, 1 burrito (170 g)	7
Functional breakfast burrito (3 pack), 1 burrito (142 g)	6
Chicken enchilada casserole, 1 cup	9
Trader Joe's	
True Thai pad see ew, ¾ cup	5
Trader Joe's Frozen	
99% fat free bean & rice burritos, 1 burrito (169 g)	7
Black bean and corn enchilada, 1 enchilada (135 g)	4
Chicken tikka masala, 1 tray (241 g)	9
Mini chicken tacos, 4 tacos (79 g)	5

	SmartPoints® value
Trader Jose's	
Handmade chicken & green chile tamales, 1 tamale (85 g)	4
Tyson	
Fajita chicken strips, 3 oz	2
Weight Watchers Smart Ones Classic Favorites	
Chicken enchiladas suiza, 1 entrée	9
Chicken Oriental, 1 entrée	7
Lemon herb chicken piccata, 1 entrée	5
Sesame noodles with vegetables, 1 entrée	8
Spicy Szechuan style vegetables, 1 entrée	8
Swedish meatballs, 1 entrée	9
Vegetable fried rice, 1 entrée	9
Weight Watchers Smart Ones Smart Anytime	
Chicken quesadilla, 1 piece	5
Weight Watchers Smart Ones Smart Creations	
Orange sesame chicken, 1 entrée	8
Teriyaki chicken and vegetables, 1 entrée	8
Thai style chicken and rice noodles, 1 entrée	8

Fish and Seafood Entrées

Healthy Choice Café Steamers	
Cajun style chicken and shrimp, 1 entrée	6
Healthy Choice Complete Meals	
Lemon pepper fish, 1 entrée	11
Lean Cuisine Culinary Collection	
Parmesan crusted fish, 1 package (255 g)	9
Shrimp Alfredo, 1 package (255 g)	6
Shrimp and angel hair pasta, 1 package (283 g)	7
Tortilla crusted fish, 1 package (226 g)	9

Fish and Seafood Entrées (cont'd)

	SmartPoints® value
Lean Cuisine Spa Collection	
Salmon with basil, 1 package (272 g)	7
Pagoda Express	
Crab rangoon, 5 pieces (85 g)	10
Weight Watchers Smart Ones Classic Favorites	
Tuna noodle gratin, 1 entrée	7
Weight Watchers Smart Ones Smart Creations	
Fish and chips, 1 entrée	9

Meat and Poultry Entrées

	SmartPoints® value
Aidells	
Chicken meatballs with teriyaki & pineapple, 3 meatballs (64 g)	4
Al Fresco	
Buffalo and blue cheese patties gourmet chicken grillers, 1 patty (98 g)	4
Meatballs, gourmet, chicken, Italian style, 4 meatballs (85 g)	4
Al Fresco All Natural	
Tomato and basil chicken meatballs, 4 meatballs (85 g)	4
Amylu	
Kickin mango chicken meatballs, 4 meatballs (75 g)	4
Atkins	
Beef merlot, 1 tray (255 g)	9
Banquet	
Boneless fried chicken, 1 entrée	18
Chicken nuggets and fries, 1 entrée	7
Barber Foods	
Stuffed chicken breasts, cordon bleu, 1 piece (140 g)	6
Stuffed chicken breasts, with rib meat, broccoli & cheese, 1 piece (140 g)	6
Bertolli	
Italian sausage and beef lasagna, 1 cup	13
Birds Eye	
Sausage and peppers skillet meal, 2 ¼ cups	10
Blake's	
Chicken and dumplings, 1 cup	10
Chicken marsala with pasta, 1 cup	4
Bob Evans	
Original sausage and gravy biscuits, ½ package (189 g)	13
Bob Evans Homestyle Recipe	
Chicken and noodles, 1 cup	5
Bremer	
Chicken pot pie, 1 pie (198 g)	14
Italian style meatballs, 6 meatballs (85 g)	8
Bryan Food Service	
Corn beef hash, 1 cup	15
Burgers by Amylu	
Caramelized onion and gouda chicken burger, 1 burger (112 g)	3
Kale & mozzarella charbroiled chicken burgers, 1 burger (112 g)	4
Butterball	
Everyday cheddar turkey burger, 1 patty (142 g)	6
Casa Di Bertacchi	
Turkey meatballs, 5 meatballs (88 g)	4
Casual Gourmet	
Chicken sausage with roasted red pepper and spinach, 1 link (90 g)	3
Coleman Organic	
Basil and roasted garlic chicken meatballs, 4 meatballs (88 g)	4
Hearty Italian chicken meatballs, 4 meatballs (88 g)	4
Cooked Perfect	
Gluten free Italian style meatballs, 3 meatballs (85 g)	8
Meatballs, turkey, 3 meatballs (85 g)	4

	SmartPoints® value
Daily Chef	
Mesquite grilled chicken fillets fully cooked, 3 oz	2
Pulled pork, 2 oz	4
Daily Chef Casa Di Bertacchi	
Italian style beef meatballs, 5 meatballs (88 g)	9
FarmRich Smokehouse	
Pulled pork bbq, ¼ cup	3
Fit & Active	
Chicken parmesan, 8 oz	6
Turkey meatballs, 6 meatballs (85 g)	4
Foster Farms	
Turkey meatballs, homestyle, 3 meatballs (84 g)	4
Fra' Mani	
Chicken marsala, 5 oz	4
Frankly Fresh	
Chicken breast burrito bowl, 1 bowl (340 g)	11
Giant	
Chicken fingers, 2 pieces (81 g)	6
Meatloaf, homestyle, 1 piece (170 g)	6
Golden Platter	
Chicken tenders, 2½ pieces (85 g)	4
Good Grains Organic	
Chicken quinoa and kale blend steamable bag (gluten free), 1 package (142 g)	4
Great Fresh Foods	
Stuffed chicken patties, 1 patty (128 g)	4
Great Value	
Popcorn chicken, ⅔ cup	4
Hamburger Helper	
Stroganoff, ½ cup	3
Ultimate beef stroganoff, ½ cup	3

	SmartPoints® value
Hamburger Helper Classic	
Cheeseburger macaroni, ⅓ cup	4
Healthy Choice	
Beef and broccoli meal, 1 entrée	8
Healthy Choice Café Steamers	
Beef merlot Entrée, 1 entrée	5
Chicken linguini with red pepper Alfredo, 1 entrée	6
Chicken margherita with balsamic, 1 entrée	8
Crustless chicken pot pie, 1 entrée	8
General Tso's spicy chicken, 1 entrée	9
Grilled basil chicken, 1 entrée	7
Grilled chicken marinara with parmesan, 1 entrée	8
Grilled chicken marsala with mushrooms, 1 entrée	7
Honey glazed turkey and potatoes, 1 entrée	7
Simply chicken and vegetable stir fry, 1 entrée	5
Simply chicken pasta primavera, 1 entrée	6
Simply grilled chicken and broccoli Alfredo, 1 entrée	4
Simply grilled chicken pesto and vegetables, 1 entrée	4
Simply lemon herb chicken, 1 entrée	7
Simply meatball marinara, 1 entrée	8
Simply southwestern style chicken, 1 entrée	5
Sweet and sour chicken, 1 entrée	12
Sweet sesame chicken, 1 entrée	10
Top chef grilled chicken pesto with vegetables, 1 entrée	8
Whiskey steak, 1 entrée	10

Meat and Poultry Entrées (cont'd)

	SmartPoints® value
Healthy Choice Complete Meals	
Chicken parmigiana, 1 entrée	10
Country fried chicken, 1 entrée	11
Homestyle salisbury steak, 1 entrée	8
Meat loaf, classic, 1 entrée	9
Turkey breast, golden roasted, 1 entrée	8
H-E-B	
Fully cooked lean burgers, 1 burger (85 g)	2
Hillshire Farm	
Grilled chicken bites, 1 package (85 g)	3
HoneySuckle White Italian Style	
Lean turkey meatballs, 3 meatballs (85 g)	4
Hormel	
Beefy mac and cheese, 1 serving (213 g)	7
Hormel Market	
Carnitas verde, 5 oz	3
Hunt's Manwich	
Original sloppy joe, ¼ cup	3
Jack Daniel's	
Pulled chicken, 4 oz	5
Jennie-O	
Turkey meatballs, Italian style, 3 meatballs (84 g)	4
Kirkland Signature	
Meatballs, 5 meatballs (90 g)	9
Kirkwood	
Cordon bleu stuffed with Swiss cheese and ham, 1 piece (142 g)	4
Kroger	
Boneless skinless chicken tenderloins, 2 tenders (136 g)	1
Chicken wing drummettes, 2 pieces (100 g)	5
Lean Cuisine	
Sweet sriracha braised beef, 1 package (212 g)	6

	SmartPoints® value
Lean Cuisine Comfort	
Cheddar bacon chicken, 1 package (226 g)	5
Chicken in sweet bbq sauce, 1 package (241 g)	9
Lean Cuisine Culinary Collection	
Baked chicken, 1 package (244 g)	7
Beef pot roast, 1 package (255 g)	6
Chicken carbonara, 1 package (255 g)	6
Chicken marsala, 1 package (230 g)	7
Chicken parmesan, 1 package (308 g)	10
Chicken pecan, 1 package (255 g)	10
Chicken with almonds, 1 package (240 g)	9
Chicken with basil cream sauce, 1 package (240 g)	6
Chile lime chicken, 1 package (251 g)	7
Glazed chicken, 1 package (240 g)	6
Glazed turkey tenderloins, 1 package (255 g)	10
Grilled chicken Caesar, 1 package (241 g)	7
Herb roasted chicken, 1 package (226 g)	4
Meatloaf with mashed potatoes, 1 package (265 g)	7
Ranchero braised beef, 1 package (233 g)	9
Roasted turkey and vegetables, 1 package (226 g)	6
Roasted turkey breast, 1 package (276 g)	10
Salisbury steak with macaroni and cheese, 1 package (269 g)	7
Steak tips portabello, 1 package (212 g)	4

	SmartPoints® value
Lean Cuisine Marketplace	
Pomegranate chicken, 1 package (212 g)	6
Spicy beef & bean enchilada, 1 package (272 g)	10
Lean Cuisine Simple Favorites	
Chicken fettuccini, 1 entrée	7
Swedish meatballs, 1 package (258 g)	8
Lean Cuisine Spa Collection	
Apple cranberry chicken, 1 package (272 g)	12
Grilled chicken primavera, 1 package (265 g)	6
Marie Callender's	
Chicken pot pies, 1 pie (284 g)	22
Pot pie, chicken, 1 cup	13
Mary Kitchen	
Corned beef hash, homestyle, 1 cup	9
Meijer	
Broccoli and cheese raw stuffed chicken breasts, 1 piece (140 g)	9
Michelina's Lean Gourmet	
Salisbury steak, 1 package (213 g)	5
Milford Valley	
Chicken cordon bleu, 1 container (142 g)	7
Nutrisystem	
Chicken pot pie, 1 package (241 g)	8
Pace Ready Meals	
Fiesta chicken and rice with green and red peppers, 1 pouch (255 g)	7
Perdue	
Popcorn chicken, 3 oz	5
Perfect Fit Meals	
Chicken parmesan with whole wheat spaghetti, 1 entrée	7
Herb crusted chicken meal, 1 package (257 g)	8

	SmartPoints® value
Pierre	
Creme brie raw stuffed chicken breasts, 1 piece (196 g)	11
Saffron Road	
Chicken enchiladas poblano, 10 oz	11
Schlereth's	
Green chile sauce with chicken medium, ¼ cup	1
Simply Balanced	
Chicken tikka masala, 1 package (255 g)	7
Stouffer's	
Chicken and dumplings, 1 cup	10
Lasagna with meat sauce, 1 serving (227 g)	11
Meatloaf, in gravy, family size, 1 loaf and gravy (156 g)	6
Trader Joe's	
Chicken soup dumplings, 1 container (170 g)	7
Fully cooked turkey meatballs, 2 meatballs (71 g)	3
Italian style turkey meatloaf topped with tomato sauce, 5 oz	6
Trader Joe's Frozen	
Butter chicken with basmati rice, 1 cup	8
Chicken fried rice, 1 cup	6
Party size mini meatballs, 6 meatballs (85 g)	7
Shepard's pie, 1 cup	4
Trader Joe's Just Sauce	
Turkey bolognese, ½ cup	2
Weight Watchers Smart Ones Smart Creations	
Chicken mesquite, 1 entrée	7
Chicken parmesan, 1 entrée	7
Chicken Santa Fe, 1 entrée	4
Chicken strips and fries, 1 entrée	9
Chicken strips with sweet potato fries, 1 entrée	8

Meat and Poultry Entrées, Weight Watchers Smart Ones Smart Creations (cont'd)

	SmartPoints® value
Chipotle lime chicken, 1 entrée	4
Creamy basil chicken with broccoli, 1 entrée	5
Crustless chicken pot pie, 1 entrée	5
Home style beef pot roast, 1 entrée	4
Homestyle turkey breast with stuffing, 1 entrée	7
Meatloaf, 1 entrée	8
Pulled pork & black beans, 1 entrée	7
Roasted chicken with herb gravy, 1 entrée	4
Salisbury steak, 1 entrée	7
Slow roasted turkey breast, 1 entrée	5
Spicy chicken strips with salt & pepper fries, 1 entrée	9
Tomato basil chicken with spinach, 1 entrée	4

Meat Substitutes Entrées

	SmartPoints® value
Boca	
All American flamed grilled veggie burger, 1 burger (71 g)	3
Original chik'n veggie patty, 1 patty (71 g)	4
Original vegan veggie burger, 1 burger (99 g)	1
Veggie burgers, original vegan, 1 burger (71 g)	1
Boca Essentials	
Chile relleno burger, 1 burger (71 g)	3
Dr. Praeger's Organic	
Harvest veggie burgers, 1 burger (113 g)	4
Dr. Praeger's Sensible Foods	
California veggie burgers, 1 burger (78 g)	3
Super greens veggie burgers, 1 burger (71 g)	3
Fit & Active	
Chickenless patties, 1 patty (71 g)	5
Foodhold USA	
Garden vegetable burger, 1 patty (71 g)	5
Gardein	
Beefless ground, ½ cup	1
Chipotle black bean burger, 1 burger (96 g)	5
Classic meatless meatballs, 2 meatballs (90 g)	3
Meatless chick'n strips, ¼ pack (98 g)	3
Gardenburger	
Veggie burgers, black bean chipotle, 1 patty (71 g)	3
Morningstar Farms	
Buffalo chik patties, 1 patty (71 g)	5
Buffalo wings, 5 wings (85 g)	6
Chik patties original, 1 patty (71 g)	4
Chik patties original veggie patties, 1 patty (71 g)	4
Chipotle black bean burger (¼ lb), 1 burger (120 g)	5
Chipotle black bean veggie burger, 1 burger (120 g)	5
Classics chikn nuggets, 4 nuggets (86 g)	5
Garden veggie burger, 1 burger (67 g)	3
Grillers crumbles, ½ cup	1
Grillers original burgers, 1 burger (64 g)	3
Grillers prime burgers, 1 burger (71 g)	4
Mediterranean chickpea burgers, 1 burger (67 g)	3
Mushroom lovers burgers, 1 burger (64 g)	3
Original burgers, 1 burger (64 g)	3
Original chik patties, 1 patty (71 g)	4
Southwest sunrise breakfast sandwiches, 1 sandwich (95 g)	6

	SmartPoints® value
Spicy black bean burger, 1 burger (67 g)	3
Spicy Indian veggie burger, 1 burger (67 g)	4
Tomato and basil pizza burgers, 1 burger (67 g)	3
Tomato and basil pizza veggie burger, 1 burger (67 g)	3
Veggie buffalo wings, 5 wings (85 g)	6
Veggie burgers, garden veggie patties, 1 burger (67 g)	3
Veggie burgers, grillers prime, 1 burger (71 g)	4
Veggie burgers, spicy black bean, 1 burger (67 g)	3
Veggie burgers, spicy black bean, value pack, 1 burger (67 g)	3
Veggie corn dogs, 1 corn dog (71 g)	5
Morningstar Farms Breakfast	
Veggie bacon strips, 2 strips (16 g)	2
Morningstar Farms Classics	
Veggie dogs, 1 link (40 g)	1
Morningstar Farms Grillers	
California turk'y veggie burger, 1 burger (64 g)	2
Veggie crumbles, ½ cup	1
Nasoya Tofubaked	
Teriyaki marinated baked tofu, 1 piece (57 g)	2
Quorn	
Chik'n cutlets, meatless & soy-free, naked, 1 cutlet (69 g)	2
Chik'n patties, meatless and soy-free, 1 patty (75 g)	4
Chik'n tenders, meatless and soy-free, 1 cup	2
Season's Choice	
Black bean chipotle burger, 1 patty (71 g)	4

	SmartPoints® value
Simply Balanced	
Smoky chipotle meatless chicken, ¾ cup	2
Trader Joe's	
Breaded turkeyless stuffed roast with gravy, 4.4 oz	5
Meatless breakfast patties, 1 patty (35 g)	2
Quinoa cowboy veggie burgers with black beans & roasted corn, 1 burger (91 g)	5
Soy chorizo, 2½ oz	4
Thai sweet chilli veggie burger, 1 burger (71 g)	4
Trader Joe's Frozen	
Meatless meatballs, 6 pieces (85 g)	3

Meat, Poultry, and Seafood Salads

Archer Farms	
Cranberry almond chicken salad, ½ cup	4
Bumble Bee	
Chicken salad with crackers, 1 package (99 g)	7
Bumble Bee Snack on the Run!	
Fat-free tuna salad with wheat crackers, 1 can (82 g)	2
Tuna salad, with crackers, 1 package (99 g)	5
Elevate Me	
Sunny Caesar salad, 1 container (156 g)	10
Good Foods	
Cranberry almond chicken salad, 1 cup	6
Reduced fat and calorie cranberry almond chicken salad, ½ cup	5
Little Salad Bar	
Chipotle chicken salad, ⅓ cup	9

Meat, Poultry, and Seafood Salads (cont'd)

	SmartPoints® value
Ready Pac Bistro	
Chicken Caesar salad, 1 container (177 g)	7
Italian style chopped salad, 1 container (149 g)	7
Sante Fe style salad, 1 container (177 g)	8
Turkey and bacon cobb salad, 1 bowl (205 g)	10
Simply Fresh Gourmet	
Santa fe style chicken salad, 1 serving (195 g)	9
StarKist	
Tuna salad, chunk light, 1 pouch (85 g)	2
StarKist Ready To Eat	
Albacore tuna salad, 1 pouch (85 g)	2
Taylor Farms Fresh Handcrafted Salads	
Bbq ranch chopped salad, ¼ package (100 g)	4
Trader Joe's	
Citrus salad with chicken (with dressing), 1 container (248 g)	8
Reduced guilt chicken salad (white meat), ½ cup	2
Wawa Grocery	
Chicken salad snack, 1 container (190 g)	8
Wawa Grocery	
Thai style chicken mango salad, 1 salad (312 g)	7

Packaged Lunches

	SmartPoints® value
Healthy Choice Café Steamers	
Chicken fresca with chardonnay, 1 entrée	5
Honey balsamic chicken, 1 entrée	6
Lean Cuisine Marketplace	
Cheese & bean enchilada verde, 1 package (226 g)	8
Mushroom & spring pea risotto, 1 package (255 g)	8
Spicy Mexican black beans & rice, 1 package (248 g)	9
Oscar Mayer P3	
Grilled snackers portable protein snack (hickory seasoned grilled chicken breast strips with sweet barbecue sauce), 1 package (76 g)	3
Portable protein pack (applewood smoked ham, cheese & cashews), 1 package (56 g)	5
Portable protein pack (chicken breast, Monterey Jack cheese & cashews), 1 package (56 g)	6
Portable protein pack chicken breast, cheddar cheese and dry roasted peanuts, 1 package (56 g)	5
Portable protein pack, smoked ham, sharp cheddar cheese and dry roasted almonds, 1 package (56 g)	5
Portable protein pack, turkey breast, cheddar cheese and dry roasted peanuts, 1 package (56 g)	5
Portable protein pack, turkey breast, marbled colby and Monterey Jack cheeses with dry roasted almonds, 1 package (56 g)	4
StarKist Charlie's Lunch Kit	
Tuna salad, with chunk light tuna in water, 1 kit (130 g)	6

Pasta and Vegetable Salads

CedarLane	
Quinoa tabouli, ½ cup	4
Cedar's	
Chickpea salad, 2 Tbsp	1
Taboule salad, fresh, party size, 2 Tbsp	1
Dole	
Cole slaw, classic, 1½ cups	0
Salad kit, Caesar, 1½ cups	5
Salad kit, light Caesar, 1½ cups	3
Salad kit, southwest, 1½ cups	5

	SmartPoints® value
Dole Chopped	
Bacon and bleu cheese salad kit, 2 cups	5
Bbq ranch salad kit, 2 cups	6
Chipotle and cheddar salad kit, 2 cups	4
Pomegranate salad kit, 1½ cups	6
Poppy seed salad kit, 1½ cups	5
Sesame Asian salad kit, 1½ cups	6
Sunflower crunch salad kit, 2 cups	7
Dole Distinctively Dole	
Salad kit, ultimate Caesar, 1½ cups	6
Eat Smart	
Sweet kale vegetable salad kit, 3 oz	6
Elevate Me	
Nutty cranberry superfood salad, 1 container (128 g)	10
Organic southwest superfood salad, 1 container (184 g)	8
Organic spinach pow salad kit, 1 container (128 g)	9
Fresh Express	
Asian chopped salad kit, 1½ cups	5
Caesar kit with Greek yogurt Caesar dressing, 2½ cups	3
Caesarlite salad kit, 2½ cups	3
Salad kit, Caesar, 2½ cups	5
Salad, broccoli salad, 1 cup	7
Southwest chopped salad kit, 1½ cups	5
Veggie lover's, 2 cups	0
Fresh Express Chopped Kit	
Sweet kale salad, 1½ cups	6
Fresh Express Early Harvest	
Salad, green & crisp, 2 cups	0
Fresh Selections	
Classic garden salad, 1½ cups	1
Classic garden salad (no dressing), 1½ cups	0
Cole slaw, 1½ cups	1

	SmartPoints® value
Hannah	
Taboule salad, ½ cup	4
H-E-B	
Sesame ginger Asian chopped salad kit, 1½ cups	6
Joseph's Mediterranean Cuisine	
Authentic taboule salad, 2 Tbsp	1
Kroger	
Cole slaw, creamy, ½ cup	7
Little Salad Bar	
Garden salad, 1½ cups	0
Marketside	
Asian chopped salad kit with dressing, 1½ cups	5
Southwest salad with dressing, ½ cup	4
Nature's Greens	
Tangy citrus kale salad kit, 3½ cups	8
Okami	
Edamame salad, ⅔ cup	4
Paisley Farm	
Five bean salad, ½ cup	4
Publix	
Baby kale salad kit, 2 cups	6
Ready Pac	
Caprese salad kit, 3 cups	6
Ready Pac Bistro	
Chef salad, 1 container (220 g)	9
Cranberry walnut salad, 1 container (128 g)	8
Pumpkin spice salad, 1 container (149 g)	12
Santa Fe style salad with ranch dressing, 1 container (177 g)	10
Spinach dijon salad, 1 container (135 g)	10
Ready Pac Foods	
Spinach wheatberry salad kit, 1 cup	6
Safeway Farms	
Cafe bowl, chicken Caesar salad, 1 container (177 g)	7

Pasta and Vegetable Salads (cont'd)

	SmartPoints® value
Signature Café	
Salad, cobb with chicken, 1 salad (305 g)	14
Simply Fresh Gourmet	
Fresh mozzarella caprese salad (with organic balsamic vinaigrette), 1 salad (155 g)	11
Taylor Farms	
Asian chopped salad kit (without dressing), 100 g	3
Caesar salad kit, 1½ cups	5
Chopped salad, southwest, 1½ cups	5
Sweet kale chopped salad, ⅓ package (100 g)	6
Taylor Farms Fresh Hand Crafted Salads	
Asian chopped salad kit with sesame ginger dressing, 1 serving (100 g)	7
Garden vegetable chopped salad with slaw dressing, 1¼ cups	6
Sweet kale chopped salad kit with poppyseed dressing, 1½ cups	7
Taylor Farms Fresh Handcrafted Salads	
Asian chopped salad with ginger dressing, 1 serving (100 g)	6
Kale chopped salad with brussels sprouts (serves 2.5), 1 serving (100 g)	4
Sweet kale chopped salad, 1 cup	6
Trader Joe's	
Kale and hemp seeds salad, 2½ cups	6
Trader Joe's Refrigerated	
Egg white salad with chives, ½ container (85 g)	1
Tuscan Garden	
Muffuletta salad, 1 oz	2
Wal-Mart Deli	
Mustard potato salad, ½ cup	7

	SmartPoints® value
Wawa Grocery	
Superfood salad, 1 salad (278 g)	8
Wegman's	
Italian chopped salad kit, 2 cups	5

Pasta Entrées

Amy's	
Vegetable lasagna, 1 serving (269 g)	12
Amy's Bowls	
3 cheese and kale bake, 1 bowl (241 g)	15
Mushroom risotto, 1 bowl (269 g)	8
Amy's Light & Lean	
Asian noodle, sweet & sour, 1 bowl (227 g)	8
Macaroni and cheese, 1 entrée	9
Pasta & veggies, 1 bowl (227 g)	6
Spaghetti Italiano, 1 bowl (227 g)	7
Spinach lasagna, 1 entrée	8
Andrea	
Low-fat large cheese ravioli, 4 pieces (123 g)	7
Annie's Homegrown	
Shells and real aged cheddar macaroni and cheese, 2½ oz	8
Annie's Homegrown Organic	
Shells & real aged cheddar macaroni & cheese unprepared, 2½ oz	8
Banquet	
Lasagna with meat sauce, 1 entrée	8
Spaghetti and meatballs, 1 entrée	10
Birds Eye Steamfresh	
Lightly sauced pasta, rotini & broccoli with cheese sauce, 2 cups	7
Pasta and broccoli with cheese sauce, 2⅓ cups	7

	SmartPoints® value
Birds Eye Steamfresh Chef's Favorites	
Couscous pasta & spinach, with olive oil & lemon sauce, lightly sauced, ½ bag (142 g)	5
Blake's	
Lasagna bake bolognese, 1 cup	8
Old fashioned mac and cheese, 1 cup	12
Bob Evans Oven Bake	
Macaroni and cheese, 1 cup	9
Boston Market	
Mac 'n cheese, 1 cup	13
Campbell's Spaghettios	
Pasta in tomato and cheese sauce, 1 cup	6
Shaped pasta in tomato and cheese sauce, 1 cup	6
Chef Boyardee	
Ravioli, beef, in tomato & meat sauce, 1 cup	8
D'orazio	
Stuffed shells, 3 shells (170 g)	12
Evol. Bowls	
Teriyaki chicken, 1 bowl (255 g)	7
Giant	
Stuffed shells, 2 pieces (113 g)	5
Great Value	
Beef ravioli, 5 oz	9
Healthy Choice Café Steamers	
100% natural tortellini primavera parmesan, 1 entrée	8
Chicken fettuccini Alfredo, 1 serving (283 g)	7
Portabella marsala pasta, 1 entrée	7
Portabella spinach parmesan, 1 entrée	7
Spaghetti and meatballs, 1 entrée	9
Healthy Choice Top Chef Café Steamers	
Ricotta & spinach ravioli & chicken marinara, 1 entrée	8

	SmartPoints® value
Jimmy Dean	
Meat supreme mac and cheese, 1 bowl (255 g)	12
Kirkland Signature	
Five cheese tortelloni with parmigiano reggiano, 1 cup	9
Knorr Pasta Sides	
Fettuccini, Alfredo, ⅔ cup	7
Fettuccini, butter & herb, ⅔ cup	7
Fettuccini, creamy chicken flavor, ⅔ cup	6
Fettuccini, parmesan, ⅔ cup	7
Kraft	
Macaroni & cheese dinner, original flavor (cup), 1 package (58 g)	7
Macaroni & cheese dinner, original flavor (unprepared), ⅓ box (70 g)	8
Original flavor macaroni and cheese dinner, 1 single cup (58 g)	7
Kraft Deluxe	
Macaroni and cheese dinner, 2% milk cheese, ¼ box (98 g)	9
Macaroni and cheese dinner, original cheddar, ¼ box (98 g)	10
Kraft Easy Mac	
Original macaroni and cheese dinner, 1 pouch (61 g)	7
Kraft Velveeta	
Bold jalapeño shells and cheese, 1 cup	11
Kroger	
Cheese ravioli, 9 pieces (145 g)	9
Lean Cuisine Culinary Collection	
Asparagus and cheese ravioli, 1 package (258 g)	9
Mushroom mezzaluna ravioli, 1 package (244 g)	9
Spinach artichoke ravioli, 1 package (255 g)	9
Lean Cuisine Marketplace	
Cheese tortellini, 1 package (219 g)	10

Pasta Entrées, Lean Cuisine Marketplace (cont'd)

	SmartPoints® value
Mac & cheese, Vermont white cheddar, 1 package (226 g)	8
Ricotta cheese & spinach ravioli, 1 package (226 g)	11
Lean Cuisine Simple Favorites	
Alfredo pasta with chicken and broccoli, 1 package (283 g)	8
Cheese ravioli, 1 package (241 g)	9
Classic five cheese lasagna, 1 package (326 g)	11
Classic macaroni and beef in tomato sauce, 1 package (269 g)	9
Fettuccini Alfredo, 1 package (262 g)	9
Five cheese rigatoni, 1 package (283 g)	11
Four cheese cannelloni, 1 package (258 g)	8
Lasagna with meat sauce, 1 package (297 g)	10
Macaroni and cheese, 1 package (283 g)	10
Spaghetti with meat sauce, 1 package (326 g)	9
Spaghetti with meatballs, 1 package (269 g)	8
Lean Cuisine Spa Collection	
Butternut squash ravioli, 1 package (280 g)	9
Louisa	
Original beef toasted breaded ravioli, 6 pieces (121 g)	11
Main Bistro St.	
Four cheese macaroni bake, ⅔ cup	7
Marie Callender's Comfort Bakes	
Mac and cheese, 1 cup	12
Market Pantry	
Cheese ravioli, 10 pieces (140 g)	9
Meijer	
Cheese tortellini, 1 cup	7
Michael Angelo's	
Three cheese baked ziti, 1 serving (312 g)	16

	SmartPoints® value
Michelina's	
Chicken and pasta marinara meal, 1 package (227 g)	7
Minute® Rice Ready to Serve	
Multi-grain rice medley, 1 cup	6
Panera Bread	
Mac and cheese (small), 1 cup	17
Pasta Prima	
Butternut and apple ravioli, 1 cup	7
Spinach and mozzarella ravioli, 1 cup	6
Peter & Pat's Pierogies	
Potato and 4 cheese pierogies, 4 pierogies (121 g)	7
Rana	
Chicken mozzarella tortelloni, 1 cup	8
Reggano Grocery	
Stroganoff pasta skillet dinner, 1 cup	3
Sam's Choice	
9 layer meat lasagna, 1 cup	12
Six cheese lasagna, 1 cup	11
Specially Selected	
Pumpkin sage ravioli, 1 cup	7
Stouffer's	
Buffalo style mac and cheese, 1 cup	8
Chicken Alfredo, family size, 1 cup	8
Classic mac and cheese mac cup, 1 cup	8
Lasagna with meat sauce family size, 1 cup	8
Macaroni & cheese, family size, 1 cup	11
Three Bridges	
Chicken and asiago cheese ravioli, 1 cup	7
Spinach and cheese ravioli, 1 cup	8
Trader Joe's	
Hatch chile mac and cheese, ½ container (170 g)	9

	SmartPoints® value
Trader Joe's Frozen	
Mushroom risotto, 1 cup	5
Reduced guilt mac & cheese, 1 container (198 g)	8
Velveeta	
Shells & cheese, 4 oz	10
Shells & cheese, 2% milk cheese, 1 package (62 g)	6
Shells & cheese, original, 1 package (68 g)	7
Weight Watchers Smart Ones Classic Favorites	
Angel hair marinara, 1 entrée	7
Creamy pasta Romano with spinach, 1 entrée	7
Creamy rigatoni with broccoli and chicken, 1 entrée	7
Fettuccini Alfredo, 1 entrée	7
Lasagna bake with meat sauce, 1 entrée	7
Lasagna florentine, 1 entrée	11
Macaroni and cheese, 1 entrée	8
Mini rigatoni with vodka cream sauce, 1 entrée	8
Pasta primavera, 1 entrée	7
Pasta with ricotta and spinach, 1 entrée	9
Ravioli florentine, 1 entrée	9
Spaghetti with meat sauce, 1 entrée	8
Three cheese macaroni, 1 entrée	9
Three cheese ziti marinara, 1 entrée	9
Traditional lasagna with meat sauce, 1 entrée	10
Weight Watchers Smart Ones Smart Creations	
Bacon macaroni & cheese, 1 entrée	9
Chicken fettuccini, 1 entrée	8
Three cheese ziti marinara with meatballs, 1 entrée	10

	SmartPoints® value
Wellsley Farms	
Grilled white chicken ravioli, 1 cup	6

Pizza

Ahold	
Crispy thin crust margherita pizza, 1 slice (140 g)	7
Amy's	
Pizza, margherita, ⅓ pizza (123 g)	8
Rice crust margherita pizza, 1 pizza (181 g)	16
Archer Farms	
Grilled pesto chicken pizza, ½ pizza (163 g)	13
Bagel Bites	
Mini bagels, cheese & pepperoni, 4 pieces (88 g)	6
Banquet	
Pizza meal with reduced fat pepperoni and macaroni and cheese sauce, 1 entrée	10
California Pizza Kitchen	
Pizza, crispy thin crust, bbq recipe chicken, ⅓ pizza (139 g)	10
Pizza, crispy thin crust, margherita, ⅓ pizza (146 g)	11
Connie's Pizza Grocery	
Sausage and uncured pepperoni pizza (serves 5), 1 slice (142 g)	12
DiGiorno	
Digiorno original rising crust supreme pizza (serves 6), 1 serving (149 g)	11
Four cheese original rising crust pizza (serves 6), 1 serving (133 g)	10
Pepperoni original rising crust pizza (serves 6), 1 serving (130 g)	10
Pizza, classic thin crust, supreme pizza, 1 serving (141 g)	10
DiGiorno Pizzeria!	
Pizza, Margherita thin, ¼ pizza (128 g)	10
DiGiorno Thin & Crispy	
Pizza, spinach and garlic, ⅓ pizza (112 g)	9

Pizza (cont'd)

	SmartPoints® value
FarmRich	
Pepperoni pizza roll ups, 2 roll ups (99 g)	9
Freschetta	
Thin and crispy crust signature pepperoni pizza, ⅓ pizza (137 g)	13
Freschetta Brick Oven	
Pizza, 5-Italian cheese, ¼ pizza (131 g)	12
Home Run Inn	
Ultra thin spicy Italian sausage and carmelized onion pizza, 1 slice (133 g)	10
Jack's	
Rising crust cheese pizza, 1 slice (142 g)	10
Jeno's Crisp 'n Tasty	
Cheese pizza, 1 pizza (141 g)	11
Combination pizza for one, 1 pizza (147 g)	12
Kashi	
Roasted vegetable traditional crust pizza, 1 pizza (153 g)	11
Kirkland Signature	
Cheese pizza, ¼ pizza (120 g)	9
Kroger	
Double pepperoni pizza, 1 slice (135 g)	11
Lean Cuisine Culinary Collection	
Deep dish spinach and mushroom pizza, 1 package (173 g)	10
Deep dish three meat pizza, 1 package (180 g)	11
Traditional deluxe pizza, 1 package (170 g)	10
Traditional four cheese pizza, 1 package (170 g)	10
Traditional pepperoni pizza, 1 package (170 g)	11
Wood fire style bbq recipe chicken pizza, 1 package (170 g)	10
Wood fire style margherita pizza, 1 package (170 g)	10
Lean Cuisine Simple Favorites	
French bread deluxe pizza, 1 pizza (173 g)	10
French bread pepperoni pizza, 1 package (148 g)	9
Lean Pockets	
Reduced fat pepperoni pizza garlic buttery seasoned crust sandwich, 1 piece (127 g)	9
Mama Mary's	
Ultra thin pizza crust, ¼ crust (43 g)	4
Marketside	
Extra large sausage and pepperoni pizza, ⅙ pizza (145 g)	14
Meat trio pizza, ¼ pizza (127 g)	10
Veggie balsamic flatbread, ½ flatbread (135 g)	13
McCain Ellios	
Pizza, cheese, 2 slices (138 g)	9
Nutrisystem	
Italian herb flatbread pizza, 1 package (106 g)	8
Palermos Primo Thin	
Pizza, ultra-thin crust, margherita pizza, ⅓ pizza (140 g)	8
Private Selection	
Margherita napolitana flatbread pizza, 1 slice (114 g)	7
Pesto and mozzarella Italian crust pizza, 1 slice (132 g)	12
Red Baron	
Pizza, classic crust, 4 cheese, ¼ pizza (146 g)	13
Red Baron Classic Crust	
Pepperoni pizza, ¼ pizza (146 g)	13
Sam's Choice	
Personal super supreme pizza, 1 pizza (235 g)	19

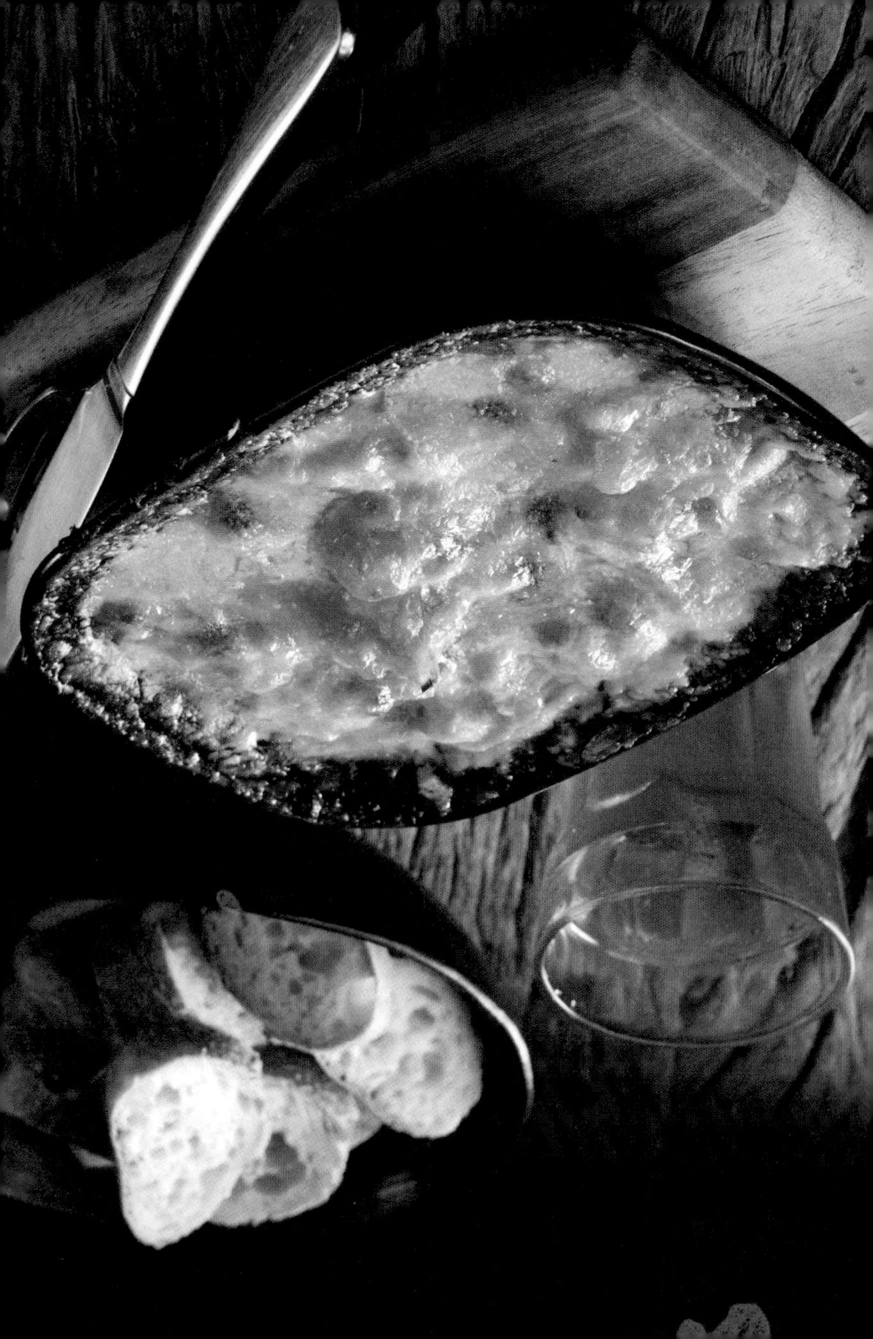

Pizza, Sam's Choice (cont'd)

	SmartPoints® value
Rising crust supreme pizza, 1 slice (150 g)	12
Thin crust 7 cheese pizza, 1 slice (134 g)	13
Screamin' Sicilian Pizza Co.	
Boss hog Italian sausage pizza (serves 5), 1 piece (142 g)	10
Signature Select	
Five cheese pizza, 1 slice (137 g)	11
Rising crust pepperoni pizza, 1 slice (144 g)	12
Ultra thin crust garlic chicken Alfredo pizza, 1 slice (121 g)	8
Smart Flour Foods	
Garden margherita pizza, ½ pizza (147 g)	11
Tombstone	
Deluxe pizza, 1 slice (128 g)	9
Pizza, original, pepperoni, ¼ pizza (146.5 g)	13
Totino's	
Cheese pizza rolls, 6 rolls (85 g)	7
Pizza, party, combination, ½ pizza (152 g)	12
Pizza, party, pepperoni, ½ pizza (145 g)	12
Totino's Pizza Rolls	
Combination pizza snacks, 6 rolls (85 g)	6
Pepperoni pizza snacks, 6 snacks (85 g)	7
Tree Tavern	
Cheese pizza, 1 slice (151 g)	12
Udi's Gluten Free	
Three cheese pizza, ½ pizza (142 g)	11
Uno	
Pizza, flatbread, bbq chicken, ½ flatbread (153 g)	10
Pizza, flatbread, margherita, ½ flatbread (130.5 g)	10

	SmartPoints® value
Weight Watchers Smart Ones Classic Favorites	
Thin crust cheese pizza, 1 pizza	9
Thin crust pepperoni pizza, 1 pizza	10
Weight Watchers Smart Ones Smart Anytime	
Brick oven style pizza pepperoni, 1 pizza	12
Cheese mini pizza, 4 pieces	8
Pepperoni mini pizzas, 1 tray	9
Wellsley Farms	
Thin crust margherita pizza, ⅓ pizza (122 g)	8

Rice and Grain Sides

Amy's Light & Lean	
Quinoa and black beans with butternut squash and chard, 1 bowl (227 g)	7
Archer Farms	
Corn and black bean quinoa blend, 1 cup	5
Birds Eye Steamfresh	
Chicken flavored rice, 1½ cups	7
Birds Eye Steamfresh Selects	
Brown & wild rice with broccoli & carrots, 1½ cups frozen	4
Brown & wild rice, with corn, carrots & peas, 1½ cups	6
Fresh frozen vegetables, long grain white rice with mixed vegetables, 1½ cups	6
Cucina & Amore	
Spicy jalapeño & roasted peppers quinoa meal, 4 oz	4
Evol.	
Quinoa and roasted veggies, 1 bowl (255 g)	9
Green Giant Just for One	
Cheesy rice and broccoli, 1 tray (120 g)	2

	SmartPoints® value
Knorr Fiesta Sides	
Spanish rice, ½ cup mix	7
Knorr Rice Sides	
Cheddar broccoli rice and pasta blend, ½ cup	7
Chicken flavor rice and pasta blend, ½ cup mix	7
Lean Cuisine Simple Favorites	
Santa fe style rice and beans, 1 package (294 g)	9
Minute	
Multi-grain medley, ½ bag (43 g)	4
Minute® Rice Ready to Serve	
Brown and wild rice mix, 1 cup	7
Near East	
Couscous mix, herbed chicken flavor, 2 oz	5
Couscous mix, parmesan, 2 oz	6
Couscous mix, wild mushroom & herb, 2 oz	5
Rice pilaf mix, original, 2 oz	5
Roasted garlic and olive oil couscous mix, 2 oz	5
Old El Paso	
Rice, Mexican, 1 cup	8
P. F. Chang's Home Menu	
Chang's signature rice, 1 cup	5
Path of Life	
Organic quinoa & kale with garlic, olive oil and sea salt, 1 cup	4
PictSweet Steam'ables	
Long grain white rice with mixed vegetables, 1 cup	4
Rice a Roni	
Rice meal, creamy four cheese flavor, ¼ cup dry	7
Rice pilaf, 2½ oz	7
Rice side, Mexican style, 2 oz dry	5
Rice, broccoli au gratin flavor, 2½ oz	8
Rice, chicken flavor (⅓ cup dry rice pasta mix & 1 tbsp seasoning mix), 2½ oz	7

	SmartPoints® value
Rice a Roni Express	
Long grain & wild rice, garlic & herb, 1 cup	8
Rice a Roni Fast Cook	
Spanish rice & vermicelli mix with Spanish style seasonings, ½ cup	6
Rice Bowl	
Cheddar broccoli rice, ½ cup	7
Rice Bowl Grocery	
New Orleans style red beans & rice, ⅓ cup	5
Rice Bowl Ready to Serve	
Whole grain brown rice pouch, 1 cup	3
Season's Choice Steam	
Kale and quinoa, 1 cup	4
Seeds of Change	
Certified organic quinoa & brown rice with garlic, 1 oz	1
Rice, brown, quinoa & whole grain, uyuni, with garlic, 1 cup	7
Simply Balanced	
Organic quinoa, ¼ cup	4
Whole grains and vegetable blend with quinoa, 1 package (255 g)	11
Suzie's	
Quinoa with olive oil, 1 cup	7
The Perfect Bite Co.	
Superfood pilaf, 1 cup	3
Uncle Ben's	
5 grain medley quinoa pilaf, 2 oz	6
Long grain & wild rice, original recipe, ¼ cup dry	6
Uncle Ben's Country Inn	
Chicken and vegetable rice, 2 oz	6
Uncle Ben's Ready Rice	
Brown basmati, 1 cup	7
Chicken flavored whole grain brown rice, 1 cup	6
Garden vegetable with peas carrots and corn, 1 cup	6
Long grain and wild rice, 1 cup	5
Rice pilaf with orzo pasta, 1 cup	6

Rice and Grain Sides, Uncle Ben's Ready Rice (cont'd)

	SmartPoints® value
Roasted chicken flavored with carrots and herbs rice, 1 cup	6
Spanish style rice, 1 cup	6
Uncle Ben's Ready Whole Grain Medley	
Brown and wild rice, 1 cup	6
Quinoa and brown rice with garlic rice, 1 cup	6
Vigo Saffron	
Yellow rice, ⅓ cup	5
Weight Watchers Smart Ones Classic Favorites	
Santa Fe style rice and beans, 1 entrée	9
Zatarains	
Yellow rice, ⅓ cup	6
Zatarains New Orleans Style	
Dirty rice, 1 cup	8
Jambalaya rice, 1 cup	9
Red beans and rice, family size, 1 cup	5

Salad Toppers

Archer Farms	
Southwestern-style tortilla strips salad topper, 2 Tbsp	1
Wonton strips salad topper, 2 Tbsp	1
Kroger	
Salad toppers, dried cranberries & honey roasted pecans, 1 Tbsp	1

Sandwiches

	SmartPoints® value
Breakfast Best	
Egg and cheese pita sandwiches, 1 sandwich (70 g)	5
Eggo	
Bacon, egg, and cheese breakfast sandwich, 1 sandwich (77 g)	7
Evol. Lean & Fit	
Chicken, apple, sausage, egg white, and cheddar breakfast sandwich, 1 sandwich (114 g)	5
Egg white, kale, roasted tomato, and goat cheese breakfast sandwich, 1 sandwich (103 g)	4
Fit & Active	
Turkey sausage breakfast sandwiches, 1 sandwich (135 g)	7
Good Food Made Simple	
Chicken chorizo cafe wrap, 1 wrap (176 g)	10
Jimmy Dean	
Applewood smoked croissant sandwiches, 1 sandwich (136 g)	7
Bacon egg and cheese biscuit, 1 biscuit (102 g)	11
Croissant sandwiches, sausage, egg & cheese, family pack, 1 sandwich (128 g)	14
Jimmy Dean Delights	
turkey sausage, egg & cheese honey wheat flatbread, 1 sandwich (116 g)	8
Applewood smoke chicken sausage egg white and cheese sandwich, 1 sandwich (136 g)	7
Applewood smoke English muffin sandwich, 1 sandwich (145 g)	7
Canadian bacon, egg white, and cheese on honey wheat English muffin sandwich, 1 sandwich (128 g)	6
Egg white with spinach & mozzarella-style cheese honey wheat flatbread, 1 sandwich (99 g)	5
Turkey sausage egg white and cheese whole grain muffin sandwich, 1 sandwich (145 g)	7
Turkey sausage, egg white & cheese croissant sandwiches, 1 sandwich (136 g)	10
Kellogg's Special K	
Flatbread breakfast sandwich, 1 sandwich (116 g)	7
Kellogg's Special K Flatbread	
Egg, spinach, and cheese medley breakfast sandwich, 1 sandwich (95 g)	6

	SmartPoints® value
Kroger	
Bacon cheeseburger, 1 burger (139 g)	14
La Favorita	
Vegetarian breakfast burritos, 1 package (168 g)	5
Lean Cuisine Culinary Collection	
Chicken club panini, 1 package (170 g)	10
Chicken ranch club flatbread melt, 1 package (184 g)	11
Chicken spinach and mushroom panini, 1 package (170 g)	9
Melt, sun dried tomato basil chicken flat bread melt, 1 package (191 g)	11
Philly style steak and cheese panini, 1 package (170 g)	10
Southwest style chicken panini, 1 package (170 g)	10
Spinach artichoke and chicken panini, 1 package (170 g)	10
Veggie egg white English muffin, 1 sandwich (106 g)	5
Lean Pockets	
Bbq recipe chicken pretzel bread sandwich, 1 piece (127 g)	8
Chicken broccoli and cheddar whole grain crust sandwich, 1 piece (127 g)	8
Chicken jalapeño cheddar pretzel bread sandwich, 1 piece (127 g)	8
Garlic chicken white pizza whole grain crust sandwich, 1 piece (127 g)	9
Ham and cheese whole grain crust sandwich, 1 piece (127 g)	9
Philly steak and cheese seasoned crust sandwich, 1 piece (127 g)	9
Roasted turkey with bacon and cheese pretzel bread sandwich, 1 piece (127 g)	9
Sausage egg and cheese seasoned crust sandwich, 1 piece (127 g)	9

	SmartPoints® value
Lean Pockets Breakfast	
Stuffed sandwiches, applewood bacon, egg & low-fat cheese, 1 piece (127 g)	9
Morningstar Farms	
Sausage egg and cheese breakfast sandwich, 1 sandwich (105 g)	6
Nutrisystem Breakfast	
Turkey, sausage, and egg muffin, 1 sandwich (125 g)	5
Oscar Mayer	
Sub kit, ham & turkey, 4 slices (57 g)	1
Philly Gourmet	
Philly cheesesteak sandwich, 1 sandwich (147 g)	11
Pierre Signatures	
Grilled chicken sandwich, 1 sandwich (113 g)	8
Sandwich Bros.	
Angus cheeseburgers flatbread pocket sandwich, 1 burger (63 g)	5
Chicken melt flatbread pocket sandwiches, 1 sandwich (70 g)	5
Chicken melts flatbread, 1 sandwich (70 g)	5
Egg and cheese flatbread pocket sandwich, 1 sandwich (70 g)	5
Egg white and turkey sausage flatbread pocket sandwich, 1 sandwich (84 g)	4
Egg white and turkey sausage flatbread pocket sandwiches, 1 sandwich (84 g)	4
Turkey sausage & cheese omelet flatbread pocket sandwich, 1 sandwich (92 g)	8
Turkey sausage and cheese flatbread pocket sandwich, 1 sandwich (63 g)	4
Smucker's	
Peanut butter and grape jelly sandwich on wheat bread, 1 sandwich (76 g)	11

Sandwiches (cont'd)

	SmartPoints® value
Smucker's Uncrustables	
Peanut butter and grape jelly sandwich, 1 sandwich (58 g)	7
Peanut butter and grape jelly sandwich, 1 sandwich (80 g)	10
Peanut butter and strawberry jam sandwich, 1 sandwich (58 g)	7
Reduced sugar peanut butter and grape spread sandwich on whole wheat bread, 1 sandwich (58 g)	6
Sandwich, reduced sugar, peanut butter & grape spread, 1 sandwich (58 g)	6
Special K	
Breakfast sandwich, flatbread, bacon, egg & cheese, 1 sandwich (95 g)	7
Breakfast sandwich, flatbread, egg with vegetables & pepper Jack cheese, 1 sandwich (95 g)	6
Breakfast sandwich, flatbread, sausage, egg & cheese, 1 sandwich (116 g)	7
Ham, egg and pepper Jack cheese flatbread breakfast sandwich, 1 sandwich (102 g)	6
Starbucks	
Egg salad deli sandwich, 1 sandwich (188 g)	14
Hot panini turkey pesto, 1 sandwich (196 g)	15
Protein bistro box, 1 package (193 g)	14
Toufayan Smart pockets	
Everything flavored pita pockets, 1 pocket (43 g)	2
Trader Joe's Refrigerated	
Tuna salad wrap in a wheat tortilla, ½ wrap (142 g)	7
Wawa	
Chicken salad and green leaf lettuce on multigrain sandwich thin, 1 sandwich (122 g)	5

	SmartPoints® value
Turkey and cheddar pinwheel wraps honey mustard dressing, 1 package (147 g)	9
Wawa Sizzli	
Turkey, sausage, egg white, and cheese on bagel, 1 sandwich (165 g)	10
Weight Watchers Smart Ones Smart Anytime	
Chicken ranchero mini wraps, 2 wraps	7
Chicken slider, 1 slider	6
Mini cheeseburger, 1 burger	6
Spicy chicken slider, 1 slider	6
Weight Watchers Smart Ones Smart Beginnings	
English muffin sandwich, Canadian style turkey bacon, 1 sandwich	6
English muffin sandwich, egg whites and cheese, 1 sandwich	6
English muffin sandwich, turkey sausage, 1 sandwich	7
English muffin sandwich, with turkey sausage, 1 sandwich	7
Smart morning wrap, egg, sausage and cheese, 2 pieces	7
White Castle	
Cheeseburgers, 2 sandwich (104 g)	11

Vegetable Sides

365 Everyday Value	
Crinkle cut sweet potato fries, 3 oz	5
Alexia	
Crispy rosemary fries with sea salt, 12 pieces (84 g)	4
Julienne fries, sweet potato, family size, 12 pieces (84 g)	5
Julienne fries, with chipotle seasoning, spicy sweet potato, 30 pieces (84 g)	6
Onion rings, 6 rings (85 g)	8

	SmartPoints® value
Organic Yukon select fries, 24 pieces (84 g)	3
Oven reds, olive oil, parmesan & roasted garlic, family size, 8 pieces (85 g)	3
Potato puffs, crispy seasoned, 14 pieces (84 g)	5
Seasoned fries, sweet potato, waffle cut, 1 cup	4
Sweet potato, crinkle cut, sea salt & pepper, 30 pieces (84 g)	5
Sweet potato, crispy bite-sized puffs, ⅔ cup	5
Sweet potato, julienne fries, 12 pieces (84 g)	5
Waffle fries, family size, 1 cup	5
Alexia Smart Classics	
Fries, crinkle cut, roasted, with sea salt, 12 pieces (84 g)	3
Fries, straight cut, roasted, with sea salt, 12 pieces (84 g)	3
Arby's	
Fries, curly, seasoned, 1⅓ cups	7
Archer Farms	
Southwest inspired corn and black bean seasoned vegetable blend, ½ cup	3
Betty Crocker	
Au gratin potatoes, ½ cup as packaged	3
Mashed potatoes, creamy butter, ⅓ cup	2
Scalloped potatoes, ½ cup	3
Birds Eye	
Teriyaki stir fry, 2 cups	7
Birds Eye Steamfresh	
Asian style frozen vegetable protein blends, 1⅔ cups	6
Broccoli, with cheese sauce, lightly sauced, 1 cup	2
Cauliflower, garlic, lightly seasoned, 1 cup	1

	SmartPoints® value
Flavor full buffalo cauliflower, 1 cup	2
Flavor full ranch broccoli, 1 cup	2
Flavor full sour cream and onion potatoes, 1 cup	5
Flavor full teryiaki broccoli, 1 cup	2
Italian style frozen vegetable protein blends, 1¾ cups	8
Southwest style frozen vegetable protein blends, 1⅔ cups	9
Birds Eye Steamfresh Chef's Favorites	
Lightly sauced creamed spinach, 1¼ cups	3
Lightly sauced roasted red potatoes and green beans, 1⅔ cups	4
Bob Evans	
Diced potatoes, seasoned home fries, 3 oz	2
Mashed potatoes, garlic, ½ cup	5
Mashed potatoes, original, 1 bowl (170 g)	7
Mashed potatoes, original, family size, ½ cup	5
Mashed potatoes, sour cream & chives, ½ cup	5
Brew City McCain	
Craft beer battered potatoes, 3 oz	6
Bush's Best	
Baked beans, country style, ½ cup	6
Baked beans, homestyle, ½ cup	5
Baked beans, maple cured bacon, ½ cup	5
Baked beans, vegetarian, ½ cup	5
Vegetarian baked beans, ½ cup	5
Buyers Best	
Shoestring French fried potatoes, 3 oz	5

Vegetable Sides (cont'd)

	SmartPoints® value
Chef's Cupboard	
Sour cream and chives mashed potatoes, ⅓ cup	2
Cleverfoodies Scramble	
Leafy greens mix, 5 Tbsp	2
Rancheros mix, ⅓ cup	1
Dee Amore Simply Baked	
French fries, never fried, ½ cup	3
Diner's Choice	
Mashed sweet potatoes, ½ cup	5
Dole Distictively Dole	
Spinach cherry almond bleu kit, 1 cup	7
Dr. Praeger's	
Gluten free sweet potato pancakes, 1 pancake (57 g)	3
Pancakes, broccoli, 1 pancake (57 g)	2
Pancakes, spinach, 1 pancake (57 g)	2
Essential Everyday	
Crinkle fries, 16 pieces (85 g)	4
Evol.	
Truffle parmesan roasted cauliflower veggie cups, 1 cup	4
Fit & Active	
Crinkle cut fries, 16 pieces (84 g)	3
Food Club	
Potatoes, yellow, diced, skin on, ½ cup	2
Gabila's	
Brooklyn's original potato knishes, 1 piece (128 g)	5
Garden Lites	
Superfood veggie cakes (gluten free), 1 cake (65 g)	3
Giant	
Instant mashed potatoes, Idaho, ⅓ cup	2
Mashed potatoes, 1 cup	4
Seasoned curly fries, 3 oz	5
Sweet potato fries, 18 pieces (85 g)	5

	SmartPoints® value
Twice baked potatoes, cheddar cheese, 5 oz	6
Golden	
Zucchini pancakes, 1 pancake (37 g)	2
Great Value	
French fried potatoes, crinkle cut, 15 pieces (84 g)	4
Fries, seasoned, 22 pieces (84 g)	5
Hash brown patties, 1 patty (64 g)	5
Potato wedges, deli style, seasoned, 8 pieces (84 g)	4
Green Giant	
Corn blend peppers and onion, ⅔ cup	3
Creamed spinach, ½ cup	3
Green Giant Just for One	
Broccoli and cheese sauce, 1 tray (120 g)	1
Green Giant Sautés	
Herb butternut squash medley, 1⅓ cups	5
Green Giant Steamers	
Baby brussels sprouts and butter sauce, ⅔ cup frozen	2
Broccoli and cheese sauce, ⅔ cup	2
Broccoli cauliflower carrots and cheese sauce, ⅔ cup	2
Broccoli spears and butter sauce, 3 spears (112 g)	2
Cauliflower and cheese sauce, ½ cup	2
Green beans and almonds, ¾ cup frozen	1
Healthy vision (mixed vegetables with rosemary butter sauce), 1 cup frozen	2
Healthy weight (mixed vegetables with butter sauce), 1 cup frozen	3
Honey glazed carrots, 1 cup	5
Niblets corn and butter sauce, boxed, ⅔ cup	4

	SmartPoints® value
Roasted red potatoes, green beans & rosemary butter sauce, 1¼ cups frozen	3
Shoepeg white corn and butter sauce, boxed, ¾ cup	4
H-E-B	
Sauced Texas style green beans, 1 cup	3
Hungry Jack	
Mashed potatoes, ⅓ cup flakes	2
Hungry Jack Easy Mash'd	
Homestyle mashed potatoes, ⅔ cup	3
Potatoes, mashed, premium homestyle, ¼ cup	3
Idahoan	
Baby reds mashed potatoes, ¼ cup	4
Buttery homestyle mashed potatoes, 1 oz	4
Buttery homestyle mashed potatoes, ¼ cup	4
Mashed potatoes, four cheese, ½ cup mix	4
Mashed potatoes, loaded baked, ¼ cup	4
Mashed potatoes, microwaveable, buttery homestyle, ¼ cup dry	4
Mashed potatoes, original, ⅓ cup mix	2
Roasted garlic mashed potatoes, ¼ cup	4
Sour cream and chives instant mashed potatoes (unprepared), ¼ cup	4
Idahoan Baby Reds	
Mashed potatoes, ¼ cup	4
Kirkland Signature	
Artichoke hearts, 2 pieces (28 g)	1
Stir fry vegetable blend, 1 cup	1
Kroger	
Country style hash browns shredded potatoes, 1 cup	2
Mashed potatoes, ½ cup	6

	SmartPoints® value
Potato nuggets, tater rounds, 11 pieces (85 g)	5
Roasted redskin potatoes, ⅔ cup	3
La Costena	
Charro beans, ½ cup	2
Lean Cuisine Simple Favorites	
Cheddar potatoes with broccoli, 1 package (290 g)	7
Stuffed cabbage, 1 package (269 g)	7
Nathan's	
French fries, crinkle cut, jumbo, 3 oz	4
Ore-Ida	
Country style hash browns, 1¼ cups	2
Country style hash browns, 1 cup	2
Crispers!, 20 pieces (84 g)	7
Crispy crowns!, 11 pieces (84 g)	6
Easy breakfast potatoes, extra crispy, ¾ cup	5
Extra crispy fast food fries, 27 pieces (84 g)	5
Golden crinkles, 12 pieces (84 g)	4
Golden fries, 14 pieces (84 g)	4
Hash browns, ⅔ cup	2
Potatoes o'brien with onions and peppers, ¾ cup	2
Seasoned crinkles, extra crispy, 13 pieces (84 g)	5
Shoestrings, 3 oz	4
Steak fries, 3 oz	3
Steak fries, 7 pieces (84 g)	3
Sweet potato fries, 22 pieces (84 g)	6
Tater tots, 9 pieces (86 g)	5
Tater tots, extra crispy, 12 pieces (86 g)	5
Tater tots, mini, 19 pieces (87 g)	5
Waffle fries, 8 pieces (84 g)	5
Zesties!, 12 pieces (84 g)	5

Vegetable Sides (cont'd)

	SmartPoints® value
Ore-Ida Easy Fries	
French fried potatoes, extra crispy, golden fries, 36 pieces (84 g)	6
Ore-Ida Extra Crispy	
Easy tater tots crispy crowns, 14 pieces (84 g)	7
Ore-Ida Golden Crinkles	
French fried potatoes, 3 oz	4
PictSweet Steam'ables	
Edamame with Asian seasoning, ½ cup	3
Spring vegetables, seasoned, ¾ cup	1
Ranch Style	
Beans, ½ cup	4
Ready Pac Ready Snax	
Snack pac, veggie, cheese & pretzel, 1 container (122 g)	6
Red Robin	
Frozen seasoned steak fries, 10 pieces (84 g)	4
Onion rings, crispy, 3 rings (94 g)	8
Reser's Fine Foods	
Steakhouse yukon gold mashed potatoes, ½ cup	6
Reser's Fine Foods Main St. Bistro	
Steakhouse mashed potatoes, ½ cup	6
Season's Choice	
Cheesy California blend, 1 cup	2
Shredded hash brown potatoes, 3 oz	2
Steamed 7 whole grains corn & peppers, 1 cup	5
Season's Choice Steam	
Asian medley, 1 cup	2

	SmartPoints® value
Simply Potatoes	
Diced potatoes, with onion, ⅔ cup	2
Mashed potatoes, ⅔ cup	6
Shredded hash browns, ½ cup	2
Sliced home fries, ⅔ cup	3
Southwest style hash browns, ⅔ cup	2
Simply Spuds Steamables	
Fingerling potatoes, 1 cup	3
Stouffer's	
Stuffed peppers, family size, 1 pepper (226 g)	7
Stouffer's Homestyle Selects	
Stuffed peppers, large size, 1 pepper (220 g)	6
Tasty Bite 1 Step 1 Minute	
Madras lentils, 5 oz	5
The Little Potato Company	
Garlic herb fresh creamer potatoes, ¼ package (114 g)	2
Garlic herb potatoes, ⅛ package (114 g)	2
Garlic parsley fresh creamer potatoes, ¼ package (114 g)	2
Savory herb seasoned creamer potatoes, ¼ package (114 g)	2
Three cheese potatoes (microwave ready), ¼ package (114 g)	3
Trader Joe's	
Cowboy caviar salsa, 2 Tbsp	1
Harvest hodgepodge eight vegetable blend, ¾ cup	1
Roasted brussels sprouts (ready to eat), ½ cup	2
Steamed lentils (ready to eat warm or cold), ½ cup	4
Vegetable masala burger, 1 burger (71 g)	4
Zucchini fries, 1 cup	4

	SmartPoints® value
Trader Joe's Frozen	
Eggplant cutlets, 3 oz	5
Handsome cut potato fries, 3 oz	4
Hashbrowns, 1 patty (64 g)	4
Mashed potatoes, 8 pieces (112 g)	3
Shredded hash browns, 3 oz	2
Vegetable fried rice, 1 cup	5
Veg-All	
Original mixed vegetables, 4 ½ oz	1
Velveeta	
Cheesy au gratin potatoes, ½ cup	6
Cheesy potatoes, hash browns, 1 serving (51 g)	5
Wegman's	
Cabbage rolls, 1 piece (198.5 g)	5
Hash brown patties, 1 piece (63 g)	4

	SmartPoints® value
Wegman's Italian Classics	
Eggplant rollatini, 3 ½ oz	6
Weight Watchers In-Meeting/ Online Products: Meal Pouches	
Tasty bite brown rice & lentils, 1 pouch	6
Tasty bite madras lentils, 1 pouch	6
Tasty bite vegetable tikka masala, 1 pouch	5
Weight Watchers Smart Ones Classic Favorites	
Broccoli and cheddar roasted potatoes, 1 entrée	6

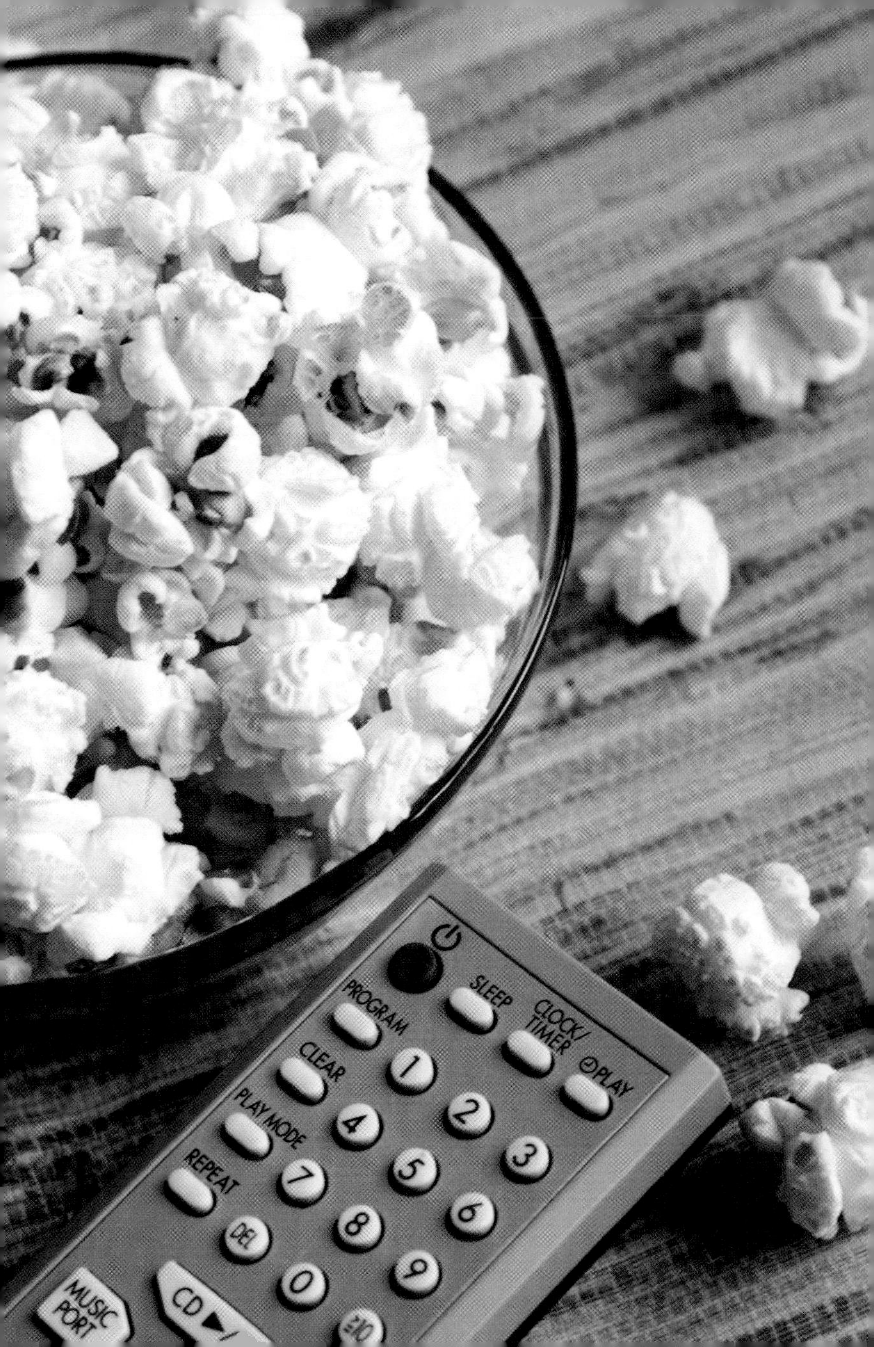
SLEEP
CLOCK/
TIMER
PROGRAM
CLEAR
PLAY
PLAY MODE
REPEAT
1
2
3
4
5
6
7
8
9
0
DEL
MUSIC
PORT
CD ▶/

snacks

	SmartPoints® value
Bagel and Pita Snacks	
Clancy's	
Sea salt bagel chips, 6 chips (28 g)	4
Food Should Taste Good	
Multigrain tortilla chips, 10 chips (28 g)	4
H-E-B	
Sea salt baked pita chips, 9 chips (28 g)	3
Maya Kaimal	
Rosemary naan chips, 9 chips (28 g)	4
New York Style	
Parmesan garlic and herb pita chips, 11 chips (28 g)	4
Stacy's	
Bagel chips, baked, simply naked, 15 chips (28 g)	4
Multigrain pita chips, 9 chips (28 g)	4
Parmesan garlic and herb pita chips, 9 chips (28 g)	4
Pita chips, 10 chips (28 g)	4
Pita chips, baked, parmesan garlic & herb, 9 chips (28 g)	4
Pita chips, baked, simply naked, 10 chips (28 g)	4
Pita chips, multigrain, 9 chips (28 g)	4
Pita chips, simply naked, 10 chips (28 g)	4
Simply cocoa pita chips, 7 chips (28 g)	5
Toasted cheddar pita chips, 7 chips (28 g)	4
Trader Joe's Grocery	
Pita chips with sea salt, 10 chips (28 g)	4
Reduced guilt multigrain pita chips w/ sesame seeds, 1 oz	3
Trader Joe's Reduced Guilt	
Pita chips with sea salt, 8 chips (28 g)	3

	SmartPoints® value
Cereal Bars and Snack Bars	
Atkins	
Blueberry Greek yogurt bar, 1 bar (48 g)	6
Chocolate chip granola bar, 1 bar (48 g)	6
Chocolate peanut butter bar, 1 bar (60 g)	8
Chocolate peanut butter pretzel bar, 1 bar (48 g)	6
Harvest trail dark chocolate peanut butter bar, 1 bar (38 g)	5
Atkins Advantage	
Caramel chocolate nut roll, 1 bar (44 g)	6
Granola bar, chocolate chip, 1 bar (48 g)	6
Granola bar, peanut butter, 1 bar (48 g)	5
Snack/light meal bar, triple chocolate, 1 bar (40 g)	5
Atkins Day Break	
Chocolate chip crisp bar, 1 bar (35 g)	4
Cranberry almond snack bar, 1 bar (35 g)	5
Peanut butter fudge crisp bar, 1 bar (37 g)	5
Atkins Endulge	
Peanut caramel cluster bar, 1 bar (34 g)	4
Treat bar, caramel nut chew, 1 bar (34 g)	5
Atkins Harvest Trail	
Dark chocolate cherry and nuts bar, 1 bar (38 g)	5
Dark chocolate peanut butter bar, 1 bar (38 g)	5
Dark chocolate sea salt caramel bar, 1 bar (38 g)	6
Balance	
Nutrition bar, peanut butter, 1 bar (50 g)	7

	SmartPoints® value
Bounce	
Coconut and macadamia natural energy ball, 1 ball (40 g)	6
Cascadian Farm	
Harvest berry chewy granola bar, 1 bar (35 g)	5
Honey roasted nut chewy bar, 1 bar (50 g)	8
Cave Man	
Dark chocolate cashew almond bar (gluten free), 1 bar (40 g)	8
Chef Robert Irvine's	
Chocolate chip cookie dough fit crunch bar, 1 bar (46 g)	6
Clif	
Energy bar, chocolate brownie, 1 bar (68 g)	10
Energy bar, chocolate chip, 1 bar (68 g)	9
Energy bar, oatmeal raisin walnut, 1 bar (68 g)	9
Energy bar, white chocolate macadamia nut, 1 bar (68 g)	9
Clif Builder's	
Protein bar, chocolate mint, 1 bar (68 g)	10
Protein bar, peanut butter, 1 bar (68 g)	10
Clif Kid	
Protein bar, chocolate, 1 bar (36 g)	5
Clif Kid Organic Z Bar	
Chocolate chip, 1 bar (36 g)	5
Iced oatmeal cookie, 1 bar (36 g)	5
Detour	
Protein bar, whey, chocolate chip caramel, 1 bar (43 g)	5
Detour Lower Sugar	
Caramel peanut whey protein bar, 1 bar (47 g)	5
Detour Simple	
Caramel peanut whey protein bar, 1 bar (85 g)	5

	SmartPoints® value
Dark chocolate sea salt almond bar, 1 bar (43 g)	5
Detour Smart	
Oatmeal bar, whole grain, blueberry, 1 bar (38 g)	4
D's Naturals	
Peanut butter cookie dough no cow bar, 1 bar (60 g)	4
Fiber One	
Blueberry streusel bar, 1 bar (40 g)	6
Oats and chocolate chewy bar, 1 bar (40 g)	6
Oats and peanut butter chewy bar, 1 bar (40 g)	5
Protein peanut butter chewy bars, 1 bar (33 g)	5
Pumpkin bar soft baked bar, 1 bar (25 g)	4
Salted caramel cheesecake bar, 1 bar (38 g)	7
Soft baked oatmeal raisin cookie, 1 bar (31 g)	5
Strawberry cheesecake bar, 1 bar (38 g)	7
Strawberry streusel bar, 1 bar (40 g)	6
Fiber One 90 Calorie	
Chocolate caramel and pretzel chewy bar, 1 bar (23 g)	4
Chocolate chewy bar, 1 bar (23 g)	4
Chocolate peanut butter chewy bar, 1 bar (23 g)	4
Lemon bar, 1 bar (25 g)	4
Orange cranberry bar, 1 bar (25 g)	4
Soft baked pumpkin bar, 1 bar (25 g)	4
Fiber One 90 Calorie Brownie	
Chocolate peanut butter, 1 brownie (25 g)	4
Fiber One Protein	
Caramel nut chewy bar, 1 bar (33 g)	5

Cereal Bars and Snack Bars, Fiber One Protein (cont'd)

	SmartPoints® value
Coconut almond chewy bar, 1 bar (33 g)	6
Cookies and creme chewy bar, 1 bar (33 g)	5
Peanut butter chewy bar, 1 bar (33 g)	5
Fit & Active	
Chocolate peanut butter protein meal bars, 1 bar (45 g)	7
Strawberry vitality cereal bar, 1 bar (23 g)	3
Fit Crunch	
Baked peanut butter bar, 1 bar (46 g)	6
Giant	
Chocolate chunk granola bars, 1 bar (24 g)	4
Goodness Knows	
Cranberry almond dark chocolate snack squares, 1 package (34 g)	6
Great Value	
Chewy granola bars, 90 calorie, chocolate chunk, 1 bar (24 g)	4
Peanut butter and dark chocolate chewy protein bar, 1 bar (40 g)	6
Trail mix granola bars, 1 bar (28 g)	5
Great Value 90 Calorie Chewy	
Chocolate chunk granola bar, 1 bar (24 g)	4
Healthy Choice	
Strawberry smoothie bar, 1 bar (67 g)	3
HMR Benefit	
Honey graham bar, 1 bar (40 g)	7
JimmyBar	
How bout dem apples clean snack bar, 1 bar (45 g)	6
Jojo	
Crispy chocolate treat bar, 1 bar (12 g)	3
Kashi	
Blackberry graham cereal bar, 1 bar (35 g)	5

	SmartPoints® value
Chewy granola bar honey almond flax, 1 bar (35 g)	4
Chewy granola bar peanut peanut butter, 1 bar (35 g)	4
Chocolate almond & sea salt with chia chewy granola bars, 1 bar (35 g)	5
Chocolate almond and sea salt chewy granola bar with chia, 1 bar (35 g)	5
Dark mocha almond chewy granola bars, 1 bar (35 g)	4
Honey oat flax crunchy granola and seed bar, 2 bars (40 g)	6
Pumpkin spice flax granola bar, 1 bar (40 g)	6
Roasted almond crunch granola bar, 2 bars (40 g)	6
Trail mix chewy granola bars, 1 bar (35 g)	5
Kashi Chewy Granola Bar	
Cherry dark chocolate, 1 bar (35 g)	4
Dark chocolate coconut, 1 bar (32 g)	5
Kashi TLC	
Cereal bars, soft-baked, ripe strawberry, 1 bar (35 g)	4
Granola bar, chewy, trail mix, 1 bar (35 g)	5
Granola bar, honey almond flax, 1 bar (35 g)	4
Granola bars, chewy, cherry dark chocolate, 1 bar (35 g)	4
Granola bars, chewy, dark mocha almond, 1 bar (35 g)	4
Granola bars, chewy, honey almond flax, 1 bar (35 g)	4
Granola bars, chewy, peanut peanut butter, 1 bar (35 g)	4
Kellogg's Nutri-Grain	
Blueberry flavored cereal bar, 1 bar (37 g)	5
Cherry almond fruit and nut bar, 1 bar (34 g)	6

	SmartPoints® value
Strawberry cereal bars, 1 bar (44 g)	6
Kellogg's Special K	
Berry medley snack bar, 1 bar (25 g)	4
Blueberry bliss snack bar, 1 bar (25 g)	4
Red berries cereal bar, 1 bar (23 g)	4
Red velvet pastry crisps, 2 crisps (25 g)	4
Salted caramel chocolate snack bars, 1 bar (25 g)	4
Salted pretzel chocolate snack bars, 1 bar (25 g)	4
Strawberry pastry crisps, 2 crisps (25 g)	4
Kellogg's Special K Chewy Nut	
Cranberry almond bar, 1 bar (33 g)	6
Kellogg's Special K Protein	
Chocolatey peanut butter granola snack bar, 1 bar (27 g)	4
Greek yogurt and fruit granola snack bar, 1 bar (27 g)	4
Strawberry meal bar, 1 bar (45 g)	7
Kellogg's Special K Protein Granola Snack Bar	
Almond honey nut, 1 bar (27 g)	4
Kind	
Almond and coconut fruit and nut bar, 1 bar (40 g)	8
Caramel almond and sea salt nuts and spices bar, 1 bar (40 g)	7
Dark chocolate nuts and sea salt nut and spice bar, 1 bar (40 g)	7
Fruit + nut bar, fruit & nut delight, 1 bar (40 g)	7
Maple glazed pecan and sea salt nuts ans spices bar, 1 bar (40 g)	7
Nuts & spices bar, dark chocolate nuts & sea salt, 1 bar (40 g)	7
Nuts & spices bars, dark chocolate cinnamon pecan, 1 bar (40 g)	7
Raspberry chia breakfast bar, 2 bars (50 g)	8

	SmartPoints® value
Kind Breakfast	
Peanut butter breakfast bar, 2 bars (50 g)	8
Kind Fruit & Nut	
Almond & coconut bar, 1 bar (40 g)	9
Blueberry vanilla cashew bar, 1 bar (40 g)	7
Kind Healthy Grains	
Dark chocolate chunk bar, 1 bar (35 g)	6
Gluten free dark chocolate chunk granola bars, 1 bar (35 g)	6
Maple pumpkin seeds with sea salt bar, 1 bar (35 g)	5
Oats and honey with toasted coconut bar, 1 bar (35 g)	6
Peanut butter berry chewy with a crunch bar (gluten free), 1 bar (35 g)	5
Peanut butter dark chocolate gluten free granola bar, 1 bar (35 g)	6
Popped dark chocolate with sea salt bar, 1 bar (35 g)	5
Vanilla blueberry granola bar, 1 bar (35 g)	5
Kind Nuts & Spices	
Caramel almond & sea salt bar, 1 bar (40 g)	7
Caramel almond and sea salt bar, 1 bar (40 g)	7
Dark chocolate mocha almond bar, 1 bar (40 g)	7
Madagascar vanilla almond bar, 1 bar (40 g)	7
Kind Plus	
Cranberry almond + antioxidants fruit and nut bar, 1 bar (40 g)	7
Dark chocolate cherry cashew and antioxidant bar, 1 bar (40 g)	7
Dark chocolate cherry cashew and antioxidants bar, 1 bar (40 g)	7
Fruit & nut bar, dark chocolate & cherry cashew, 1 bar (40 g)	7

Cereal Bars and Snack Bars, Kind Plus (cont'd)

	SmartPoints® value
Peanut butter dark chocolate and protein bar, 1 bar (40 g)	7
Protein bar, peanut butter dark chocolate, 1 bar (40 g)	8
Walnut macadamia meal bars, 1 bar (40 g)	6
Kind Popped	
Dark chocolate with sea salt granola bar (gluten free), 1 bar (35 g)	5
Kind Snack Bars Nuts & Spices	
Dark chocolate nuts and sea salt bar, 1 bar (40 g)	7
Kirkland Signature	
Chocolate chips soft and chewy granola bar, 1 bar (24 g)	4
Kroger	
Oats and chocolate chewy bars, 1 bar (40 g)	5
Sweet and salty almond granola bars, 1 bar (35 g)	6
Larabar	
Apple pie fruit and nut bar, 1 bar (45 g)	8
Cashew cookie fruit and nut bar, 1 bar (48 g)	9
Cherry pie fruit and nut bar, 1 bar (48 g)	9
Chocolate chip cookie dough fruit and nut bar, 1 bar (45 g)	9
Peanut butter chocolate chip fruit and nut bar, 1 bar (45 g)	9
Peanut butter cookie flavored fruit and nut bar, 1 bar (48 g)	9
Snickerdoodle bar, 1 bar (45 g)	8
Life Choice	
Peanut butter chocolate chip energy bar, 1 bar (50 g)	10
Life Choice Protein	
Double chocolate high protein bar, 1 bar (45 g)	5
Luna	
Berry Greek yogurt high protein bar, 1 bar (45 g)	6

	SmartPoints® value
Caramel nut brownie whole nutrition bar for women, 1 bar (48 g)	7
Chocolate peppermint stick nutrition bar for women, 1 bar (48 g)	7
Dark chocolate hazelnut bar, 1 bar (42 g)	6
Dark chocolate mocha almond nutrition bar, 1 bar (42 g)	6
Nutrition bar, chocolate dipped coconut, 1 bar (48 g)	7
Nutrition bar, for women, nutz over chocolate, 1 bar (48 g)	6
Nutrition bar, lemon zest, 1 bar (48 g)	7
Peanut butter chocolate chunk bar, 1 bar (42 g)	6
Protein bar, chocolate peanut butter, 1 bar (45 g)	7
S'mores whole nutrition bar for women, 1 bar (48 g)	7
Luna Protein	
Chocolate chip cookie dough bar, 1 bar (45 g)	7
Chocolate coconut almond bar, 1 bar (45 g)	7
Chocolate salted caramel high protein bar, 1 bar (45 g)	7
Mariani	
Honey bar, 1 bar (40 g)	7
Medifast	
Caramel crunch bar, 1 bar (32 g)	3
Chocolate crunch bar, 1 bar (32 g)	3
Chocolate mint crunch bar, 1 bar (32 g)	3
Cookie dough chewy bar, 1 bar (36 g)	4
Oatmeal raisin crunch bar, 1 bar (32 g)	3
Peanut butter chocolate chip chewy bar, 1 bar (36 g)	3
Peanut butter crunch bar, 1 bar (32 g)	3

	SmartPoints® value
Smore crunch bar, 1 bar (32 g)	4
Millville	
Blueberry pastry crisps, 2 crisps (25 g)	4
Chocolate chip chewy dipped chocolatey covered granola bars, 1 bar (31 g)	7
Dark chocolate cherry trail mix chewy granola bars, 1 bar (35 g)	5
Millville Crispy Rice Treats	
Original crispy marshmallow squares, 1 bar (22 g)	4
MusclePharm	
Chocolate peanut butter cup bar, 1 bar (63 g)	6
Combat crunch chocolate chip cookie dough bar, 1 bar (63 g)	6
MusclePharm Combat Crunch	
Chocolate cake protein bar, 1 bar (63 g)	6
Nature Valley	
Almond dark chocolate nut crips bar, 1 bar (25 g)	5
Blueberry almond soft baked protein granola bites, 3 pieces (45 g)	6
Chew bars, protein, peanut, almond & dark chocolate, 1 bar (40 g)	6
Cinnamon brown sugar soft baked oatmeal squares, 1 bar (35 g)	6
Crunchy granola bars, oats 'n dark chocolate, 2 bars (42 g)	7
Dark chocolate granola thins, 1 pouch (17 g)	3
Granola bars, chewy, trail mix, dark chocolate cherry, 1 bar (35 g)	6
Granola bars, crunchy, oats 'n honey, 2 bars (42 g)	7
Granola bars, sweet & salty nut, dark chocolate, peanut & almond, 1 bar (35 g)	7

	SmartPoints® value
Honey peanut and almond protein chewy bar, 1 bar (40 g)	6
Peanut butter dark chocolate chewy protein bar, 1 bar (40 g)	6
Roasted peanut & honey simple nut bar, 1 bar (33 g)	6
Salted caramel peanut nut crisp bar, 1 bar (25 g)	5
Soft baked blueberry oatmeal squares, 1 bar (35 g)	6
Soft baked honey almond granola bites, 3 pieces (45 g)	6
Sweet and salty dark chocolate peanut and almonds bar, 1 bar (35 g)	7
Sweet and salty nut granola bars, cashew, 1 bar (35 g)	7
Trail mix bars, chewy, fruit & nut, 1 bar (35 g)	6
Nature Valley Crunchy	
Granola bars, peanut butter, 2 bars (42 g)	7
Oats 'n honey granola bars, 2 bars (42 g)	7
Pecan crunch granola bars, 2 bars (42 g)	7
Nature Valley Protein	
Salted caramel nut chewy bar, 1 bar (40 g)	6
Nature Valley Soft Baked	
Cinnamon brown sugar oatmeal squares, 1 bar (35 g)	6
Peanut butter oatmeal squares, 1 bar (35 g)	6
Nature Valley Sweet & Salty Nut	
Chocolate pretzel nut granola bars, 1 bar (35 g)	6
Granola bars, almond, 1 bar (35 g)	7
Granola bars, peanut, 1 bar (35 g)	7
Nature's Bakery	
Apple cinnamon fig bar, ½ package (28 g)	4
Raspberry fig bar, ½ package (28 g)	4

Cereal Bars and Snack Bars, Nature's Bakery (cont'd)

	SmartPoints® value
Stone ground whole wheat fig bar, 1 bar (28 g)	4
Whole wheat blueberry fig bar, ½ bar (28 g)	4
NuGo	
Peanut butter chocolate bar, 1 bar (50 g)	6
Vanilla yogurt bar, 1 bar (50 g)	6
Nutri-Grain	
Cereal bar, apple cinnamon, 1 bar (37 g)	5
Cereal bar, blueberry, 1 bar (37 g)	5
Cereal bar, cherry, 1 bar (37 g)	5
Cereal bar, mixed berry, 1 bar (37 g)	5
Cereal bar, raspberry, 1 bar (37 g)	5
Cereal bar, strawberry, 1 bar (37 g)	5
Nutrisystem	
Apple strudel bar, 1 package (43 g)	6
Cinnamon bun bar, 1 bar (40 g)	5
Fudge graham bar, 1 package (50 g)	7
Nutrisystem Breakfast	
Harvest nut bar, 1 bar (40 g)	5
Peanut butter granola bar, 1 bar (40 g)	6
Nutrisystem Lunch	
Trail mix bar, 1 bar (50 g)	7
Oh Yeah!	
Birthday cake bar, 1 bar (60 g)	6
Lemon cake one bar, 1 bar (60 g)	6
Peanut butter pie one bar, 1 bar (60 g)	6
Victory chocolate chip cookie dough bar, 1 bar (65 g)	5
Oh Yeah! One	
Chocolate chip cookie dough bar, 1 bar (60 g)	4
Oh Yeah! Victory	
Peanut butter chip bar, 1 bar (65 g)	5

	SmartPoints® value
Pearson's	
Salted nut rolls, 1 bar (92 g)	18
Perfectly Simple	
Bing cherry and almond bar, 1 bar (40 g)	7
Peppermint bark protein bar, 1 bar (40 g)	7
Roasted cashew and dark chocolate bar, 1 bar (40 g)	7
Post	
Strawberry breakfast biscuits bar, 4 biscuits (50 g)	8
Power Crunch	
Protein energy bar, original, French vanilla creme, 1 bar (40 g)	7
Protein energy bar, peanut butter creme, 1 bar (40 g)	7
Power Crunch Original	
Chocolate mint protein energy bar, 1 bar (40 g)	7
PowerBar Protein Plus	
Chocolate peanut butter bar, 1 bar (60 g)	7
PowerBar Triple Threat	
Caramel nut brownie energy bar, 1 bar (50 g)	7
Premier Protein	
Chocolate peanut butter bar, 1 bar (72 g)	8
Naturally sweetened whey protein, 1 scoop (46 g)	3
Publix	
No sugar added fudge bars, 2 bars (76 g)	2
Pure Protein	
Chewy chocolate chip bar (gluten free), 1 bar (50 g)	5
Chocolate deluxe bar (gluten free), 1 bar (50 g)	5
Chocolate peanut butter bar, 1 bar (50 g)	5
Chocolate peanut butter bar (gluten free), 1 bar (50 g)	5

	SmartPoints® value
Chocolate peanut caramel (gluten free), 1 bar (50 g)	5
Cranberry almond cashew bar, 1 bar (53 g)	6
Dark chocolate coconut bar (gluten free), 1 bar (50 g)	5
Tropical fruit macadamia nut bar, 1 bar (53 g)	6
Pure Protein High Protein Bar	
Chocolate deluxe, 1 bar (50 g)	5
Quaker	
Caramel coconut chewy girl scouts granola bars, 1 bar (24 g)	4
Cranberry almond breakfast flats bars, 3 bars (40 g)	7
Golden raisin cinnamon breakfast flats, 3 bars (40 g)	6
Thin mints chewy granola bar, 1 bar (24 g)	4
Quaker Breakfast Flats	
Banana honey nut breakfast bar, 3 bars (40 g)	6
Golden raisin cinnamon bar, 3 bars (40 g)	6
Quaker Chewy	
25% less sugar chocolate chip granola bar, 1 bar (24 g)	4
Banana chocolate chip bar, 1 bar (24 g)	4
Banana chocolate chip granola bar, 1 bar (24 g)	4
Caramel apple bar, 1 bar (24 g)	4
Chocolate chip granola bar, 1 bar (24 g)	4
Low-fat oatmeal raisin granola bar, 1 bar (24 g)	3
Peanut butter chocolate chip granola bar, 1 bar (24 g)	4
S'mores granola bar, 1 bar (24 g)	4
Quaker Chewy 25% Less Sugar	
Peanut butter chocolate chip granola bar, 1 bar (24 g)	4

	SmartPoints® value
Quaker Chewy 90 Calories	
Low-fat chocolate chunk granola bar, 1 bar (24 g)	4
Quaker Oats Chewy	
Chocolate chip granola bar, 1 bar (24 g)	4
Quest Bar	
Banana nut muffin protein bar, 1 bar (60 g)	4
Double chocolate chunk protein bar, 1 bar (60 g)	4
Lemon cream pie flavor protein bar, 1 bar (60 g)	4
Lemon cream pie protein bar, 1 bar (60 g)	4
Mixed berry bliss protein bar, 1 bar (60 g)	4
Natural protein bar, banana nut muffin, 1 bar (60 g)	4
Protein bar, apple pie, 1 bar (60 g)	4
Protein bar, chocolate brownie flavor, 1 bar (60 g)	4
Protein bar, chocolate chip cookie dough, 1 bar (60 g)	4
Protein bar, chocolate peanut butter flavor, 1 bar (60 g)	4
Protein bar, cinnamon roll flavor, 1 bar (60 g)	4
Protein bar, coconut cashew flavor, 1 bar (60 g)	4
Protein bar, cookies & cream flavor, 1 bar (60 g)	4
Protein bar, double chocolate chunk flavor, 1 bar (60 g)	4
Protein bar, mint chocolate chunk, 1 bar (60 g)	5
Protein bar, natural, lemon cream pie, 1 bar (60 g)	4
Protein bar, peanut butter supreme, 1 bar (60 g)	5
Protein bar, s'mores flavor, 1 bar (60 g)	4

Cereal Bars and Snack Bars, Quest Bar (cont'd)

	SmartPoints® value
Protein bar, strawberry cheesecake flavor, 1 bar (60 g)	4
Protein bar, vanilla almond crunch, 1 bar (60 g)	4
Protein bar, white chocolate raspberry flavor, 1 bar (60 g)	5
Pumpkin pie flavored coated protein bar (gluten free), 1 bar (60 g)	6
Smores protein bar, 1 bar (60 g)	4
Rice Krispie Treats The Original	
Crisp rice cereal and marshmallow square, 1 bar (22 g)	4
Rice Krispies	
Crispy marshmallow squares, original size bars, 1 bar (22 g)	4
Crispy marshmallow squares, the original, 1 bar (22 g)	4
Rice Krispies Treats	
Crispy marshmallow squares, holiday color, 1 bar (22 g)	4
Marshmallow squares, crispy, the original, value pack, 1 bar (22 g)	4
Original crispy marshmallow square, 4 bars (44 g)	3
The original crispy marshmallow squares, 1 bar (22 g)	4
Rice Krispies Treats Scotcheroos	
Crispy marshmallow squares, chocolate and butterscotch, 1 piece (25 g)	5
Simple Truth	
Mint chocolate protein bar, 1 bar (50 g)	5
Skinny Cow Blissful Truffle	
Milk chocolate candy bar, 1 bar (22 g)	7
Skinnygirl	
Chocolate chip cookie dough protein bar, 1 bar (39 g)	4

	SmartPoints® value
South Beach Diet	
Good to go bars, peanut butter, 1 bar (35 g)	5
Snack bars, whipped peanut butter, 1 bar (28 g)	4
Southern Grove 100 Calorie Packs	
Natural almond and walnut mix, 1 package (16 g)	3
Special K	
Cereal bar, chocolatey pretzel, 1 bar (22 g)	4
Chocolate caramel protein bar, 1 bar (45 g)	7
Granola bars, protein & fiber, chocolatey peanut butter, 1 bar (27 g)	4
Protein meal bar, chocolatey chip, 1 bar (44 g)	7
Protein meal bar, double chocolate, 1 bar (45 g)	7
Strawberry cereal bar, 1 bar (23 g)	4
Special K Protein	
Chocolate peanut butter meal bar, 1 bar (45 g)	7
Meal bar, chocolate peanut butter, 1 bar (45 g)	7
Meal bar, strawberry, 1 bar (45 g)	7
Special K Protein Granola Bars	
Dark chocolate granola, 1 bar (27 g)	4
Stabilyze	
Dark chocolate coconut cashew bar, 1 bar (50 g)	7
Sunbelt Bakery	
Apple spice chewy granola bar, 1 bar (27 g)	5
Banana harvest granola bars, 1 bar (25 g)	5
Chewy chocolate chip granola bars, 1 bar (30 g)	6

	SmartPoints® value
Chewy oats and honey granola bars, 1 bar (27 g)	5
Peanut sweet and salty chewy granola bar, 1 bar (30 g)	6
Think Thin	
Chocolate almond brownie lean protein and fiber bar, 1 bar (40 g)	5
High protein bar, chocolate fudge, 1 bar (60 g)	6
Peanut butter protein bites, 8 pieces (44 g)	6
Protein bar, white chocolate chip, 1 bar (60 g)	6
Unwrapped salted caramel protein bites, 8 pieces (44 g)	6
Think Thin High Protein Bar	
Brownie crunch, 1 bar (60 g)	6
Chunky peanut butter, 1 bar (60 g)	6
Chunky peanut butter chocolate, 1 bar (60 g)	6
Creamy peanut butter, 1 bar (60 g)	6
Think Thin Lean Protein & Fiber	
Chocolate almond brownie protein bar, 1 bar (40 g)	5
Chunky chocolate peanut protein bar, 1 bar (40 g)	5
Salted caramel protein bar, 1 bar (40 g)	5
Salted caramel bar, 1 bar (40 g)	5
Trader Joe's	
Dark chocolate nuts and sea salt bar, 1 bar (40 g)	7
Dark chocolate walnut peanut fig and date bar, 1 bar (40 g)	6
This "fig walks into a bar..." cereal bars, 1 bar (37 g)	5
Trader Joe's Fiberful	
Rolled oats and chocolate chips granola bars, 1 bar (35 g)	4

	SmartPoints® value
Trader Joe's Grocery	
Rolled oats & chocolate chips fiberful granola bars, 1 bar (35 g)	4
Vega Sport	
Chocolate peanut butter protein bar, 1 bar (60 g)	9
Weight Watchers In-Meeting/ Online Products: Breakfast Squares	
Cranberry almond yogurt, 1 bar	5
Dark chocolate nut, 1 bar	5
Weight Watchers In-Meeting/ Online Products: Mini Bars	
Caramel macchiato, 1 bar	2
Chocolate caramel, 1 bar	2
Chocolate pretzel blast, 1 bar	2
Mint cookie crisp, 1 bar	2
Peanut butter cookie explosion, 1 bar	3
So-good salted caramel, 1 bar	3
Sprinkle me pink, 1 bar	3
Weight Watchers In-Meeting/ Online Products: Snack Bars	
Peanut butter trail mix, 1 bar	4
Sweet & salty toffee twist, 1 bar	4
Wild Roots	
Trail mix bars, 1 bar (40 g)	7
World Gourmet Sensible Portions	
100 calorie bar, cinna-swirl, 1 bar (30 g)	4
Zone Perfect	
Nutrition bars, all-natural, double dark chocolate, 1 bar (45 g)	8
Zone Perfect Classic	
Nutrition bars, all-natural, chocolate peanut butter, 1 bar (50 g)	8
Zone Perfect Dark	
Nutrition bar, dark chocolate almond, 1 bar (45 g)	7

Cheese Snacks

	SmartPoints® value
Cheetos	
Cheese flavored snack puffs, 13 puffs (28 g)	5
Crunchy flavored cheese snacks, 21 pieces (28 g)	5
Flamin hot crunchy cheese snacks, 21 pieces (28 g)	5
Flamin' hot flavored oven baked snack, 34 pieces (28 g)	4
Cheetos Baked!	
Crunchy cheese flavored snacks, 34 pieces (28 g)	3
Cheetos Crunchy	
Cheddar jalapeño cheese flavored snack, 21 pieces (28 g)	5
Cheese flavored snacks, 21 pieces (28 g)	5
Cheetos Oven Baked	
Crunchy cheese flavored snacks, 1 single bag (21.25 g)	3
Cheetos Puffs	
Cheese flavored snacks, 13 pieces (28 g)	5
Cheetos Simply Natural	
White cheddar puffed corn snacks, 32 pieces (28 g)	5
Cheez Doodles	
Cheese flavored corn snacks, puffed, 23 pieces (28 g)	5
Crunchy cheese flavored corn snacks, ½ cup	5
Puffed baked cheese flavored corn snacks, 23 pieces (28 g)	5
Cheez-It	
Baked cheese snacks, crisps, cheddar crunch, 36 crackers (32 g)	5

	SmartPoints® value
Chester's	
Flamin hot flavor fries, 33 pieces (28 g)	5
Puffcorn, cheese, 3 cups	5
Clancy's	
Crunchy cheese curls, 1 cup	4
Great Value	
Cheese puffs, 1 oz	5
Handi Snacks Ritz	
Crackers 'n cheese dip, 1 pack (27 g)	3
Herr's	
Cheese balls, 31 balls (28 g)	5
Laughing Cow	
Creamy Swiss with classic breadsticks, 1 pack (35 g)	4
Market Pantry	
Cheddar cheeseballs, 1½ cups	5
Nutrisystem	
Cheese puffs, 1 package (33 g)	4
Pepperidge Farm Goldfish	
Cheddar baked snack crackers, 55 pieces (30 g)	4
Sargento Balanced Breaks	
Natural sharp cheddar cheese with cashews and cranberries, 1 tray (43 g)	7
Natural sharp white cheddar cheese, sea salted cashews & golden raisin medley, 1 tray (43 g)	7
Simply Chex	
Cheddar snack, 1 pouch (26 g)	4
Smithfield Ready, Snack, Go!	
Roasted turkey breast and hot pepper cheese, 1 roll (43 g)	3
Trader Joe's Grocery	
Baked cheese crunchies, 33 pieces (28 g)	4
Reduced fat cheese puffs, 1 serving (28.35 g)	4

	SmartPoints® value
Utz	
Cheese balls, 32 balls (28 g)	4
Utz Cotton Tails	
White cheddar cheese ball snack, 1 oz	6
Wawa Grocery	
Black forest ham & cheddar cheese on a pretzel sandwich thin, 1 package (122 g)	6
Weight Watchers In-Meeting/ Online Products: Crunchy Snacks	
Cheddar twists, 1 pouch	2
Nacho cheese supreme, 1 pouch	2

Chips and Snacks, Other

Aldi	
Lemon poppy almond sweet crisps, 4 pieces (15 g)	2
Andy Capp's	
Hot fries, 1 bag (24 g)	4
Bare Fruit	
Fuji red apple chips, ½ cup	5
Beanitos	
Bean chips, white bean with sea salt, restaurant style, 1 oz	4
Betty Crocker	
Chex mix brand snack, traditional, 1 bag (47 g)	7
Breaking News	
Himalayan pink salt lentil chips, 16 chips (28 g)	3
Calbee	
Wasabi ranch snapea crisps, 22 pieces (28 g)	3

	SmartPoints® value
Cheetos	
Crunchy cheese flavored snacks, 21 pieces (28 g)	5
Flamin' hot crunchy cheese flavored snacks, 21 pieces (28 g)	5
Puffs cheese flavored snacks, 13 pieces (28 g)	5
Cheetos Puffs	
Flamin hot cheese flavored snacks, 13 pieces (28 g)	5
Cheetos Sweetos	
Cinnamon sugar puffs, 1 package (28 g)	5
Cheez Doodles	
Jalapeño cheddar poppers, 1 bag (35 g)	6
Cheez-It	
Snack mix, ½ cup	4
Cheez-It 100 Calorie Right Bites	
Snack mix, 1 pouch (21 g)	3
Chex Mix Muddy Buddies	
Peanut butter and chocolate covered chex, 1 pouch (17 g)	3
Snack mix, peanut butter & chocolate, ⅓ cup	6
Chex Mix The Original	
Traditional snack mix, ½ cup	4
Creative Snacks Co.	
Vanilla almond granola, ⅔ cup	8
Dang	
Original recipe toasted coconut chips, 1 bag (20 g)	6
Eatsmart Naturals	
Sea salt garden veggie sticks, 2 cups	4

Chips and Snacks, Other (cont'd)

	SmartPoints® value
Enlightened	
Mesquite bbq roasted broad beans, 1 package (28 g)	2
Sriracha roasted broad beans, 1 oz	2
First Street	
Honey and oats almonds granola, ½ cup	9
Food Should Taste Good	
Multigrain bean chips, 10 chips (28 g)	4
Fresh Gourmet	
Wonton strips, authentic, 2 Tbsp	1
Frollicks	
Sea salt crunchy chickpeas, ¼ cup	4
Funyuns	
Onion flavored rings, 13 pieces (28 g)	4
Fusia Asian Inspirations	
Crunchy rice rolls, 1 roll (10 g)	2
Garden Fresh Gourmet	
Salted kettle style tortilla strips, 13 strips (28 g)	4
Garden Lites	
Italian veggie bites, 4 veggie bites (85 g)	4
Gardetto's	
Original recipe snack mix, ½ cup	5
gimME	
Wasabi roasted seaweed snacks, ½ package (5 g)	1
Glico	
Pocky sticks, 1 pouch (40 g)	8
Good Health	
Mickey shaped veggie chips, 35 chips (28 g)	4

	SmartPoints® value
Gourmet Basics	
Classic sea salt smart fries, 50 sticks (28.3 g)	3
Ideal Protein	
Vanilla crispy square, 1 square (42 g)	4
J.R. Dippers	
Cheese dip and pretzel sticks, 1 serving (19 g)	2
Jayone	
Honey cinnamon crunchy rice snack, 1 rice snack (10 g)	1
Kellogg's Special K	
White cheddar flavored popcorn chips, 25 chips (28 g)	4
Kellogg's Special K Popped Delights	
Cocoa with fudge drizzle popped snacks, 1 pouch (11.76 g)	3
Kettle	
Real sliced sweet potatoes (chips), 13 chips (28 g)	6
Kim's Magic Pop	
Magic pop, 1 piece (5 g)	0
LiveGfree	
Applewood smoked bbq rice thins, 20 crackers (30 g)	4
Salt and vinegar rice thins, 20 rice thins (30 g)	4
LuLu	
Salted plantain chips, ½ bag (31.7 g)	6
Lundberg	
Rice chips, sea salt, 9 chips (28 g)	4
Market Basket	
Vanilla almond granola, ¼ cup	3
Mrs. Thinsters	
Blueberry waffle crisps, 1 oz	5

	SmartPoints® value
Munchies	
Cheese fix snack mix, ¾ cup	4
Nabisco 100 Calorie Packs	
Baked snacks, ritz snack mix, 1 package (22 g)	3
Nice!	
Wasabi peas, ⅓ cup	3
Pasta Chips	
Marinara pasta snack, 1 oz	3
Pepperidge Farm Goldfish	
Honey mustard and pretzel mix, 43 pieces (30 g)	4
Pirate's Booty	
Aged white cheddar baked rice and corn puffs, 1 oz	4
Pop Chips	
Barbeque potato snacks, 20 chips (28 g)	4
Crazy hot chips, 1 bag (20 g)	2
Popped chip snack, cheddar & sour cream potato, 22 chips (28 g)	4
Popped chip snack, sour cream & onion potato, 22 chips (28 g)	4
Sea salt potato snack, 23 chips (28 g)	4
Smooth cheddar rice chips, 23 chips (28 g)	4
Veggie chips, hint of olive oil, 23 chips (28 g)	3
Pringles Stix	
Honey butter flavored baked snack sticks, 1 pack (17 g)	3
Pizza flavored baked snack sticks, 1 pack (17 g)	3

	SmartPoints® value
Quest Protein Chips	
Bbq flavor, 1 bag (32 g)	2
Cheddar & sour cream flavor, 1 bag (32 g)	2
Sea salt, 1 bag (32 g)	2
Sour cream & onion flavor, 1 bag (32 g)	2
Rice Works	
Sea salt gourmet rice snacks, 10 chips (28 g)	4
Riceworks	
Sea salt and black sesame wildrice crisps, 10 chips (28 g)	4
Ritz	
Toasted chips, dairyland cheddar, 14 chips (28 g)	4
Toasted chips, main street original, 16 chips (28 g)	4
Toasted chips, sweet home sour cream & onion, 14 chips (28 g)	4
Robert's American Gourmet	
Pirate's booty with aged white cheddar, ½ oz	2
Sabra	
Classic hummus with pretzels, 1 container (128 g)	12
Roasted garlic hummus with pretzels, 1 container (128 g)	11
Roasted red pepper hummus with pretzels, 1 container (128 g)	11
Savanna Orchards Gourmet	
Rice cracker and nut blend, ⅓ cup	4
Sensible Portions Garden Veggie Straws	
Apple straws, cinnamon, 38 straws (28 g)	4
Garden veggie straws with zesty ranch, 1 bag (28 g)	4

Chips and Snacks, Other (cont'd)

	SmartPoints® value
Sensible Portions Puffs	
Baked cheddar corn snack, 1 bag (28 g)	4
Simple Truth Organic	
Sweet onion roasted seaweed snack, 1 pack (5 g)	1
Simply 7	
Barbeque quinoa chips, 20 chips (28 g)	3
Cheddar quinoa chips, 20 chips (28 g)	3
Sea salt lentil chips, 31 chips (28 g)	4
Sea salt quinoa chips, 20 chips (28 g)	4
SimplyNature	
Green pea crisps (baked pea snack), 1 oz	3
Skippy	
Double peanut butter p.b. bites, 10 pieces (30 g)	7
Pretzel p.b. bites, 15 pieces (30 g)	7
Slimfast 100 Calorie Snacks	
Cinnamon bun swirl drizzled crisps, 1 pack (28 g)	4
Peanut butter chocolate snack bites, 1 package (23 g)	5
Sour cream and onion baked crisps, 1 package (28 g)	3
Snapz	
Organic apple crisps with 100% natural cheese puffs, 1 package (13 g)	2
Somersaults	
Cinnamon crunch sunflower seed snack, 14 pieces (30 g)	5
Dutch cocoa, 14 pieces (30 g)	4
Pacific sea salt, 14 pieces (30 g)	4

	SmartPoints® value
Southern Grove	
Chocolate flavored yogurt covered raisins, ¼ cup	9
Special K	
Cracker chips, cheddar, 1 package (25 g)	3
Cracker chips, cheddar, 25 chips (30 g)	4
Sea salt cracker chips, 1 package (25 g)	3
White cheddar popcorn chips, 25 chips (28 g)	4
Stacy's	
Fire roasted jalapeño pita chips, 9 chips (28 g)	4
Pita crisps, simply naked, 13 chips (28 g)	4
Stonefire	
Original naan crisps, 15 crisps (28 g)	4
SunChips	
Garden salsa flavor chips, 15 chips (28 g)	5
Garden salsa multigrain snacks, 1 package (43 g)	7
Harvest cheddar multigrain snacks, 1 package (43 g)	7
Multigrain snacks, original, 16 chips (26 g)	5
Original multigrain snacks, 1 package (43 g)	7
Sunshine Cheez-It 100 Calorie Right Bites	
Extra cheddar party mix, 1 pouch (21 g)	3
Party mix, 1 pouch (21 g)	3
Taylor Farms	
Protein punch snack tray, 1 container (185 g)	12

	SmartPoints® value
Think Thin	
Salted caramel unwrapped protein bites (gluten free), 8 pieces (44 g)	6
Tom's	
Nacho rings corn snacks, 30 rings (28 g)	5
Trader Joe's	
Cinnamon apple snack sticks, 38 sticks (28 g)	5
Kettle popped sweet & salty whole grain popcorn chips, 1 oz	3
Sweet plantain chips, 12 chips (28 g)	5
Wasabi roasted seaweed snack, ½ package (5 g)	1
Trader Joe's Grocery	
Roasted seaweed snack, ½ package (5 g)	1
Wegman's	
Sea salt crunchy rice chips, 10 chips (28 g)	4
Wegman's Food You Feel Good About	
Sea salt get poppin' potato snacks, 24 chips (28 g)	3
Weight Watchers In-Meeting/ Online Products: Crunchy Snacks	
Popped cinnamon flavored snacks, 1 pouch	2
Popped sea salt hummus chips, 1 pouch	2
Weight Watchers In-Meeting/ Online Products: Hummus Snack Packs	
Classic hummus, 1 pack	3
Roasted red pepper, 1 pack	3
Welch's	
Concord grape pb&j bite size snacks, 1 pouch (22.7 g)	5

	SmartPoints® value
Wheat Thins	
Toasted chips, great plains multigrain, 13 chips (28 g)	4
Toasted chips, veggie, 1 pack (47 g)	7
Wheat Thins Popped	
Chips, popped, barbecue, 24 chips (30 g)	4
Sour cream and onion popped chips, 26 chips (30 g)	4
Whisps	
Parmesan cheese crisps, 15 crisps (18 g)	3
Wild Garden	
Roasted garlic hummus and sea salt quinoa chips, 1 pack (64 g)	3
Wild Roots	
Red quinoa and chia wild chips, 7 chips (28 g)	4

Corn Chips

Barcel	
Takis, fuego, 14 pieces (28 g)	5
Bugles	
Baked crispy corn snacks, original flavor, 1½ cups	4
Original corn chip snack food, 1 pouch (42 g)	10
Frito Lay	
The original corn chips, 32 chips (28 g)	5
Fritos	
Chili cheese flavored corn chips, 31 chips (28 g)	5
Original corn chips, 1 oz	5
Original corn chips, 32 chips (28 g)	5
The original corn chips, 32 chips (28 g)	5

Corn Chips (cont'd)

	SmartPoints® value
Fritos Flavor Twists	
Honey bbq corn snacks, 23 pieces (28 g)	5
Honey bbq flavored corn snacks, 23 chips (28 g)	5
Fritos Scoops!	
Corn chips (party size), 10 chips (28 g)	5
PopCorners	
Popped corn chips, kettle, 1.1 oz package, 1 package (32 g)	4
Popped corn chips, sea salt, 1 oz	4
Popped corn chips, sea salt, 1.1 oz package, 1 package (32 g)	4
Popped corn chips, white cheddar, 1 serving (32 g)	4
White cheddar flavored popped corn chips, 18 chips (28 g)	4
Ritz	
Salsa verde toasted corn chips, 13 chips (28 g)	5
Ritz Bits	
Original toasted corn chips, 14 chips (28 g)	5
Tostitos Scoops!	
Fajita corn chips, 10 chips (28 g)	4
Xochitl	
Corn chips, Mexican style, 1 oz	4
Corn chips, stone-ground, salted, 1 oz	4

Crackers

	SmartPoints® value
34 Degrees	
Crispbread, cracked pepper, 19 crackers (30 g)	3
Crispbread, natural, 19 crackers (30 g)	4
Crispbread, whole grain, 9 crackers (15 g)	1
Toasted onion savory crisps, 9 crackers (15 g)	1
Ak Mak	
Sesame crackers, 5 crackers (28 g)	3
Annie's	
Cheddar bunnies, 51 crackers (30 g)	4
Annie's Homegrown	
Cheddar bunnies baked snack crackers, 1 packet (28 g)	4
Arnold	
Special bread, rye, seedless, melba thin, 2 slices (41.3 g)	4
Austin	
Cheese crackers with peanut butter, 1 package (26 g)	4
Crackers, peanut butter, 1 package (26 g)	4
Back To Nature	
Crackers, organic, stoneground wheat, 5 crackers (16 g)	2
Crispy wheat crackers, 17 crackers (30 g)	4
Honey graham sticks, 1 pouch (28 g)	4
Barnum's Animals Snak-Saks	
Crackers, 17 crackers (31 g)	5
Blue Diamond Artisan Nut-Thins	
Cracker snacks, natural, flax seeds, 13 crackers (30 g)	4
Cracker snacks, natural, multi-seeds, 13 crackers (30 g)	4
Blue Diamond Natural Nut-Thins	
Cracker snacks, nut & rice, almond, hint of sea salt, 17 crackers (30 g)	4
Cracker snacks, nut & rice, almond, smokehouse, 16 crackers (30 g)	4
Blue Diamond Nut-Thins	
Cracker snacks, country ranch, 16 pieces (30 g)	4
Cracker snacks, Honey cinnamon, 17 crackers (30 g)	4
Cracker snacks, nut & rice, 16 crackers (30 g)	4

	SmartPoints® value
Cracker snacks, nut & rice, cheddar cheese, 16 crackers (30 g)	4
Cracker snacks, nut & rice, pecan, 16 crackers (30 g)	4
Cambridge Fit & Active	
Reduced fat wheat crackers, 18 crackers (29 g)	4
Carr's	
Crackers, rosemary, 4 crackers (16 g)	2
Crackers, whole wheat, 2 pieces (17 g)	3
Table water crackers (variety pack), 4 crackers (14 g)	2
Table water crackers, with cracked pepper, 5 crackers (17 g)	2
Cheese Nips	
Cheddar baked snack crackers, 29 crackers (30 g)	4
Cheez-It	
Baked snack crackers, 27 crackers (30 g)	5
Baked snack crackers, cheddar Jack, 25 crackers (30 g)	4
Baked snack crackers, hot & spicy, 25 crackers (30 g)	5
Baked snack crackers, Italian four cheese, 25 crackers (30 g)	5
Baked snack crackers, reduced fat, 29 crackers (30 g)	4
Baked snack crackers, reduced fat, white cheddar, 25 crackers (30 g)	4
Baked snack crackers, white cheddar, 25 crackers (30 g)	5
Extra toasty baked snack crackers, 27 crackers (30 g)	5
The amazing spider man 2 (variety pack), 1 pouch (29 g)	4

	SmartPoints® value
Cheez-It Grooves	
Crispy cracker chips, sharp white cheddar, 18 cracker chips (29 g)	4
Hot and spicy cheddar crispy cracker chips, 18 cracker chips (29 g)	4
Original cheddar crispy cracker chips, 18 pieces (29 g)	4
Zesty cheddar ranch crispy cracker chips, 18 cracker chips (29 g)	4
Cheez-It Reduced Fat	
Baked snack crackers, 29 crackers (30 g)	4
Chicken in a Biskit	
Baked snack crackers, original, 12 crackers (31 g)	5
Club	
Crackers, minis, original, 17 crackers (15 g)	2
Crackers, multi-grain, 4 crackers (14 g)	2
Crackers, original, 4 crackers (14 g)	2
Crackers, reduced fat, 5 crackers (16 g)	2
Crunchmaster	
5 seed multi-grain oven baked crackers (gluten free), 14 crackers (30 g)	4
6-seed multi-grain crackers (gluten free), 14 crackers (30 g)	4
Crackers, multi-grain, white cheddar, 15 crackers (30 g)	4
Crackers, multi-seed, original, 15 crackers (30 g)	4
Crackers, multi-seed, rosemary + olive oil, 14 crackers (30 g)	4
Crackers, multi-seed, sea salt, 16 crackers (30 g)	4
Crackers, rice, artisan four cheese, 15 crackers (30 g)	4
Original multi-seed crackers, 7 crackers (14 g)	2

Crackers (cont'd)

	SmartPoints® value
Dare	
Crackers, original, 4 crackers (18 g)	3
Dare Breton	
Crackers, multigrain, 3 crackers (16 g)	3
Dare Grainsfirst	
Whole grain crackers, 4 crackers (18 g)	2
Diamond Bakery	
Crackers, soda, 4 crackers (15 g)	2
Doctor Kracker	
Flatbreads, klassic 3 seed, 1 flatbread (25 g)	3
Eat Smart Naturals 100 Calorie Pack	
Crisps, garden veggie, potato, tomato & spinach, 1 package (21 g)	3
Finn Crisp	
Rye crispbread, 3 pieces (18 g)	2
Firehook	
Garlic thyme Mediterranean baked crackers, 1 oz	3
Multigrain flax Mediterranean baked crackers, 1 oz	3
Food Club	
Rice cakes, caramel corn, 1 cake (13 g)	2
Frito Lay Munchies	
Peanut butter sandwich crackers, 1 package (40 g)	7
Goldfish	
Baked snack crackers, saltine original, 55 pieces (30 g)	4
Crackers, baked snack, pizza, 55 pieces (30 g)	4
Parmesan baked snack crackers, 60 pieces (30 g)	4
Snack crackers, baked, cheddar, 55 pieces (30 g)	4
Snack crackers, baked, whole grain, cheddar, 55 pieces (30 g)	4

	SmartPoints® value
Team goldfish baked snack crackers, American cheese, 55 pieces (28 g)	4
Goldfish Colors	
Snack crackers, baked, cheddar, 55 pieces (30 g)	4
Goldfish Flavor Blasted	
Crackers, baked snack, xtra cheddar, 51 pieces (30 g)	4
Snack crackers, baked, xtra cheddar, 1 pouch (26 g)	4
Great Value	
Baked buttery crackers, 5 crackers (16 g)	3
Crackers, saltine, 5 crackers (15 g)	2
Crackers, unsalted tops, 5 crackers (15 g)	2
Soup and oyster crackers, 37 crackers (15 g)	2
Honey Maid	
Graham crackers, squares, 4 squares (27 g)	5
Honey Maid Teddy Grahams	
Birthday cake graham snacks, 24 pieces (30 g)	5
KA-ME	
Rice crunch crackers, plain, 19 crackers (33 g)	3
Rice crunch crackers, sesame, 19 crackers (33 g)	3
Kashi TLC	
Pita crisps, original 7 grain, with sea salt, 11 crisps (30 g)	4
Snack crackers, original 7 grain, 15 crackers (30 g)	4
Keebler	
Cheese and peanut butter sandwich crackers, 1 package (39 g)	6
Crackers, export sodas, 3 crackers (14 g)	2

	SmartPoints® value
Entertainment crackers, 5 crackers (16 g)	3
Original graham snacks, 1 package (28 g)	5
Toast and peanut butter sandwich crackers, 1 package (39 g)	7
Keebler Club	
Crackers, minis, multi-grain, 17 crackers (15 g)	2
Multi-grain crackers, 4 crackers (14 g)	2
Original crackers, 4 crackers (14 g)	2
Reduced fat crackers, 5 crackers (16 g)	2
Keebler Town House	
Cinnamon sugar pita oven baked crackers, 6 crackers (15 g)	2
Rosemary and olive oil focaccia crackers, 3 crackers (14 g)	2
Tuscan cheese focaccia crackers, 3 crackers (15 g)	3
Keebler Town House Pita	
Mediterranean herb oven baked crackers, 6 crackers (16 g)	2
Sea salt oven baked crackers, 6 crackers (15 g)	2
Kellogg's Special K Cracker Chips	
Salt and vinegar crispy snacks, 25 chips (30 g)	4
Sour cream and onion baked snack, 1 pack (25 g)	3
Kirkland Signature	
Crackers, 3 crackers (18 g)	3
Krispy	
Original saltine crackers, 5 crackers (15 g)	2
Kroger	
Baked cheese bits crackers, 28 crackers (30 g)	5
Baked original flavour oyster crackers, 19 crackers (15 g)	2

	SmartPoints® value
Crackers, oyster, 19 crackers (15 g)	2
Peanut butter and cheese sandwich crackers, 1 package (39 g)	7
Saltines, original, 5 crackers (14 g)	2
Thin and crispy wheat saltines, 5 crackers (14 g)	2
Lance	
Bite size gluten free sandwich crackers, 12 crackers (28 g)	5
Captain's wafers, 4 crackers (13 g)	2
Real peanut butter toasty crackers, 6 crackers (36.5 g)	6
Toastchee, rich 'n creamy peanut butter, reduced fat, 1 package (39 g)	6
Lance Captain's Wafers	
Cream cheese and chives filled crackers, 1 package (39 g)	7
Peanut butter and honey filled crackers, 1 package (39 g)	7
Lance Toast Chee	
Peanut butter crackers, 6 crackers (43 g)	7
Real peanut butter crackers, 6 crackers (43 g)	7
Lance Toasty	
Crackers, peanut butter, 1 package (35 g)	6
Lance Whole Grain	
Peanut butter cracker sandwiches, 6 crackers (43 g)	7
LiveGfree	
Garlic parmesan cheese crackers, 28 crackers (28 g)	4
Market Pantry	
Cheese squares baked snack crackers, 28 crackers (30 g)	5
Peanut butter sandwich crackers, 6 crackers (35 g)	6

Crackers (cont'd)

	SmartPoints® value
Mary's Gone Crackers	
Crackers, organic, herb, 13 crackers (30 g)	4
Crackers, organic, original, 13 crackers (30 g)	4
Crackers, organic, super seed, 13 crackers (30 g)	5
Lightly salted thins crackers, 12 crackers (30 g)	5
Original wholegrain crackers, 13 crackers (30 g)	4
Milton's	
Crackers, baked, original multi-grain, 2 crackers (16 g)	2
Crispy sea salt baked crackers, 14 crackers (30 g)	4
Milton's Craft Bakers	
Gluten free crispy sea salt baked crackers, 14 crackers (30 g)	4
Milton's Gluten Free	
Crackers, baked, crispy sea salt, 14 crackers (30 g)	4
Nabisco	
Crackers, saltine, original, 5 crackers (15 g)	2
Even thinner wheat thins crackers, 22 crackers (30 g)	5
Premium saltine crackers, 5 crackers (16 g)	2
Saltine crackers, original premium, 5 crackers (16 g)	2
Veggie blend good thins, 26 pieces (30 g)	4
Nabisco Sociables	
Crackers, baked savory, 5 crackers (14 g)	2
Nice!	
Saltine crackers, 5 crackers (15 g)	2
Old London	
Melba snacks, roasted garlic, 4 pieces (15 g)	1
Melba snacks, sea salt, 4 pieces (15 g)	1

	SmartPoints® value
Melba snacks, whole grain, 4 pieces (15 g)	1
Melba toast, classic, 3 pieces (17 g)	2
Melba toast, whole grain, 3 pieces (18 g)	2
P$$t...	
Oyster crackers, 38 crackers (15 g)	2
Pamela's	
Cinnamon grahams crackers, 2 pieces (36 g)	8
Pepperidge Farm Goldfish	
Baby baked cheddar snack crackers, 89 pieces (30 g)	4
Baked pretzel crackers, 1 oz	4
Cheddar baked snack crackers, 55 pieces (30 g)	4
Snack crackers, baked, pretzel, 43 pieces (30 g)	4
Vanilla cupcake baked graham snacks, 1 package (11 g)	2
Whole grain pretzel baked snack crackers, 43 pieces (30 g)	3
Premium	
Crackers, saltine, original, minis, 17 crackers (15 g)	2
Crackers, saltine, unsalted tops, 5 crackers (16 g)	2
Crackers, soup & oyster, 22 crackers (15 g)	2
Saltine crackers, original, 5 crackers (16 g)	2
Premium Rounds	
Saltine crackers with whole grain topped with sea salt, 6 crackers (15 g)	2
Red Oval Farms	
Crackers, wheat, stoned wheat thins, 2 crackers (14 g)	2

	SmartPoints® value
Red Oval Farms Stoned Wheat Thins	
Snack crackers, mini, 19 crackers (30 g)	4
Rice Thins Gluten Free	
Original thin rice snacks, 18 pieces (31 g)	4
Sea salt and pepper thin rice snacks, 13 pieces (30 g)	4
White cheddar thin rice snacks, 13 pieces (30 g)	4
Ritz	
Bacon flavor crackers, 5 crackers (16 g)	3
Cracker sandwiches, cheese, 1 package (38 g)	7
Cracker sandwiches, peanut butter, 1 pack (39 g)	7
Crackers, baked with whole wheat, fresh stacks, 5 crackers (15 g)	2
Crackers, hint of salt, 5 crackers (16 g)	3
Crackers, reduced fat, 5 crackers (15 g)	2
Crackers, whole wheat, 5 crackers (15 g)	2
Roasted vegetable crackers, 5 crackers (16 g)	3
Whole wheat crackers, 5 crackers (15 g)	2
Ritz Bits	
Cracker sandwiches, cheese, 1 package (28 g)	6
Ritz Fresh Stacks	
Original crackers, 5 crackers (16 g)	3
Roundy's	
Cheddar cheese oven baked rice crisps, 9 pieces (15 g)	2
Ryvita	
Whole grain rye crispbread, dark rye, 1 slice (10 g)	1
Whole grain rye crispbread, sesame rye, 1 crispbread (10 g)	1

	SmartPoints® value
Savoritz	
6 cracker assortment, 3 crackers (15 g)	2
Garden vegetable crackers, 3 pieces (15 g)	2
Garlic and chive pita crackers, 9 crackers (28 g)	3
Multigrain pita crackers, 9 crackers (28 g)	3
Oyster crackers, 37 crackers (15 g)	2
Reduced fat cheese crackers, 32 crackers (30 g)	4
Wheat round crackers, 5 crackers (15 g)	2
Savoritz 4 Kids	
Mini peanut butter sandwich crackers, 12 crackers (30 g)	6
Savoruz	
White cheddar cheese crackers, 25 crackers (30 g)	5
Sesmark Rice Thins	
Crackers, rice, brown rice, 17 crackers (30 g)	3
Crackers, rice, sesame, 16 crackers (30 g)	4
ShopRite	
Soup and chili oyster crackers, 38 crackers (15 g)	2
Snack Factory Pretzel Crisps	
Pretzel crisps, original, deli style, 11 crackers (28 g)	3
Special K	
Cracker chips, honey barbecue, 25 chips (30 g)	4
Cracker chips, sour cream & onion, 25 chips (30 g)	4
Crackers, multi-grain, 24 crackers (30 g)	4
Starbucks Coffee	
Dark chocolate covered grahams, 1 cookie (28 g)	7

Crackers (cont'd)

	SmartPoints® value
Sunshine Cheez-It	
Baked snack crackers, 1 pouch (29 g)	4
Suzie's	
Crackers, puffed, corn, quinoa & sesame, 3 cakes (13 g)	1
THINaddictives	
Cranberry almond thins, 1 package (23 g)	4
Toasteds	
Buttercrisp lightly toasted crackers, 5 crackers (16 g)	3
Crackers, sesame, 5 crackers (16 g)	3
Harvest wheat lightly toasted crackers, 5 crackers (16 g)	2
Tops	
Thin wheats, reduced fat, 16 crackers (29 g)	4
Town House	
Crackers, light buttery, original, 5 crackers (16 g)	3
Original light and buttery crackers, 5 crackers (16 g)	3
Reduced fat light buttery crackers, 6 crackers (15 g)	2
Town House Flatbread Crisps	
Italian herb crackers, 8 crackers (15 g)	2
Roasted garlic crackers, 8 crackers (15 g)	2
Sea salt and olive oil crackers, 8 crackers (15 g)	2
Town House Flip Sides	
Original pretzel crackers, 5 crackers (15 g)	2
Trader Joe's	
12 grain mini snack crackers, 22 crackers (30 g)	4
Bit size everything crackers, 14 crackers (30 g)	4
Classic original water crackers, 4 crackers (15 g)	2

	SmartPoints® value
Fig & olive crisps, 11 crackers (30 g)	3
Golden rounds crackers, 9 crackers (30 g)	4
Honey graham crackers, 2 sheets (31 g)	5
Multigrain pita bite crackers, 8 crackers (28 g)	3
Multiseed with soy sauce savory thin mini rice crackers, 1 oz	3
Original savory thin mini crackers, 1 oz	3
Pita bite crackers with sea salt, 9 crackers (28 g)	3
Raisin rosemary crisps, 10 pieces (30 g)	3
Roasted gorgonzola flavored oven crisp crackers, 31 crackers (30 g)	4
Savory thin mini edamame crackers, 38 chips (28 g)	3
Soup & oyster crackers, 14 crackers (15 g)	2
Stone ground wheat crackers, 4 crackers (30 g)	3
Trader Joe's Reduced Guilt	
Wheat crisps, 14 crackers (30 g)	4
Woven wheats wafers, 8 crackers (32 g)	3
Triscuit	
Balsamic vinegar & basil crackers, 6 crackers (28 g)	4
Balsamic vinegar & basil crackers, 6 crackers (28 g)	4
Brown rice and wheat sweet potato and sea salt crackers, 6 crackers (30 g)	4
Crackers, cracked pepper & olive oil, 6 crackers (28 g)	3
Crackers, fire roasted tomato & olive oil, 6 crackers (28 g)	3
Crackers, garden herb, 6 crackers (28 g)	3

	SmartPoints® value
Crackers, hint of salt, 6 crackers (28 g)	3
Crackers, original, 6 crackers (28 g)	3
Crackers, reduced fat, with sea salt, 7 crackers (30 g)	3
Crackers, roasted garlic, 6 crackers (28 g)	3
Crackers, rosemary & olive oil, 6 crackers (28 g)	3
Crackers, rye with caraway seeds, 6 crackers (28 g)	3
Crackers, wheat, baked whole grain, reduced fat, 7 crackers (29 g)	3
Dill sea salt and olive oil crackers, 6 crackers (28 g)	3
Mediterranean style olive crackers, 6 crackers (28 g)	3
Reduced fat crackers made with whole wheat, 7 crackers (30 g)	3
Smoked gouda crackers, 6 crackers (28 g)	4
Triscuit Brown Rice	
Crackers, sea salt & black pepper, 6 crackers (29 g)	4
Roasted red pepper crackers, 9 crackers (29 g)	4
Triscuit Thin Crisps	
Brown rice and wheat crackers sour cream and chive, 7 crackers (30 g)	4
Brown rice wasabi and soy sauce crackers, 10 crackers (30 g)	4
Crackers, original, 15 crackers (30 g)	4
Crackers, parmesan garlic, 14 crackers (29 g)	4
Valley Produce Company	
Parmesan cheese crackerthins, 6 crackers (10 g)	1
Van's	
Baked crackers, crispy whole grain, say cheese!, 30 crackers (30 g)	4

	SmartPoints® value
Wasa	
Crispbread, fiber, 1 slice (10 g)	1
Crispbread, flax seed, 2 slices (19 g)	2
Crispbread, hearty, 1 slice (14 g)	2
Crispbread, light rye, 2 slices (18 g)	2
Crispbread, sourdough, 1 slice (11 g)	1
Crispbread, whole grain, 1 slice (12 g)	1
Multi grain crispbread, 1 slice (15 g)	2
Wasa Crisp'n Light	
7 grains crackerbread, 3 slices (18 g)	2
Crackerbread, wholesome wheat, 3 slices (18 g)	2
Way Better	
Sprouted barley crackers, 14 crackers (28 g)	3
Westminster Bakers Co.	
Oyster crackers, 1 package (14 g)	2
Saltines, 2 crackers (7.5 g)	1
Wheat Thins	
Crackers, oven baked, toasted pita, garlic herb, 14 crackers (30 g)	4
Crackers, oven baked, toasted pita, original, 15 crackers (30 g)	4
Crackers, reduced fat, 16 crackers (29 g)	4
Garden valley veggie toasted chips, 13 chips (28 g)	4
Original whole grain crackers, 16 crackers (31 g)	5
Reduced fat whole grain crackers, 16 crackers (29 g)	4
Snacks, multigrain, 14 pieces (31 g)	4
Snacks, original, 16 pieces (31 g)	5
Snacks, ranch, 15 pieces (30 g)	5

Crackers, Wheat Thins (cont'd)

	SmartPoints® value
Snacks, reduced fat, 16 pieces (29 g)	4
Snacks, sundried tomato & basil, 15 pieces (30 g)	5
Wheat thins, original, 16 pieces (31 g)	5
Wheat Thins Big	
Whole grain crackers, 11 crackers (31 g)	5
Wheat Thins Fiber Selects	
Garden vegetable whole grain snacks, 15 pieces (30 g)	4
Wild California	
Apricot ginger twice baked crisps, 1 oz	3
Zesta	
Saltine crackers, original, 5 crackers (16 g)	2
Saltine crackers, whole wheat, 5 crackers (15 g)	2

Fruit and Nut Mixes

	SmartPoints® value
180 Degrees Snacks	
Blueberry pomegranate clusters, ½ cup	5
Archer Farms	
Monster mix cookie snack bites, 4 pieces (31 g)	7
Fresh Gourmet	
Cranberries & glazed walnuts, ½ Tbsp	1
Great Grains	
Granola snack mix, 1 pouch (40 g)	6
Kar's	
Unsalted raisin almond cashew mix, ¼ cup	5
Orchard Valley Harvest	
Cranberry almond cashew trail mix, 1 package (28 g)	5
Planters Holiday	
Brittle nut medley, 3 Tbsp	6
Power Up	
Antioxidant mix, 1 oz	5
Quaker Real Medleys	
Dark chocolate cranberry almond granola clusters, ⅓ cup	5
Salad Pizazz	
Raspberry cranberry walnut frisco, 1 Tbsp	1
Sargento Balanced Breaks	
pepper Jack natural cheese with peanuts & raisins, 1 serving (43 g)	7
Sunkist	
Strawberry banana blend trail mix, 1 oz	5

Fruit Snacks

	SmartPoints® value
Annie's Homegrown	
Summer strawberry organic bunny fruit snacks, 1 pouch (23 g)	3
Betty Crocker	
Fruit flavored snacks, 1 pouch (23 g)	4
Dole	
Dark chocolate banana dippers, 4 slices (44 g)	5
Strawberry fruit snacks, 21 pieces (28 g)	6
Fiber One	
Mixed berry fruit flavored snacks, 1 pouch (23 g)	3
Fit & Active	
Assorted fruit flavored snacks, 1 package (18 g)	1
Fit & Active	
Raspberry fruit strips, 1 fruit strip (14 g)	2
Florida's Natural	
Fruit snacks, 1 pouch (21 g)	4
Fruit Gushers	
Fruit flavored snacks, assorted, value pack, 1 pouch (25 g)	4

	SmartPoints® value
Fruit Roll Ups	
Fruit flavored snacks, assorted flavors, variety pack, 1 roll (14 g)	2
Kellogg's	
Disney frozen fruit flavored snacks, 1 pouch (22 g)	3
Kellogg's Fruity Snacks	
Mixed berry flavored fruit snacks, 1 pouch (22 g)	3
Market Pantry	
Mixed fruit snacks, 14 pieces (30 g)	5
Mott's	
Mango peach applesauce pouch, 1 pouch (90 g)	4
Mott's Medleys	
Fruit flavored snacks, assorted fruit, 1 pouch (23 g)	4
Ocean Spray	
Blueberry craisins, ¼ cup	6
Raisinets	
Classic milk chocolate California raisins, ¼ cup	10
Simply Balanced	
Freeze dried peach slices, 1 package (50 g)	11
Fruit strips, strawberry, 1 strip (14 g)	2
Welch's	
Fruit snacks, mixed fruit, value pack, 1 pouch (26 g)	4
Welch's Fruit Snacks	
Island fruits flavored fruit snack, 1 packet (25.5 g)	4
Mixed fruit, 1 bag (14 g)	2

Jerky

	SmartPoints® value
Butterball	
Smoked turkey snack sticks, 3 sticks (30 g)	2
Chef's Cut	
Honey barbecue chicken jerky, 1 oz	2
Field Trip	
Cracked pepper turkey jerky, 1 oz	1
Golden Island Gourmet Snacks	
All natural Korean barbecue recipe pork jerky, 1 oz	3
Jack Link's	
Barbecue beef jerky, 1 oz	2
Chicken strips snack, 1 pack (23 g)	2
Original beef steak, 1 package (23 g)	1
Original turkey snack sticks, 1 stick (23 g)	2
Prime rib seasoning tender cuts, 1 oz	1
Teriyaki beef jerky, 1 oz	2
Jack Link's Meat Snacks	
Korean bbq recipe pork flame grilled jerky, 1 oz	3
Original beef jerky, 1 oz	2
Original beef steak tender bites, 1 oz	2
Reduced sodium original beef jerky, 1 oz	2
Sweet and hot beef jerky, 1 oz	2
Jack Link's Original	
Beef jerky, 1 oz	2
Turkey jerky, 1 oz	2
Jack Link's Premium Cuts	
Beef jerky, original, 1 oz	1
Beef jerky, peppered, 1 oz	1
Beef steak, original, 1 steak (28 g)	1
Jack Link's Small Batch	
Original no. 11 handcrafted beef jerky, 1 oz	1

Jerky (cont'd)

	SmartPoints® value
Kirkland Signature	
Extra thick cut steak strips, 1 oz	1
Krave	
Jerky, pork, black cherry barbecue seasoned, 1 oz	2
Market Pantry	
Turkey sausage snack sticks, 1 stick (16 g)	1
Oberto	
Original beef jerky, 1 oz	2
Oberto All Natural	
Original beef jerk, 1 oz	2
Oh Boy! Oberto	
Beef jerky, original, 1 oz	2
Teriyaki beef jerky, 1 oz	2
Old Wisconsin	
Turkey bites, turkey sausage, 6 pieces (30 g)	2
Turkey sausage snack sticks, 1 stick (25 g)	2
Pacific Gold	
Original beef jerky, 1 package (35 g)	2
Teriyaki beef jerky, 1 package (35 g)	2
Perky Jerky	
Ultra premium turkey jerky, 1 oz	2
Shaffer	
Smoked venison snack stick, original flavor, 1 oz	1
Simms	
Beef sausage snack stick, 1 stick (16 g)	2
Original beef jerky, 1 oz	2
Slim Jim	
Smoked snack stick, 1 stick (28 g)	5
Smoked snack sticks, original, 4 pieces (32 g)	6
Slim Jim Giant Slim	
Snack stick, smoked, original, 1 package (28 g)	5

	SmartPoints® value
Smartfood Delight	
White cheddar popcorn, 3 ½ cups	4
Trader Joe's	
Original turkey jerky, 1 oz	1
Trader Joe's Grocery	
Natural turkey jerky original, 1 oz	1
Natural turkey jerky teriyaki, 1 oz	1
Turkey Perky Jerky	
Original turkey jerky, 1 oz	1

Nuts

Aldi	
Chopped walnuts, ¼ cup	6
Archer Farms	
Almonds, raw, unsalted, ¼ cup	5
Lightly salted roasted almonds, ¼ cup	5
Lightly salted roasted cashews, ¼ cup	5
Unsalted raw mixed nuts, ¼ cup	5
Betty Crocker	
Pecans halves and pieces, ¼ cup	7
Blue Diamond Almonds	
Honey roasted almonds, 28 almonds (28 g)	5
Lightly salted almonds, 28 almonds (28 g)	5
Lightly salted almonds made with sea salt, 1 oz	5
Oven roasted almonds with sea salt, 28 almonds (28 g)	5
Roasted salted almonds, 28 almonds (28 g)	5
Roasted salted almonds, value pack, 28 almonds (28 g)	5
Salted caramel flavored almonds, 28 almonds (28 g)	5
Smokehouse almonds, value pack, 28 almonds (28 g)	5
Toasted coconut almonds, 28 almponds (28 g)	5

	SmartPoints® value
Wasabi & soy sauce almonds, 1 oz	5
Whole natural almonds, 1 oz	5
Whole natural almonds, grab & go bags, 1 bag (18 g)	3
Whole natural almonds, value pack, 24 almonds (28 g)	5
Blue Diamond Bold	
Almonds, habanero bbq, 28 almonds (28 g)	5
Almonds, salt 'n vinegar, 28 almonds (28 g)	5
Almonds, wasabi & soy sauce, 28 almonds (28 g)	5
Almonds, wasabi & soy sauce, value pack, 28 almonds (28 g)	5
Blue Diamond Low Sodium	
Lightly salted sea salt almonds, 1 oz	5
Blue Diamond Nut-Thins	
Cracker snacks, pepper Jack cheese, 16 crackers (30 g)	4
Daily Chef	
Fancy pecan halves, ¼ cup	6
Emerald	
100 calorie packs dry roasted almonds, 1 package (17.5 g)	3
Cocoa roast almonds, ¼ cup	5
Dill pickle cashews 100 calorie packs, 1 package (18 g)	3
Salt & pepper cashews, 1 package (17.5 g)	3
Smoked almonds, ¼ cup	5
Emerald 100 Calorie Pack	
Cocoa roast almonds, 1 pack (18 g)	3
Dill pickle cashews, 1 pack (17.5 g)	3
Halves and pieces cashew, 1 pack (18 g)	3
Natural walnuts and almonds, 1 pack (16 g)	3
Smoked almonds, 1 pack (16 g)	3
Vanilla roast almonds, 1 pack (18 g)	3

	SmartPoints® value
Fisher	
Glazed pecans, ¼ cup	6
Pecan halves (10 oz stand-up bag), 1 oz	6
Fresh Gourmet	
Almonds, sliced, toasted, 1 Tbsp	1
Oven roasted sliced almonds, 1 Tbsp	1
Pecan pieces, honey roasted, 2 tsp	1
Walnut pieces, glazed, 2 tsp	1
Galil	
Roasted chestnuts, 1¾ oz	4
Garden Fresh Gourmet	
Harvest nut blend, 1 packet (14 g)	3
Gold Emblem	
Honey roasted mixed nuts, ¼ cup	5
Great Value	
Cashews roasted and salted with sea salt, ¼ cup	5
Harvested for You	
Gluten free Italian style meatballs, ¼ cup	6
Hoody's	
Cinnamon toasted almonds, 11 pieces (28 g)	6
Deep south praline pecans, 17 pieces (28 g)	7
Kar's	
Roasted salted almonds, 1 package (28 g)	5
Kirkland Signature	
Almonds, ¼ cup	5
Cashew clusters with almonds and pumpkin seeds, 1 oz	5
Dry roasted sea salt almonds, ¼ cup	5
Extra fancy mixed nuts, ¼ cup	6

Nuts, Kirkland Signature (cont'd)

	SmartPoints® value
Extra fancy unsalted mixed nuts, 1 oz	5
Super extra-large peanuts, 3 Tbsp	5
Whole fancy Indian cashews, 1 oz	6
Whole fancy unsalted cashews, 16 pieces (28 g)	5
Kroger	
Hot and spicy peanuts, ¼ cup	5
Lightly salted mixed nuts, ¼ cup	5
Lance	
Dill pickle peanuts, 1 package (39 g)	7
Lance Fresh	
Roasted salted peanuts, 1 package (31.9 g)	6
Nature's Eats	
Shelled walnuts, 1 oz	6
Nature's Harvest	
Sea salted almonds, 32 almonds (28 g)	5
Nice!	
Whole natural almonds, ⅓ cup	7
Nut Harvest	
Honey roasted nut mix, 3 Tbsp	6
Salted in shell pistachios, 1 package (25 g)	4
Planters	
Cashew, halves & pieces, 43 pieces (28 g)	5
Deluxe mixed nuts, 20 pieces (28 g)	5
Dry roasted honey roasted peanuts, 39 pieces (28 g)	5
Dry roasted peanuts, 1 oz	5
Dry roasted peanuts, lightly salted, 1 oz	5
Fancy whole cashews with sea salt, 18 pieces (28 g)	5
Mixed nuts, unsalted, 30 pieces (28 g)	5
Peanuts, cocktail, 35 pieces (28 g)	5

	SmartPoints® value
Peanuts, honey roasted, 39 pieces (28 g)	5
Peanuts, salted, 1 package (28 g)	5
Stadium peanuts, roasted in-shell salted, 19 pieces (28 g)	5
Planters Nut-rition	
Heart healthy mix, 1 pack (42 g)	8
Wholesome nut mix, 18 pieces (28 g)	5
Poindexter Nut Company	
Chopped pieces walnuts, ¼ cup	6
Walnuts halves and pieces, ¼ cup	6
Sconza	
Pumpkin pie almonds, ¼ cup	10
Simple Truth	
Pecans pieces, ¼ cup	7
Raw almonds, ¼ cup	5
Snak Club	
Almonds, raw, 22 pieces (30 g)	5
Southern Grove	
Deluxe mixed nuts, ¼ cup	5
Deluxe mixed nuts with sea salt, ¼ cup	5
Deluxe whole cashews no salt, 19 pieces (28 g)	5
Deluxe whole cashews with sea salt, 19 pieces (28 g)	5
Mixed nuts, 1 oz	5
Roasted and salted pistachios, 1 package (43 g)	4
Shelled pistachios with sea salt, ¼ cup	5
Trader Joe's	
Cinnamon roasted almonds, ¼ cup	6
Dry roasted and salted almonds, ¼ cup	5
Dry roasted and unsalted almonds, ¼ cup	5
Organic raw almonds, ¼ cup	5
Raw fancy mixed nuts, ¼ cup	5
Raw sliced almonds, ¼ cup	5

	SmartPoints® value
Raw slivered almonds, ¼ cup	5
Unsalted dry toasted slivered almonds, ¼ cup	5
Trader Joe's Grocery	
Candied pecans, 1 oz	7
Candied walnuts, ¼ cup	7
Just a handful of dry roasted unsalted almonds, 1 bag (35 g)	6
Organic raw almonds, ¼ cup	5
Trader Joe's Nuts	
Raw whole cashews, ¼ cup	5
Roasted and salted marcona almonds with rosemary, ¼ cup	5
Unsalted dry toasted pecan pieces, ¼ cup	7
Walgreen's	
Pistachios, in shells, 28 pieces (18 g)	3
Wellsley Farms	
Roasted and salted almonds, ¼ cup	5
Roasted and salted pistachios, ½ cup	5
Wonderful	
Lightly salted pistachios (with shells), ½ cup	5
Pistachios, roasted & salted, 1.5 oz package, 1 package (43 g)	4
Roasted and salted pistachios (with shells), ½ cup	5

Popcorn

	SmartPoints® value
365 Everyday Value	
Organic classic salted popcorn, 3 cups	4
Act II	
94% fat free butter microwave popcorn, 3 Tbsp unpopped	4
94% fat free butter popcorn, 6½ cups	4
Butter lovers microwave popcorn, 4½ cups	4
Microwave popcorn, butter lovers, 2 Tbsp unpopped	5
Aldi	
Caramel popcorn drizzled with white and dark chocolate coating, 1 oz	6
Angie's Boom Chicka Pop	
Lightly sweet popcorn, 3¼ cups	4
Lightly sweet popcorn, 3¼ cups	4
Popcorn, sea salt, 1 package (17 g)	3
Popcorn, sea salt, 4 cups	4
Sea salt popcorn, 4 cups	4
Sweet & salty kettle corn, 2 cups	5
Sweet and salty kettle corn, 2 cups	5
Sweet and salty kettle corn popcorn, 1 package (28 g)	5
White cheddar popcorn, 2½ cups	5
Annie's Homegrown	
Organic white cheddar popcorn, 1 packet (18 g)	4
Annie's Homegrown Organic	
White cheddar popcorn, 2¼ cups	6
Archer Farms	
White chocolate peppermint caramel corn clusters, ½ cup	7
Brim's Snack Foods	
Premium butter flavor popcorn, 3 cups	6
White cheddar popcorn, 3 cups	6
Buddha Bowl Foods	
Avocado licious popcorn, 3 cups	4
Himalaya pink popcorn, 1 package (25 g)	4
Cape Cod	
Salted caramel popcorn, 3 cups	4
Sea salt popcorn, 4 cups	4
Clancy's	
Sweet and salty kettle corn, 2 cups	5

Snacks

Popcorn (cont'd)

	SmartPoints® value
Cousin Willie's	
Buttery explosion microwave popcorn, 2 Tbsp	5
Movie theater butter microwave popcorn, 2 Tbsp	5
Sea salt mauve popcorn, 4 ½ cups	4
Cracker Jack	
Caramel coated popcorn & peanuts, the original, 3 pack, 1 package (28 g)	5
Holiday sugar cookie popcorn, ½ cup	5
Deep River Snacks	
Organic popcorn with sea salt, 1 bag (18 g)	3
Essential Everyday	
Popcorn, white kernel, unpopped, 3 Tbsp	4
Fit & Active	
Butter flavor microwave popcorn, 3 Tbsp unpopped	4
Butter microwave popcorn unpopped, 1 bag (35 g)	4
From the Kitchen of Cooking Light Magazine	
Simply sea salt popcorn gluten free, 4 cups	4
G. H. Cretors	
Chicago mix popcorn, 1 ¼ cups	6
Good Health	
Popcorn, half naked, with a hint of olive oil, 4 cups	4
Great Value	
White cheddar popcorn, 3 ½ cups	4
Jenny's	
Cheese popcorn, 2 ½ cups	5
Jiffy Pop	
Microwave popcorn, light butter, 2 Tbsp	3

	SmartPoints® value
Jolly Time	
Kinda sweet...kinda salty pre-popped pop corn, 1 serving	4
White cheddar pre-popped pop corn, 1 serving	4
Sea salted pre-popped pop corn, 1 serving	3
Jolly Time Healthy Pop	
Butter flavor, 3 pack, 1 serving	3
Butter flavor, 6 pack, 1 serving	3
Butter flavor, 12 pack dispenser, 1 serving	3
Butter flavor, 24 pack, 1 serving	3
Butter flavor, 30 pack, 1 serving	3
Butter flavor, 100 calorie bags, 4 pack, 1 serving	3
Butter flavor, 100 calorie bags, 10 pack, 1 serving	3
Butter flavor, low sodium, 100 calorie bags, 4 pack, 1 serving	3
Caramel apple, 3 pack, 1 serving	3
Crispy white, 3 pack, 1 serving	3
Crispy white, 6 pack, 1 serving	3
Kettle corn, 3 pack, 1 serving	3
Kettle corn, 6 pack, 1 serving	3
Kettle corn, 100 calorie bags, 4 pack, 1 serving	3
Kettle corn, 100 calorie bags, 10 pack, 1 serving	3
Kirkland Signature	
Microwave popcorn, unpopped, 2 Tbsp	7
Movie theater butter microwave popcorn, 2 Tbsp	7
Kroger	
94% fat free butter flavoured popcorn mini bag, 1 bag (34 g)	4
94% fat free microwave popcorn, 2 Tbsp	3
Lesserevil Buddha Bowl Foods	
Himalayan pink popcorn, 3 cups	4

	SmartPoints® value
Lindt	
Sweet popcorn, 1 stick (39 g)	11
Meijer	
Fat free butter microwave popcorn, 2 Tbsp	3
Nutrisystem	
White cheddar popcorn, 1 package (28 g)	4
Old Dutch	
Cheddar cheese popcorn, 2 ½ cups	5
White cheddar flavored popcorn, 2 ½ cups	5
Orville Redenbacher's	
Classic bag movie theater butter popcorn, 2 Tbsp	6
Gourmet popping corn, white corn, 3 Tbsp	3
Movie theater butter gourmet popping corn, 2 Tbsp	6
Original gourmet popping corn, 3 Tbsp	3
Original gourmet popping corn, 3 Tbsp	3
Smartpop butter gourmet popping corn, 3 Tbsp	3
Orville Redenbacher's Gourmet Naturals	
Popping corn, gourmet, classic butter & sea salt, 2 Tbsp unpopped	4
Popping corn, gourmet, simply salted, 2 Tbsp unpopped	4
Orville Redenbacher's Pop Up Bowl	
Butter flavor gourmet popping corn, 4 cups popped	7
Gourmet popping corn, butter, smart pop, microwave, 3 Tbsp	3
Light butter popping corn, 5 ½ cups popped (31 g)	4

	SmartPoints® value
Orville Redenbacher's SmartPop!	
94% fat free butter flavored microwavable popcorn (unpopped), 1 serving (37 g)	3
Butter flavored popped corn, 1 bag (33 g)	3
Gourmet popping corn, butter, single serve bags, 1 bag (33 g)	3
Gourmet popping corn, kettle korn, single serve bags, 1 bag (33 g)	3
Kettle korn, pop up bowl, 3 Tbsp unpopped	4
Popping corn, gourmet, 94% fat free, mini bags, butter, 1 bag (35 g)	3
Sweet and salty kettle corn, 94% fat free, 1 bag (33 g)	3
Orville Redenbacher's SmartPop! Pop Up Bowl	
Gourmet popping corn, kettle korn, 3 Tbsp	4
Popping corn, gourmet, butter, 3 Tbsp	3
Pop Weaver	
Popcorn, light butter, 1 bag unpopped (61 g)	7
Popcorn, Indiana	
Chicago style caramel and cheese popcorn, 1 cup	6
Movie theater popcorn, 2 cups	5
Sweet and salty kettlecorn, 2 cups	5
Popcorn, Indiana Fit	
Sea salt popcorn, 3 ½ cups	4
Popcorn, Indiana Original	
Movie theater popcorn, 2 cups	5
PopCorners	
Sweet chili popped corn chips gluten free, 1 oz	4

Popcorn (cont'd)

	SmartPoints® value
Popcornopolis	
Caramel corn popcorn, 1 oz	7
Kettle corn gourmet popcorn, 1½ oz	8
Nearly naked gourmet popcorn, 1 package (16 g)	3
Organic white cheddar popcorn, 1 oz	7
Pop-Secret	
Homestyle butter popcorn, 3 cups	5
Homestyle microwave popcorn, 2 Tbsp unpopped	1
Homestyle popcorn, 2 Tbsp	6
Kettle corn popcorn, 3 cups	5
Popcorn, premium, movie theater butter, 3 Tbsp	6
Pop-Secret 100 Calorie Pop	
Microwave popcorn, premium, butter, snack size, 1 bag (35 g)	4
Premium butter popcorn snack bag prepared, 1 bag (32 g)	3
Premium kettle corn snack bag prepared, 1 bag (31 g)	3
Premium popcorn, homestyle, 3 Tbsp	3
Simple Truth Organic	
Low sodium popcorn, 3½ cups	4
Sea salt and black pepper popcorn, 3¼ cups	4
Skinnygirl	
Butter and sea salt popcorn, 6 cups (42.5 g)	5
Lime and salt microwave popcorn, 6 cups (42.5 g)	5
SkinnyPop	
Black pepper popcorn, 4 cups	5
Popcorn, 3¾ cups	5
Popcorn 100 calorie bag, 1 package (18 g)	3
Popcorn, skinny pack, 1 package (18 g)	3
Popcorn, ultra lite, 3½ cups	5

	SmartPoints® value
Popcorn, ultra lite, white cheddar flavor, 3½ cups	5
Popcorn, xl skinny, 3¾ cups	5
Ultra light white cheddar popcorn, 3½ cups	5
Ultra lite white cheddar popcorn, 1 oz	5
Smartfood	
Movie theater butter popcorn, 1 oz	5
Popcorn, white cheddar cheese, 1¾ cups	5
Spicy jalapeño ranch popcorn, 2 cups	5
Sweet and salty kettle corn popcorn, 1 oz	6
Smartfood 100 Calorie	
Popcorn, white cheddar, 1 package (18 g)	3
Smartfood Delight	
Popcorn, air popped, white cheddar, 3½ cups	4
Sea salt popcorn, 1 oz	4
Sea salt, air popped popcorn, 1 oz	4
Sea salted caramel popcorn, 3¾ cups	4
White cheddar popcorn, 3½ cups	4
Smartfood Ready To Go Snacks	
White cheddar flavored popcorn, 1 package (17.8 g)	3
Snak King	
Popcorn, caramel, ¾ cup	5
Trader Joe's	
94% fat free microwave popcorn, 1 bag (40 g)	4
Lite kettle corn, 1 oz	4
Organic popping corn, 3 Tbsp	4

	SmartPoints® value
Trader Joe's Grocery	
Organic popcorn with olive oil, 2 cups	4
Reduced guilt air-popped popcorn, 2½ cups	3
World's puffiest white cheddar corn puffs, 2½ cups	4
World's puiffiest sour cream & onion corn puffs, 2½ cups	4
Vic's Corn Popper	
Lite half salt white popcorn (100 calorie bag), 1 package (20 g)	3
Wegman's Organic	
Olive oil and himalayan salt popcorn, 3 cups	3
White cheddar popcorn, 3 cups	4
Wise	
Sea salt air popped popcorn, 3 cups	4
White cheddar popcorn, 3 cups	4

Pork Skins and Rinds

Baken-ets	
Fried pork skins, hot 'n spicy, 9 pieces (14 g)	2
Hot n spicy chicharrones, 9 pieces (14 g)	2
Traditional chicarrones fried pork skins, 9 pieces (14 g)	2
Barcel	
Pork rinds, chicharron, ½ oz	2
Mac's	
Bar b q chicharrones pork skins, ½ oz	2
Bar b q flavored chicharrones, ½ oz	2
Rudolph's	
Bold and spicy bbq pork rinds, ½ oz	2

Potato Chips

	SmartPoints® value
7-Select	
Reduced fat kettle style original potato chips, 18 chips (28 g)	4
Boulder Canyon	
Sea salt kettle cooked potato chips, 14 chips (28 g)	4
Cape Cod	
Kettle cooked potato chips, 1 package (21.3 g)	3
Reduced fat kettle cooked potato chips, 19 chips (28 g)	4
Sea salt and vinegar kettle cooked potato chips, 18 chips (28 g)	4
Clancy's	
Sea salt and cracked pepper kettle chips, 12 chips (28 g)	4
Sour cream and onion baked potato crisps, 14 crisps (28 g)	4
Dutch Crunch	
Jalapeño and cheddar kettle chips, 15 chips (28 g)	5
Essential Everyday	
Sriracha kettle chips, 12 chips (28 g)	4
Fresh Finds	
Mesquite barbecue kettle cooked gourmet potato chips, 14 chips (28 g)	5
Good Health Natural Foods	
Kettle style avocado potato chips, 1 oz	4
Great Value	
Ripple potato chips, 22 chips (28 g)	5
H-E-B	
Tuscan garden baked ridged chips, 17 chips (28 g)	3
Herr's	
Potato popped chips, 1 bag (43 g)	5
Jimmy John's Jimmy Chips	
Regular potato chips, 18 chips (28 g)	5

Snacks

Potato Chips (cont'd)

	SmartPoints® value
Jimmy John's Thinny Chips	
Crunchy and salty reduced-fat potato chips, 1 oz	4
Kettle	
Lightly salted krinkle cut potato chips, 13 chips (28 g)	5
Olive oil real sliced potatoes baked potato chips, 20 chips (28 g)	4
Potato chips, 40% reduced fat, sea salt, 13 chips (28 g)	4
Potato chips, sea salt, 13 chips (28 g)	5
Kirkland Kettle	
Lightly salted krinkle cut chips, 1 oz	5
Lay's	
Baked potato crisps (variety pack), 1 package (31.8 g)	4
Barbecue chips (2.75 oz bag), 15 chips (28 g)	5
Classic potato chips, 15 chips (28 g)	5
Classic potato chips (2.75 oz bag), 15 chips (28 g)	5
Kettle cooked cream cheese and chive potato chips, 6 chips (28 g)	4
Korean barbecue chips, 15 chips (28 g)	5
Lightly salted potato chips, 15 chips (28 g)	5
Lightly salted potato chips, 15 chips (28 g)	5
Olive oil and herbs kettle cooked potato chips, 18 chips (28 g)	5
Original wavy potato chips, 11 chips (28 g)	5
Potato chips, barbecue flavored, 1 package (28 g)	5
Potato chips, classic, 1 package (28 g)	5

	SmartPoints® value
Salt & vinegar potato chips, 17 chips (28 g)	5
Salt and vinegar potato chips, 17 chips (28 g)	5
Sea salted thick cut potato chips, 1 package (39 g)	6
Smoked gouda and chive potato chips, 17 chips (28 g)	5
Sour cream & onion potato chips, 17 chips (28 g)	5
Sour cream and onion potato chips, 17 chips (28 g)	5
Wavy organic sea salted potato chips, 11 chips (28 g)	5
Lay's Baked!	
Cheddar & sour cream potato crisps, 1 package (32 g)	5
Lay's Classic	
Potato chips, 15 chips (28 g)	5
Lay's Kettle Cooked	
40% less fat jalapeño cheddar potato chips, 16 chips (28 g)	4
Jalapeño flavored potato chips, 15 chips (28 g)	5
Jalapeño potato chips, 15 chips (28 g)	5
Mesquite bbq potato chips, 18 chips (28 g)	5
Original potato chips, 16 chips (28 g)	5
Original potato chips (40% less fat), 18 chips (28 g)	4
Sea salt & cracked pepper potato chips, 18 chips (28 g)	5
Sea salt & vinegar potato chips, 18 chips (28 g)	5
Lay's Kettle Cooked Lattice Cut	
Aged cheddar and black pepper lattice cut potato chips, 13 chips (28 g)	5

	SmartPoints® value
Lay's Oven Baked	
Barbecue potato crisps, 1 package (32 g)	5
Original potato chips, 18 crisps (28 g)	4
Original potato crisps, 1 package (32 g)	4
Sour cream and onion potato crisps, 1 package (32 g)	4
Lay's Simply	
Sea salted thick cut potato chips, 15 chips (28 g)	5
Lay's Stax	
Original potato crisps, 12 crisps (28 g)	5
Lay's Wavy	
Original potato chips, 11 chips (28 g)	5
Original potato chips, 11 chips (28 g)	5
Metro Deli	
Hickory barbeque kettle cooked potato chips, 21 chips (43 g)	7
Mikesell's	
Groovy reduced fat potato chips, 17 chips (28 g)	4
Miss Vickie's	
Jalapeño kettle cooked potato chips, 1 mini bag (39 g)	7
Potato chips, kettle cooked, sea salt & vinegar, 1 package (38.9 g)	7
Potato chips, simply sea salt, original recipe, 1 package (39 g)	7
Potato chips, smokehouse bbq, 1 package (39 g)	7
One Potato Two Potato	
Sweet potato chips, 14 chips (28 g)	5

	SmartPoints® value
Pop Chips	
Barbeque potato popped chip snack, 1 bag (23 g)	3
Crazy hot potato chips, 20 chips (28 g)	4
Original potato popped chip snack, 1 bag (23 g)	3
Popped chip snack, barbeque, 1 bag (23 g)	3
Popped chip snack, sea salt & vinegar potato, 22 chips (28 g)	4
Potato chips, barbeque, 18 chips (23 g)	3
Potato chips, original, 18 chips (23 g)	3
Sea salt and vinegar potato chips, 22 chips (28 g)	4
Sea salt potato chips, 23 chips (28 g)	4
Sour cream and onion popped chip snack, 22 chips (28 g)	4
Tangy barbeque potato ridges, 20 chips (28 g)	4
Pop Chips Ridges	
Cheddar and sour cream potato chips, 9 chips (28 g)	4
PopCrinkles	
Sweet bbq popped potato crinkles, 1 oz	4
Pringles	
Bbq potato crisps, 15 crisps (28 g)	5
Cheddar cheese flavored potato crisps, 15 crisps (28 g)	5
Lightly salted potato crisps, 16 crisps (28 g)	5
Original potato crisps, 16 crisps (28 g)	5
Potato crisps, cheddar cheese, 15 crisps (28 g)	5
Potato crisps, reduced fat, original, 16 crisps (28 g)	5

Potato Chips, Pringles (cont'd)

	SmartPoints® value
Potato crisps, reduced fat, sour cream & onion, 16 crisps (28 g)	5
Salt and vinegar potato crisps, 1 oz	5
Sour cream and onion fat free potato crisps, 15 crisps (28 g)	2
Sour cream and onion potato crisps, 1 tub (19 g)	4
Sour cream and onion potato crisps, 15 crisps (28 g)	5
Pringles 100 Calorie Pack	
Original potato crisps, 16 crisps (28 g)	5
Original reduced fat potato crisps, 1 oz	5
Sour cream and onion potato crisps, 1 tub (18 g)	3
Pringles Original	
Potato crisps, 1 tub (18 g)	3
Ruffles	
Cheddar and sour cream flavored potato chips, 1 package (43 g)	8
Cheddar and sour cream oven baked chips, 11 chips (28 g)	4
Cheddar and sour cream potato chips, 11 chips (28 g)	5
Original potato chips, 12 chips (28 g)	5
Potato chips, reduced fat, 13 chips (28 g)	4
Reduced fat potato chips, 13 chips (28 g)	4
Ruffles Baked!	
Cheddar and sour cream potato crisps, 1 package (32 g)	4
Cheddar and sour cream potato crisps, 10 chips (28 g)	4
Original potato crisp, 9 crisps (28 g)	4

	SmartPoints® value
Ruffles Natural	
Potato chips, reduced fat, sea salted, 15 chips (28 g)	4
Slimfast	
Mesquite bbq baked crisps, 1 bag (28 g)	3
Mesquite bbq baked snacks, 1 oz	3
Sour cream and onion baked crisps, 1 bag (28 g)	3
SunChips	
French onion multigrain snacks, 15 chips (28 g)	5
Garden salsa multigrain snacks, 15 chips (28 g)	5
Harvest cheddar multigrain snacks, 15 chips (28 g)	5
Trader Joe's	
Kettle style organic potato chips, 14 chips (28 g)	4
Sriracha potato chips, 13 chips (28 g)	5
Trader Joe's Grocery	
Barbecue popped potato chips, 20 chips (28 g)	4
Trader Joe's Reduced Guilt	
Lightly salted kettle cooked potato chips, 12 chips (28 g)	4
Utz	
Potato chips, 20 chips (28 g)	5
Potato chips, ripple cut, family size, 20 chips (28 g)	5
Wegman's Get Poppin'	
Sea salt crispy potato snacks, 1 oz	3
Weight Watchers In-Meeting/ Online Products: Crunchy Snacks	
Popped barbeque potato crisps, 1 pouch	2
Popped salt & vinegar potato crisps, 1 pouch	2

	SmartPoints® value
Wellsley Farms	
All natural sea salt kettle cooked potato chips, 14 chips (28 g)	4
Wheat Thins	
Sea salt popped chips, 27 chips (30 g)	4
Sour cream & onion popped chips, 26 chips (30 g)	4
Wise	
Kettle cooked jalapeño potato chips, 13 chips (28 g)	5
Kettle cooked potato chips 40% reduced fat, 19 chips (28 g)	4
Original kettle cooked potato chips, 13 chips (28 g)	5
Ridged sour cream and onion potato chips, 15 chips (28 g)	5
Zapp's	
New Orleans kettle style potato chips, 1 package (56.7 g)	10
Potato chips, 1 package (42.5 g)	7

Pretzels

	SmartPoints® value
365 Everyday Value	
Crunchy pretzel twists, 16 twists (28 g)	3
Organic mini pretzel twists, 1 oz	3
Anderson	
Pretzels, peanut butter filled, 10 pretzels (30 g)	5
Archer Farms	
Chocolate covered pretzels, 11 pretzels (40 g)	8
Pumpkin spice pretzels, 8 pretzels (40 g)	10
Bachman	
Pretzels, pretzel stix, 1 oz	3
Clancy's	
Everything pretzel slims, 1 oz	3
Honey wheat pretzels, 7 pieces (28 g)	4
Old fashioned pretzel minis, 17 pieces (28 g)	3
Original baked pretzel slims, 1 oz	3
Original pretzel flats, 13 pieces (28 g)	3
Pretzel rods, 3 pieces (28 g)	3
Pretzel sticks, old fashioned, 32 pieces (28 g)	3
Clover Valley	
Mini pretzel twists, 17 twists (28 g)	3
Pretzel sticks, 32 pieces (28 g)	3
Combos	
Baked cheddar cheese pretzel snacks, ⅓ cup	5
Creative Snacks Co.	
Milk chocolate peppermint pretzels, 9 pretzels (40 g)	9
Flipz	
Chocolate covered pretzels, milk chocolate covered, 8 pieces (28 g)	6
Food Lion	
Baked pretzel sticks, 42 pretzels (30 g)	3
Glutino Gluten Free	
Pretzel sticks, 33 pretzels (30 g)	5
Pretzel twists, 24 pretzels (30 g)	5
Great Value	
Fat free pretzel sticks, 1 serving (30 g)	3
Honey wheat braided pretzel twists, 1 serving (30 g)	4
H.K. Anderson	
Original peanut butter filled pretzel nuggets, 10 pieces (30 g)	5
Hannaford	
Mini pretzels, 18 pretzels (30 g)	3
H-E-B	
Low-fat pretzel sticks, 39 pretzels (28 g)	3
Herr's	
Pretzels, extra thin, one pounder, 9 pretzels (28 g)	3

Pretzels (cont'd)

	SmartPoints® value
Hy-Vee	
Pretzel sticks, 32 pieces (28 g)	3
Tiny twists pretzels, 17 pieces (28 g)	3
Keebler	
Pretzel thins, 6 crackers (15.6 g)	2
Pretzel thins, parmesan herb, 6 crackers (15.6 g)	2
Kellogg's Special K	
Fudge dipped pretzels, 1 pouch (21 g)	5
White fudge dipped, 1 pouch (21 g)	5
Kroger	
Braided twist honey wheat pretzels, 9 pretzels (28 g)	4
Mini peanut butter filled pretzels, 28 pretzels (30 g)	4
Pretzel sticks, 48 pretzels (28 g)	3
Pretzel waffles, 17 pretzels (28 g)	3
Tiny pretzel twists, 21 pretzels (28 g)	3
LiveGfree	
Gluten free mini twists pretzels, 19 pieces (28 g)	3
Gluten free pretzel sticks, 32 pieces (28 g)	3
Market Pantry	
Peanut butter filled pretzels, 10 pretzel bites (30 g)	4
Medifast	
Cinnamon pretzel sticks, 1 package (29 g)	3
Honey mustard pretzel sticks, 1 packet (29 g)	3
Meijer	
Pretzels, stix, 51 pretzels (30 g)	3
Pretzels, tiny twists, 19 pretzels (30 g)	3

	SmartPoints® value
Mikesell's	
Pretzel sticks, 32 pieces (28 g)	3
Nice!	
Yogurt covered pretzels, 6 pieces (30 g)	8
Nutrisystem	
Milk chocolate flavored pretzels, 1 package (30 g)	6
Pennysticks	
Braided pretzels, honey wheat, 18 pretzels (28 g)	3
Philly's Finest	
Soft pretzels, baked, 1 pretzel (146.5 g)	8
Pretzel Crisps	
Buffalo wing deli style pretzel crackers, 10 crackers (28 g)	3
Honey mustard and onion crisps, 10 crackers (28 g)	3
Original deli style pretzel crisps, 11 crackers (28 g)	3
Pretzel crisps, cheddar, minis, 35 crackers (28 g)	3
Pretzel crisps, deli style, everything, 11 crackers (28 g)	3
Pretzel crisps, original, minis, 42 crackers (28 g)	3
Sea salt and cracked pepper crisps, 10 crackers (28 g)	3
Pretzel Crisps Minis	
Gluten free original thin crunchy pretzel crackers, 42 crackers (28 g)	3
Publix	
Peanut butter pretzels, 10 pieces (31 g)	4
Rold Gold	
Garlic parmesan pretzel thins, 13 pretzels (28 g)	4
Honey wheat braided pretzel twists, 8 pretzels (28 g)	3

	SmartPoints® value
Original pretzel thins, 14 pieces (28 g)	3
Pretzels, rods, 3 pretzels (28 g)	3
Pretzels, sticks, 53 pretzels (28 g)	3
Pretzels, thins, 9 pretzels (28 g)	3
Pretzels, tiny twists, 1 package (28 g)	3
Pretzels, tiny twists, cheddar flavored, 20 pretzels (28 g)	3
Pretzels, tiny twists, honey mustard, 20 pretzels (28 g)	3
Tiny twists pretzels, 18 pretzels (28 g)	3
Seyfert's	
Extra dark extra salty beer pretz-o's pretzels, 15 pretzels (28 g)	3
ShopRite	
Pretzels, mini, fat free, 19 pretzels (30 g)	3
Simply Nature	
Everything pretzel slims, 1 oz	3
Original pretzel slims, 1 oz	3
Snack Factory	
Classic pretzel crisps, 11 crackers (28 g)	6
Everything pretzel crisps, 11 crackers (28 g)	3
Garlic parmesan pretzel crisps, 10 crackers (28 g)	3
Honey mustard and onion pretzel crisps, 10 crackers (28 g)	3
Pretzel snacks, thin crunchy, original, 11 crisps (28 g)	3
Snack Factory Pretzel Crisps	
Buffalo wing pretzel crackers, 10 crackers (28 g)	3
Dark chocolate crunch pretzel snacks, 5 pieces (28 g)	6
Garlic parmesan pretzel crackers, 10 crackers (28 g)	3

	SmartPoints® value
Pretzel crackers, deli style, everything, 11 crackers (28 g)	3
Pretzel crackers, deli style, garlic parmesan, 10 crackers (28 g)	3
Pretzel crackers, deli style, original, 11 crackers (28 g)	3
Snack Fresh	
Beef cheese & pretzel bites, 2 oz	8
Snappers	
Gourmet caramel & pretzel treats with dark chocolate and sea salt caramel, 3 pieces (40 g)	7
Snyder of Berlin	
Super thin pretzels, 10 pieces (28 g)	3
Snyder's 100 Calorie Pack	
Mini pretzels, 1 mini bag (26 g)	3
Pretzel sticks, 1 serving (26 g)	3
Pretzels, snaps, 1 package (26 g)	3
Snyder's Gluten Free	
Pretzel sticks, 40 sticks (30 g)	4
Snyder's of Hanover	
Butter snap pretzels, 24 pretzels (30 g)	3
Everything pretzel pieces, ⅓ cup	4
Honey mustard & onion pretzel pieces, ⅓ cup	5
Honey wheat braided twists, 7 twists (30 g)	4
Mini pretzels (single serve), 1 package (14 g)	1
Nibblers, sourdough, the pounder, 16 nibblers (30 g)	3
Old fashioned dipping sticks, 14 sticks (30 g)	3
Peanut butter filled pretzels, 10 pieces (28 g)	4
Pretzel poppers, original, 21 pretzels (30 g)	3
Pretzel rods, 3 pretzels (30 g)	3
Pretzel snaps, 24 pretzels (30 g)	3
Pretzels, mini, the pounder, 20 minis (30 g)	3

Pretzels, Snyder's of Hanover (cont'd)

	SmartPoints® value
Pretzels, nibblers, sourdough, 16 nibblers (33 g)	3
Unsalted mini pretzels, 20 minis (30 g)	3
Snyder's of Hanover Gluten Free	
Hot buffalo wing pretzel sticks, 29 sticks (30 g)	4
Snyder's the Pounder	
Pretzels, sticks, 28 sticks (30 g)	3
Sproutzels	
Honey wheat pretzels, 1 oz	4
Stacy's Simple Naked	
Pretzel thins, 13 pieces (28 g)	3
Super Pretzel	
Baked soft pretzels, 1 pretzel (71.4 g)	5
Pretzel bites, baked, soft, 5 bites (53 g)	4
Soft pretzels, baked, 1 pretzel (64 g)	4
The Snack Factory Pretzel Crisps Minis	
Original pretzel crackers, 42 pieces (28 g)	3
Trader Joe's	
Assorted chocolate covered pretzel rods, 1 piece (26 g)	5
Honey wheat pretzel sticks, 10 sticks (30 g)	4
Multi-grain pretzel nuggets with sesame seeds, 22 pretzels (28 g)	3
Peanut butter filled pretzels, 11 pieces (30 g)	5
Peanut butter filled pretzels with no salt on the pretzel, 11 pieces (30 g)	5
Pretzel slims, 23 pretzels (28 g)	3
Trader Joe's Grocery	
Pretzel slims everything, 23 pieces (28 g)	3

	SmartPoints® value
Uncle Ray's	
Mini pretzels, 21 pretzels (31 g)	4
Unique Pretzels	
Pretzel shells, 12 pretzels (28 g)	3
Unique Pretzels Splits	
Pretzels, extra dark, 3 pretzels (28 g)	3
Utz	
Country store pretzel stix, 5 pieces (28 g)	3
Gourmet pretzel blend, 8 pretzels (28 g)	3
Pretzel rods, old fashioned, 3 pretzels (30 g)	3
Pretzels, extra thin, the pounder, 10 pretzels (28 g)	3
Pretzels, nuggets, sourdough, 10 pretzels (28 g)	3
Pretzels, sourdough hard, old fashioned, 1 pretzel (23 g)	3
Sourdough specials pretzels, 5 pieces (28 g)	3
Utz Specials	
Pretzels, extra dark, the pounder, 5 pretzels (28 g)	3
Pretzels, sourdough, the pounder, 5 pretzels (28 g)	3
Wege of Hanover	
Pretzel o's pretzels, 15 pretzels (28 g)	3
Weight Watchers In-Meeting/ Online Products: Crunchy Snacks	
Original mini pretzel thins, 1 pouch	2

Rice and Corn Cakes

	SmartPoints® value
Bamboo Lane	
Crunchy rice roller, 1 roller (12.5 g)	2
Rice rollers, 1 roll (10 g)	2
Clancy's Fit & Active	
Rice snacks, 8 chips (15 g)	2
Coco Lite	
Pop cakes, multigrain, 1 piece (5 g)	0
Pop cakes, multigrain, 6 pieces (30 g)	3
Eating Right for Calorie Counting	
White cheddar rice cakes, 1 rice cake (11 g)	1
Element	
Dark chocolate rice cakes, 1 rice cake (17 g)	3
Fit & Active	
Chocolate rice snacks, 7 chips (15 g)	2
Ranch rice snacks, 9 rice snacks (16 g)	2
Rice snacks, 8 mini cakes (15 g)	2
Forrelli	
Thin multigrain rice cakes, 1 slice (5 g)	1
Giant	
Rice cakes, apple cinnamon, 1 cake (12 g)	2
Rice cakes, fat free, unsalted, multigrain, 1 cake (10 g)	1
Rice cakes, lightly salted, plain, 1 cake (10 g)	1
H-E-B	
Caramel rice cakes, 1 cake (13 g)	2

	SmartPoints® value
Jayone	
Crunchy white rice roll (gluten free), 1 stick (10 g)	2
Kellogg's Special K Popped Delights	
Cocoa with fudge drizzle, 1 pouch (12 g)	3
Kim's Magic Pop	
Cheddar cheese flavor popped grain snack, 1 piece (5 g)	0
Wheat and brown rice onion snack cakes, 1 cake (5 g)	0
Wheat and brown rice strawberry snack cakes, 1 cake (5 g)	0
Kim's Magic Pop All Natural	
Multigrain cakes, 1 piece (5 g)	0
Kroger	
Cheddar flavored mini rice cakes, 9 mini cakes (16 g)	2
Rice cakes, low sodium, 1 cake (9 g)	1
Rice cakes, white cheddar flavored, 1 cake (11 g)	1
Lieber's	
Sea salt rice cakes, 1 slice (5 g)	1
Lucerne Foods	
Caramel corn rice cakes, 1 rice cake (13 g)	2
Lundberg	
Lightly salted brown rice cakes, 1 cake (19 g)	2
Lightly salted organic rice cake, 1 cake (19 g)	2
Rice cakes, cinnamon toast, 1 cake (21 g)	3
Lundberg Eco-Farmed	
Rice cakes, honey nut, 1 cake (21 g)	2

Rice and Corn Cakes (cont'd)

	SmartPoints® value
Lundberg Organic	
Rice cakes, wild rice, lightly salted, 1 cake (19 g)	2
Salt-free brown rice cakes, 1 cake (19 g)	2
Lundberg Thin Stackers	
Organic brown rice lightly salted rice cakes, 4 cakes (28 g)	3
Red rice and quinoa puffed grain cakes, 4 cakes (28 g)	3
Popped	
Rice snacks, apple cinnamon, 13 mini cakes (30 g)	5
Rice snacks, ranch, 1 bag (19 g)	2
Rice snacks, ranch, 17 mini cakes (30 g)	4
Publix	
Fat free caramel rice snacks, 8 pieces (15 g)	2
Fat free salt free rice cakes, 1 cake (10 g)	1
Ranch rice snacks, 9 rice snacks (16 g)	2
Quaker	
Apple cinnamon rice cakes, 1 cake (13 g)	2
Butter popped corn rice cake, 1 cake (9 g)	1
Caramel corn rice cake, 1 cake (13 g)	2
Chocolate crunch rice cake, 1 cake (15 g)	2
Lightly salted rice cakes, 1 cake (9 g)	1
Salt free rice cake, 1 cake (9 g)	1
White cheddar rice cake, 1 cake (11 g)	1

	SmartPoints® value
Quaker Popped	
Bbq flavor rice snacks, 1 mini bag (19 g)	2
Butter popcorn rice crisps, 18 mini cakes (30 g)	5
Buttered popcorn flavored rice snacks, 18 mini cakes (30 g)	4
Caramel corn flavor rice snacks, 13 mini cakes (30 g)	4
Cheddar cheese flavor rice snacks, 1 mini bag (19 g)	3
Cheddar cheese flavor rice snacks, 18 mini cakes (30 g)	4
Chocolate flavor rice snacks, 13 mini cakes (30 g)	4
Garlic parmesan rice crisps (gluten free), 18 pieces (30 g)	4
Kettle corn rice snacks, 15 mini cakes (30 g)	4
Ranch flavor rice snacks, 17 mini cakes (30 g)	4
Sour cream and onion rice snacks, 18 mini cakes (30 g)	4
Sweet chili flavor rice snacks, 18 mini cakes (30 g)	4
Real Foods	
Corn thins, multigrain, 2 slices (12 g)	1
Corn thins, organic, original, 2 slices (12 g)	1
Corn thins, sesame, 2 slices (14 g)	1
Right for Calorie Counting	
Apple cinnamon rice cakes (gluten free), 1 cake (13 g)	2
ShopRite	
Rice cakes, fat free, whole grain, popped corn, white cheddar, 1 cake (11 g)	1

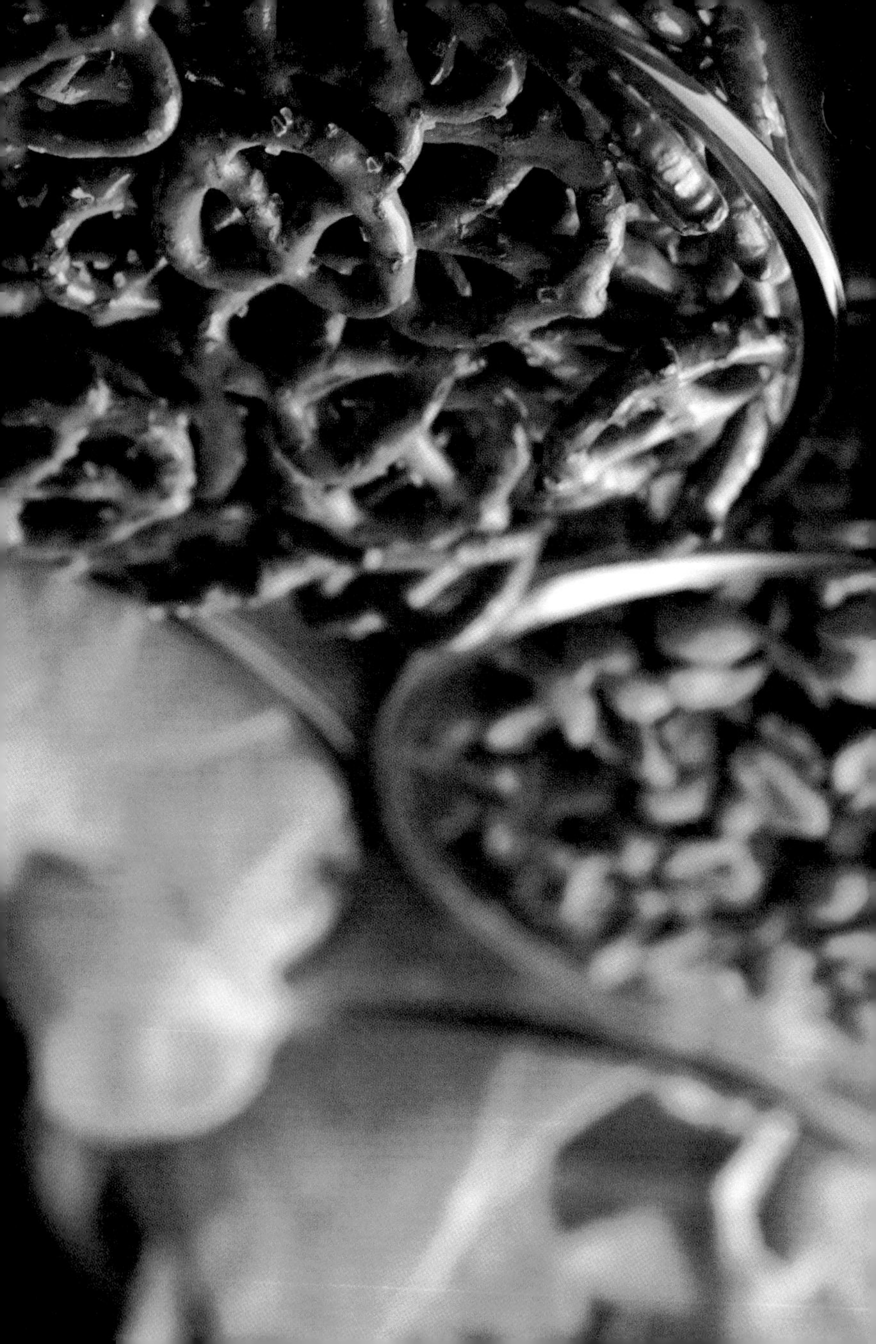

Rice and Corn Cakes (cont'd)

	SmartPoints® value
Simply Nature	
Unsalted rice cakes, 1 rice cake (10 g)	1
Stew Leonard's	
Rice cakes, 1 rice cake (5 g)	0
Stop & Shop	
Chocolate mini rice cakes, 7 chips (15 g)	2
Suzie's	
Quinoa and sesame all natural puffed crackers, 1 cake (15 g)	1
Thin cakes, brown rice, 4 cakes (17 g)	2
Wild RiceWorks	
Sea salt and black sesame gourmet wildrice crisps, 10 chips (28 g)	4
Woodstock Mini Me's	
Dark chocolate coating organic rice bites, 6 pieces (21 g)	4

Seeds

	SmartPoints® value
365 Everyday Value Organic	
Finely ground flaxseed, 2 Tbsp	2
Barlean's	
Flax chia coconut blend, 1½ Tbsp	2
Bob's Red Mill Grains-Of-Discovery	
Whole seed chia, 1 Tbsp	2
Carrington Farms	
Organic chia seeds, 2 Tbsp	2
David	
Original sunflower seeds, 1 package (23 g)	4
Garden of Life	
Flax and chia seed, 2 Tbsp	2
Great Value	
Roasted and salted sunflower seeds, ¼ cup	6
Hodgson Mill	
Flax seed, milled, 2 Tbsp	2
Manitoba Harvest	
Hemp seeds, shelled, raw, 3 Tbsp	5
Nature's Harvest	
Dry roasted & salted pumpkin seeds, ⅓ cup	3
Lightly salted dry roasted pepitas, ¼ cup	6
Nature's Intent	
Organic chia seeds, 3 Tbsp	4
Nature's Path	
Chia seeds, 2½ Tbsp	4
Nutiva	
Chia seed, 1 Tbsp	2
Coconut superseed blend, 1 Tbsp	2
Premium Gold	
Flaxseed, 2 Tbsp	2
Premium Orchard	
Pumpkin seeds roasted with sea salt, ¼ cup	3
Southern Grove	
Honey roasted sunflower kernels, ¼ cup	5
Spectrum	
Chia seed, ground, 2 Tbsp	2
Spectrum Essentials	
Chia seed, 1 Tbsp	2
Organic premium flaxseed ground, 2 Tbsp	2
Trader Joe's	
Flax seed with blueberries, 2 Tbsp	3
Golden roasted flax seed (whole seeds), 2 Tbsp	3
Organic chia seed, 2 Tbsp	4
Raw shelled hemp seed, 1 tsp	1
Trader Joe's Grocery	
Chia seeds, ½ oz	2

Snack and Trail Mixes

	SmartPoints® value
Archer Farms	
Zen party trail mix, ⅓ cup	4
Bear Naked	
Cacao and cashew butter granola, ¼ cup	4
Cinnamon and sunflower butter granola, ⅓ cup	5
Cascadian Farm Organic	
Honey almond and chia granola, ⅓ cup	5
Cheez-It	
Sriracha snack mix, ½ cup	4
Chex Mix	
Snack mix, bold party blend, ½ cup	4
Snack mix, cheddar, ½ cup	4
Snack mix, sweet 'n salty, honey nut, ½ cup	4
Gardetto's	
Reduced fat snack mix, ½ cup	4
Great Value	
Cajun trail mix, ¼ cup	5
Rocky road trail mix, ¼ cup	8
Harvest Stone	
Gluten free bold crispy snack mix, ½ cup	4
Kar's	
Sweet and salty mix, 1 package (57 g)	12
Sweet n salty mix, 1 package (57 g)	11
Keystone	
Party mix snack mix, 1 oz	5
Kind Healthy Grains	
Cinnamon oat clusters with flax seeds, ⅓ cup	4
Oats & honey clusters with toasted coconut, ⅓ cup	5
Peanut butter whole grain clusters, ⅓ cup	4
Vanilla blueberry clusters with flax seeds, ⅓ cup	4
Kirkland Signature	
Trail mix, 3 Tbsp	6
Trail mix with m&m candies, 3 Tbsp	6
Market Pantry	
Knapsack trail mix, ¼ cup	6
Nature Valley	
Granola crunch, ¼ cup	4
Oats n honey granola crunch, ¼ cup	4
Sargento Balanced Breaks	
Natural sharp cheddar cheese, sea salted cashews & cherry juice infused dried cranberries, 1 tray (43 g)	7
Natural sharp white cheddar cheese, sea salted cashews & golden raisin medley, 1 tray (43 g)	7
Natural white cheddar cheese, sea salted roasted almonds & dried cranberries, 1 tray (42 g)	7
pepper Jack natural cheese, honey roasted peanuts & raisins, 1 tray (43 g)	7
Simple Truth Organic	
Pomegranate blueberry chia granola clusters, 1 oz	4
Southern Grove	
Mountain trail mix, ¼ cup	6
Trail mix with rainforest alliance certified cocoa, ¼ cup	7
Utz Select	
Pub mix, ½ cup	4
Wegman's Organic	
Pumpkin flax granola, ¼ cup	5

Tortilla Chips

	SmartPoints® value
365 Everyday Value	
Organic yellow corn lightly salted tortilla strips, 10 strips (28 g)	4
7-Select	
Sweet chili corn tortilla chips, 12 chips (35 g)	5
Calidad	
Mexican restaurant style corn tortilla chips, 15 chips (28 g)	5
Tortilla chips, 12 chips (28 g)	5
Central Market	
Blue corn tortilla chips, 14 chips (28 g)	4
Charley's Chips	
Fresh tortilla chips, 8 chips (28 g)	5
Clancy's	
Big dipper tortilla chips, 10 pieces (28 g)	4
White rounds tortilla chips, 11 chips (28 g)	4
Daily Chef	
White corn tortilla chips, 14 chips (28 g)	4
Don Pancho Authentic Mexican Food	
Blue sesame tortilla chips, 12 chips (28 g)	4
Donkey	
Tortilla chips, authentic, salted, 8 chips (28 g)	4
Doritos	
Cool ranch flavored tortilla chips, 12 chips (28 g)	5
Cool ranch tortilla chips, 12 chips (28 g)	6
Nacho cheese flavored tortilla chips, 1 package (31.8 g)	5
Nacho cheese flavored tortilla chips, 11 chips (28 g)	4
Nacho cheese tortilla chips, 11 chips (28 g)	4
Spicy nacho flavored tortilla chips, 12 chips (28 g)	4
Spicy sweet chili flavored tortilla chips, 11 chips (28 g)	4
Toasted corn tortilla chips, 13 chips (28 g)	4
Wild white nacho tortilla chips, 12 chips (28 g)	4
Doritos Jacked	
Ranch dipped hot wings tortilla chips, 6 chips (28 g)	4
El Milagro	
Tortilla chips, Mexican kitchen style, salted, 1 oz	4
Food Should Taste Good	
Multigrain tortilla chips, 10 chips (28 g)	4
Sweet potato tortilla chips, 1 oz	4
Fresh Gourmet	
Sante fe style tortilla strips, 2 Tbsp	1
Tortilla strips, lightly salted, 2 Tbsp	1
Tortilla strips, tri-color, 2 Tbsp	1
Garden Fresh Gourmet	
Kettle style blue corn tortilla chips, 11 chips (28 g)	4
Garden of Eatin'	
Blue corn tortilla chips, 11 chips (28 g)	4
Multi-grain tortilla chips, sea salt with flax seeds, 16 chips (28 g)	4
Tortilla chips, blue, party size, 1 oz	4
Tortilla chips, red hot blues, 15 chips (28 g)	4

	SmartPoints® value
Giant	
Tri color tortilla strips, 2 Tbsp	1
Go! Smart	
Multi grain corn tortilla chips, 12 chips (35 g)	5
Great Value	
Bite size tortilla chips, 22 chips (28 g)	5
Stadium style yellow corn tortilla chips, 8 chips (28 g)	4
Hy-Vee	
Bite size white corn tostados round tortilla chips, 20 chips (28 g)	4
Juanita's	
Tortilla chips, 13 tortillas (28 g)	5
Tortilla chips, fiesta bag, 13 chips (28 g)	5
Kirkland Signature	
Organic tortilla chips, 11 chips (28 g)	4
Kroger	
Tortilla chips, traditional, 12 chips (28 g)	5
La Favorita	
Tortilla chips, yellow corn, 10 chips (28 g)	2
Late July	
Sea salt by the seashore multigrain tortilla chips, 9 chips (28 g)	4
Late July Organic	
Sea salt by the seashore multigrain tortilla chips, 9 chips (28 g)	4
Sea salt restaurant style tortilla chips, 10 chips (28 g)	4

	SmartPoints® value
Mission®	
Restaurant style tortilla rounds, 10 chips (28 g)	4
Restaurant style tortilla strips, 12 chips (28 g)	4
Tortilla chip rounds, 10 chips (28 g)	4
Old Dutch	
Restaurant style original tortilla chips, 9 chips (30 g)	5
Restaurante style tostados yellow corn tortilla chips, 11 chips (30 g)	5
On the Border	
Tortilla chips, 7 chips (28 g)	5
Tortilla chips, cantina thins, 14 chips (28 g)	4
Pueblo Lindo	
Restaurant style tortilla triangles, 14 chips (28 g)	4
RW Garcia MixtBag	
Gluten free veggie tortilla chips, 15 chips (28 g)	4
Santitas	
Tortilla chips, 9 chips (28 g)	4
Tortilla chips, triangles, 9 chips (28 g)	4
Simply Balanced	
Spinach corn tortilla chips, 11 chips (28 g)	4
Simply Nature	
Organic yellow corn tortilla chips, 25 chips (28 g)	4
Simply Tostitos Scoops!	
Organic tortilla chips, 13 chips (28 g)	4
Snyder's of Hanover	
Reduced fat white corn tortilla chips (family size), 13 chips (28 g)	4

Tortilla Chips (cont'd)

	SmartPoints® value
Tostitos	
Baked scoops, 16 chips (28 g)	4
Bite size tortilla chips, 24 chips (28 g)	4
Cantina chipotle thins, 13 chips (28 g)	5
Crispy rounds tortilla chips, white corn, 13 chips (27 g)	4
Hint of lime tortilla chips, 6 Chips (28 g)	5
Original restaurant style tortilla chips, 7 Chips (28 g)	4
Tortilla chips, multigrain, 8 chips (28 g)	5
Tortilla chips, restaurant style, 7 chips (28 g)	4
Tostitos Baked!	
Tortilla chips, scoops!, 14 chips (28 g)	4
Tostitos Cantina	
Thin and crispy tortilla chips, 15 chips (28 g)	5
Traditional tortilla chips, 7 chips (28 g)	5
Tostitos Rolls	
Rolled tortilla chips, 15 chips (28 g)	5
Tostitos Scoops!	
Tortilla chips, 13 chips (28 g)	4
Tortilla chips, multigrain, 12 chips (28 g)	4
Tostitos Simply	
Organic blue corn tortilla chips, 6 chips (28 g)	4
Trader Joe's	
Nacho cheese tortilla chips, 1 oz	4
Salted tortilla chips, 10 chips (28 g)	4
Salted tortilla chips made with stone ground yellow corn, 1 oz	4

	SmartPoints® value
Soy and flaxseed tortilla chips, 15 chips (28 g)	4
Sweet potato tortilla chips, 9 chips (28 g)	4
Unsalted organic white corn tortilla chips, 14 chips (28 g)	4
Veggie and flaxseed tortilla chips, 7 chips (28 g)	4
Trader Joe's Grocery	
Organic white corn tortilla chips, 14 chips (28 g)	4
Quinoa & black bean infused tortilla chips, 8 chips (28 g)	4
Trader Joe's Organic	
Blue corn tortilla chips, 12 chips (28 g)	4
Yellow corn tortilla chip rounds, 9 chips (28 g)	4
Trader Joe's Reduced Guilt	
Organic white corn tortilla chips, 14 chips (28 g)	3
Trader Jose's	
Baked blue corn tortilla chips - salted, 18 chips (28 g)	3
Way Better Simply Sprouted	
Tortilla chips, simply sweet potato, 11 chips (28 g)	4
Wild Harvest	
Spicy blue corn tortilla chips, 12 chips (28 g)	4

Vegetable and Soy Chips

A&G	
Veggie sticks, 1⅔ cups	5
Beanitos	
Simply pinto bean with sea salt bean chips, 12 chips (28 g)	4
Calbee	
Black pepper snapea crisps, 1 package (50 g)	6

	SmartPoints® value
Calbee Harvest Snaps	
Black pepper snapea crisps, 22 pieces (28 g)	3
Onion thyme lentil snaps, 24 pieces (28 g)	3
Tomato basil lentil snaps snack, 24 pieces (28 g)	3
Calbee Snapea Crisps	
Original lightly salted green pea crisps, 22 pieces (28 g)	3
Central Market	
Tangy ranch veggie straws, 38 straws (28 g)	4
Central Market H-E-B	
Veggie straws, 38 straws (28 g)	4
Clancy's Original	
Vegetable chips, 1 oz	4
CVS	
Veggie chips, 1 oz	4
Fresh Finds	
Cheddar veggie straws, 1 oz	4
Gluck	
Jalapeño veggie sticks, 70 sticks (28 g)	4
Good Health	
Jalapeño veggie straws, 40 straws (28 g)	4
Good Health Enjoy Being Good	
Sea salt veggie straws, 40 straws (28 g)	4
Good Health Natural Foods	
Veggie chips, 1 oz	4
Veggie stix, 1 oz	4
Harvest Snaps	
Lightly salted baked original green pea crisps, 22 pieces (28 g)	3

	SmartPoints® value
Hi I'm Skinny	
Skinny sticks, multi-grain sweet onion, 34 sticks (28 g)	4
Skinny sticks, sweet potato, 34 sticks (28 g)	4
Skinny sticks, veggie tortilla, 34 sticks (28 g)	4
Mediterranean Snack Food	
Chips, baked lentil, sea salt, 22 chips (28 g)	3
Nature's Promise Naturals	
Vegetable sticks, natural, 1 oz	4
Pirate's Booty	
Aged white cheddar baked rice and corn puffs, 1 bag (14 g)	2
Pop Chips	
Mediterranean herb veggie chips, 23 chips (28 g)	3
Sea salt veggie chips, 23 chips (28 g)	3
Sensible Portions Garden Veggie Chips	
Cheddar cheese flavored potato crisps, 14 pieces (28 g)	5
Sour cream & onion flavored potato crisps, 14 pieces (28 g)	5
Veggie chips, garden, sea salt, 38 chips (28 g)	4
Sensible Portions Garden Veggie Straws	
Cheddar cheese, 1 bag (28 g)	4
Garden veggie straws with sea salt, 38 straws (28 g)	4
Veggie straws, garden, variety pack (sea salt flavor), 1 bag (28 g)	4
Zesty ranch vegetable and potato snack, 1 bag (28 g)	4
Simple Truth Free From 101	
Natural vegetable chips, 20 chips (28 g)	4

Vegetable and Soy Chips (cont'd)

	SmartPoints® value
Snapea Crisps	
Lightly salted baked original green pea crisps, 1 oz	3
Lightly salted green pea crisps, 22 pieces (28 g)	3
Snyder's EatSmart Naturals	
Garden veggie crisps, potato, tomato & spinach, 21 chips (28 g)	4
SunChips	
Farmhouse ranch veggie harvest chips, 14 chips (28 g)	4
Tomato basil and cheese veggie harvest chips, 15 chips (28 g)	4
Terra	
Mediterranean real vegetable chips, 14 chips (28 g)	5
Original vegetable chips, 14 chips (28 g)	5
Sweet potato chips, 17 chips (28 g)	5
Vegetable chips, exotic, original, 14 chips (27 g)	5
The Better Chip	
Spinach & kale whole grain chips, 10 chips (28 g)	4
The Daily Crave	
Aged white cheddar lentil chips, 16 chips (28 g)	3
The Good Bean	
Sea salt crispy crunchy chickpeas, 1 oz	3
Trader Joe's	
Seasoned kale chips, ½ package (28 g)	4
Veggie sticks potato snacks, 50 sticks (28 g)	4
Trader Joe's Contemplates	
Inner peas snack, 22 pieces (28 g)	4
Trader Joe's Grocery	
Crunchy curls, 31 pieces (28 g)	4
Roasted plantain chips, 20 chips (28 g)	5
Veggie chips, 26 chips (28 g)	5

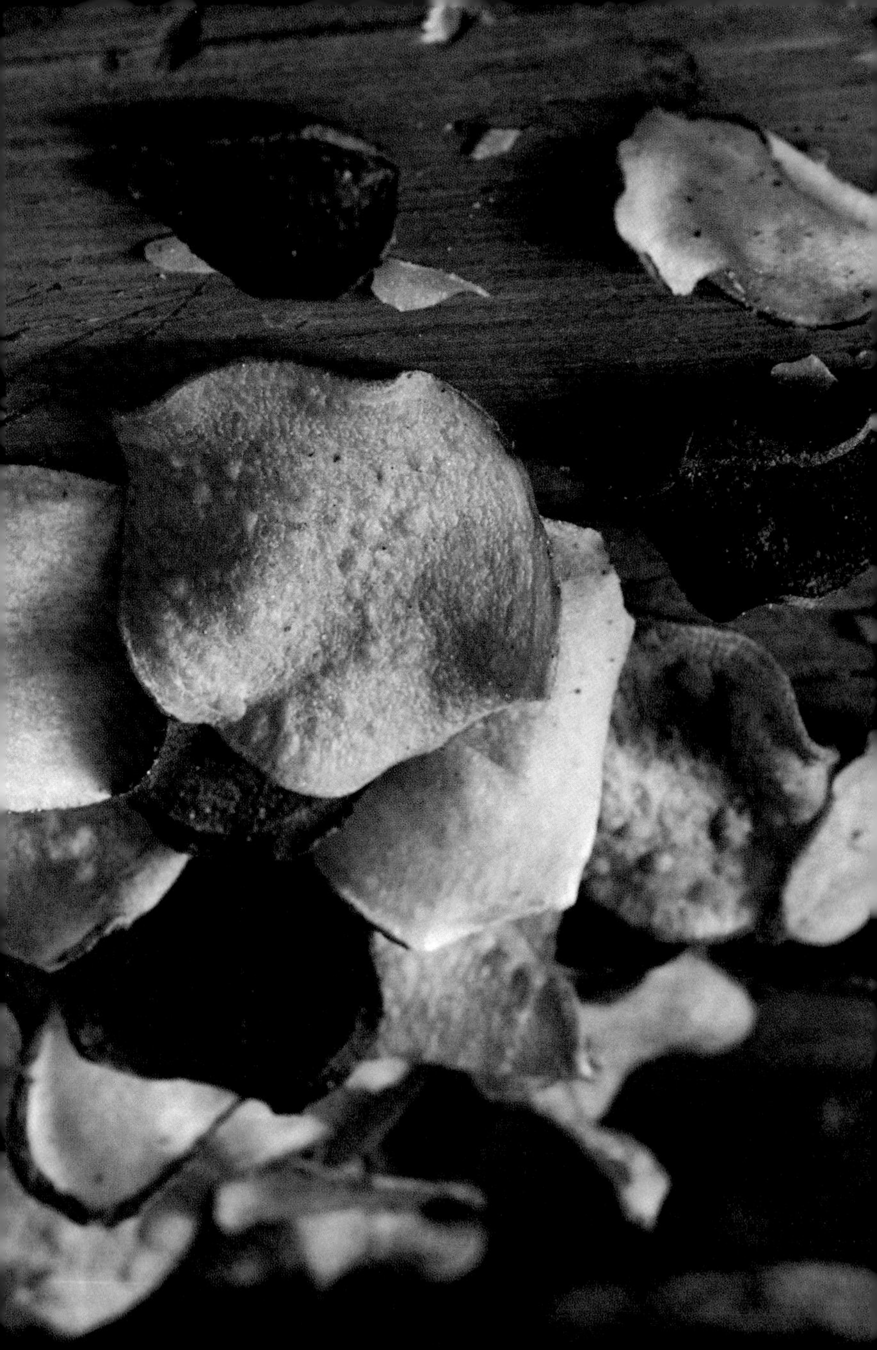

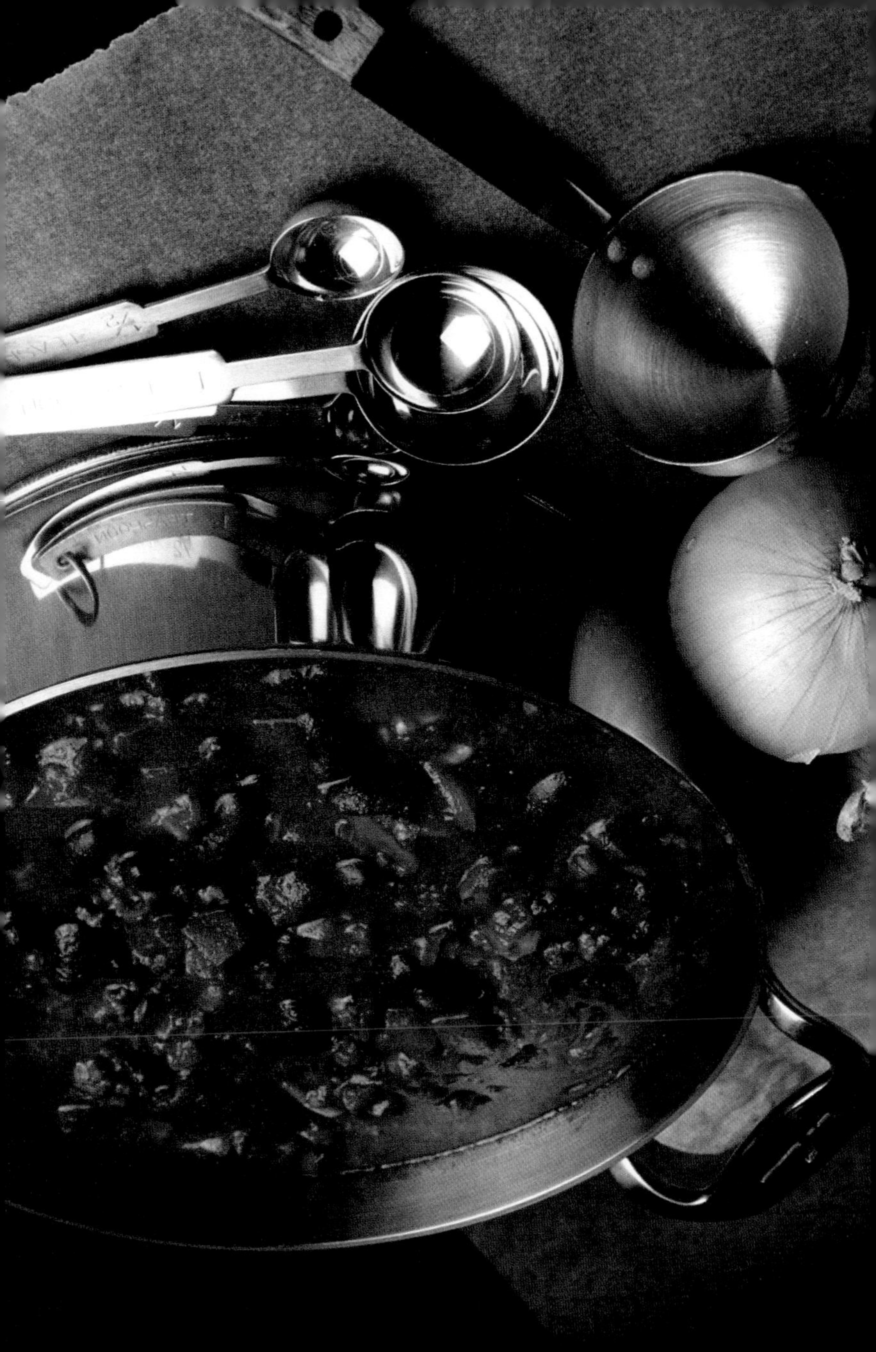

soups, stews & chili

	SmartPoints® value
Beef Soups	
Annie Chun's	
Soup bowl, Vietnamese pho, 1 bowl (170 g)	8
Campbell's	
Condensed beef with vegetables and barley soup, ½ cup	3
Condensed vegetable beef soup, ½ cup	3
Soup, vegetable beef, 1 cup	2
Campbell's Chunky	
Chili beef & bean roadhouse, 1 cup	7
Sirloin burger with country vegetables soup, 1 cup	5
Campbell's Chunky Healthy Request	
Soup, sirloin burger with country vegetables, 1 cup	4
Campbell's Home Style	
Soup, Italian-style wedding, light, 1 cup	2
Maruchan	
Soup, ramen noodle, beef flavor, ½ block (43 g)	6
Nissin Cup Noodles	
Beef flavor ramen noodle soup, 1 container (71 g)	11
Progresso	
Chef's select beef burgundy soup, 1 cup	4
Progresso Light	
Beef pot roast soup, 1 cup	2
Savory beef barley vegetable soup, 1 cup	2
Progresso Rich & Hearty	
Beef pot roast with country vegetables soup, 1 cup	3
Savory beef barley vegetable soup, 1 cup	3
Progresso Traditional	
Beef barley soup, 1 cup	4

	SmartPoints® value
Signature Café	
Soup, stuffed pepper with beef, 1 cup	4
Bouillon, Broth, and Stocks	
Campbell's	
Broth k-cup pods and noodle packets, 1 serving (18.9 g)	2
Swanson	
Broth, chicken, 1 cup	0
Chicken broth, 1 cup	0
Unsalted cooking chicken stock, 1 cup	0
Vegetable cooking stock, 1 cup	1
Trader Joe's	
Low sodium organic vegetable broth, 1 cup	1
Miso ginger broth, 1 cup	0
Organic free range chicken broth, 1 cup	1
Chicken Soups	
Bear Creek	
Soup mix, chicken noodle, chicken flavored, ¼ cup dry	4
Campbell's	
Chicken broth and noodle soup, 1 serving (18.9 g)	2
Chicken noodle soup, 1 cup	2
Classic chicken noodle soup, 1 cup	2
Condensed chicken noodle soup, ½ cup	2
Condensed cream of chicken soup, ½ cup	4
Condensed homestyle chicken noodle soup, ½ cup	2
Cream of chicken condensed soup, ½ cup	2
Soup, homestyle chicken noodle, 1 cup	2

	SmartPoints® value
Campbell's Chunky	
Chicken corn chowder soup, ½ cup	4
Classic chicken noodle soup, 1 cup	3
Creamy chicken and dumplings soup, 1 cup	5
Savory chicken with white and wild rice soup, 1 cup	3
Campbell's Chunky Healthy Request	
Soup, chicken noodle, 1 cup	3
Soup, grilled chicken & sausage gumbo, 1 cup	4
Campbell's Fresh Brewed Soup	
Homestyle chicken broth soup mix k-cup and noodles, 1 serving (18.9 g)	2
Southwest style chicken broth and noodle mix k-cup, 1 k-cup	2
Campbell's Healthy Request	
Condensed cream of chicken soup, ½ cup condensed	2
Condensed soup, chicken noodle, ½ cup	2
Campbell's Home Style	
Mexican-style chicken tortilla soup, 1 cup	4
Soup, chicken noodle, light, 1 cup	2
Campbell's Select Harvest Healthy Request	
Soup, savory chicken and brown rice, 1 cup	3
Campbell's Soup on the Go	
Chicken and star shaped pasta soup, 1 container (305 g)	2
Chef's Cupboard	
Chunky chicken and dumplings soup, 1 cup	5
Clover Valley	
Chicken noodle soup, ½ cup	2

	SmartPoints® value
Full Circle	
Chicken noodle soup, 1 cup	2
Healthy Choice	
Old fashioned soup, chicken noodle, pre-priced, 1 cup	2
Homemade Gourmet	
Fiesta soup trio soup mixes, 2½ tsp	1
Kirkland Signature	
Chicken tortilla soup, 1 cup	4
Lipton	
Noodle soup with real chicken broth, 2 Tbsp	2
Lipton Cup-a-Soup	
Instant soup, chicken noodle with white meat, 1 envelope (13 g)	1
Instant soup, cream of chicken flavor, 1 envelope (17 g)	2
Lipton Soup Secrets	
Noodle soup mix with real chicken broth, 2 Tbsp	1
Soup, chicken noodle, with diced white chicken meat, 3 Tbsp	2
Soup, noodle, 2 Tbsp	2
Maruchan	
Chicken flavor instant lunch, 1 container (64 g)	10
Chicken flavor ramen noodle soup, ½ package (43 g)	6
Mrs. Grass	
Soup mix, noodle soup, ¼ carton (18 g)	2
Nissin Cup Noodles	
Soup, ramen noodle, chicken flavor, 1 container (64 g)	11
Nissin Top Ramen	
Ramen noodle soup, chicken flavor, 1½ oz	6
Nutrisystem Lunch	
Chicken noodle soup, 1 container (213 g)	3

Chicken Soups (cont'd)

	SmartPoints® value
Panera Bread	
Gluten free low-fat chicken tortilla soup, 1 cup	3
Low-fat chicken noodle soup (grocery store), 1 cup	3
Low-fat chicken tortilla soup, 1 cup	3
Panera Bread Grocery	
Chicken kale and sweet potato soup, 1 cup	3
Chicken tortilla soup, 1 container (284 g)	4
Progresso	
Light chicken and vegetables with rosemary soup, 1 cup	2
Light creamy roasted chicken with herb dumplings soup, 1 cup	3
Progresso Heart Healthy	
Chicken and wild rice reduced sodium soup, 1 cup	2
Chicken noodle reduced sodium soup, 1 cup	2
Progresso Light	
Chicken and cheese enchilada flavor soup, 1 cup	3
Chicken and dumpling soup, 1 cup	2
Chicken corn chowder soup, 1 cup	3
Chicken noodle soup, 1 cup	2
Chicken pot pie style soup, 1 cup	3
Chicken vegetable rotini soup, 1 cup	2
Creamy chicken Alfredo with pasta, 1 cup	3
Roasted chicken and vegetable soup, 1 cup	2
Santa fe style chicken soup, 1 cup	2

	SmartPoints® value
Progresso Rich & Hearty	
Chicken and homestyle noodles soup, 1 cup	3
Chicken corn chowder soup, 1 cup	7
Creamy roasted chicken wild rice soup, 1 cup	4
Progresso Traditional	
99% fat free chicken noodle soup, 1 cup	3
Chicken and herb dumplings soup, 1 cup	3
Chicken and orzo with lemon soup, 1 cup	2
Chicken and sausage gumbo soup, 1 cup	4
Chicken and wild rice soup, 1 cup	3
Chicken barley soup, 1 cup	2
Chicken noodle soup, 1 cup	3
Chicken rice with vegetables soup, 1 cup	3
Chicken tortilla soup, 1 cup	3
Hearty chicken and rotini soup, 1 cup	3
Homestyle chicken soup with vegetables and pearl pasta, 1 cup	3
Trader Joe's Refrigerated	
Chicken, barley and vegetable soup, 1 cup	3

Chili

Chilli Man	
Chili, with beans, 1 cup	10
Chili, with beans, lean beef, 1 cup	8
Hormel	
Chili, no beans, 1 cup	7
Turkey chili with beans, 1 cup	6
Turkey chili with no beans, 1 cup	4

	SmartPoints® value
Marie Callender's	
White chicken chili with beans, 1 cup	7
Nutrisystem Dinner	
Chili with beans, 1 container (213 g)	7
Panera Bread Grocery	
Turkey chili with beans, 1 container (340 g)	8
Stagg Chili	
Steak house reserve chili with beans, 1 cup	9
Tabatchnick	
Vegetarian chili, 1 pouch (213 g)	5
Trader Joe's Grocery	
Turkey chili with beans, 1 cup	7

Seafood Soups

Authentic Asia	
Shrimp wonton soup, with noodles, Chinese-style, 6 oz	7
Giant	
Maryland crab soup, 1 cup	3
Legal Sea Foods Grocery	
Alaskan king crab and sweet corn chowder, 1 cup	10
Progresso Light	
New England clam chowder soup, 1 cup	3
Progresso Traditional	
Manhattan clam chowder soup, 1 cup	3
New England clam chowder soup, 1 cup	6

Stews

Otria	
Beef stew, thick & hearty, 1 cup	7

	SmartPoints® value

Turkey Soups

Blount Seafood	
Turkey sausage and kale soup, 1 cup	4

Vegetable and Other Soups

365 Everyday Value	
Organic rustic vegetable soup, 1 cup	3
Amy's	
Soups, organic, chunky vegetable, 1 cup	2
Amy's Light in Sodium	
Organic lentil vegetable soup, 1 cup	5
Amy's Organic	
Lentil vegetable soup, 1 cup	5
Soups, split pea, 1 cup	3
Annie's Homegrown	
Creamy carrot & bunny pasta soup, 1 cup	5
Back To Nature	
Reduced sodium minestrone with farro soup, 1 cup	5
Bear Creek	
Soup mix, creamy potato, ¼ cup dry	5
Soup mix, minestrone, ⅓ cup dry	3
Boulder Organic!	
Butternut squash soup with sage, 8 oz	4
Campbell's	
Condensed bean with bacon soup, ½ cup	5
Condensed vegetarian vegetable soup, ½ cup	3
Cream of mushroom condensed soup, ½ cup	3
Double noodle condensed soup, ½ cup	3

	SmartPoints® value
Soup, condensed, cream of mushroom, ½ cup	3
Soup, condensed, tomato, ½ cup	4
Tomato soup, 1 cup	5
Campbell's Chunky	
Hearty bean and ham with natural smoke flavor soup, 1 cup	5
Campbell's Condensed	
98% fat free cream of mushroom soup, ½ cup	2
Campbell's Home Style	
Italian style wedding soup, 1 cup	3
Campbell's Soup on the Go	
Classic tomato soup, 1 container (305 g)	6
CedarLane	
Chopped tomato and vegetable soup with quinoa, 1 cup	3
CedarLane Organic	
Chopped vegetable and barley soup, 1 cup	2
Chef's Cupboard	
Butternut squash and red pepper gourmet soup, 1 cup	4
Cream of mushroom condensed soup, ½ cup	3
Dr. Mcdougall's	
Organic black bean lower sodium soup, 1 cup	4
Food Should Taste Good	
Carrot ginger bisque soup, 1 cup	4
Fresh Foods Market	
Thai style chicken coconut curry soup, 1 cup	12

	SmartPoints® value
Hurst's HamBeens	
15 bean soup, Cajun, ½ cup	3
Idahoan	
Creamy potato soup, ⅓ cup	10
Imagine Organic	
Creamy tomato basil soup, 1 cup	3
Lipton Cup-a-Soup	
Instant soup, spring vegetable, 1 envelope (13 g)	1
Lipton Soup Secrets	
Extra noodle soup mix, 3 Tbsp	2
Nissin Cup Noodles	
Chicken flavor cup noodles, 1 cup	11
Pacific Organic	
Soup, creamy tomato, 1 cup	4
Soup, roasted red pepper & tomato, 1 cup	5
Panera Bread	
Baked potato soup, 1 cup	9
Broccoli cheddar soup, 1 cup	11
Organic tomato bisque, 1 cup	5
Progresso	
Artisan hearty pasta e fagioli soup, 1 cup	7
Progresso Heart Healthy	
Creamy tomato basil soup, 1 cup	5
Italian style wedding with meatballs reduced sodium soup, 1 cup	2
Southwest style black bean and vegetable soup, 1 cup	3

	SmartPoints® value
Progresso Light	
Creamy potato with bacon and cheese soup, 1 cup	3
Italian style meatball soup, 1 cup	3
Savory vegetable barley soup, 1 cup	2
Vegetable soup, 1 cup	2
Zesty southwestern style vegetable soup, 1 cup	2
Progresso Rich & Hearty	
Loaded potato with bacon soup, 1 cup	6
Progresso Traditional	
Beef and vegetable soup, 1 cup	4
Chickarina soup (chicken soup with meatballs), 1 cup	4
Italian style wedding soup, 1 cup	3
Split pea with ham soup, 1 cup	4
Turkey noodle soup, 1 cup	2
Progresso Vegetable Classics	
99% fat free lentil soup, 1 cup	3
99% fat free minestrone soup, 1 cup	3
French onion soup, 1 cup	2
Garden vegetable soup, 1 cup	3
Hearty tomato soup, 1 cup	5
Lentil soup, 1 cup	4
Macaroni and bean soup, 1 cup	5
Minestrone soup, 1 cup	3
Vegetable soup, 1 cup	2
Vegetarian vegetable with barley soup, 1 cup	3

	SmartPoints® value
Signature Café	
Broccoli and cheesy cheddar soup, 1 cup	10
White bean and kale soup, 1 cup	3
Sushi Chef	
Clear soup, traditional Japanese style, 1 package (9 g)	1
Thai Kitchen	
Tom yum soup, hot & sour, 7 oz	2
Trader Joe's	
Butternut squash soup, 1 cup	3
Trader Joe's Grocery	
Butternut squash soup, 1 cup	3
Carrot ginger soup, 1 cup	3
Organic creamy tomato soup, 1 cup	4
Organic tomato and roasted red pepper soup, 1 cup	4
Trader Ming's	
Chicken and vegetable wonton soup, 1 bowl (305 g)	6

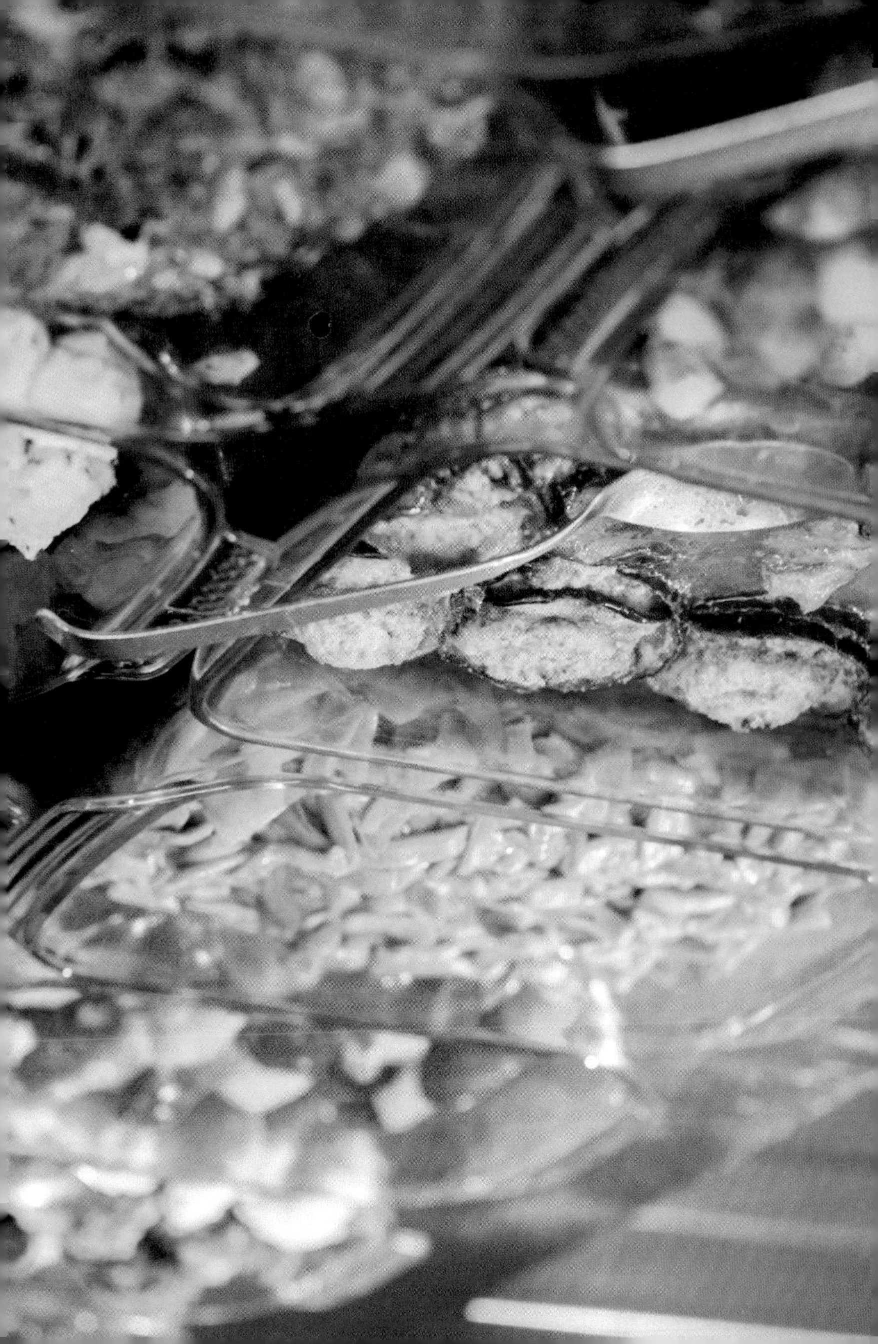

vegetables

Beans

	SmartPoints® value
Birds Eye Steamfresh	
Cut green beans, ⅔ cup	0
Green beans, cut, ⅔ cup	0
Birds Eye Steamfresh Premium Selects	
Green beans, whole, 1 cup	0
Bush's Best	
Black beans, ½ cup	3
Black beans, reduced sodium, ½ cup	3
Black beans, seasoned recipe, ½ cup	3
Hot sauce pinto beans in chili sauce, ½ cup	3
Pinto beans, ½ cup	2
Dakota's Pride	
Chick peas, ½ cup	3
Great northern beans, ½ cup	2
Pinto beans, ½ cup	3
Del Monte Fresh Cut	
Blue lake cut green beans, ½ cup	0
French style green beans, ½ cup undrained	0
Green beans, cut, no salt added, ½ cup	0
Enlightened	
Sea salt roasted broad beans, 1 package (28 g)	2
Glory Foods Seasoned Country Style	
String beans, ½ cup	1
Goya	
Blacks beans, premium, ½ cup	2
Kidney beans, red, ½ cup	2
Goya Prime Premium	
Chick peas, garbanzos, canned, ½ cup	2

	SmartPoints® value
Great Value	
Baby lima beans, 3 oz	3
Black beans, ½ cup	3
Blackeye peas, ½ cup	3
Pinto beans, ½ cup	2
Green Giant	
Cut green beans, ½ cup	0
Kroger	
Black beans, ½ cup	3
French style green beans, 1 cup	1
Vegetarian refried beans, ½ cup	4
Libby's	
Cut green beans, ½ cup	0
Old El Paso	
Refried beans, fat free, ½ cup	2
Refried beans, fat free, spicy, ½ cup	3
Refried beans, traditional, ½ cup	3
Refried beans, vegetarian, ½ cup	2
PictSweet Deluxe Sides	
Edamame, with sea salt, 1 carton (170 g)	3
Rosarita	
Refried beans, green chile & lime, ½ cup	2
Refried beans, low-fat, black, ½ cup	3
Refried beans, traditional, ½ cup	3
Refried beans, traditional, no fat, ½ cup	3
Refried beans, vegetarian, ½ cup	3
Sunny Select	
Cut green beans no salt added, ½ cup	0
Taco Bell	
Refried beans, original, ½ cup	3
Trader Joe's	
Fat free traditional style refried beans, ½ cup	3

	SmartPoints® value
Beets	
Aunt Nellie's	
Beets, pickled, sliced, 4 slices (29 g)	1
Pickled beets, 1 cup	4
Trader Joe's	
Steamed and peeled baby beets, 2 baby beets (85 g)	0
Broccoli	
Birds Eye Steamfresh	
Broccoli florets, premium selects, 1 cup	0
Birds Eye Steamfresh Selects	
Fresh frozen vegetables, broccoli cuts, 1 cup	0
Green Giant Steamers	
Broccoli florets, 1¼ cups	0
Tuscan seasoned broccoli, 1¼ cups frozen	2
Marketside	
Broccoli florets, 1½ cups	0
Brussels Sprouts	
Birds Eye Steamfresh	
Brussels sprouts, ¾ cup	0
Evol.	
Balsamic brussels sprouts, 1 package (127 g)	4
Green Giant Steamers	
Brussels sprouts with sea salt and cracked pepper, ¾ cup frozen	2
Cabbage	
King's Kimchi	
Korean marinated cabbage, spicy, 2 oz	0

	SmartPoints® value
Carrots	
Bolthouse Farms	
Baby carrot snack bag, 1 package (56 g)	1
Carrot chips, 3 oz	0
Carrots, premium sweet petites, 3 oz	0
Bolthouse Farms Hop	
Baby carrots, 3 oz	0
Bunny Luv	
Organic peeled baby carrots, 3 oz	0
Crispak	
Baby carrots, 3 oz	2
Del Monte	
Carrot sticks, 3 oz	0
Fresh Selections by Kroger	
Petite carrots, 3 oz	0
Great Value	
Crinkle cut carrots, ⅔ cup	1
Green Giant	
Baby cut carrots, 14 carrots (91 g)	0
Grimmway Farms	
Baby carrots, 3 oz	0
Krispak	
Carrot petites, 25 pieces (85 g)	0
Kroger Fresh Selections	
Baby carrots, 3 oz	0
Simple Truth Organic	
Cut & peeled baby carrots, 1 cup	0
Cauliflower	
Green Giant	
Cauliflower crumbles, ¼ cup	0
Trader Giotto's	
Organic riced cauliflower, ⅓ package (113 g)	0
Trader Joe's	
Riced cauliflower, ⅓ package (113 g)	1

	SmartPoints® value
Celery	
Del Monte	
Celery sticks, 4 oz	0
Corn	
Birds Eye Steamfresh	
Corn, super sweet, ⅔ cup	3
Super sweet corn, ½ cup	2
Del Monte	
Corn, whole kernel, no salt added, ½ cup undrained	2
Del Monte Fresh Cut	
Golden sweet whole kernel corn, ½ cup undrained	2
Great Value	
Cream style sweet corn, 4 ½ oz	4
Golden sweet whole kernel corn, 4 ½ oz	2
Green Giant	
Whole kernel sweet corn, canned, ½ cup	2
Libby's	
Sweet corn, whole kernel, ½ cup	3
Lowes Foods	
Golden sweet creamed corn, ½ cup	4
Edamame	
Archer Farms	
Edamame, ½ cup	3
Imperial Gourmet	
Edamame, 1 bag (226 g)	3
Madame Edamame	
Organic edamame, 1 bag (255 g)	4
PictSweet Steam'ables	
Edamame, seasoned, with sea salt, ½ cup	3

	SmartPoints® value
Private Selection	
Mukimame, ½ cup	3
Seapoint Farms	
Dry roasted edamame, lightly salted, ¼ cup	3
Hearts of Palm	
SunPix	
Crisp & zesty hearts of palm, ¼ cup	0
Lentils	
Tasty Bite	
Madras lentils Indian cuisine, ½ pack (143 g)	5
Lettuce and Leafy Greens	
Dole	
50 50 spring mix and baby spinach, 3 cups	0
Chopped romaine salad blends, 2 cups	0
Classic romaine, 1 ½ cups	0
Romaine, leafy, 2 cups	0
Salad, butter bliss, 1 ½ cups	0
Shredded lettuce, 1 ½ cups	0
Spring mix, 3 cups	0
Spring mix baby lettuces, 3 oz	0
Summer salad kit, 3 ½ oz	5
Earthbound Farm	
Organic half and half spring mix and baby spinach, 2 cups	0
Organic spring mix, 3 oz	0
Romaine hearts, 2 cups	0
Earthbound Farm Deep Green Blends	
Power greens mix, 2 cups	0

	SmartPoints® value
Earthbound Farm Organic	
Baby spinach, 2 cups	0
Half spring mix & half baby spinach, 2 cups	0
Power deep green blends, 2 cups	0
Fresh Express	
50/50 mix of spring mix and baby spinach, 1 package (142 g)	0
American salad, 2 cups	0
Baby kale mix, 1 package (141 g)	1
Hearts of romaine, 2 cups	0
Italian salad, 2½ cups	0
Leafy green romaine, 2 cups	0
Salad, greener European salad blend with iceberg, romaine & green leaf, 2½ cups	0
Seasonal blend of mixed greens, spring mix, 3 cups	0
Sweet butter salad, 2 cups	0
Fresh Selections	
Hearts of romaine, 2 cups	1
Garden Cuts	
Green leaf lettuce, 3 oz	0
Giant	
Romaine salad, crisp romaine lettuce, 2½ cups	0
Glory Foods	
Collard greens, seasoned southern style, ½ cup	1
Kroger Fresh Selections	
Field greens, 1½ cups	0
Little Salad Bar	
Italian salad, 1½ cups	0
Spring mix, 1 package (141 g)	0
Sweet butter lettuce, 2½ cups	0

	SmartPoints® value
Marketside	
Butter lettuce salad, 1½ cups	0
Field greens salad, 1½ cups	0
Organic half and half salad mix, ½ package (85 g)	0
Spring mix, 4½ cups	0
Spring mix salad, 3 cups	0
Marketside Organic	
Half and half mix baby spinach and spring mix, 2 cups	0
Organic Girl	
50% spring mix and 50% baby spinach, 2 cups	0
Super greens, 3 cups	0
Ready Pac	
Organic spring mix, 4½ cups	0
Taylor Farms	
Organic power greens kale medley, 2 cups	0
Superfood power greens, 1 cup	1
Taylor Farms Organic	
Power greens baby spinach and baby kale, 3 oz	0
Wholesome Garden	
Organic spring mix, 3 cups	0

Mixed Vegetables

America's Choice	
California blend mixed vegetables, 3 oz	0
Birds Eye	
Fresh frozen deluxe vegetables, broccoli and cauliflower, 1 cup	0
Mixed vegetables, classic, 3 cups	2
Oriental stir fry with Asian sauce, 1 cup	2
Birds Eye Recipe Ready	
Tri color pepper and onion blend, ¾ cup	0

Mixed Vegetables (cont'd)

	SmartPoints® value
Birds Eye Steamfresh	
Broccoli & cauliflower, 3 cups	0
Broccoli, carrots, sugar snap peas & water chestnuts, ¾ cup	0
Broccoli, cauliflower, & carrots, 3 cups	0
Fresh frozen mixed vegetables, ⅔ cup	2
Gold and white corn carrots asparagus mixtures, ⅔ cup	2
Lightly seasoned Asian medley, 1 cup	2
Mixed vegetables selects, ⅔ cup	2
Vegetables, fresh frozen, baby broccoli blend, 1 cup	2
Daily Chef	
Normandy blend, steamable, 1 cup	0
Dole	
American blend, 1½ cups	0
Lettuce, classic iceberg, 1½ cups	0
Dole Chopped	
Summer garden blend salad, 1½ cups	0
Flav-R-Pac	
Northwest vegetable blend, 1 cup	0
Fresh Express	
Iceberg garden salad, 1½ cups	0
Fresh Express Veggie Medley	
Farmers garden salad, 2 cups	0
Great Value	
California style vegetable mix broccoli carrots and cauliflower, ⅔ cup	0
Mixed vegetables, steamable, 3 cups	0

	SmartPoints® value
Green Giant Fire Roasted	
Root vegetables with red onions, ¾ cup	2
Zucchini carrots and onion, ¾ cup	0
Green Giant Steamers	
Garden vegetable medley, 1 cup frozen	2
Teriyaki vegetables, 1¼ cups	2
Kirkland Signature	
Normandy style vegetable blend, 1 cup	0
Kroger Meal-Ready Sides	
Vegetables, stir-fry, 1 cup	0
Kroger Value Recipe Beginnings	
3 pepper and onion blend, 1 cup	0
Mann's	
Broccoli cole slaw, 3 oz	0
Meijer	
Peas and carrots, ⅔ cup	0
Ore-Ida	
Potatoes O'Brien with onions and peppers, ¾ cup	2
Path of Life	
Garbanzo and lentils, ½ package (142 g)	6
PictSweet Steam'ables	
Broccoli florets, cauliflower and carrots, 1 cup	0
Private Selection	
Vegetable medley, broccoli, cauliflower, carrots, 3 oz	0
Season's Choice Steam	
Frozen mixed vegetables, ½ cup	2
Simply Enjoy	
Mixed vegetables, grilled, 3 oz	2

	SmartPoints® value
Trader Joe's	
Broccoli and kale slaw, 1½ cups	8
Cruciferous crunch collection mixed greens, 3 cups	0
Dolmas, 4 dolmas (110 g)	4
Fire roasted bell peppers and onions, ¾ cup	0
Healthy 8 chopped veggie mix, ¾ cup	0
Veg-All Steam Supreme	
Mixed vegetables, original, 3 cups	2
Wellsley Farms Organic	
Mixed vegetables, 1 cup	2

Mushrooms

Giorgio	
Fresh mushrooms, 3 oz	0
Great Value	
Mushrooms pieces & stems, 1 serving (115 g)	0
Happy Harvest	
Mushrooms pieces and stems, ½ cup	0
Monterey Mushrooms	
Whole mushrooms, 3 oz	0

Okra

Old South	
Okra, pickled, mild, 2 pods (28 g)	0

Onions

French's	
French fried onions, 2 Tbsp	2
French's	
Original French fried onions, 2 Tbsp	2
Fresh Gourmet	
Lightly salted crispy onions, 1½ Tbsp	1
Onions, crispy, garlic pepper, 1½ Tbsp	1
Birds Eye Steamfresh	
Sweet peas selects, ⅔ cup	2
Bush's Best	
Peas, blackeye, ½ cup	2
Calbee Harvest Snaps	
Caesar snapea crisps, 22 pieces (28 g)	3
Giant	
Petite peas, ⅔ cup	0
Green Giant	
Sweet peas, ½ cup	2
Hapi	
Wasabi peas, hot, 55 pieces (28 g)	4
Le Sueur	
Very young small sweet peas, ½ cup	2
Mann's	
Stringless sugar snap peas, 1 cup	1
Market Pantry	
Frozen sweet peas, ⅔ cup	2
Trappey's	
Black eye peas, ½ cup	3

Peppers

Bell View	
Red peppers, sweet, 1 oz	1
Del Destino	
Fire roasted red peppers, 1 piece (130 g)	2
Mighty Minis	
Sweet mini peppers, 3½ pieces	0

Peppers (cont'd)

	SmartPoints® value
Pero Family Farms	
Mini sweet peppers, 3 ½ pieces	0
Signature Brands	
Mini peppers, 3 peppers (85 g)	1
Tuscan Garden	
Mild pepper rings, 1 oz	0
Vlasic Deli Style	
Banana pepper rings, mild, 12 pepper rings (28 g)	0

Potatoes

	SmartPoints® value
Express Bake PotatOH!	
Russet potato, small, 1 potato (170 g)	4
Fifth Generation	
Sweet potato, 1 potato (130 g)	4
Harvest Club	
Potatoes, yukon gold, 1 potato (148 g)	3
Healthy Fresh Produce	
Microwaveable sweet potato, 1 potato (130 g)	5
MountainKing Steakhouse Roasters	
Prime fingerling potatoes, 5 potatoes (148 g)	3
Ore-Ida Steam n' Mash	
Potatoes, cut russet, ¾ cup	2
SunLite	
Potatoes, 1 potato (148 g)	2
The Little Potato Company	
Blushing belle potatoes, 6 potatoes (148 g)	3
Dynamic duo fresh creamer potatoes, 5 potatoes (148 g)	3
Terrific trio creamer potatoes, 6 potatoes (148 g)	3
The Little Potato Company Dynamic Duo	
Fresh creamer potatoes, 5 potates (148 g)	3
Trader Joe's	
Sweet potato wedges, 3 oz	3

Pumpkin

	SmartPoints® value
Meijer	
100% pure pumpkin, ½ cup	0

Seaweed and Sea Vegetable

	SmartPoints® value
Kirkland Signature	
Roasted seasoned seaweed (serves 5), 1 serving (3.4 g)	1

Spinach

	SmartPoints® value
Dole	
Baby spinach, 3 cups	0
Fresh Express	
Baby kale & spinach juicing greens, 3 cups	0
Baby spinach, 1 package (142 g)	0
Salad, spinach & arugula, 2 cups	0
Spinach, 2 cups	0
Green Giant Steamers	
Frozen chopped spinach, ¾ cup frozen	0
Kroger Fresh Selections	
Baby spinach, 2 cups	0
Little Salad Bar	
Spinach, 3 cups	0
Marketside	
Organic baby spinach, 4 ½ cups	0
Organic Girl	
Baby spinach, 3 cups	0
Trader Joe's	
Organics baby spinach, 1 cup	1

	SmartPoints® value
Squash and Zucchini	
Trader Joe's	
Cut butternut squash, ¾ cup	0
Tomato Paste and Puree	
Hunt's	
Sauce, tomatoes, ¼ cup	0
Tomato paste, 2 Tbsp	1
Tomato sauce, ¼ cup	0
Tomatoes	
Bella Sun Luci	
Sun dried tomatoes with olive oil and Italian herbs, ⅔ oz	3
Cherubs	
Heavenly salad tomatoes, ½ package (149 g)	0
Great Value	
Fire roasted diced tomatoes, ½ cup	1
Hunt's	
Fire roasted diced tomatoes with garlic, ½ cup	0
Tomatoes, diced, basil, garlic & oregano, ½ cup	2
Kroger	
Grape tomatoes, 1 cup	1
Mutti	
Tomatoes, baby roma, ½ cup	0
Nature Sweet	
Cherubs salad tomatoes, 1 cup	0
NatureSweet Sunbursts	
Sweet golden tomatoes, 1 tomato (212 g)	0

	SmartPoints® value
Ro-Tel	
Diced tomatoes & green chilies, mild, ½ cup	0
Diced tomatoes & green chilies, original, ½ cup	0
Santa Sweets	
Grape tomato, 3 oz	1
Sweet potatoes, 1 potato (130 g)	5
Yucca	
Goya	
Yuca, 2 pieces (199 g)	3

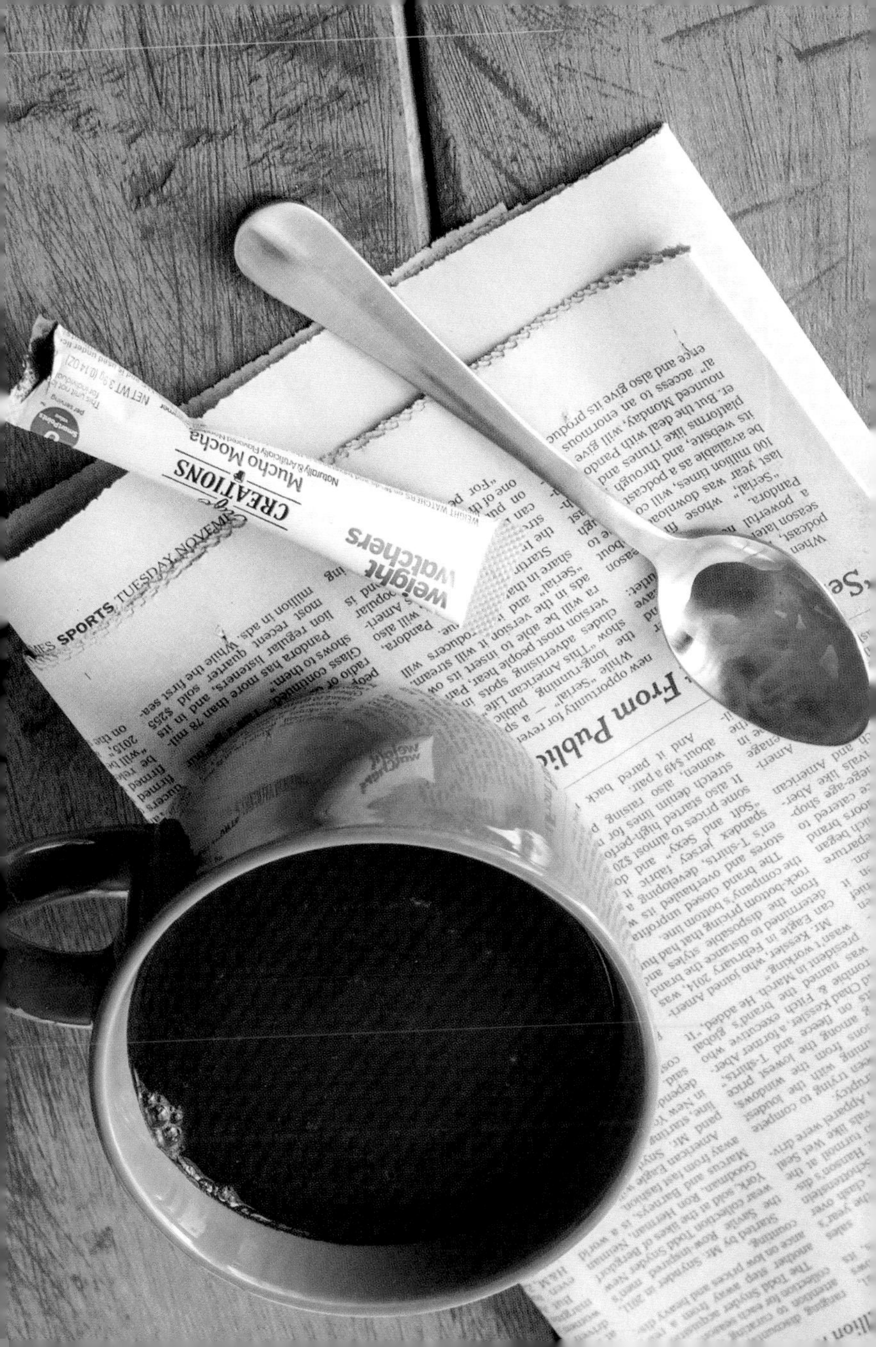
weight watchers
CREATIONS
Mucho Mocha
SPORTS TUESDAY

weight watchers

food products

	SmartPoints® value
Frozen Novelties	
Weight Watchers	
Dark chocolate mint bars, 1 bar	3
Dark chocolate raspberry bars, 1 bar	3
Giant chocolate fudge bars, 1 bar	4
Snack size chocolate fudge bars, 1 bar	2
Snack size cookies & cream bars, 1 bar	4
Snack size divine triple chocolate bars, 1 bar	4
Snack size double caramel swirl cones, 1 cone	4
Snack size English toffee crunch bars, 1 bar	4
Snack size mocha latte bars, 1 bar	2
Snack size peanut butter caramel candy bars, 1 bar	4
Snack size salted caramel bars, 1 bar	4
Snack size vanilla fudge swirl cones, 1 cone	4
Cheese	
Weight Watchers Cheese Shreds	
Reduced fat Mexican style blend, ⅓ cup	3
Weight Watchers Cheese Singles	
Reduced fat cheese singles, 1 slice	2
Reduced fat pepper jack singles, 1 slice	1
Weight Watchers Cheese Snacks	
Light jalapeño string cheese, 1 stick	1
Natural light mozzarella string cheese, 1 stick	1
Natural reduced fat colby jack cheese stick, 1 stick	2
Reduced fat mild cheddar cheese sticks, 1 stick	2

	SmartPoints® value
Weight Watchers Cream Cheese	
Reduced fat cream cheese spread, 1 portion cup	3
Reduced fat whipped cream cheese spread, 2 Tbsp	3
Cereal	
Weight Watchers	
Oat clusters with almonds cereal, ¾ cup	4
Chocolate Candy	
Weight Watchers by Whitman's	
Bite size dark chocolates, 1 pouch	5
Bite size red velvet chocolates, 1 pouch	5
Caramel bite size covered in milk chocolate, 1 pouch	6
Caramel chocolates, 3 pieces	8
Caramel with crispies chocolates, 3 pieces	7
Chocolate mousse dark chocolates, 3 pieces	6
Coconut chocolates, 3 pieces	7
English toffee chocolate candies, 3 pieces	6
Mint patties dark chocolate candies, 3 pieces	6
Pecan crown bite size chocolates, 1 pouch	6
Pecan crowns chocolates, 3 pieces	7
In-Meeting/Online Products	
Weight Watchers Café Creations	
Mucho mocha, 1 packet	0
Pumpkin spice, 1 packet	0
Vanilla bean, 1 packet	0
Weight Watchers Candies	
Blackberry sugar free candies, 8 candies	1

	SmartPoints® value
Citrus drops sugar free candies, 11 candies	1
Cherry & grapefruit drops sugar free candies, 11 candies	1
Strawberry sugar free candies, 8 candies	1
Weight Watchers Crunchy Snacks	
Cheddar twists, 1 pouch	2
Nacho cheese supreme, 1 pouch	2
Original mini pretzel thins, 1 pouch	2
Popped barbeque potato crisps, 1 pouch	2
Popped cinnamon flavored snacks, 1 pouch	2
Popped salt & vinegar potato crisps, 1 pouch	2
Popped sea salt hummus chips, 1 pouch	2
Weight Watchers Snack Bars	
Sweet & salty toffee twist, 1 bar	4
Peanut butter trail mix, 1 bar	4
Weight Watchers Breakfast Squares	
Cranberry almond yogurt, 1 bar	5
Dark chocolate nut, 1 bar	5
Weight Watchers Mini Bars	
Caramel macchiato, 1 bar	2
Chocolate caramel, 1 bar	2
Chocolate pretzel blast, 1 bar	2
Mint cookie crisp, 1 bar	2
Peanut butter cookie explosion, 1 bar	3

	SmartPoints® value
So-good salted caramel, 1 bar	3
Sprinkle me pink, 1 bar	3
Weight Watchers Hummus Snack Packs	
Classic hummus, 1 pack	3
Roasted red pepper, 1 pack	3
Weight Watchers Meal Pouches	
Tasty bite brown rice & lentils, 1 pouch	6
Tasty bite madras lentils, 1 pouch	6
Tasty bite vegetable tikka masala, 1 pouch	5
Weight Watchers Oatmeal	
Apple cinnamon, 1 container	3
Blueberry vanilla, 1 container	3
Maple brown sugar, 1 container	3
Strawberry 'n' cream, 1 container	3
Weight Watchers Smoothies	
Creamy chocolate, 1 slim pack	2
French vanilla, 1 slim pack	2
Salted caramel super smoothie, 1 slim pack	3
Triple berry super smoothie, 1 slim pack	3
Weight Watchers Water Enhancers	
Berry pomegranate, 2 ml	0
Southern sweet tea, 2 ml	0
Pink punch, 2 ml	0
Weight Watchers Cocktail Mixers	
Cosmopolitan city, 3 fl oz	0
Margarita mambo, 3 fl oz	0

NOTE: The Weight Watchers line of food products is continuously being revised to meet your needs and help you follow the Weight Watchers program. So although the information for the products listed here was current at the time this guide was compiled, you might find that things are different once a product is purchased. Always check product packaging for the latest information, including SmartPoints values, when you purchase one of these products.

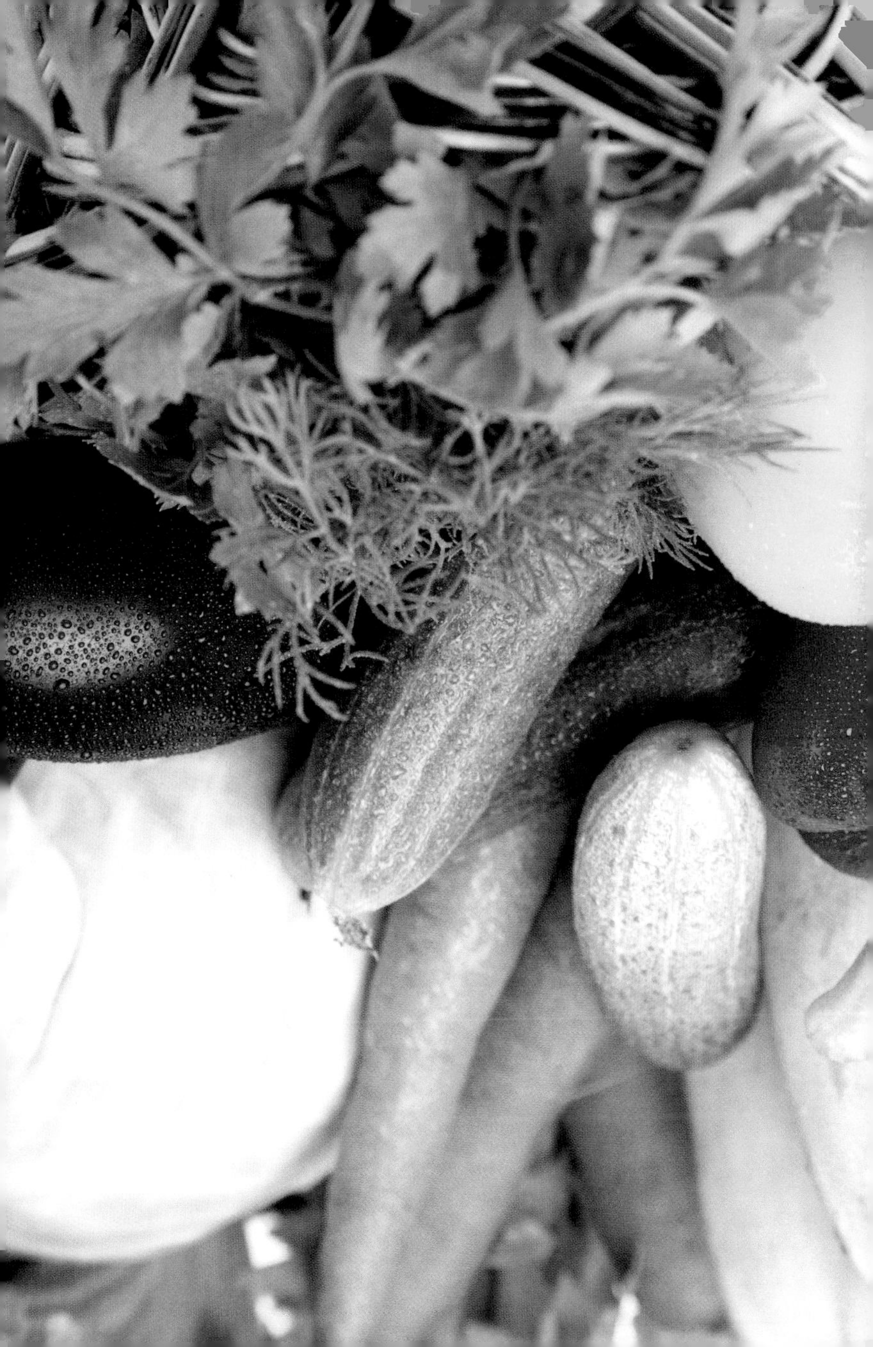

index

A

B

C

D

E

F

G

H

I

J

K

L

M

N

O

P